Anesthesia

Edited by

MAY C. M. PIAN-SMITH, MD, MS

Co-Chief, Division of Obstetric Anesthesia
Department of Anesthesia and Critical Care
Massachusetts General Hospital;
Assistant Professor
Department of Anesthesia
Harvard Medical School
Boston, MA

LISA LEFFERT, MD

Co-Chief, Division of Obstetric Anesthesia
Department of Anesthesia and Critical Care
Massachusetts General Hospital;
Instructor
Department of Anesthesia
Harvard Medical School
Boston, MA

CAMBRIDGE
UNIVERSITY PRESS

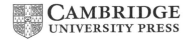

CAMBRIDGE UNIVERSITY PRESS

Cambridge, New York, Melbourne, Madrid, Cape Town, Singapore, São Paulo, Delhi

Cambridge University Press
32 Avenue of the Americas, New York, NY 10013-2473, USA

www.cambridge.org
Information on this title: www.cambridge.org/9780521709392

First published 2007

Printed in the United States of America

A catalog record for this publication is available from the British Library.

Library of Congress Cataloging in Publication Data

Obstetric anesthesia / [edited by] May C.M. Pian-Smith, Lisa Leffert.
  p.   ;   cm.
ISBN-13: 978-0-521-70939-2 (pbk.)
ISBN-10: 0-521-70939-3 (pbk.)
1. Anesthesia in obstetrics – Handbooks, manuals, etc.   I. Pian-Smith,
May C. M., 1959–   II. Leffert, Lisa, 1962–
[DNLM: 1. Anesthesia, Obstetrical – methods – Handbooks.
2. Pharmaceutical Preparations – Handbooks. WO 231 O14 2007]
RG732.O2634   2007
617.9′682–dc22   2007016913

ISBN   978-0-521-70939-2 paperback

Cambridge University Press has no responsibility for
the persistence or accuracy of URLs for external or
third-party Internet Web sites referred to in this publication
and does not guarantee that any content on such
Web sites is, or will remain, accurate or appropriate.

Every effort has been made in preparing this book to provide accurate and
up-to-date information that is in accord with accepted standards and practice at
the time of publication. Nevertheless, the authors, editors, and publisher can
make no warranties that the information contained herein is totally free from
error, not least because clinical standards are constantly changing through
research and regulation. The authors, editors, and publisher therefore disclaim
all liability for direct or consequential damages resulting from the use of
material contained in this book. Readers are strongly advised to pay careful
attention to information provided by the manufacturer of any drugs or
equipment that they plan to use.

NOTICE

Because of the dynamic nature of medical practice and drug selection and dosage, users are advised that decisions regarding drug therapy must be based on the independent judgment of the clinician, changing information about a drug (e.g., as reflected in the literature and manufacturer's most current product information), and changing medical practices.

While great care has been taken to ensure the accuracy of the information presented, users are advised that the authors, editors, contributors, and publisher make no warranty, express or implied, with respect to, and are not responsible for, the currency, completeness, or accuracy of the information contained in this publication, nor for any errors, omissions, or the application of this information, nor for any consequences arising therefrom. Users are encouraged to confirm the information contained herein with other sources deemed authoritative. Ultimately, it is the responsibility of the treating physician, relying on experience and knowledge of the patient, to determine dosages and the best treatment for the patient. Therefore, the author(s), editors, contributors, and the publisher make no warranty, express or implied, and shall have no liability to any person or entity with regard to claims, loss, or damage caused, or alleged to be caused, directly or indirectly, by the use of information contained in this publication.

Further, the author(s), editors, contributors, and the publisher are not responsible for misuse of any of the information provided in this publication, for negligence by the user, or for any typographical errors.

CONTENTS

PART TWO. OBSTETRIC ANESTHESIA FORMULARY

Contents

Preface

Obstetric Anesthesia is a definitive, comprehensive and yet easily navigated reference for all anesthesia practitioners caring for parturients. With chapters written by Harvard anesthesia residents and fellows, it has been carefully edited and updated by faculty mentors and reflects the practice at our affiliated institutions.

The formatting was designed to offer rapid access to information, and thus is suited as a convenient reference on the labor floor. The first section focuses on the pharmacology, physiology and delivery of anesthesia as they relate to pregnancy. The second section offers both medical theory, as well as practical steps for the management of patients with co-existing disease (relevant physiology, pathology, obstetric management and anesthetic management). The third section focuses on the management of obstetric emergencies (physiology, pathology, step-by-step management and potential complications). We also include sections on anesthesia for non-delivery surgery and strategies for managing adverse outcomes such as neurologic complications and risk management. Finally, the book includes a detailed formulary of common medications, emphasizing indications, contraindications, and maternal and fetal effects of the drugs.

Obstetric Anesthesia is the result of a huge collaborative effort involving our trainees and our faculty colleagues. We thank the authors for their hard work and the contagious enthusiasm that they brought to the task. Indeed, it is working in this wonderful community that makes our clinical and teaching jobs so rewarding; thus it was not surprising that this writing project, too, was stimulating and enjoyable. This book is a reflection of the intellectual curiosity, high standards and dedication to patient care that characterize this amazing team.

We also acknowledge gratefully the important administrative assistance of Linda Patten.

May C. M. Pian-Smith and Lisa Leffert

PART ONE

Obstetric Anesthesia

ACHONDROPLASIA

STEPHEN PANARO, MD
EDWARD MICHNA, MD

FUNDAMENTAL KNOWLEDGE

- Inherited disorder of bone metabolism that results in short stature, a small maxilla, large mandible & spinal abnormalities
- Lumbar lordosis & thoracic kyphosis are increased.
- The small vertebral pedicles & short anteroposterior & transverse diameters of the vertebral canal can result in spinal stenosis, which can worsen w/ age as scoliosis worsens & osteophytes form.

STUDIES

- Physical exam
- Lumbosacral spine films may add information.

MANAGEMENT/INTERVENTIONS

- Cervical mobility may be diminished; combined w/ other facial abnormalities, this may make intubation difficult.
- Regional anesthesia may be technically difficult but is not contraindicated.
- Because of the pt's short stature & spinal stenosis, the dosage for a single-shot spinal may be difficult to estimate.
- Insertion of an epidural or spinal catheter may be a better alternative to a single-shot spinal to allow careful titration of anesthetic.

CAVEATS/PEARLS

- Consider using an epidural or spinal catheter instead of a single-shot spinal, which may be difficult to dose appropriately.
- Prepare for a difficult intubation if decreased cervical mobility or facial anomalies are present.

CHECKLIST

- Physical exam, lumbosacral spine films

ACROMEGALY

GRACE C. CHANG, MD, MBA; ROBERT A. PETERFREUND, MD, PhD;
AND STEPHANIE L. LEE, MD, PhD

FUNDAMENTAL KNOWLEDGE

Definition

- Rare disfiguring & disabling disease caused by growth hormone hypersecretion
- Usually due to growth hormone-secreting anterior pituitary adenoma

Epidemiology

- Prevalence 50–60 cases per million population
- Equal distribution btwn genders
- Very rare for acromegalic women to become pregnant because of impaired gonadotropic axis; 60% of acromegalic women are amenorrheic
- <100 pregnancies reported in women w/ acromegaly

Signs/Symptoms

- Headache
- Papilledema
- Visual disturbances
- Enlargement of tongue & epiglottis
- Increased length of mandible
- Overgrowth of soft tissues of upper airway
- Hoarseness or change in voice
- Stridor
- Peripheral neuropathy
- Diabetes mellitus
- Systemic hypertension
- Ischemic heart disease
- Osteoarthritis/osteoporosis
- Thick & oily skin
- Skeletal muscle weakness

Changes Associated w/ Pregnancy

- During early pregnancy, growth hormone (GH) is secreted by pituitary.
- In 2nd trimester, placenta starts producing variant of GH.
- GH levels continue to increase throughout pregnancy, peaking in 3rd trimester.

- Placental GH induces maternal hepatic IGF-1 production, which inhibits pituitary GH secretion.
- Serum IGF-1 levels increase in 2nd half of pregnancy.
- Conflicting evidence that pregnancy worsens pituitary macroadenoma growth; some case reports of worsening of symptoms during pregnancy; others showed improvement.
- In acromegalic women, pituitary GH secretion persists throughout pregnancy.

Maternal Complications
- Diabetes mellitus
- Hypertension
- Heart disease

Fetal/Neonatal Complications
- Newborns of untreated mothers have greater mean birthweights than newborns of treated mothers.

STUDIES
- Plasma GH concentration >3 ng/mL
- Failure of plasma GH concentration to decrease 1–2 hours after administration of 75–100 g glucose
- Pituitary MRI w/ gadolinium for pituitary mass

MANAGEMENT/INTERVENTIONS
- Transsphenoidal surgical excision of pituitary adenoma is definitive treatment.
  - ➤ May be required during pregnancy if pt has symptoms of tumor expansion or signs & symptoms not relieved by medical mgt
  - ➤ Perform surgery in 2nd trimester: surgery in 1st trimester associated w/ increased risk of spontaneous abortion; surgery in 3rd trimester may cause premature labor
- Medical mgt
  - ➤ Dopamine agonists
    - Bromocriptine or Dostinex; however, dopamine agonist treatment is successful in only 10% of cases
    - Dopamine agonists are more effective on tumors w/ GH & prolactin co-secretion.
  - ➤ Somatostatin analogs
    - Octreotide, octreotide LAR, lanreotide
    - Normalization of GH/IGF in 40–60% of pts
    - Limited experience during pregnancy

➤ GH receptor antagonists
  • Pegvisomant: no reported pregnancies on this medication
■ Radiotherapy
  ➤ Takes a long time to work
  ➤ High incidence of hypopituitarism

Anesthetic Management
■ Thorough evaluation of airway
  ➤ Acromegalic pts have higher incidence of difficult intubation.
  ➤ Distorted facial anatomy & increased length of mandible may lead to difficult mask airway.
  ➤ Enlargement of tongue & epiglottis & overgrowth of soft tissue in upper airway can lead to obstruction.
  ➤ Pt may require smaller endotracheal tube than normal because of subglottic narrowing & enlargement of vocal cords.
  ➤ Nasal turbinate enlargement may make nasal intubation difficult.
  ➤ Pt may require awake fiberoptic intubation.
■ Use non-depolarizing muscle relaxants sparingly, especially if skeletal muscle weakness exists.
■ Both regional anesthesia & general anesthesia can be used safely.
■ Anticipate difficulty placing epidural or spinal because of skeletal changes.
■ Document pre-op neuropathies & carefully pad all pressure points.
■ Carefully monitor blood glucose, especially if pt has diabetes mellitus or glucose intolerance.

CAVEATS/PEARLS
■ Pt may have various airway issues; anticipate difficult intubation if general anesthetic is required.

CHECKLIST
■ Thorough preanesthetic evaluation, especially for hypertension, coronary artery disease, diabetes mellitus
■ Thorough airway evaluation
■ Anticipate difficult mask ventilation & intubation; may require fiberoptic bronchoscope.
■ Monitor blood glucose.

ACUTE FATTY LIVER OF PREGNANCY (AFLP)

LAWRENCE WEINSTEIN, MD
DOUG RAINES, MD

FUNDAMENTAL KNOWLEDGE

Epidemiology
- Approximate prevalence: 1/7,000 to 1/16,000 pregnancies
- Disorder of late pregnancy, w/ most cases diagnosed btwn 35 & 37 weeks gestation

Pathogenesis
- Exact causal mechanisms are unknown, but there seems to be an association of AFLP w/ maternal long-chain 3-hydroxyacyl CoA dehydrogenase deficiency (LCHAD).
  - Long-chain 3-hydroxyacyl CoA dehydrogenase is an enzyme that is involved in mitochondrial beta-oxidation of fatty acids. It is thought that in mothers w/ this deficiency, fatty acid metabolites from the fetus & placenta can build up & overwhelm the mother's mitochondrial oxidation pathways. These metabolites can be hepatotoxic, & their accumulation is thought to be a possible causative mechanism for AFLP.
- Some evidence suggests a link between AFLP & pre-eclampsia.
  - There can be hepatic involvement in pre-eclampsia (HELLP syndrome).
  - Pre-eclampsia is often seen concurrently in pts w/ AFLP.
  - Liver biopsies in pre-eclamptic women w/ & w/o liver dysfunction both show microvesicular fat infiltration, suggesting that AFLP may be at the severe end of a pathologic spectrum encompassing pre-eclampsia, HELLP syndrome & AFLP.

Clinical Manifestations
- AFLP occurs late, near term in the 3rd trimester.
- Symptoms of nausea, vomiting, lethargy, malaise & headache can be part of a prodromal period in AFLP.
- Pt may report RUQ abdominal pain.
- Jaundice or bleeding is sometimes the initial presentation.
- Hepatic encephalopathy can be a late finding.
- In contrast to intrahepatic cholestasis of pregnancy, pruritus is NOT a common symptom in AFLP.
- Over half of pts w/ AFLP have pre-eclampsia as well during their course.
- Coagulopathy & progression to DIC are possible in AFLP.

Diagnosis

- Diagnosis is usually made clinically through examination of symptoms & lab values (see "*Studies*").
- Work up the pt for pre-eclampsia & HELLP syndrome, since they are so often associated w/ AFLP.
  - ➤ HELLP syndrome consists of hemolysis, elevated liver enzymes & low platelet count.
- Imaging studies are not needed to diagnose AFLP but may be helpful to rule out other pathology, such as hepatic infarct or hematoma.

STUDIES

Laboratory Data & Studies

- Serum transaminases are generally elevated in the neighborhood of 300–500 IU/L. Values may be as high as 1,000 but rarely exceed that.
- Alkaline phosphatase levels are markedly elevated (can be 10× normal).
- Leukocytosis w/ a left shift is a common but nonspecific finding.
- Hypoglycemia is common secondary to impaired hepatic gluconeogenesis.
- Acute renal failure may be a component of AFLP, w/ resultant rises in creatinine & BUN.
- If there has been progression to DIC, then thrombocytopenia is seen, along w/ elevations in PT & aPTT & a decrease in fibrinogen.
- Liver biopsy demonstrates microvesicular fatty infiltration of pericentral hepatocytes. There is also hepatocellular necrosis, portal inflammation & cholestasis. Biopsy is rarely needed to make the diagnosis & is in fact often contraindicated secondary to low platelets or abnormal coagulation studies.

MANAGEMENT/INTERVENTIONS

- The ultimate treatment for AFLP is fetal delivery as soon as safely possible. Prompt attention is necessary because progressive hepatic failure & fetal death can occur within days.
- There is no evidence suggesting an advantage of cesarean delivery over prompt vaginal delivery.
- Prior to delivery, the pt should be stabilized, w/ attention to correcting metabolic & coagulation abnormalities.
  - ➤ Glucose infusion for hypoglycemia
  - ➤ Correction of coagulopathy w/ FFP, platelets or cryoprecipitate as needed (to avoid massive intrapartum hemorrhage). This is particularly important if neuraxial spinal/epidural anesthesia

is planned, because of the potential for a devastating epidural hematoma in a pt w/ coagulopathy &/or low platelets.

➤ If acute renal failure complicates the clinical picture, dialysis can be necessary.

■ Be aware of the renal status & potassium, & adjust your anesthetic plan accordingly (avoid potassium-containing replacement fluids if the pt is retaining K+, avoid succinylcholine if K+ is elevated).

■ In the case of hepatic encephalopathy, blood ammonia levels should be obtained & lactulose given if appropriate.

➤ If the encephalopathy is sufficiently bad to impair respiration, then mechanical ventilation in an ICU setting may be necessary.

■ For either vaginal delivery or cesarean delivery, establish large-bore IV access in anticipation of the need for fluid resuscitation & administration of blood products.

■ Be aware of intra-operative losses & have rapid access to appropriate replacement fluids & blood products.

■ An arterial line can be an appropriate monitor to assist in frequent sampling of blood for Hct & coagulation studies & also to provide close BP monitoring should vasopressors become necessary.

■ In the operating environment, especially if general anesthesia is required, it may be prudent to keep the pt warm to minimize coagulopathy.

■ Anesthetic mgt for AFLP, & indeed for all liver disease of pregnancy, should be guided by the symptoms & manifestations of the liver process. Various manifestations will have differing effects on physiology & choice of anesthetic technique.

➤ If pt is coagulopathic, see the section on *"General Concepts."*

➤ If pt is cirrhotic, see sections on *"General Concepts," "Cirrhosis," "Portal Hypertension," "Ascites," "Hepatic Encephalopathy."*

■ For general discussion of regional & general anesthesia considerations, see the section on *"General Concepts."*

CAVEATS/PEARLS

■ AFLP is a rare but potentially devastating disorder of pregnancy.

■ Presents in 3rd trimester

■ Lab abnormalities are prominently elevated alkaline phosphatase, w/ a less marked rise in serum transaminases. Coagulation studies may also be abnormal, w/ potential for DIC.

■ After diagnosis, treatment is maternal stabilization & delivery as soon as safely possible.

➤ Anesthetic mgt should be guided by OB criteria & physiologic manifestations of the disease process.

➤ Special attention to coagulation status, as it has important implications for regional anesthesia & peripartum hemorrhage
➤ The maternal condition usually improves within 24 hours of delivery, w/ continued recovery over the next week.
• There is generally no long-term liver dysfunction for survivors.

CHECKLIST
■ Know OB plan.
■ Degree of pt's compromise will dictate need for invasive monitoring, ICU care.
■ Beware of coagulopathy, renal failure.

ACUTE GLOMERULONEPHRITIS

JOSHUA WEBER, MD
PETER DUNN, MD

FUNDAMENTAL KNOWLEDGE
■ Immunologic response to infection, usually group A beta-hemolytic streptococcal (although can be initiated by other bacterial or viral infections), that damages renal glomeruli
■ Acute glomerulonephritis is rare during pregnancy.
■ 3 urinary patterns are seen: focal nephritic, diffuse nephritic, nephrotic.

STUDIES
Lab tests commonly ordered to evaluate renal function in pregnancy include:
■ Creatinine
■ BUN
■ Electrolytes
■ Creatinine clearance
■ CBC
■ Urinalysis typically shows hematuria, proteinuria & red cell casts.
■ In addition, consider:
■ Renal biopsy

Focal nephritic
■ Inflammatory lesions in less than half of glomeruli
■ Urinalysis shows red cells, +/− red cell casts, & mild proteinuria.

Diffuse nephritic
■ Affects most or all glomeruli

- Heavy proteinuria
- +/− renal insuffiency

Nephrotic
- Heavy proteinuria
- Few red cell casts

MANAGEMENT/INTERVENTIONS

Medical/OB mgt of acute glomerulonephritis:
- Treatment of acute glomerulonephritis depends on the underlying etiology.
- For decreased renal function:
  - Increased frequency of prenatal visits (q2 wks in 1st & 2nd trimesters, then q1 week)
  - Monitoring: monthly measurements of serum creatinine, creatinine clearance, fetal development, BP
  - Erythropoietin may be used for maternal anemia.
  - Preterm delivery is considered for worsening renal function, fetal compromise or pre-eclampsia.
  - Renal biopsy is considered if rapid deterioration in renal function occurs prior to 32 weeks gestation.
  - If glomerulonephritis is responsive to steroids, these should be continued during pregnancy.
  - See "*Parturients on Dialysis*" for dialysis mgt.

Anesthetic mgt of pts w/ acute glomerulonephritis
Pre-op
- Evaluate degree of renal dysfunction & hypertension.
- Evaluate for anemia & electrolyte abnormalities.

Intraoperative mgt
- Monitors: standard monitoring + fetal heart rate (FHR) +/− arterial line +/− CVP
- Limit fluids in pts w/ marginal renal function to prevent volume overload.
- Use strict aseptic technique, as uremic pts are more prone to infection.
- Careful padding/protection of dialysis access is important.
- Consider promotility agents, as uremic pts may have impaired GI motility.

Regional anesthesia
- Uremia-induced platelet dysfunction leads to increased bleeding time.

- Pts may have thrombocytopenia from peripheral destruction of platelets.
- Increased toxicity from local anesthetics has been reported in pts w/ renal disease, but amide & ester local anesthetics can be used safely.
- Contraindications to regional technique: pt refusal, bacteremia, hypovolemia, hemorrhage, coagulopathy, neuropathy

General anesthesia

- Uremic pts may have hypersensitivity to CNS drugs due to increased permeability of blood-brain barrier.
- Uremia causes delayed gastric emptying & increased acidity, leading to increased risk of aspiration pneumonitis (consider sodium citrate, H2-receptor blocker, metoclopramide).
- Hypoalbuminemia leads to increased free drug concentration in drugs that are bound to albumin (ie, thiopental).
- Succinylcholine is relatively contraindicated, as it causes approx. 1-mEq/L increase in serum potassium, which may precipitate cardiac dysrhythmias.
- Use caution w/ drugs dependent on renal excretion (gallamine, vecuronium, pancuronium) & clearance (mivacurium, rocuronium).

CAVEATS & PEARLS

- Succinylcholine is relatively contraindicated, as it causes approx. 1-mEq/L increase in serum potassium, which may precipitate cardiac dysrhythmias.
- Use caution w/ drugs dependent on renal excretion (gallamine, vecuronium, pancuronium) & clearance (mivacurium, rocuronium).
  - ➤ Cisatracurium is a good muscle relaxant for pts w/ renal dysfunction, as its clearance is independent of renal function (Hoffman degradation).
  - ➤ Standard doses of anticholinesterases are used for reversal of neuromuscular blockade.
  - ➤ Consider whether pt is likely to have platelet dysfunction (secondary to uremia) or significant peripheral neuropathy before doing regional anesthetic.

CHECKLIST

- Check OB plan for pt.
- Document degree of renal dysfunction.
- Be prepared to manage hypertension.

ACUTE INTERSTITIAL NEPHRITIS

JOSHUA WEBER, MD
PETER DUNN, MD

FUNDAMENTAL KNOWLEDGE

Acute interstitial nephritis is usually characterized by development of acute renal failure after starting a known offending drug.

Causes

- Drugs: antibiotics, NSAIDs
- Infection
- Sarcoidosis
- Systemic lupus
- Idiopathic

Presentation

- Rash
- Fever
- Eosinophilia

STUDIES

Lab tests commonly ordered to evaluate renal function in pregnancy include:

- Creatinine
- BUN

Expect acute elevations in BUN & creatinine

- Electrolytes
- Creatinine clearance
- CBC
- Urinalysis will show white cells, red cells & white cell casts.

In addition to labs commonly evaluated in pregnancy, the following tests may be performed:

- Decreased urine output
- Eosinophilia in serum
- Renal biopsy
- Gallium scan (high false-negative rate)

MANAGEMENT/INTERVENTIONS

Medical/OB mgt of AIN

- Trial of corticosteroids (improvement usually seen in 1–2 weeks)

Increased frequency of prenatal visits (q2 wks in 1st & 2nd trimesters, then q1 week)

- Monitoring: monthly measurements of serum creatinine, creatinine clearance, fetal development, BP
- Erythropoietin may be used for maternal anemia.
- Preterm delivery is considered for worsening renal function, fetal compromise or pre-eclampsia.
- Renal biopsy is considered if rapid deterioration in renal function occurs prior to 32 weeks gestation.

Anesthetic mgt in pts w/ renal dysfunction

Pre-op

- Evaluate degree of renal dysfunction & hypertension.
- Evaluate for anemia & electrolyte abnormalities.
- Intraoperative mgt:
- Monitors: standard monitoring + fetal heart rate (FHR) +/− arterial line +/− CVP
- Limit fluids in pts w/ marginal renal function to prevent volume overload.

Regional anesthesia

- Increased toxicity from local anesthetics has been reported in pts w/ renal dysfunction, although esters & amides can be used safely.
- Contraindications to regional technique: pt refusal, bacteremia, significant hypovolemia, severe hemorrhage, coagulopathy, potentially preexisting neuropathy

General anesthesia

- Succinylcholine may be relatively contraindicated, as it causes approx. 1-mEq/L increase in serum potassium, which may precipitate cardiac dysrhythmias.
- Use caution w/ drugs dependent on renal excretion (gallamine, vecuronium, pancuronium) & clearance (mivacurium, rocuronium).

CAVEATS & PEARLS

- Trial of corticosteroids (improvement usually seen in 1–2 weeks) may be indicated.
- Succinylcholine may be relatively contraindicated, as it causes approx. 1-mEq/L increase in serum potassium, which may precipitate cardiac dysrhythmias.
- Use caution w/ drugs dependent on renal excretion (gallamine, vecuronium, pancuronium) & clearance (mivacurium, rocuronium).

TVO 56 79

■ Cisatracurium is a good muscle relaxant for pts w/ renal dysfunction, as its clearance is independent of renal function (Hoffman degradation).

■ Standard doses of anticholinesterases are used for reversal of neuromuscular blockade.

■ Consider whether pt is likely to have platelet dysfunction (secondary to uremia) or significant peripheral neuropathy before doing regional anesthetic.

CHECKLIST
■ Check OB plan for pt.
■ Document degree of renal dysfunction.
■ Be prepared to manage hypertension.

ACUTE TUBULAR NECROSIS

JOSHUA WEBER, MD
PETER DUNN, MD

FUNDAMENTAL KNOWLEDGE
■ Acute tubular necrosis (ATN) is an *intrarenal* cause of acute renal failure in pregnancy. Characterized by renal vasoconstriction, which leads to a 50% decrease in blood flow

Pathogenesis
■ Ischemia: hypotension leads to decreased blood flow, which damages medullary cells
■ Toxins: cause damage to proximal tubules

Causes of ATN
■ Trauma/rhabdomyolysis
■ Renal ischemia from septic/hemorrhagic/hypovolemic shock
■ Nephrotoxic drugs
■ Amniotic fluid embolism
■ Intrauterine fetal death

STUDIES
■ Creatinine (may see acute elevation)
■ BUN (may see acute elevation)
■ BUN/creatinine ratio 10:1
■ Electrolytes
■ Creatinine clearance

- CBC
- Urinalysis
- Decreased urine output
- Urinalysis -> brown epithelial cell casts
- Urine osmolality <350 mOsm/kg water
- Urine sodium >40 mEq/L
- Fractional sodium excretion (FENa) >1%
- Urinary/plasma creatinine <20

MANAGEMENT/INTERVENTIONS

Medical/OB mgt of ATN

- Rule out DIC.
- For decreased renal function
  - Increased frequency of prenatal visits (q2 wks in 1st & 2nd trimesters, then q1 week)
  - Monitoring: monthly measurements of serum creatinine, creatinine clearance, fetal development, BP
  - Erythropoietin may be used for maternal anemia.
  - Preterm delivery is considered for worsening renal function, fetal compromise or pre-eclampsia.
  - Renal biopsy is considered if rapid deterioration in renal function occurs prior to 32 weeks gestation.
  - See "*Parturients on Dialysis*" for dialysis mgt.

Anesthetic mgt for pts w/ new-onset renal dysfunction

Pre-op

- Evaluate degree of renal dysfunction & hypertension.
- Evaluate for anemia & electrolyte abnormalities.

Intraoperative mgt

- Monitors: standard monitoring + fetal HR +/− arterial line +/− CVP
- Limit fluids in pts w/ marginal renal function to prevent volume overload.

Regional anesthesia

- Uremia-induced platelet dysfunction leads to increased bleeding time.
- Pts may have thrombocytopenia from peripheral destruction of platelets.
- Increased toxicity from local anesthetics has been reported in pts w/ renal disease, but amide & ester local anesthetics can be used safely.
- Contraindications to regional technique: pt refusal, bacteremia, hypovolemia, hemorrhage, coagulopathy, neuropathy

General anesthesia

- Uremic pts may have hypersensitivity to CNS drugs due to increased permeability of blood-brain barrier.
- Uremia causes delayed gastric emptying & increased acidity, leading to increased risk of aspiration pneumonitis (consider sodium citrate, H2-receptor blocker, metoclopramide).
- Hypoalbuminemia leads to increased free drug concentration of drugs that are bound to albumin (ie, thiopental).
- Succinylcholine is relatively contraindicated, as it causes approx. 1-mEq/L increase in serum potassium, which may precipitate cardiac dysrhythmias.
  - ➤ Use caution w/ drugs dependent on renal excretion (gallamine, vecuronium, pancuronium) & clearance (mivacurium, rocuronium).

CAVEATS & PEARLS

- BUN >18 & creatinine >0.8 are signs of renal dysfunction in pregnancy.
- Goals are to maintain renal perfusion & euvolemia.
- ATN may require diuretics, vasopressors & alkalinization.

CHECKLIST

- Check OB plan for pt.
- Document degree of renal dysfunction.
- Beware of electrolyte imbalances.

ADRENAL INSUFFCIENCY

GRACE C. CHANG, MD, MBA; ROBERT A. PETERFREUND, MD, PhD; AND STEPHANIE L. LEE, MD, PhD

FUNDAMENTAL KNOWLEDGE

See *"Hypercortisolism."*

Physiology

- Results from inadequate basal or stress level of plasma cortisol
- Diagnosis is imperative, as failure to initiate treatment can be fatal.

Epidemiology

- Rare endocrine condition; even more rare in pregnancy

Signs/Symptoms

- Weakness

- Altered consciousness, progressing from inattention to delirium to coma
- Malaise
- Slow respiration
- Nausea/vomiting
- Hypoglycemia
- Hypotension
- Hypothermia
- Bradycardia
- Cyclical fever
- Abdominal pain

Etiology
- Drugs (etomidate, ketoconazole, abrupt cessation of glucocorticoids or Megace therapy)
- Preexisting conditions that inhibit synthesis of steroid can suppress normal corticosteroid response & lead to adrenal insufficiency.
- Infections
- Tumors
- Adrenal hemorrhage
- Coagulopathy
- Postpartum pituitary necrosis (Sheehan's syndrome)

Complications
- Pregnancy & live birth can be expected in 87% of treated pts, compared w/ 54% of untreated pts.

STUDIES
- Initial tests should evaluate levels of ACTH & TSH.
- Use provocative tests such as ACTH (cosyntropin) test to provoke responses of cortisol & aldosterone.
- Plasma cortisol in nonpregnant pts should rise at least 12 mcg/dL above baseline, increase 2–3× over baseline & exceed 18 mcg/dL, & reach a maximal level at 60 minutes.
- Normal range of aldosterone: 7–35 ng/dL
- Primary adrenal insufficiency: baseline aldosterone levels are low & there is no response to cosyntropin
- Secondary adrenal insufficiency: baseline aldosterone levels may be low or normal, but then should rise to at least 4 ng/dL at 30 minutes after injection
- Check TSH w/ free T4 level in secondary adrenal insufficiency to exclude other pituitary deficiencies.

- Autoimmune primary adrenal insufficiency is associated w/ primary hypothyroidism.

MANAGEMENT/INTERVENTIONS
- Hormone replacement therapy depends on type & extent of lesion & degree of hormone deficit.
- In acute severe adrenal crisis, give 100 mg hydrocortisone IV, w/ gradual taper (50 mg every 8 hours over 1–2 days), & then oral administration of usual steroid replacement.
- Use aggressive IV hydration w/ D5 to prevent hypoglycemia.
- Correct thyroid deficiency w/ L-thyroxine.
- Consider mineralocorticoid replacement w/ fludrocortisone, although secondary adrenal insufficiency does not require mineralocorticoid therapy.
- Adrenal insufficiency requires continued replacement of corticosteroid throughout pregnancy, w/ stress doses at delivery (50–100 mg IV q8h or as continuous infusion).
- During stressful events, such as labor, increased doses of corticosteroids are required to prevent adrenal crisis.

Anesthetic Management
- Both general & regional anesthesia can be safely used.
- Epidural anesthesia is recommended to decrease stress response from labor.
- Aggressive volume replacement
- Monitor urine output closely; decreased renal blood flow is associated w/ adrenal insufficiency.
- Give stress-dose steroids (100 mg hydrocortisone IV) pre-op, or prior to labor or C-section, or if sudden hypotension occurs.
- In life-threatening adrenal insufficiency, treat w/ hydrocortisone 100 mg IV bolus or continuous IV infusion of hydrocortisone, 10 mg/hr.
  ➤ Invasive monitoring w/ arterial line & pulmonary artery catheter may be advisable.
- Use IV & inhalational anesthetics carefully, since they can cause myocardial depression & hypotension.
- Carefully monitor electrolytes; adrenal insufficiency is associated w/ hyponatremia, hypokalemia, hypoglycemia.
- Pt may have reduced non-depolarizing muscle relaxant requirement.
- Monitor muscle blockade carefully w/ peripheral nerve stimulator.
- Avoid etomidate, as it is associated w/ adrenal suppression.

CAVEATS/PEARLS

- Adrenal insufficiency is associated w/ skeletal muscle weakness; pt may require less non-depolarizing neuromuscular blocking agents.
- Adrenal insufficiency w/ fever & abdominal pain can mimic an abdominal infectious process.

CHECKLIST

- Give stress-dose steroids (100 mg hydrocortisone IV) pre-op, during labor & prior to C-section. With prolonged labor, continue with hydrocortisone 50–100 mg IV q8h.
- Monitor hemodynamics & fluid status closely.
- Be prepared to manage adrenal crisis.
- Monitor electrolytes closely.
- Use non-depolarizing neuromuscular blocking agents judiciously.

ALCOHOLIC HEPATITIS

LAWRENCE WEINSTEIN, MD
DOUG RAINES, MD

FUNDAMENTAL KNOWLEDGE

- Alcoholic hepatitis is characterized by acute or chronic inflammation & hepatic necrosis.
- Often reversible, but may be a precursor to chronic alcoholic cirrhosis
- Presentation can range from an asymptomatic pt w/ hepatomegaly to a critically ill person w/ a fulminant course.
- Physical symptoms & signs include abdominal pain, fever, ascites, jaundice & encephalopathy.
- Recent heavy drinking, hepatomegaly, jaundice & anorexia strongly support diagnosis.

STUDIES

- Elevated transaminases
  - ➤ AST is usually elevated to a greater extent than ALT.
- Elevated alkaline phosphatase
- Bilirubin elevated in >50% of pts
- PT can be elevated w/ advanced hepatocellular compromise. High elevations in PT correlate w/ increased mortality; see the section on "General Concepts."
- Serum albumin decreased

- Macrocytic anemia may be present secondary to dietary deficits of folate & vitamin B12.
- Thrombocytopenia is seen in about 10% of pts.
- Liver biopsy is diagnostic & shows macrovesicular fat, neutrophilic infiltration, hepatic necrosis & Mallory bodies.
- Ultrasound can be useful to rule out biliary obstruction.

MANAGEMENT/INTERVENTIONS

- Abstinence from alcohol is essential. Pts should be provided w/ nutritional support (especially folate & thiamine).
- Corticosteroids may be of benefit in reducing short-term mortality.
- For pts w/ alcoholic hepatitis specifically, a history of alcohol use may have resulted in alcoholic cardiomyopathy w/ compromised ventricular function. For discussion of mgt of the parturient w/ cardiomyopathy, see *"Valvular Disease"* chapter.
- As w/ all liver disease pts, anesthetic decisions should be guided by the symptoms & manifestations of the liver process. Various manifestations will have differing effects on physiology & choice of anesthetic technique for labor or delivery.
  - ➤ If pt is coagulopathic, see the section on *"General Concepts."*
  - ➤ If pt is cirrhotic, see sections on *"General Concepts," "Cirrhosis," "Portal Hypertension," "Ascites," "Hepatic Encephalopathy."*
  - ➤ For general discussion of regional & general anesthesia considerations, see the section on *"General Concepts."*

CAVEATS/PEARLS

- Alcoholic hepatitis can be suspected in pts w/ elevated aminotransferases & a history of excessive alcohol use.
- Treatment is mostly supportive, w/ abstinence from alcohol being essential.
- Anesthetic decisions are based on physiologic manifestations present at time of surgery or delivery.
- Cardiac function may be compromised from long-term alcohol abuse; an echocardiogram may be prudent in this population.

CHECKLIST

- Watch for other alcohol-related complications, including those of withdrawal.
- Check coagulation status prior to initiation of regional anesthesia.

AMNIOTIC FLUID EMBOLUS (AFE)

JASON JENKINS, MD
LEE WESNER, MD

FUNDAMENTAL KNOWLEDGE

Incidence, morbidity, mortality

- While rare overall, true incidence is unknown due to difficulty in diagnosis. Clinical or fatal episodes occur in 1:8,000 to 1:80,000 pregnancies.
- High mortality: 80%, frequently within 5 hours of onset
- Only 15–25% of survivors remain neurologically intact.

Risk factors

- No specific risk factors other than pregnancy have been identified at this time.

Etiology

- Remains uncertain. Cardiovascular collapse does not appear to be due to an embolic process, as previously thought. Humoral mechanisms are currently suspected, & prognosis appears worse w/ meconium-stained amniotic fluid. Evidence does not support hypertonic uterine contractions as causative.

Clinical presentation

- General: classically described as sudden & profound cardiopulmonary collapse in a pregnant pt after an unexpected episode of dyspnea & restlessness. May occur throughout pregnancy, labor & immediate post-partum period.
- Cardiovascular: hypotension & tachycardia progressing to arrhythmias & cardiac arrest. Fatal right ventricular (RV) failure early due to pulmonary vasospasm, followed by left ventricular (LV) failure. Low cardiac output.
- Pulmonary: dyspnea, hypoxia, wheezing or bronchospasm, pulmonary edema, cough, ARDS
- Neurologic: anxiety, restlessness, headache, unconsciousness, convulsions
- Hematologic: consumptive coagulopathy progressing to disseminated intravascular coagulation (DIC). Severe DIC may lead to exsanguinating hemorrhage.
- Fetal: bradycardia, hypotension. Perinatal mortality near 80%, <40% of survivors neurologically intact.

STUDIES

AFE is primarily a clinical diagnosis of exclusion. Do not delay CPR for confirmatory studies.

Lab tests
- Hematologic: overall picture of coagulopathy
  - Thrombocytopenia
  - Decreased fibrinogen
  - Elevated d-dimer or fibrinogen split products
  - Prolonged PT or PTT
- ABGs may show metabolic acidosis.
- PA blood smear: presence of squamous cells is not diagnostic.

Imaging
- Ultrasound
  - Echocardiography: may see LV or RV dysfunction, possibly pulmonary hypertension
- Radiographic
  - Angiography, CT, V-Q scans useful in eliminating other diagnoses

Monitoring
- Standard noninvasive monitors (oximetry, ECG, etc.)
- Invasive monitoring guides fluid mgt.
  - Pulmonary artery (PA) line: monitor cardiac output, filling pressures, obtain mixed venous blood samples. Pulmonary hypertension often resolves by the time PA monitoring begins.
  - Arterial line: useful for pressure monitoring & frequent blood sampling

MANAGEMENT/INTERVENTIONS

General principles
- Treatment is generally supportive & symptom-directed. Since most pts are previously young & healthy, prompt & aggressive resuscitative measures are appropriate.

Cardiovascular
- Vascular
  - Volume: rapid volume infusion to optimize preload
  - Systemic vasopressors (eg, phenylephrine) to support systemic perfusion
  - Pulmonary vasodilators (eg, NO, prostacyclin) may be useful adjuncts, but few data exist for their use in AFE.

> Diuretics may be required to treat pulmonary edema following major volume infusion.

- Cardiac
  > Inotropic support (eg, dopamine, dobutamine) is often needed to treat cardiogenic shock.
  > Full or partial cardiopulmonary bypass, though rare, has been used successfully.
  > Afterload reduction may be required to promote cardiac output, but must be balanced carefully w/ need to maintain systemic perfusion.

Pulmonary

- Goal is providing maximal oxygenation, & almost all pts require emergent endotracheal intubation. Initial hypoxia may be severe enough to result in permanent neurologic injury.
- Ventilatory support can be challenging, requiring CPAP or PEEP. ARDS can develop in severe cases, further complicating mgt. ECMO may be beneficial in the direst cases.

Hematologic

- PRBCs to treat massive hemorrhage often associated w/ AFE
- Platelets as appropriate for thrombocytopenia
- FFP is generally used for coagulopathy, but cryoprecipitate may be useful if volume overload is concerning.

Neurologic

- Maintain perfusion pressure & oxygenation. Hypoxic neurologic insult is common & devastating.

Fetal

- Prompt cesarean delivery may assist maternal survival.
- Perimortem delivery may allow fetal survival.

CAVEATS/PEARLS

- AFE is devastating, not preventable & not predictable. It is a diagnosis of exclusion & must be considered quickly.
- Some suggest "anaphylactoid syndrome of pregnancy" & feel embolus is misnomer.
- Epithelial cells in maternal serum nondiagnostic for AFE, but presence of vernix/lanugo on PA blood smear may support diagnosis.
- Anaphylaxis-like picture in AFE; may consider epinephrine/corticosteroids if other modalities fail.
- Pulmonary hypertension may resolve before placement of PA catheter.

■ Cardiopulmonary bypass, embolectomy, inhaled pulmonary vaso–dilators uncommon but successful use reported.

CHECKLIST
■ High index of suspicion; consider & treat early.
■ Cardiovascular support: volume, pressors, inotropes
■ Pulmonary support: intubation & ventilation
■ Hematologic treatment: large volumes of blood products
■ Prompt fetal delivery

AMYOTROPHIC LATERAL SCLEROSIS (ALS)

MEREDITH ALBRECHT, MD
MICHELE SZABO, MD

FUNDAMENTAL KNOWLEDGE

Definition
■ Progressive neurodegenerative motor neuron disease

Epidemiology
■ Progressive respiratory paralysis; median survival 3–5 years
■ Incidence 1–3 per 100,000
  Males > females
■ Sporadic but 5–10% familial (autosomal dominant)

Pathophysiology
■ Pathologic hallmark: death of both lower motor neurons (anterior horn cells) & upper motor neurons (corticospinal)
■ Sensory apparatus is unaffected.

Clinical Manifestations
■ Variable depending on degree of upper or lower motor neuron involvement
■ Sensory, bowel, bladder & cognitive function are spared.

Effect of Pregnancy on ALS
■ Mainly unaffected, although can increase respiratory compromise

Effect of ALS on Pregnancy & the Fetus
■ ALS does not appear to have any effect on the fetus/pregnancy.
■ Can increase the incidence of instrumented deliveries due to lack of muscle strength

STUDIES

History & Physical
- Muscle weakness
- Hyperreflexia
  - ➤ Fasciculations
- Muscle atrophy
- History of bulbar weakness
- History of respiratory involvement

Imaging
- MRI
- Contrast myelography

Other
- Pulmonary function tests to assess baseline respiratory status

MANAGEMENT/INTERVENTIONS

Medical Treatment
- Supportive
- Physical therapy
- Riluzole (glutamate antagonist): modest lengthening of trach-free survival
- Celecoxib (COX-2 inhibitor) & minocycline (tetracycline antibiotic) have been used.

Anesthesia
- Predelivery assessment
  - ➤ Evaluate respiratory status prior to & during labor.
  - ➤ Determine presence of bulbar weakness and increased risk for aspiration.
  - ➤ Document preexistent weakness.
- General anesthesia
  - ➤ Suggested if severe respiratory dysfunction exists
  - ➤ Increased incidence of aspiration; aspiration prophylaxis is recommended
  - ➤ Increased sensitivity to muscle relaxants
  - ➤ Avoid succinylcholine due to risk of hyperkalemia & rhabdomyolysis.
- Regional anesthesia
  - ➤ Epidural can be used w/o decreased neurologic function.
  - ➤ Spinal anesthesia: conflicting reports; has been associated w/ worsened neurologic function post-op in a few cases, but also no decrease in neurologic function in other cases.

CAVEATS & PEARLS
- Progressive neurodegenerative disease affecting both upper & lower motor neurons,
- Hallmarks are motor weakness & hyperreflexia.
- Pregnancy contributes to increased respiratory compromise.
- Bulbar paralysis increases risk of aspiration
- Increased sensitivity to muscle relaxants
- Avoid succinylcholine.
- May require post-op ventilation
- Regional anesthesia has been used without altering baseline neurologic function.

CHECKLIST
- Document preexisting neurologic dysfunction.
- Carefully assess pulmonary status at start of & during labor.
- Pulmonary function tests are recommended if pulmonary involvement is present.
- Aspiration prophylaxis
- General anesthesia if severe respiratory dysfunction present
- Avoid succinylcholine.

ANEMIA

JEANNA VIOLA, MD
JANE BALLANTYNE, MD

FUNDAMENTAL KNOWLEDGE
- Anemia = a low erythrocyte count; it can be further classified as macrocytic, normocytic or microcytic.
- Causes vary from nutritional deficiency to disorders of hemoglobin production.
- Common diagnosis in pregnancy, usually due to hemodilutional state or deficiency of iron and/or folate
- Certain pts may have chronic anemia that precedes pregnancy: pts w/ renal disease or those taking drugs that impair erythropoiesis (certain anti-rheumatologic therapy).
- Most parturients tolerate anemia well.

STUDIES
- Hemoglobin, Hct, MCV
- Further studies are directed at determining the cause of anemia.

➤ Microcytic anemia: iron, ferritin, TIBC levels; consider hemoglobin electrophoresis to diagnose thalassemia

➤ Macrocytic anemia: check folate, vitamin B12 levels

➤ Normocytic anemia: may be a combination of nutritional deficiencies

MANAGEMENT/INTERVENTIONS

■ Transfusion of PRBCs usually not warranted

➤ Guide decision to transfuse by evidence of poor hemodynamic status, severe symptoms of anemia (shortness of breath, dyspnea on exertion, flow murmur), active bleeding or hemolysis.

➤ Weigh benefits of transfusion against risks of clerical error, bacterial or viral infection or transfusion reaction.

■ Give oxygen to pts w/ Hgb <8 during delivery.

■ Maintain a warm environment for pts w/ cold agglutinin-induced hemolytic anemia.

■ If anemia exists as part of pancytopenia, pt may also require a platelet transfusion or antibiotics for neutropenia-induced infections.

■ Regional anesthesia is not contraindicated unless the anemia is associated w/ a thrombocytopenia or coagulopathy.

CAVEATS AND PEARLS

■ Most parturients compensate for the anemia well.

■ Regional anesthesia is not contraindicated unless there is a concomitant thrombocytopenia or coagulopathy.

CHECKLIST

■ Check CBC to assess severity of anemia & to rule out other cytopenias.

■ Evaluate how well the pt has compensated for the anemia:

➤ Shortness of breath?

➤ Dyspnea on exertion?

➤ Presence of flow murmur?

■ Administer supplemental oxygen.

Send blood sample for type & cross if transfusion may be warranted.

ANESTHESIA FOR CESAREAN DELIVERY

DRAGOS DIACONESCU, MD
JEAN MARIE CARABUENA, MD

FUNDAMENTAL KNOWLEDGE

Cesarean delivery: the delivery of a fetus by surgical incision through the abdominal wall & uterus

Incidence: In 2002, 26.1% of deliveries in the U.S. were via cesarean delivery. This has increased in recent years due to the lower rates of vaginal birth after cesarean delivery (VBAC), among other factors.

Common indications
- Prior cesarean delivery (about 35%)
- Dystocia or cephalopelvic disproportion (30%)
- Breech presentation (12%)
- Non-reassuring fetal heart rate tracings (9%)

Morbidity/mortality
- About 80% of cases of anesthesia-related maternal deaths occurred during cesarean deliveries.
- The case fatality rate associated w/ general anesthesia is about 15 times higher than w/ regional techniques.
- The increased use of regional anesthesia for cesarean delivery has led to a significant decrease in anesthesia-related maternal mortality.

Surgical considerations
- Preferably performed by lower uterine incision (less blood loss, lower incidence of rupture during next pregnancies). Classic uterine incision is rarely used but is necessary in some pts (more blood loss, introduces need for a repeat cesarean delivery w/ subsequent pregnancies).
- Operative time varies according to obstetrician & clinical situation; usually 20–90 minutes, longer for classic incision.
- Usual blood loss 800–1,000 mL; may be more w/ repeat cesarean delivery, classic incision on uterus, previous abdominal surgery, multiple gestation, placenta accreta, abruption, etc.

Anesthetic considerations
- Anesthesia choices: spinal, epidural, combined spinal epidural, general, local.

- Special concerns: airway, full stomach, placental transfer of medications, pre-existing conditions (obstetric or medical), potential for blood loss
- Requires constant communication w/ obstetric care provider, nurses & other personnel

Classification (based on the level of urgency)
- **Elective:** scheduled at a time to suit the maternity unit and/or the OB floor
- **Emergency:** not performed on a scheduled basis
  - Stable: Fetal & maternal physiology is stable, but surgery is required before destabilization occurs
  - Urgent: Maternal and/or fetal physiology is unstable but is not immediately life-threatening to either of them
  - Emergent (stat): Pt has a condition that is immediately life-threatening to mother or fetus

Indications
- **Elective**
  - Mother's request
  - Deteriorating maternal medical illness (cardiac or pulmonary disease)
  - Maternal infection w/ HIV
  - Active genital herpes simplex virus infection in mother
  - Previous classic cesarean delivery
  - Previous myomectomy or uterine or vaginal reconstruction
  - Cervical cancer
  - Mechanical obstruction to vaginal birth (large leiomyoma or condyloma acuminata, severely displaced pelvic fracture)
  - Placenta previa
  - Suspected placenta accreta
  - Fetopelvic disproportion
  - Transverse or oblique lie
  - Most breech presentations
  - High-order multiple pregnancy
  - Fetal macrosomia
  - Fetal bleeding diathesis

Controversial
- Twin pregnancy
- Maternal hepatitis C infection

- Severe preeclampsia/eclampsia remote from term
- Certain fetal congenital abnormalities (gastroschisis, neural tube defects)
- Previous cesarean delivery (see "*Management of TOLAC or VBAC*")
  - ➤ **Stable**
    - Chronic uteroplacental insufficiency
    - Abnormal fetal presentation w/ ruptured membranes but not in labor
    - Dysfunctional uterine activity
  - ➤ **Urgent**
    - Failure to progress in labor
    - Active herpes w/ rupture of membranes
    - Non-bleeding placenta previa in labor
    - Cord prolapse w/o fetal distress
    - Variable FHR decelerations w/ prompt recovery & normal FHR variability
  - ➤ **Stat**
    - Agonal fetal distress (prolonged severe fetal bradycardia, late FHR decelerations w/ no FHR variability)
    - Cord prolapse w/ fetal distress
    - Massive hemorrhage (placenta previa, abruption, etc.)
    - Ruptured uterus

Anesthesia effects on the neonate
- Some studies have concluded that regional or general anesthesia does not cause significant changes in the fetal acid-base status as long as maternal hypotension & hypoxia are avoided.
- There is disagreement among studies as to whether general anesthesia is associated w/ lower 1-min Apgar scores.
- Inhalational agents cause only mild fetal depression when given in doses <1 MAC & if delivery occurs <10 minutes from induction.
- Uterine incision-to-delivery (U-D) interval >3 minutes is associated w/ a higher incidence of low fetal blood pH & Apgar scores.
- In some studies, w/ general anesthesia, induction-to-delivery (I-D) interval >8 minutes is associated w/ a higher incidence of low fetal blood pH & Apgar scores.
- Induction agents in usual doses & local anesthetics given spinally or epidurally have minimal effects on the fetus. Benzodiazepines & opiates may cause fetal depression & their use is minimized before the delivery. Muscle relaxants do not cross the placenta.

FHR monitoring

- Used by obstetricians as an indicator of fetal status, although it has a relatively low positive-predictive value for abnormal fetal condition. The false-positive rate can be as high as 50%.
- An external Doppler placed on the abdomen can provide continuous monitoring of the fetal heart rate & pattern. A fetal scalp electrode may be placed on the baby's head to obtain a more accurate tracing. Normal FHR is 120–160 bpm w/ good beat-to-beat variability. Long-term variability is also considered.
- The tracing can be within normal limits (as above) or suggestive of fetal compromise (non-reassuring). Non-reassuring FHR (late decelerations, deep variable decelerations, fetal tachycardia w/ loss of beat-to-beat variability, fetal bradycardia, undulating baseline, etc.) may prompt emergency delivery or further testing.
- Fetal scalp blood sampling may clarify a suspicion of compromised fetal well-being. A fetal scalp pH > 7.25 is normal, whereas a pH < 7.20 requires rapid delivery.
- The severity of the fetal compromise indicated by the abnormal FHR determines the urgency of the situation & the anesthetic choice.
- For chronic fetal distress (IUGR, etc.) the anesthetic choice of choice is regional, whereas acute severe fetal distress may require general anesthesia.
- Non-reassuring FHR may resolve or improve w/ certain maneuvers (maternal position change, adjustment of oxytocin, treatment of hypotension, etc.). Frequent monitoring & communication w/ the obstetric team may obviate the need for emergency induction of general anesthesia.

STUDIES

- Antepartum anesthesia consultation is recommended in some cases:
  - ➤ Massive obesity
  - ➤ Asthma requiring medications
  - ➤ Severe hypertensive disease
  - ➤ Maternal coagulopathy
  - ➤ Serious medical or obstetrical conditions
  - ➤ History of anesthetic complications
  - ➤ Severe facial or neck edema
  - ➤ Extremely short stature

➤ Decreased mobility of the neck, difficulty opening the mouth
➤ Anatomic abnormalities of face, mouth, neck or jaw
■ Past medical/surgical history, anesthetic history
■ Physical exam, airway exam
■ Hemoglobin
■ Type & screen; cross-match if significant loss of blood is anticipated
■ Coagulation times (PT, PTT, fibrinogen) & platelet count if pre-eclampsia, heavy maternal bleeding, abruptio placentae or preexisting bleeding diathesis
■ Check any recent imaging studies (previous ultrasound, MRI, etc.) to clarify any abnormalities that may affect the anesthetic plan (e.g., uterine or placental abnormalities).
■ Other studies as indicated from history & physical

MANAGEMENT/INTERVENTIONS

Preparation for Anesthesia

■ **NPO status**
➤ In the uncomplicated parturient, no solid food for at least 6, preferably 8 hours prior to elective cesarean delivery. Clear liquids can be ingested until 2 hours before surgery.
➤ Laboring women should avoid solid food & restrict their oral intake to clear liquids.
➤ All parturients are considered "full stomach" regardless of their NPO status.

■ **Pt education, anxiolysis & reassurance**
➤ A concise explanation of the anesthetic procedure & common side effects during & immediately after placement helps allay fears in most pts.
➤ Constant reassurance as the regional anesthetic is evolving is also helpful.
➤ Benzodiazepines & opiates in small doses can be given for severe anxiety (midazolam IV 0.5–2 mg, diazepam IV 2–5 mg, fentanyl IV 25–50 mcg). Amnesia & fetal depression are risks.
➤ Support person (e.g., the father of the baby) present during cesarean delivery under regional anesthesia provides reassurance & emotional support.

■ **Prophylactic IV fluid before induction**
➤ Was found to reduce the incidence of maternal hypotension & to improve uteroplacental perfusion
➤ Up to 15–20 mL/kg of crystalloid (Ringer's lactate, normal saline) in pts receiving regional anesthesia

> Avoid glucose or dextrose in the IV fluids because it causes maternal hyperinsulinemia w/ resultant fetal hypoglycemia in early postpartum.

> Colloids may be better than crystalloids because they remain in the intravascular space for a longer time, but they are more expensive & can alter the blood rheology & platelet function.

> Generally, the prophylactic administration of IV fluids should not delay the induction of anesthesia in cases that require immediate cesarean delivery.

■ **Prevention of acid aspiration**

> All parturients are considered at risk for aspiration regardless of the planned anesthetic.

> Oral non-particulate antacids (sodium citrate 30 mL), given 15–30 minutes prior to induction, increase the pH of the gastric contents. Avoid particulate antacids because they may cause pulmonary injury similar to that caused by gastric acid, if aspirated.

> Metoclopramide (10 mg IV) increases gastric emptying, acts as an antiemetic & increases the tone of the lower esophageal sphincter.

> Intravenous H2-receptor antagonists or proton pump inhibitors combined w/ sodium citrate cause a greater increase in the gastric pH if administered at least 30 minutes before intubation.

> Empty the stomach w/ an orogastric tube in all pts receiving general anesthesia.

■ **Supplemental oxygen**

> Indicated in cases of emergency cesarean delivery when the fetus and/or the mother is in distress.

> No documented benefit was found in neonates of healthy parturients having an elective cesarean delivery.

■ **Maternal positioning during & before cesarean delivery**

> In the supine position the gravid uterus compresses the aorta & inferior vena cava, leading to decreased venous return, uterine artery perfusion & cardiac output.

> Maintain left uterine displacement by placing a wedge (folded or rolled blankets) under the pt's right hip.

Monitoring during anesthesia

■ Standard monitors (noninvasive BP, EKG, pulse oximeter), urine output

■ Capnograph & temperature for general anesthesia

- Consider an arterial line for severe preeclampsia or massive blood loss.
- Consider central pressure monitoring as maternal condition warrants (e.g., significant maternal heart disease).

Choice of anesthetic
- Consider the indication for surgery, the urgency of the procedure, maternal coexisting disease & maternal preference. The anesthetic plan should be discussed w/ the obstetrician.
- Regional anesthesia is the preferred technique for both elective & emergency surgery due to its safety profile. A sensory level of T4 is desirable.
  - Spinal anesthesia
    - First-choice anesthetic technique for elective cesarean delivery
    - Good choice for many emergency cesarean deliveries due to rapid onset & simplicity
    - Negligible maternal risk of systemic local anesthetic toxicity or local anesthetic depression of the infant
    - Rapid onset of sympathetic blockade may result in abrupt hypotension w/ reduced uteroplacental perfusion.
    - Less ideal technique in pts w/ severe respiratory compromise, due to blockade of the thoracoabdominal segments.
    - May not provide long enough anesthesia if surgery lasts >90–120 minutes
  - Continuous spinal anesthesia
    - Not a first-line technique due to the high incidence of post-dural puncture headache w/ the 17- or 18-gauge needle/20-gauge catheter
    - Feasible technique in cases of accidental dural puncture if the catheter has threaded into the spinal space & CSF can be easily aspirated
    - Spinal drugs can be given in small doses to the desired effect, minimizing exaggerated BP changes. In addition, respiratory changes are less severe since the level is easier to control.
    - May be the technique of choice in select complicated obstetric pts; evaluate the risk:benefit ratio.
  - Epidural anesthesia
    - Slower onset, higher incidence of failed block & technically more involved than spinal anesthesia

- Less ideal in emergency cesarean delivery when time is of the essence
- Requires higher doses of local anesthetic that may be associated w/ significant maternal & fetal toxicity if injected intravascularly
- Severe hypotension or weakness of respiratory muscles can often be avoided or better addressed due to the incremental administration of drugs.
- A labor epidural w/ a demonstrable level can be extended to provide anesthesia for emergency cesarean delivery, thus obviating the need for general anesthesia.

➤ Combined spinal epidural anesthesia (CSE)
- Combines the advantages of spinal anesthesia (speed of onset, reliability) w/ the utility of an epidural catheter (ability to extend the duration of anesthesia by administering additional epidural drug)
- Preferred for elective cesarean deliveries when the anticipated surgical time is expected to be longer
- Technically more involved & may be more time-consuming than spinal anesthesia, thus limiting its use in an emergency situation

■ Contraindications to regional anesthesia
➤ Absolute: severe, uncorrected hypovolemia, anticoagulants or bleeding diathesis, severe aortic or mitral stenosis, increased intracranial pressure, infection at the site of injection
➤ Relative: uncooperative pt, preexisting neurologic deficits, stenotic valvular heart lesions, severe spinal deformity

■ General anesthesia
➤ The most reliable & rapid means of achieving adequate anesthesia for emergency stat cesarean delivery
➤ Should be reserved for cases in which adequate anesthesia cannot be achieved w/ regional techniques in a timely manner
➤ The overall risk of maternal mortality w/ general anesthesia is $17\times$ higher than w/ regional anesthesia; most deaths are due to airway problems.
➤ If the airway cannot be secured in a timely manner, the safety of the mother takes priority over delivery of the fetus.
➤ Urgency of delivery & the severity of fetal distress should always be weighed against the maternal risks of general anesthesia. Most emergency cesarean deliveries can be safely done under a regional technique.

> In pts w/ recognized difficult airway, placement of an epidural catheter early in labor provides a partial block that can be promptly extended if emergency delivery is required.
> Other indications: coagulopathy or other conditions that preclude the use of a regional technique, inadequate regional anesthesia or maternal refusal of regional anesthesia

■ Local anesthesia
> Very rarely employed as the sole anesthetic technique
> Involves local infiltration w/ large amounts of local anesthetic w/ high risk of systemic toxicity
> Indications: when rapid administration of regional or general anesthesia is not possible (severe coagulopathy & a known difficult airway); selected pts w/ extremely debilitating diseases; anesthesia personnel are not available
> Can be used as an adjuvant in pts w/ incomplete spinal or epidural anesthesia

■ Anesthetic options
> Elective cesarean delivery: spinal, epidural or CSE anesthesia, general anesthesia
> Emergency stable & urgent cesarean deliveries: spinal or extended epidural anesthesia, general anesthesia
> Emergent (stat) cesarean deliveries: general anesthesia or extended epidural (if a preexistent T10 or higher sensory level is present)

Anesthetic management
■ **Elective cesarean delivery w/ regional anesthesia**
1. Check NPO status.
2. Clarify maternal, fetal & obstetric issues w/ obstetrician.
3. Administer IV fluids.
4. Administer sodium citrate 30 ml PO, metoclopramide 10 mg IV.
5. Apply standard monitors.
6. Consider supplemental O_2 by face mask or nasal prongs.
7. Place pt in sitting or lateral decubitus position.
   Spinal
   • Should be administered in the surgical suite on the operative table
   • L3–L4 lumbar puncture w/ a 24- to 27-gauge non-cutting spinal needle
   • Medications: hyperbaric solution of bupivacaine (10–15 mg); may add fentanyl 10–25 mcg (to increase the intensity &

duration of the block) & preservative-free morphine 0.2–0.3 mg (for up to 24 hours postop analgesia)

Combined spinal epidural

- Should be administered in the surgical suite on the operative table
- Identify epidural space at L3–L4 w/ standard epidural needle. Use the spinal needle-through-epidural needle technique for dural puncture.
- Medications: same as above
- Remove the spinal needle & thread the epidural catheter.
- If the block is patchy or the pt becomes uncomfortable as the surgery is prolonged, the catheter can be tested w/ 3 mL of 2% lidocaine w/ epinephrine 1:200,000 w/ sodium bicarbonate (1 mEq/10 mL lidocaine). Additional local anesthetic can then be titrated to pt comfort.

Epidural

- May be administered outside the surgical suite (slower onset)
- Place L2–L3 or L3–L4 epidural catheter.
- Administer local anesthetic (lidocaine or bupivacaine) in 3- to 5-mL aliquots while monitoring maternal BP & ensuring fetal well-being.
  - 15–20 mL 2% lidocaine w/ epinephrine 1:200,000 w/ sodium bicarbonate (1 mEq/10 mL lidocaine)
  - 15–20 mL 0.5% bupivacaine (may add 0.05 mEq sodium bicarbonate/10 mL bupivacaine for a faster onset). Beware of potential for precipitation if more sodium bicarbonate is used.
  - Other adjuvants
    - Fentanyl 50–100 mcg (to increase intensity & duration of the block)
    - Preservative free morphine 3–5 mg (to prolong postop analgesia up to 24 hours)
8. Place pt supine on operative table, maintain uterine displacement & treat hypotension aggressively.
9. Reassure the pt as the numbing effects of the regional anesthetic evolve.
10. Clarify the level of anesthesia prior to incision.

■ **Elective cesarean delivery w/ general anesthesia**
  1. Check NPO status.
  2. Clarify maternal, fetal & obstetric issues w/ obstetrician.

3. Administer IV fluids.
4. Administer sodium citrate 30 mL PO & metoclopramide 10 mg IV (consider H2 antagonist or proton pump inhibitor 30 minutes before induction).
5. Apply standard monitors.
6. Place pt supine, maintaining left uterine displacement.
7. OR personnel can proceed w/ surgical prep & drape (minimizes induction-delivery interval).
8. If difficult airway is not suspected, proceed w/ denitrogenation 3–5 minutes 100% O_2 face mask.
9. Ensure proper pt positioning (elevation of the shoulders, "sniffing" position).
10. Rapid sequence induction w/ cricoid pressure
    • Medications: propofol 2 mg/kg or thiopental 4 mg/kg or ketamine 1 mg/kg & succinylcholine 1–1.5 mg/kg.
11. Intubation w/ a smaller cuffed ETT (6.5, 7.0). A short-handled laryngoscope can make intubation easier. Surgery can begin after confirmation of the proper placement of the ETT.
12. Maintenance on 50% nitrous oxide, oxygen & up to 0.5 MAC of volatile anesthetic. Avoid hyperventilation as it reduces uterine blood flow. Minimize IV narcotics until after delivery.
13. Aspirate gastric contents w/ an orogastric tube.
14. Administer intermediate-acting muscle relaxant if necessary.
15. After delivery, the nitrous oxide can be increased & the volatile decreased or discontinued to facilitate uterine involution. Administer opioids & consider benzodiazepines to prevent awareness.
16. At the end of the surgery, reverse muscle relaxants if necessary, remove orogastric tube & extubate when pt is awake.

■ **Emergency (stable, urgent, stat) cesarean delivery w/ regional anesthesia de novo**
1. Clarify maternal, fetal & obstetric issues w/ obstetrician as well as the urgency of the surgery.
2. Anesthetic of choice is spinal for more stable conditions, general for stat conditions.
3. Principles & procedure of spinal & general anesthesia as listed above
4. Clarify fetal-well being on arrival to operative suite.

■ **Emergency (stable, urgent, stat) cesarean delivery w/ pre-existing regional labor epidural**
➤ Clarify w/ obstetrician the fetal status & the urgency of delivery.

Stable cesarean delivery

1. Administer sodium citrate 30 mL PO & metoclopramide 10 mg IV.
2. Supplemental O_2 by face mask or nasal prongs
3. Check the level of existing blockade.
4. Administer supplemental IV fluids.
5. Monitor maternal BP & FHR as epidural is reinforced.
6. Medications:
   - Administer local anesthetic (lidocaine or bupivacaine) in 3- to 5-mL aliquots while monitoring maternal BP & ensuring fetal well-being.
   - 15–20 mL 2% lidocaine w/ epinephrine 1:200,000 w/ sodium bicarbonate (1 mEq/10 mL lidocaine)
   - 15–20 mL 0.5% bupivacaine (may add 0.05 mEq sodium barcarbonate/10 mL bupivacaine for a faster onset). Beware of potential for precipitation if more sodium bicarbonate is used.
   - Other adjuvants:
     - Fentanyl 50–100 mcg (to increase intensity & duration of the block)
     - Preservative-free morphine 3–5 mg (to prolong postoperative analgesia up to 24 hour).
7. Maintain uterine displacement & aggressively treat hypotension.
8. Transfer to the surgical suite, reapply standard monitors, maintain supplemental oxygen & uterine displacement & ensure fetal well-being.
9. Clarify the level of anesthesia prior to incision.

Urgent cesarean delivery

1. Steps 1 through 4 as above, but do not delay the administration of anesthesia to give the fluid bolus.
2. Monitor maternal BP & FHR as epidural is reinforced.
3. Medications
   - Administer local anesthetic (lidocaine or chloroprocaine) in 5-mL aliquots while monitoring maternal BP & ensuring fetal well-being.
   - 15–20 mL 2% lidocaine w/ epinephrine 1:200,000 w/ sodium bicarbonate (1 mEq/10 mL lidocaine)
   - 15–20 mL 3% 2-chloroprocaine w/ sodium bicarbonate (1 mEq/10 mL chloroprocaine)
   - Other adjuvants:

- Fentanyl 50–100 mcg (to increase intensity & duration of the block)
- Preservative-free morphine 3–5 mg (to prolong postop analgesia up to 24 hours)

4. Monitor BP & fetal status.
5. Transfer to OR; maintain uterine displacement.
6. Clarify the level of anesthesia prior to incision.

Emergent (stat) cesarean delivery

1. Administer sodium citrate 30 ml PO & metoclopramide 10 mg IV if readily available & call for someone to assist w/ the multiple tasks ahead.
2. Administer IV fluids & rapidly (over 2–3 minutes) reinforce epidural w/ 15–20 mL 3% 2-chloroprocaine in 5-mL aliquots as pt is being transferred to the surgical suite.
3. With rapid epidural bolus administration, maintain communication w/ the pt to ensure maternal well-being.
4. Maintain uterine displacement & re-apply supplemental oxygen on transfer to operative table (ensure that airway position is ideal).
5. Quickly apply standard monitors & assess level of anesthesia while FHR is being reassessed & the surgical prep is being done.
6. Can administer ketamine IV 10–20 mg (if not contraindicated) as the block is evolving, but be prepared for general anesthesia as a backup if regional block is insufficient.
7. If difficult intubation is suspected, consider awake intubation despite fetal depression.
8. If difficult intubation is not suspected, proceed w/ general anesthesia as outlined above.
9. Chloroprocaine can affect the onset & efficacy of epidural narcotics & amide local anesthetics. Redose the epidural after the delivery w/ 5–10 mL 2% lidocaine w/ epinephrine 1:200,000 & sodium bicarbonate (1 mEq/10 mL lidocaine) to maintain an established level of anesthesia.

Intraoperative mgt

- ■ **Difficult airway**
  - ➤ See "*General Anesthesia and Management of the Difficult Airway.*"
- ■ **Shortness of breath**
  - ➤ Mild dyspnea is common after the administration of the regional anesthetic & is caused by the high level of anesthesia concomitant

w/ the decreased pulmonary reserve w/ a gravid uterus. This usually improves after delivery. Recheck the sensory level, oxygen saturation, BP & heart rate. Oxygen & reassurance will usually suffice.

➤ In rare cases of total spinal or high spinal w/ severe respiratory compromise, consider gentle assistance w/ a fitted mask in the awake pt.

➤ Intubate if the pt is obtunded or adequate oxygenation cannot be maintained w/ spontaneous breathing.

■ **Hypotension**

➤ Defined as 20–30% decrease in BP or a systolic BP < 100 mm Hg. Hypertensive pts may need a higher BP to maintain uterine perfusion.

➤ Common side effect of regional anesthesia due to sympathetic blockade; more common in women who are not in labor than in women who are in labor

➤ May lead to decreased uteroplacental perfusion w/ non-reassuring FHR & fetal acidosis; pt may report nausea

➤ Measure BP every 1–2 minutes & aggressively treat it until it stabilizes.

➤ Prevention
  • IV boluses of fluid
  • Left uterine displacement
  • Prophylactic administration of ephedrine 25–50 mg IM before spinal anesthesia or 5–10 mg IV immediately after intrathecal injection has a questionable efficacy.

➤ Treatment
  • Ensure adequate uterine displacement.
  • IV boluses of fluid
  • Administration of supplemental O_2
  • Ephedrine (5- to 10-mg boluses IV)
  • Phenylephrine in small doses (25–50 mcg IV) is considered safe in healthy parturients having elective cesarean delivery. It may be indicated in conditions in which ephedrine-induced tachycardia is less desirable or in cases of refractory hypotension. Vasoconstriction w/ uteroplacental insufficiency may be of concern w/ large doses.

■ **Nausea & vomiting**

➤ Nausea that occurs immediately after a regional anesthetic is a very sensitive indicator of hypotension & should be treated as above. Visceral pain or neuraxial opioids (especially long-acting) are other causes of nausea in the peripartum period.

➤ Maintain adequate BP.
➤ Other medications
  • Ondansetron IV 1–4 mg
  • Metoclopramide IV 10–20 mg
  • If nausea is a side effect of the opioids: naloxone IV 40–160 mcg or nalbuphine IV 2.5–5 mg
  • Transdermal scopolamine (after the delivery) has a prolonged antiemetic effect.

■ **Failed block/Inadequate anesthesia**
➤ The failed block (complete absence or patchy sensory or motor blockade) is more common w/ epidural than w/ spinal anesthesia. When it occurs, the regional anesthetic procedure can be repeated, but if time is important, general anesthesia is required.
➤ During the surgery, pt may experience some abdominal discomfort even w/ adequate regional anesthesia. Severe discomfort & pain are common w/ incomplete (patchy) epidural block & can be treated with:
  • Ketamine IV in 10- to 20-mg increments
  • Opioids after delivery of the fetus
  • Induction of general anesthesia if pain cannot be controlled

■ **Antibiotic prophylaxis**
➤ Substantially reduces the risk of postop fever, endometritis, wound & urinary tract infection
➤ Optimal time of administration (after the cord is clamped vs. preop) is not known; currently is administered immediately after the cord clamping.
➤ Cefazolin (1 or 2 g IV) is most commonly used.

■ **Uterine atony**
➤ Uterine involution & increasing uterine tone significantly reduce the bleeding after delivery.
➤ Intravenous oxytocin is routinely given once the fetus is born & the cord is clamped (10–20 units oxytocin in 1,000 mL crystalloid, administered IV at 40–80 mU/min). Side effects: maternal hypotension & tachycardia.
➤ Communicate w/ obstetrician to clarify uterine tone. Verbally confirm each drug & preferred route of administration.
➤ If uterine atony & bleeding persists:
  • Methylergonovine: 0.2 mg IM or in cases of life-threatening uterine hemorrhage 0.2 mg IV over 1 minute or longer. Side effects: severe hypertension, esp. w/ IV administration.

- 15-methyl prostaglandin F2-alpha: 250 mcg IM or intramyometrially. Side effects: tachycardia, hypertension, bronchoconstriction, fever & vomiting.

■ **Shortness of breath after delivery**
  ➤ May be the result of venous air embolism. Found to occur subclinically in >60% of pts undergoing cesarean delivery. It is associated w/ chest pain, oxygen desaturation, hypotension & even cardiac arrest in severe cases.
  ➤ Mild symptoms can be treated w/ supplemental oxygen, IV fluid bolus, flooding the surgical field & slight reverse Trendelenburg (places the heart above the level of the surgical field).
  ➤ In severe cases, adequate circulatory & ventilatory support is warranted. May consider rapid insertion of a central venous catheter to aspirate air or hyperbaric oxygen therapy if cerebral air embolism is suspected.

■ **Shoulder pain**
  ➤ Blood within the peritoneum may trigger transient referred shoulder pain. Reassurance will usually suffice. Ensure adequate hemostasis & stability of maternal vital signs. IV opioids may be given to relieve severe discomfort.

■ **Shivering**
  ➤ Shivering is uncontrollable & can be considerable & quite disturbing to the parturient.
  ➤ Thermogenic & non-thermogenic factors may be involved (pain, labor, cold room, cold IV fluids, regional/general anesthesia).
  ➤ Use warm IV fluids. A warm blanket & verbal reassurance may reduce anxiety & help pt feel better. IV opioids may be given after delivery for persistent shivering.

CAVEATS & PEARLS

Advantages of elective cesarean delivery over vaginal birth include:

■ A known endpoint to the pregnancy, facilitating issues related to work, childcare, etc.
■ Possible reduction in the risk of pelvic floor injury & its sequelae (incontinence, prolapse)
■ Avoidance of post-term pregnancy & prevention of stillbirth
■ Avoidance of potential intrapartum problems (hypoxia, meconium aspiration, cord prolapse, etc.) & of perinatal transmission of maternal infections (HIV, herpes simplex virus, hepatitis B)
■ Reduction of fetal complications related to vaginal birth (cranial or clavicle fractures, brachial plexus injuries, etc.) & possible reduction in perinatal mortality

Complications
- **Surgery-related**
  - ➤ Infection
  - ➤ Bladder & bowel injury
  - ➤ Pulmonary thromboembolism
  - ➤ Venous air embolism
  - ➤ Amniotic fluid embolism
- **Anesthesia-related**
  - ➤ Inability to oxygenate & ventilate the pt
  - ➤ Pulmonary aspiration
  - ➤ Local anesthetic toxicity
  - ➤ Cardiovascular instability
  - ➤ Nausea/vomiting
  - ➤ Post-dural puncture headache
  - ➤ Postop respiratory depression
  - ➤ Epidural hematoma
  - ➤ Nerve damage

CHECKLIST
1. Close communication w/ obstetrician is essential for choosing the appropriate anesthetic technique.
2. Antepartum anesthesia consultation is ideal for the high-risk pt.
3. Pt education & constant reassurance are vital components of complete anesthetic care.
4. For all pts in the surgical suite, attention should be given to the position of the airway, regardless of the anesthetic technique used. This ensures that w/ an unforeseen need for general anesthesia, optimal positioning is already addressed.
5. All obstetric pts are considered "full stomach" regardless of the time of last oral intake & are at risk for pulmonary aspiration.
6. Pts who are at increased risk for complications associated w/ general anesthesia should have epidural catheters placed early in labor.
7. FHR abnormalities may resolve; frequent monitoring may obviate the need for rapid induction of general anesthesia.
8. Spinal or epidural anesthesia is preferred to general anesthesia because regional anesthesia is associated w/ much lower maternal mortality.
9. Hypotension is very common during regional anesthesia & should be promptly treated to prevent fetal distress.
10. The incidence of failed intubation in parturients is 10x higher than in the non-obstetric population.

11. When general anesthesia is induced, if the airway is difficult to secure, the safety of the mother takes priority over the delivery of the fetus.
12. Neuraxial administration of long-acting narcotics (e.g., morphine) places the pt at risk for late respiratory depression. Close monitoring for up to 24 hours after administration is required.

ANESTHESIA FOR NON-OBSTETRIC SURGERY IN THE PREGNANT PATIENT

NISHA GUPTA, MD
RICHARD A. STEINBROOK, MD

FUNDAMENTAL KNOWLEDGE

■ Up to 2% of pregnant women in the U.S. undergo non-obstetric surgery.
■ Surgical conditions common to the maternal age group include appendicitis, cholelithiasis, ovarian cysts & torsion, breast tumor, trauma & cervical incompetence.
■ In caring for a pregnant pt, take into consideration both maternal safety & fetal well-being.

Maternal Considerations

Pregnancy affects virtually every organ system in the mother. The following are major physiologic changes having anesthetic implications.

Respiratory changes

■ Decreased functional residual capacity by 20%
■ Increased oxygen consumption
■ Increased alveolar ventilation (normal PCO_2 is approx. 32–35 mm Hg at term)
■ Increased reported incidence of difficult intubations

Cardiovascular changes

■ Increased blood volume
  ➤ By 10% during the 1st trimester
  ➤ By 30% during the 2nd trimester
  ➤ By 45% during the 3rd trimester
■ Increased cardiac output (CO)
  ➤ By 35–40% at end of 1st trimester
  ➤ By 50% during 2nd trimester
  ➤ No further increase during 3rd trimester

- Decreased systemic & pulmonary vascular resistances
- Presence of hyperdynamic flow murmurs on physical exam
- ECG changes (eg, left axis deviation) due to enlargement & cephalad rotation of the heart
- Aortocaval compression by gravid uterus in supine position

GI changes
- Decreased lower esophageal sphincter tone
- Increased intragastric pressure
- Increased gastric acid secretion
- Increased risk for gastroesophageal reflux

Hematologic changes
- Physiologic anemia (baseline hemoglobin approx. 11–12 g/dL by mid-gestation)
- Hypercoagulability

Neurologic changes
- Decreased MAC for inhalational agents by 25–40%
- Decreased local anesthetic requirement by 30% for regional blockade

Fetal Considerations
With regard to the fetus, the anesthesiologist's primary goals are to avoid teratogens, recognize the risk of preterm labor & prevent fetal asphyxia.

Teratogenicity
- The fetus is most vulnerable to teratogens during the 1st trimester, when organogenesis takes place.
- W/ the exception of cocaine, no anesthetic agent has been identified as a human teratogen.
  - Risks of cocaine in human pregnancy
    - Fetal growth retardation
    - Placental abruption
    - Uterine rupture
  - Regarding benzodiazepines
    - Use became controversial after several studies in the 1970s reported an association between 1st- trimester diazepam use & oral cleft anomalies.
    - Subsequently, large cohort & case-control investigations have shown no increased risk w/ benzodiazepine therapy.
    - No evidence suggests that a single benzodiazepine dose given preoperatively to a pregnant pt would be harmful to the fetus.
  - Regarding nitrous oxide
    - Despite being a weak teratogen in rodents, nitrous oxide has not shown adverse effects in human pregnancy.

- A cautious approach would be to avoid nitrous oxide during the 1st trimester, to administer it at concentrations of 50% or less, and to limit its use during long operations.

■ Drugs w/ long history of safe use during pregnancy include:
  ➤ Thiopental
  ➤ Opiates
  ➤ Inhalational agents
  ➤ Muscle relaxants
  ➤ Local anesthetics

Preterm labor & delivery

■ Epidemiologic studies of non-obstetric surgery during pregnancy report an increased incidence of abortion & preterm delivery.

■ Lowest risk occurs when surgery takes place during 2nd trimester & does not involve uterine manipulation.

■ Evidence does not support that any particular anesthetic agent or technique influences the risk of preterm labor.

Fetal asphyxia

Intra- & perioperative factors that can compromise fetal oxygenation include:

■ Maternal hypotension

■ Maternal hypoxia

■ Maternal hypocarbia causing maternal alkalosis
  ➤ Leads to decreased umbilical blood flow due to vasoconstriction
  ➤ Leads to decreased release of oxygen to fetus at placenta due to leftward shift of maternal oxyhemoglobin dissociation curve

■ Maternal hypercarbia leads to fetal respiratory acidosis &, if severe, fetal myocardial depression.

■ Uterine contractions

■ Intra-abdominal surgical manipulation & retraction

STUDIES

Pregnancy testing if diagnosis is uncertain

Perioperative fetal heart rate (FHR) monitoring

■ For gestations <24 weeks, consider pre-op & post-op documentation of fetal heart tones.

■ For gestations >24 weeks, consider intraoperative FHR monitoring.
  ➤ Loss of beat-to-beat variability occurs w/ anesthetic meds.
  ➤ Fetal decelerations, however, may indicate need to optimize intrauterine environment (eg, by ensuring adequate maternal BP & oxygenation, instituting tocolysis or repositioning surgical retraction).

➤ May not be feasible in urgent situations or during abdominal procedures
➤ Requires personnel skilled at FHR interpretation
➤ Has not been shown to improve fetal outcomes

Perioperative monitoring of uterine activity considered for gestations >24 weeks

MANAGEMENT/INTERVENTIONS

Pre-op mgt

- Obtain obstetric consultation regarding:
  ➤ Perioperative FHR monitoring (see "Studies")
  ➤ Perioperative tocolysis
    • Use is controversial. Side effects of terbutaline & ritodrine include cardiac arrhythmias & pulmonary edema, & it is unclear whether prophylactic tocolysis improves outcome.
    • Some recommend monitoring of uterine contractions intraoperatively (when technically feasible) & post-op, w/ the institution of tocolytic therapy if appropriate.
- Discuss w/ pt her concerns regarding anesthetic risks to fetus & pregnancy.
- If no increased risk to mother, consider delaying surgery until 2nd trimester to minimize or eliminate fetal exposure to drugs during 1st trimester.
- Starting at 18–20 weeks gestation, consider pt as having a "full stomach" & administer aspiration prophylaxis [some combination of a non-particulate antacid (eg, sodium citrate 30 mL PO), metoclopramide (10 mg IV) & H2-receptor antagonist (eg, ranitidine 50 mg IV)].
- Administer anxiolytics (eg, midazolam 1–2 mg IV) & analgesics (eg, fentanyl 50–100 mcg IV) as necessary to treat maternal anxiety & pain.

Intraoperative mgt

- Primary goals are to maintain maternal BP & oxygenation.
- Standard monitors include ECG, BP, pulse oximetry, end-tidal CO2 & temp.
- Regional anesthesia
  ➤ Consider regional if appropriate for maternal condition & surgical procedure.
  ➤ Advantages
    • Minimizes drug transfer to fetus

- Provides good post-op analgesia, reducing need for sedating meds & allowing for earlier mobilization
- Does not cause changes in FHR variability
➤ Prevent hypotension w/ sufficient preload & lateral uterine displacement.
➤ Treat hypotension w/ ephedrine boluses (5–15 mg IV) as necessary.
➤ Reduce regional local anesthetic dose by approximately 30% compared w/ nonpregnant pts.
- General anesthesia
  ➤ Adequate preoxygenation prior to induction is essential, since pregnant pts are prone to desaturate rapidly during periods of apnea.
  ➤ Starting at 18–20 weeks gestation, consider pregnant pts as having a "full stomach" & use rapid sequence induction w/ cricoid pressure.
  ➤ If difficult intubation is anticipated, consider awake fiberoptic intubation & have emergency airway supplies readily available.
  ➤ Reduce volatile anesthetic concentration by approx. 40% compared w/ nonpregnant pts.
- No matter what anesthetic technique is used, remember that the greatest risk to the fetus is from maternal hypoxia, hypotension & hypoventilation, which can compromise fetal blood flow & oxygenation.
  ➤ Identify & treat common causes of hypoxia, which are the same as for nonpregnant pts (including laryngospasm, airway obstruction, improperly positioned endotracheal tube, hypoventilation).
  ➤ Correct maternal hypotension w/ appropriate treatments:
    - Lighten anesthesia for deep general anesthetic
    - Vasopressors for sympathectomy secondary to regional anesthetic
    - Fluid for hypovolemia
    - Lateral uterine displacement for aortocaval compression
  ➤ Maintain normal maternal PCO_2 w/ adequate ventilation.

Post-op mgt
- Continue monitoring of FHR & uterine activity.
- Encourage early mobilization, since pregnant pts are at higher risk for thromboembolic complications.

Special considerations

- Laparoscopy
  - ➤ Once considered contraindicated during pregnancy but now becoming increasingly common as alternative to laparotomy in pregnant pts
  - ➤ Advantages
    - Smaller, less painful incisions, reducing need for sedating analgesics post-op
    - Earlier post-op mobilization
  - ➤ Pregnant pts are particularly susceptible to effects of CO_2 insufflation:
    - Hypercarbia secondary to CO_2 absorption, decreased pulmonary compliance & inadequate ventilation
    - Hypoxia from further decreases in FRC
    - Hypotension from increased intra-abdominal pressure & sudden position changes
  - ➤ Recommendations
    - Use open technique for trocar insertion.
    - Minimize insufflation pressures (no higher than 12–15 mm Hg).
    - Make position changes gradually.
    - Maintain lateral uterine displacement.
    - Adjust ventilation to maintain end-tidal CO_2 around 32 mm Hg.
- Neurosurgery
  - ➤ Conditions such as aneurysm or AVM repair may be required during pregnancy.
  - ➤ FHR monitoring during induced hypotension may be useful in evaluating intrauterine environment.
  - ➤ Hypotensive agents such as esmolol, hydralazine, nitroprusside, nitroglycerin & inhalational agents have been used successfully in pregnant pts.
  - ➤ Remember that hyperventilation shifts the maternal oxyhemoglobin dissociation curve to the left, thereby decreasing oxygen release to the fetus. However, this maneuver may still be necessary for optimal care of the mother.
  - ➤ During endovascular procedures, the fetus should be shielded from radiation.

CAVEATS & PEARLS

- Defer elective surgery until after delivery, when maternal physiologic changes have returned to normal.

- For essential surgery, consider delaying until after 1st trimester, if possible, to minimize fetal exposure to drugs.
- For emergency surgery, proceed w/ optimal care for mother, taking into account physiologic changes of pregnancy.
- Above all, for the safety of the mother & fetus, avoid maternal hypotension & hypoxia.

CHECKLIST
- Obstetric consultation
- Aspiration prophylaxis & rapid sequence induction
- Lateral uterine displacement

ANKYLOSING SPONDYLITIS

STEPHEN PANARO, MD
EDWARD MICHNA, MD

FUNDAMENTAL KNOWLEDGE
See "*Autoimmune Disease.*"
- Systemic rheumatic disorder characterized by chronic inflammatory arthropathy of both the axial skeleton & the large peripheral joints; progresses to fibrosis, ossification & ankylosis
- Typically there is progressive flexion & fusion of the spine & fixation of the rib cage.
- Prevalence of ankylosing spondylitis in women is 0.3% to 0.6%.
- Wide range of symptoms
  - Initial signs typically begin in the 20s and progress slowly over years.
  - Although cervical involvement can occur early, it more commonly presents after the child-bearing years (classic chin-on-chest deformity).
  - Extra-articular manifestations of ankylosing spondylitis are rare in pregnancy but can include cardiovascular complications of aortic insufficiency & conduction abnormalities (more commonly AV conduction delays leading to complete heart block).
  - Pulmonary complications usually occur late in the disease process & include pulmonary fibrosis & restrictive lung disease.
  - Systemic manifestations include fever, fatigue, weight loss, uveitis & anemia.
  - Neurologic complications include cauda equina syndrome, peripheral nerve lesions & vertebrobasilar insufficiency.

STUDIES

- Careful & directed history & physical exam; few pts will have manifestations that complicate anesthetic mgt during child-bearing years
  - ➤ Attention to history of TMJ dysfunction, cervical spine involvement & cardiopulmonary manifestations
- Lumbosacral radiographs

MANAGEMENT/INTERVENTIONS

- See *"Autoimmune Disease."*
- Pt may be taking aspirin or NSAIDs chronically. In most instances, the use of these meds is not a contraindication to regional anesthesia.
- Epidural or spinal anesthesia: Consider the paramedian approach, as ossification of the interspinal ligaments or osteophyte formation may make placement of the epidural challenging
- "Early" epidural placement is reasonable given anticipated difficulty w/ placement.
- Consider awake fiberoptic intubation if pt requires general anesthesia & has significant involvement of cervical spine, TMJ & cricoarytenoids.

CAVEATS/PEARLS

- Spinal rigidity & deformity as well as extra-articular manifestations are rare in young pts.
- Although women w/ ankylosing spondylitis often report chronic back pain, which itself is a risk factor for post-partum back pain, the overall risk of complications w/ regional anesthesia is minimal.
- Ossification of the interspinal ligaments or osteophyte formation may make placement of an epidural challenging.
- Consider awake fiberoptic intubation if pt requires general anesthesia & has significant involvement of cervical spine, TMJ & cricoarytenoids.

CHECKLIST

- Examine the airway. Be prepared for potential awake fiberoptic intubation.
- Establish an early epidural.

ANKYLOSING SPONDYLITIS, BACK PROBLEMS

AUGUST CHANG, MD
MIRIAM HARNETT, MD

FUNDAMENTAL KNOWLEDGE

Definition
- Chronic, progressive inflammatory disease involving the sacroiliac & synovial joints of the spine

Epidemiology
- Prevalence: 0.3–0.6% of women
- Peak age of onset btwn 15 & 29 years of age
- Male: female 3:1

Clinical manifestations
- Fibrosis, ossification & ankylosis occur, leading to the characteristic radiographic finding of "bamboo spine."
- Generally confined to hips & spine
- Extra-articular manifestations
  - Systemic
    - Fever
    - Weight loss
    - Fatigue
  - Cardiac
    - Aortitis
    - Aortic insufficiency
    - Conduction disorders
  - Pulmonary
    - Restrictive lung disease
    - Interstitial fibrosis
  - Neurologic
    - Peripheral neuropathies
    - Cauda equina syndrome
    - Vertebrobasilar insufficiency
  - Hematologic
    - Anemia
  - Urologic
    - Prostatitis
  - Ophthalmic
    - Uveitis

Effect of pregnancy on AS
- No significant change during pregnancy
- Active AS during conception increases the risk of postpartum flare of anterior uveitis, peripheral arthritis

Effect on pregnancy & fetus
- Higher incidence of C-section
- AS is reported to be the indication for C-section in 58% of these pts

STUDIES
History & Physical
- Airway: examine for indicators of potentially difficult intubation
  - Limited neck range of motion, complete cervical fusion in flexed position
  - If disease has been present >16 years, 75% of pts have cervical ankylosis & high risk of cervical fractures
  - TMJ involvement may significantly limit mouth opening
  - Cricoarytenoid involvement increases risk of trauma to vocal cords
- Cardiac
  - Aortic insufficiency due to proximal aortitis
  - Mitral valve involvement, but usually only in pts w/ disease >15 years
- Pulmonary
  - Restrictive pattern due to involvement of costovertebral angle & fixation of thoracic cage
  - Pulmonary fibrosis
- Musculoskeletal: examine back & hip anatomy
- Neurologic: evaluate for peripheral neuropathies

Imaging
- Cervical spine radiograph
- Chest radiograph

Other
- ECG
- Pulmonary function testing in all pts

MANAGEMENT/INTERVENTIONS
Medical treatment
- Aspirin/NSAIDs

➤ No evidence of teratogenicity
➤ No need for prophylactic cessation, but pregnancy should be closely monitored
➤ Recommend discontinuation during 3rd trimester because of:
  • Inhibitory effect on platelets & hemostasis
  • Increased risk of fetal CNS hemorrhage
  • Possible premature closure of ductus arteriosus
  • Possible compromised fetal renal perfusion & abnormal amniotic fluid dynamics
  • Possible factor in necrotizing enterocolitis (NEC)
➤ Sulfasalazine
  • No evidence of teratogenicity or difference in fetal outcome
➤ Corticosteroids
  • No demonstrated benefit in AS

Anesthesia
■ General anesthesia
  ➤ Awake fiberoptic intubation is recommended for pts w/ significant cervical spine disease
■ Regional anesthesia
  ➤ Establish early epidural due to potential difficulties w/ emergent induction of general anesthesia
  ➤ Regional technique may be difficult due to ossification of interspinous ligaments & limitation of flexion of lumbar vertebrae

CAVEATS & PEARLS
■ Anticipate potentially difficult airway due to possible involvement of cervical spine, TMJ & cricoarytenoids
■ Take care to avoid high regional block, particularly in pts w/ significant restrictive lung disease
■ May need to consider paramedian instead of midline approach due to ossification of interspinous ligaments & limitation of flexion of lumbar vertebrae

CHECKLIST
■ Thorough airway exam
■ Immediate availability of special airway equipment: laryngeal mask airway, fiberoptic laryngoscope, transtracheal jet ventilation, emergency cricothyrotomy kit
■ Document presence of preexisting cauda equina syndrome & peripheral neuropathies prior to general or regional anesthesia
■ Establish early epidural

ANTEPARTUM ASSESSMENT

ANJALI KAIMAL, MD
LORI BERKOWITZ, MD

FUNDAMENTAL KNOWLEDGE

■ Perinatal mortality rate in U.S. has fallen steadily since 1965. According to the National Center for Health Statistics Definition, rate in 1997 was 7.3/1,000.

■ To determine a strategy for antepartum monitoring, the risk of perinatal mortality must be determined for a specific clinical scenario.

■ Antepartum deaths may be divided into 4 categories:
1. Chronic asphyxia (multiple origins)
2. Congenital malformations
3. Superimposed complications of pregnancy (abruption, infection, Rh disease)
4. Deaths of unexplained cause

■ Antenatal surveillance is designed to identify those at risk for poor outcome.

■ Although no current data are available describing etiologies of fetal deaths in the U.S., available studies suggest that 30% of antepartum deaths may be attributed to asphyxia, 30% to maternal complications, 15% to congenital malformations & chromosomal abnormalities & 5% to infections. At least 20% are unexplained.

■ Anecdotal experience suggests that antepartum fetal assessment can affect the frequency & causes of antenatal fetal deaths. Unfortunately, few of the tests commonly used today have been subjected to prospective, randomized evaluation.

■ Indications for antepartum fetal monitoring:
1. High risk for uteroplacental insufficiency
   a. Prolonged pregnancy
   b. Diabetes
   c. Hypertension
   d. Previous stillbirth
   e. Suspected IUGR
   f. Advanced maternal age
   g. Multiple gestation w/ discordant growth
   h. Antiphospholipid antibody syndrome
2. Suspected IUGR
3. Decreased fetal activity

4. Oligohydramnios
5. Routine antepartum surveillance

STUDIES

Maternal assessment of fetal activity

■ During the third trimester, the fetus makes about 30 gross body movements per hour. Approx. 70–80% of these are perceptible by the mother.

■ Periods of fetal activity are generally approximately 40 minutes, w/ quiet periods lasting 20 minutes.

■ Fetal movement peaks btwn 9 pm & 1 am, when maternal glucose levels are falling.

■ Presence of fetal movements is a reassuring sign of fetal health. Absence of fetal movement requires further evaluation before a determination of fetal status can be made.

■ Maternal ability to perceive fetal activity may be influenced by many factors, including maternal habitus, placental location, amniotic fluid volume, maternal position & duration of fetal movements.

■ There is a wide range of normal fetal activity. Generally, 10 movements in 2 hours is considered a reassuring result.

Fetal heart rate assessment

See "*Non-reassuring Fetal Heart Rate Tracing*" chapter.

■ FHR assessment consists of identifying patterns indicative of fetal well-being & patterns that may be associated w/ adverse neonatal outcomes.

■ Reassuring patterns:
  ➤ Baseline FHR 120–160 bpm
  ➤ Absence of FHR decelerations: Mild, transient episodes of hypoxia lead to bradycardia, either as variable or late decelerations depending on the etiology (cord compression or fetoplacental insufficiency)
  ➤ Age-appropriate fetal heart accelerations: Advancing gestational age is associated w/ increased frequency & amplitude of fetal heart rate increases. Before 30 weeks' gestation, accelerations are typically 10 bpm for 10 seconds as opposed to 15 bpm for 15 seconds. Hypoxemia leads to a loss of the normal sympathetic response to movement & accelerations are absent.
  ➤ Normal FHR variability: FHR variability results from sympathetic & parasympathetic nervous system input. Parasympathetic

influence increases w/ gestational age, so absence of variability is abnormal after 28 weeks.

- Nonreassuring patterns:
  - ➤ Late decelerations: In this case, the nadir of the deceleration occurs after the peak of the contraction. Mild late decelerations are a response to hypoxia. Repetitive late decelerations with absent variability are particularly concerning.
  - ➤ Variable decelerations: Intermittent mild or moderate variable decelerations w/ a quick return to baseline likely result from cord compression & are not worrisome. In contrast, deep, repetitive, severe variables can be associated w/ a fall in pH.
  - ➤ Absent variability: Loss of variability is thought to result from cerebral hypoxia & acidosis & signifies that the compensatory mechanisms to maintain adequate oxygenation to the brain have failed.
- Distress patterns:
  - ➤ Severe bradycardia: FHR <100 bpm for a prolonged time in the absence of drugs, heart block, or hypothermia
  - ➤ Tachycardia w/ diminished variability, esp. when associated w/ other nonreassuring patterns or in the absence of maternal fever

Nonstress test
- A nonstress test is performed by monitoring the FHR using an external monitor.
- A reassuring heart rate tracing has a baseline of 120–160 bpm, the absence of decelerations, presence of age-appropriate accelerations & normal variability.
- The presence of accelerations almost always indicates a non-acidotic fetus.
- Nonstress tests can be performed as soon as the fetal cardiac & neurologic systems are mature enough to demonstrate accelerations: as early as 26–28 weeks, more reliably at 32 weeks.
- A test is reactive is there are at least 2 accelerations of 15 bpm above the baseline lasting 15 seconds in a 20-minute period.
- The stillbirth rate after a reactive nonstress test is approximately 1.9/1,000. A reactive nonstress test or a negative contraction stress test has been associated with fetal survival for 1 week in more than 99% of cases.

Contraction stress test or oxytocin challenge test
- Uterine contractions cause a reduction in blood flow to the intervillous space. Therefore, a fetus w/ inadequate placental reserve will

demonstrate late decelerations due to hypoxia in response to frequent contractions.

■ A contraction stress test should be performed on Labor & Delivery or an Antenatal Diagnostic Unit as there is a small but real risk of need for immediate delivery for fetal distress.

■ FHR is monitored for 10–20 minutes to provide a baseline. If adequate contractions are not occurring spontaneously, they can be induced by nipple stimulation or infusion of oxytocin. Adequate contractions are defined as at least 3 moderate-intensity contractions in 10 minutes, w/ each contraction lasting 40–60 seconds.

■ Fetal & uterine monitoring is continued until contractions return to baseline.

■ Results:
  ➤ Negative: Adequate contractions, no late decelerations
  ➤ Positive: Late decelerations w/ >50% of the contractions, w/o excessive uterine activity
  ➤ Suspicious: Inconsistent late decelerations
  ➤ Hyperstimulation: Uterine contractions more frequently than every 2 minutes or lasting >90 seconds, or 5 contractions in 10 minutes. If no late decelerations are seen, test is negative.
  ➤ Unsatisfactory: Quality of fetal heart tracing is inadequate for interpretation, or adequate contractions are not obtained.

■ Contraindications to contraction stress test: conditions w/ increased risk for preterm labor, contraindications to contractions such as prior classic cesarean section or uterine surgery, placental abruption, placenta previa

■ The stillbirth rate after a negative contraction stress test is 0.3/1,000.

Biophysical profile

■ The BPP consists of assessment of 5 biophysical variables: fetal movement, fetal tone, fetal breathing, amniotic fluid volume & nonstress testing.

■ Each component is given a score of 0 or 2 points depending on if criteria are met:
  ➤ Fetal movement: 2 points if 2 or more discrete body or limb movements in 30 minutes
  ➤ Fetal tone: 2 points if one or more episodes of extension of a fetal extremity or fetal spine with return to flexion
  ➤ Fetal breathing: 2 points for one or more episodes of rhythmic breathing movements of at least 20 seconds within 30 minutes

➤ Amniotic fluid: 2 points if there is a single pocket of fluid measuring at least 2 cm vertically
➤ Nonstress test: 2 points if reactive

■ Any given variable reflects the integration of CNS signals. The presence of normal biophysical activity virtually ensures functional integrity of the regulatory systems.

■ Progressive loss of brain regulation leads to loss of reactivity, fetal breathing, fetal movement, fetal tone & amniotic fluid, in a reverse ontologic order.

■ The modified BPP consists of amniotic fluid & nonstress test, with complete testing for those with an abnormal result.

■ The risk of fetal demise within 1 week of a normal BPP is 0.8/1,000.

■ A BPP of 8/10 or 10/10 is equally predictive as long as the points are not deducted for amniotic fluid volume.

■ The BPP may be falsely depressed by corticosteroid administration; these changes are transient & usually return to normal by 48–96 hours after steroid administration. Neonatal outcome is not affected.

Doppler ultrasonography

■ Umbilical artery flow can be examined w/ Doppler velocimetry.

■ In fetuses w/ placental vasculopathy, impedance in the placental bed should be increased, leading to decreased diastolic flow.

■ Results are described w/ a quotient of systolic to diastolic flow; <3.0 is considered normal after 28 weeks.

■ This is generally used in combination with the BPP and nonstress test, esp. in pregnancies complicated by IUGR, preeclampsia or oligohydramnios.

MANAGEMENT/INTERVENTIONS

Maternal assessment of fetal activity

■ Maternal perception of decreased fetal activity should lead to a nonstress test.

Nonstress test

■ Mgt of a nonreactive nonstress test depends on the clinical context & gestational age; either further fetal evaluation or delivery is indicated.

■ The false-positive rate of a nonreactive nonstress test may be as high as 50%, so in the setting of a preterm gestation, additional testing is useful to prevent an unnecessary iatrogenic preterm delivery.

■ Repetitive late decelerations or severe variable decelerations generally require prompt delivery by cesarean section.

Contraction stress test

■ A positive contraction stress test indicates decreased fetal reserve & is associated w/ abnormal FHR patterns in labor.

■ An equivocal or suspicious test is also associated w/ abnormal FHR patterns in labor. The presence of repetitive late decelerations generally requires prompt delivery, often by cesarean section.

Biophysical profile

■ BPP mgt protocol:
> BPP 10/10: Normal infant; repeat testing weekly as indicated
> BPP 8/10: Normal infant as long as amniotic fluid volume is normal; repeat as indicated
> BPP 6/10: Suspect chronic asphyxia, repeat testing in 4–6 hours, deliver for oligohydramnios
> BPP 4/10: Suspect chronic asphyxia. If >36 weeks or mature fetal lungs, deliver. If <36 weeks, repeat in 24 hours; if repeat <4, deliver.
> BPP 0–2/10: Strong suspicion of chronic asphyxia. Extend testing to 120 minutes. If persistent score <4, deliver if viable.

Doppler ultrasonography

■ A high Doppler index, absent end-diastolic flow and reversed end-diastolic flow are associated w/ an increased likelihood of poor perinatal outcome.

■ Depending on the gestational age, these findings should prompt delivery or more intensive fetal monitoring.

CAVEATS/PEARLS

■ Antepartum monitoring is designed to identify those at risk for asphyxia, as well as those w/ congenital anomalies.

■ Few of the tests used for antepartum assessment have been subjected to prospective, randomized evaluation.

■ The fetus makes about 30 gross body movements an hour during the third trimester. Fetal movement peaks btwn 9 pm & 1 am.

■ FHR assessment consists of identifying patterns of fetal well-being & patterns that may be associated w/ adverse neonatal outcomes.

■ A baseline of 120–160, the absence of decelerations, the presence of accelerations & normal heart rate variability are reassuring.

■ Persistent late decelerations, variable decelerations & absent variability are nonreassuring patterns.

■ Severe bradycardia or tachycardia w/ absent variability indicates fetal distress.

- BPP consists of ultrasound assessment of fetal movement, fetal tone, fetal breathing & amniotic fluid in combination w/ a nonstress test. Scores of 8/10 or 10/10 require no further intervention.
- Umbilical artery flow can be a useful adjunct to other modes of testing.
- Mgt of abnormal test results depends on the clinical scenario & gestational age.

CHECKLIST
- Identify fetuses at risk for asphyxia.
- Initiate appropriate testing.
- Obtain additional testing as necessary to confirm fetal well-being.

Proceed w/ delivery or plan for repeat testing based on gestational age, test results & clinical scenario.

ANTIPHOSPHOLIPID SYNDROME

AUGUST CHANG, MD
MIRIAM HARNETT, MD

FUNDAMENTAL KNOWLEDGE

Definition

- Antiphospholipid syndrome (APS) is a hypercoagulable state defined by recurrent miscarriage &/or late pregnancy loss in the presence of antiphospholipid antibodies (aPLs)
- Primary APS occurs in pts **without** SLE or other connective tissue disease
- Secondary APS occurs in pts w/ SLE or other connective tissue disease

Epidemiology

- Prevalence is unknown because the accepted diagnostic criteria are new & subject to frequent revision & debate

Pathophysiology

- Two most common aPLs associated w/ recurrent pregnancy loss, thromboembolism, thrombocytopenia
  - ➤ Lupus anticoagulant (LA): identified by abnormal coagulation assay & confirmed w/ a mixing test
    - Misnomer resulting from its prolongation of phospholipid-dependent clotting studies in vitro

- No true anticoagulant activity in vivo; actually promotes thrombosis
- Present in 34% of pts w/ SLE
- Only 35% of pts w/ LA have SLE
➤ Anticardiolipin (aCL): measured by ELISA
  - Present in 44% of pts w/ SLE
  - Antibodies may be induced in HIV-1-positive pts, but this does not appear to lead to APS

Clinical manifestations

▦ Most serious complication is thrombosis
  ➤ 70% venous
  ➤ Mostly in lower extremities
▦ Placental pathology: thrombosis of placental & decidual vessels, infarction
▦ Pulmonary embolism, myocardial infarction, TIA/CVA, amaurosis fugax may also occur
▦ Autoimmune thrombocytopenia & anemia linked to APS
▦ Renal insufficiency
▦ Pulmonary hypertension
▦ Diagnostic clinical criteria for APS
  1. One or more unexplained deaths of morphologically normal fetus (documented by ultrasound or direct fetal exam) at or beyond gestational age of 10 weeks
  2. One or more premature births of morphologically normal neonate at or before gestational age of 34 weeks due to severe pre-eclampsia or eclampsia, or severe placental insufficiency
  3. Three or more unexplained consecutive spontaneous abortions before the gestational age of 10 weeks w/ the exclusion of maternal anatomic/hormonal & parental chromosomal causes

Effect on pregnancy & fetus

▦ Increased risk of APS-related pregnancy loss, preeclampsia 16–50% & IUGR attributed to defective embryonic implantation

STUDIES

History & Physical

▦ Evaluate for signs & symptoms of thromboembolism & pulmonary hypertension

Other

▦ Antiphospholipid antibodies
▦ Coagulation studies & platelet count

- Exclusion of anatomic, hormonal, chromosomal abnormalities as factors in recurrent pregnancy loss

MANAGEMENT/INTERVENTIONS

Medical treatment: focus is on anticoagulation

- Aspirin
  - No evidence of teratogenicity
  - Should be started as soon as pregnancy test is positive
  - Discontinue at 36th week of gestation to avoid:
    - Premature closure of ductus arteriosus
    - Inhibitory effect on platelets & hemostasis
    - Increased risk of fetal CNS hemorrhage
- Heparin or LMWH
  - No evidence of teratogenicity
  - Should be started as soon as intrauterine pregnancy confirmed
  - Times to peak & half-life are shortened in pregnancy, so BID dosing is recommended
  - Chronic unfractionated heparin therapy is associated w/ maternal osteopenia/osteoporosis, but LMWH is associated w/ significantly less risk of bone loss
- Corticosteroids
  - No evidence of teratogenicity
  - Inactivation by placental 11-beta-OH-dehydrogenase results in low fetal levels of active drug
  - May precipitate gestational diabetes mellitus & hypertension
- Longer-term adverse effects
  - Osteoporosis
  - GI ulceration
  - Impaired immunity
  - Adrenal suppression
- IVIG & hydroxychloroquine
  - Under investigation

Anesthesia

- Hold morning dose of heparin when induction of labor or C-section is planned
- Hold anticoagulants & check for normalization of coagulation studies prior to regional technique
- Ideally, wait 24 hours since last dose of LMWH prior to regional technique

- If regional technique is requested in a pt still taking LMWH, may perform Hep test (anti-factor Xa activity)
  - ➤ Proceed if normal
  - ➤ If abnormal, wait until normalization; may prescribe pt-controlled anesthesia w/ fentanyl +/− ketamine in the meantime
- Recommend frequent neurologic evaluations for the first 6–12 hours after a regional technique for early detection of epidural hematoma formation

CAVEATS & PEARLS

- Coagulopathy &/or thrombocytopenia may contraindicate regional anesthetic until corrected
- Increased risk for thromboembolic phenomena: DVT, pulmonary embolism, myocardial infarction, TIA/CVA, placental thrombosis
- Lupus anticoagulant (LA) is a misnomer because it has no true anticoagulant activity in vivo & actually promotes thrombosis

CHECKLIST

- Hold anticoagulants, check platelet count & check for normalization of coagulopathy prior to administering regional anesthetic
- Hold morning dose of heparin when induction of labor or C-section is planned
- Frequent neurologic evaluations for the first 6–12 hours after a regional technique are recommended for early detection of epidural hematoma formation

---

AORTIC REGURGITATION

MATTHEW CIRIGLIANO, MD
DWIGHT GEHA, MD

FUNDAMENTAL KNOWLEDGE

- Multiple etiologies exist for aortic regurgitation (AR).
- Disease processes may lead to the destruction of the aortic valve. The etiology of AR is rheumatic heart disease in 75% of cases. Women w/ AR secondary to rheumatic heart disease often have a diseased mitral valve as well. Isolated AR is more often than not secondary to a process other than rheumatic heart disease. Infective endocarditis is another process that may lead to the destruction of the aortic valve w/ AR.

- Congenital deformities of the aortic valve may result in AR. Pts w/ a ventricular septal defect can develop a prolapse of an aortic cusp (15% of pts w/ a ventricular septal defect). Congenital fenestrations may be present. A bicuspid aortic valve may have isolated AR. Bicuspid aortic valve is highly associated w/ aortic root abnormalities leading to aortic root & annular dilatation.

- Several different processes may lead to widening of the aortic annulus, resulting in AR. Severe hypertension may widen the aortic annulus, leading to progressive AR. Syphilis, via cellular infiltration & scarring of the media of the thoracic aorta, may lead to aortic dilation, aortic annulus dilation & AR. Cystic medial necrosis may lead to widening of the ascending aorta & aortic annulus, which in turn leads to AR. Pts w/ Marfan syndrome may develop widened aortic annulus w/ AR. Idiopathic dilation of the aorta widens the aortic annulus & results in AR. In pts w/ aortic dissection, retrograde dissection may involve the aortic annulus & cause AR.

- Regurgitation leads to L ventricular dilatation & L ventricular hypertrophy, which eventually may promote L ventricular systolic dysfunction, diastolic dysfunction & myocardial ischemia. When the aortic valve leaflets fail to oppose due to leaflet, annulus or cusp deformity, blood regurgitates into the L ventricle from the aorta during diastole. The L ventricle dilates to accommodate the extra volume from regurgitation. As the L ventricle dilates, wall stress increases. Over time, the L ventricle hypertrophies to compensate for the increased wall stress (afterload). As the L ventricle hypertrophies, it becomes less compliant. With decreased compliance comes increased L ventricular end-diastolic pressures for a given L ventricular volume. L ventricular end-diastolic pressure may reach upwards of 40 mmHg. Increased L ventricular end-diastolic pressures may lead to subendocardial ischemia. An increased L ventricular end-diastolic pressure may promote increased L atrial pressure & its concomitant issues.

- Initially, a competent mitral valve protects the pt from pulmonary manifestations of increased ventricular end-diastolic volume & pressure. Eventually, L ventricular pressure may exceed L atrial pressure toward the end of diastole, causing premature closing of the mitral valve or diastolic mitral regurgitation. Increased L atrial pressure may lead to pulmonary edema & atrial arrhythmias.

- The decreased systemic vascular resistance (SVR) that accompanies pregnancy unloads the heart & may improve ventricular function in the setting of AR.

■ There may come a time when the heart cannot sufficiently balance increased L ventricular volume, L ventricular pressure & L ventricular hypertrophy to yield the necessary cardiac output. The heart rate will increase to augment cardiac output. The increased heart rate may lead to myocardial ischemia. Increased myocardial oxygen demand accompanies an increased heart rate. At baseline, there is decreased coronary flow during diastole in the pt w/ AR, for the pressure gradient falls quickly: there is less time w/ a sufficient pressure head to enable coronary flow. An increased heart rate means less time is spent in diastole. Heart failure may ensue. This is most likely to occur in the parturient during labor & delivery.

■ In the healthy parturient, cardiac output increases up to 60% from prepregnancy values during labor & delivery. Immediately after delivery, intravascular volume increases dramatically as the uterus contracts; the heart may be unable to accommodate the large increase in blood volume. Immediately after delivery, compression of the inferior vena cava decreases, which facilitates venous return.

STUDIES

■ Several sources of information or studies may be used to arrive at a diagnosis of AR.

➤ The history may provide evidence of cardiac dysfunction resulting from AR. The history may reveal symptoms consistent w/ L ventricular overload & dysfunction: exertional dyspnea & other symptoms of diminished cardiac reserve; orthopnea; paroxysmal nocturnal dyspnea; pounding sensation in the head and/or chest, especially when supine; diaphoresis; peripheral edema; congestive hepatomegaly; ascites.

• Symptoms of L ventricular failure are more common than symptoms of myocardial ischemia, but these symptoms may occur & should be elicited: chest pain, anginal symptoms, excessive pounding of the heart on the chest wall, coronary insufficiency.

• A history of symptoms consistent w/ L atrial volume overload causing pulmonary edema suggests that a pt may have involvement of the L atrium due to equalization of pressures or concomitant mitral valve disease. Pt may report dyspnea or orthopnea. Pt may report hemoptysis (occurs secondary to rupture of dilated bronchial veins), blood-tinged sputum secondary to pulmonary edema. Pt may report chest pain or palpitations.

➤ Auscultation may reveal evidence of AR.
  • Three murmurs are associated w/ AR:
    • High-pitched, blowing decrescendo murmur that occurs during diastole due to regurgitant blood through the aortic valve into the L ventricle
    • Systolic murmur secondary to increased forward flow across the aortic valve
    • Austin Flint murmur: This is a low-pitched murmur that occurs during diastole. The murmur occurs secondary to the incomplete opening of the mitral leaflets due to elevated L ventricular filling pressures.
  • An S_3 gallop may be present if pt has developed heart failure.
➤ Palpation may reveal evidence of AR.
  • A widened pulse pressure may be detected via palpation of the pulse. The pulse is bounding w/ a rapid upstroke & quick collapse ("water hammer pulse"). The cardiac impulse is hyperdynamic. A diastolic thrill may be palpated at the L sternal border, third intercostal space.
➤ EKG may reveal evidence of a dilated L ventricle diseased by AR: L axis deviation, increased QRS voltage. Voltage criteria for L ventricular hypertrophy include R wave in AVL >12 mm; R wave in I >15 mm; sum of the S wave in V_1 or V_2 plus R wave in V_5 or V_6 equal to or greater than 35 mm.
➤ EKG may reveal evidence of a dilated L atrium if disease is far progressed.
  • Atrial enlargement, characterized by:
    • A wide P wave in lead II that lasts >0.12 seconds
    • Deeply inverted terminal component in lead V_1
  • Atrial fib
  • R ventricular hypertrophy, characterized by:
    • Tall R waves in V_1 though V_3
    • Deep S waves in leads I, L, V_5 & V_6
    • R axis deviation
➤ Chest x-ray may reveal evidence of AR: cardiomegaly, L atrial enlargement, pulmonary edema.
➤ Echocardiography is the best study for evaluating & characterizing AR. The lesion can be examined in real-time to determine the mechanism. Leaflet morphology can be evaluated. Severity of aortic insufficiency can be assessed. The valve area can be calculated if mixed aortic stenosis & AR exist. A gradient can be estimated for prognostication if mixed aortic stenosis & AR exist.

- Echocardiography is indicated when a diastolic murmur, a continuous murmur or a loud systolic murmur is auscultated; when the murmur is associated w/ symptoms or when the murmur is associated w/ an abnormal EKG.
- Few sources of information or studies may be used to offer a prognosis for how the pregnant pt w/ AR will fare.
  - Pts are considered high risk when the L ventricular end-systolic diameter is >50 mm or the ejection fraction is <50%.
  - According to the American College of Cardiology/American Heart Association guidelines, pts predicted to have a high risk of abnormal outcomes are those w/ an abnormal functional capacity & those w/ L ventricular dysfunction.
  - The American College of Cardiology & the American Heart Association have classified maternal & fetal risk during pregnancy based on the type of valvular abnormality in conjunction w/ the New York Heart Association functional class.
    - NYHA functional classification for congestive heart failure:
      - Class I: Pts have no limitation of activities, no symptoms from ordinary activities.
      - Class II: Pts have slight, mild limitation of activity; pts are comfortable w/ mild exertion.
      - Class III: Pts have marked limitation of activity; they are comfortable only at rest.
      - Class IV: Any physical activity brings discomfort; symptoms occur at rest.
    - Associated w/ low maternal & fetal risk: AR in the setting of NYHA class I or II & normal L ventricular function
    - Associated w/ high maternal & fetal risk: AR w/ NYHA class III or IV symptoms; AR in the setting of pulmonary hypertension; AR in the setting of depressed L ventricular function (ejection fraction <40%)

MANAGEMENT/INTERVENTIONS

Medical mgt

- Time course for evaluation by a cardiologist
  - During pregnancy, women w/ valvular heart disease should be evaluated once each trimester for presence or worsening of symptoms & if there is a change in symptoms to assess for any deterioration in maternal cardiac status.
  - The American College of Cardiology & the American Heart Association recommend that women w/ high-risk cardiac lesions undergo full evaluation prior to & during pregnancy.

- During the antepartum period, treatment goals for the pt w/ mild or moderate symptoms focus on:
  - Treatment of volume overload to avoid or treat pulmonary edema:
    - Diuretic therapy w/ a loop or thiazide diuretic
    - Titrate diuretics to avoid hypovolemia & uteroplacental hypoperfusion.
    - Avoid excessive salt intake, which will increase intravascular volume.
  - Treat L ventricular systolic dysfunction:
    - Digoxin to increase contractility
    - Afterload reduction w/ vasodilators:
      - Hydralazine dilates arterioles, but not veins; associated reflex tachycardia is tolerated well by the pt w/ AR.
      - Avoid ACE inhibitors (unsafe for pregnancy; associated w/ IUGR, premature deliveries, neonatal renal failure, anemia, limb defects, patent ductus arteriosus).
    - Avoid bradycardia:
      - An increase in diastolic time will increase L ventricular filling & thus the regurgitant volume per cardiac cycle. Atrial fib should be aggressively treated, as the loss of the atrial contraction will decrease atrial emptying & may lead to pulmonary congestion. Atrial fib w/ hemodynamic instability and/or pulmonary edema requires cardioversion. Atrial fib w/o hemodynamic instability should be rate-controlled pharmacologically.
        - Beta blockers are safe for use in pregnancy.
        - Digoxin depresses atrioventricular conduction & thus an excessively high ventricular rate & is safe for use in pregnancy.
        - Calcium channel blockers block activated & inactivated calcium channels in the sinoatrial & atrioventricular node. Peripheral vasodilation is a side effect. They are safe for use in pregnancy.
        - Cardioversion often is performed when pharmacologic therapy fails to control the ventricular response to atrial fib.
      - Medications that have a suppressive effect on atrial fib may have been prescribed to the parturient in the antepartum period.
        - Procainamide, a sodium channel blocking drug (class I), may cause direct myocardial depression & may reduce

peripheral vascular resistance. It is safe for use in pregnancy.

- Quinidine, a sodium channel blocking drug (class I), depresses the pacemaker rate, depresses conduction & excitability & has alpha receptor-blocking properties & may cause vasodilatation & a reflex increase in sinoatrial node rate. It is safe for use in pregnancy.
- Amiodarone, a blocker of sodium, potassium & calcium channels, suppresses supraventricular & ventricular arrhythmias. It may cause peripheral vascular dilation through alpha-blocking effect & may cause bradycardia. It is *not* listed as safe for use in pregnancy due to the risk of hypothyroidism in the fetus as well as IUGR & prematurity.
- Pts in atrial fibrillation will need to be anticoagulated.
- When the onset of atrial fib cannot be determined, the pt should not be cardioverted until she has been anticoagulated for a sufficient period of time as determined by her cardiologist (unless she is hemodynamically unstable).

■ Surgery during pregnancy usually is indicated for pts w/ refractory NYHA class III or IV symptoms.

Obstetric mgt of the pt w/ AR

■ AR is often tolerated well during pregnancy; labor & delivery often proceed w/o complication.

■ C-section is performed only when there are obstetrical indications for such a mode of delivery.

■ The American College of Cardiology/American Heart Association Guidelines for the mgt of pts w/ valvular heart disease recommend that antibiotic prophylaxis be provided for the pt w/ aortic regurgitation to prevent endocarditis.

■ Recommendations are that antibiotic prophylaxis be provided for dental procedures & certain respiratory, GI & GU procedures, as listed in the ACC/AHA guidelines. Antibiotic prophylaxis for endocarditis is not recommended for routine vaginal delivery or C-section.

■ Anesthetic mgt should avoid conditions that exacerbate AR & facilitate conditions that improve the symptoms of AR. Maintain a normal to increased heart rate to decrease diastolic time. This will decrease the time during diastole for regurgitation into the L ventricle. Administer agents that have a favorable side effect profile & avoid agents with an unfavorable side effect profile in relation to heart rate (ephedrine instead of phenylephrine; meperidine may be the preferred opioid; although ketamine is not associated w/ bradycardia, it is associated w/ increased SVR & as such would not offer a favorable side effect profile).

- Aggressively treat atrial fib (maintain normal sinus rhythm). Cardioversion is always indicated if new-onset atrial fib causes hemodynamic instability. Treat rapid ventricular rate: IV beta blockers, IV calcium channel blockers, IV (careful: narrow therapeutic window!)

➤ Maintain cardiac output. Maintain normal to increased heart rate to avoid L ventricular volume overload. Maintain venous return. Avoid aortocaval compression; maintain L uterine displacement. Avoid insufficient intravascular volume while avoiding volume overload. If a central venous catheter is in situ, optimize the central venous pressure to allow for sufficient systolic BP while avoiding pulmonary edema. If a pulmonary artery catheter is in situ, optimize pulmonary capillary wedge pressure to maximize cardiac output while avoiding pulmonary edema. Avoid an increase in pulmonary vascular resistance: avoid pain, hypoxia, hypercarbia, acidosis. Boluses of oxytocin, methylergonovine & 15 methyl prostaglandin F2-alpha may result in increased pulmonary vascular resistance.

- Maintain a decreased afterload. An increase in SVR may increase the regurgitant fraction & may decrease cardiac output. The decrease in SVR associated w/ pregnancy benefits pts w/ this lesion. Avoid uterine compression of the aorta, as this may increase SVR.

- Neuraxial anesthesia will provide a decrease in SVR. Neuraxial anesthesia is well tolerated by pts w/ AR. Early administration during labor prevents a pain-mediated increase in SVR. Maintain (but do not increase) SVR during the onset of sympathetic blockade w/ epidural administration of local anesthetic. General anesthesia w/ a volatile agent will provide a decrease in SVR & is well tolerated by the parturient w/ AR. *Isoflurane* & *sevoflurane* decrease SVR the most of the volatile agents. Halothane produces myocardial depression much more than a decrease in SVR & is a poor choice if other volatile agents are available.

- Pharmacologic agents may be necessary to decrease SVR: sodium nitroprusside; hydralazine (dilates arterioles & not veins; reflex increase in heart rate is a favorable side effect for the parturient w/ AR); nitroglycerin (use w/ caution as this agent will cause uterine relaxation). Avoid ACE inhibitors until after delivery as they are associated w/ several adverse fetal effects.

CAVEATS/PEARLS

- AR is usually well tolerated by the parturient. The increased heart rate & the increased intravascular volume that accompany pregnancy are favorable to the pt w/ AR. The decreased SVR that accompanies pregnancy is also favorable to the pt w/ AR.
- Early administration of epidural analgesia during labor prevents a pain-mediated increase in SVR, which may exacerbate AR.
- For a general anesthetic, halothane should not be the first choice of volatile agent as it is a direct myocardial depressant & it sensitizes the myocardium to catecholamines.
- Hydralazine is an excellent choice for afterload reduction, as it is associated w/ an increase in heart rate, which may benefit the pt w/ AR.
- Avoid ACE inhibitors for afterload reduction until after delivery as they are associated w/ several adverse fetal effects.
- Nitroglycerin will provide afterload reduction, but it may cause deleterious uterine relaxation.

CHECKLIST

- Ascertain if the pt has had symptoms of pulmonary congestion or heart failure during pregnancy.
- Review meds that the pt may be taking for rate control, atrial fib suppressive therapy & symptoms of heart failure.
- Obtain echocardiographic data to characterize severity of AR if there has been a significant change in the pt's symptoms.
- Pt is high risk if she has AR w/ NYHA class III or IV symptoms; aortic valve disease resulting in pulmonary hypertension; or aortic valve disease w/ L ventricular systolic dysfunction.
- Women who are at high risk should have invasive monitoring during labor & delivery, as this is the period w/ the greatest magnitude in change w/ regard to hemodynamics.
- If GU procedures are to be performed other than routine vaginal delivery or C-section, administer prophylactic antibiotics to prevent endocarditis from bacteremia.
- C-section is performed only when there are obstetrical indications for such a mode of delivery.
- During anesthetic mgt, maintain normal to increased heart rate to avoid L ventricular volume overload. Maintain venous return &

decreased afterload. Consider epidural labor analgesia for vaginal delivery. Consider epidural anesthesia for cesarean delivery. Consider isoflurane, sevoflurane & desflurane rather than halothane for general anesthesia. Consider vasodilators as necessary, but avoid ACE inhibitors.

AORTIC STENOSIS

MATTHEW CIRIGLIANO, MD
DWIGHT GEHA, MD

FUNDAMENTAL KNOWLEDGE

■ Aortic stenosis (AS) may be congenital or rheumatic in origin. In pregnant women, the most common cause of AS is a congenital bicuspid aortic valve. Progressive fibrosis & calcification of the congenitally abnormal valve renders it stenotic.

■ Rheumatic heart disease is another cause of AS in women of childbearing age. Disease occurs after fusion of the commissures; there is scarring & eventual calcification of the cusps.

■ Severe AS is poorly tolerated during pregnancy.

■ A stenotic aortic valve due to anatomic distortion alters the normal physiology of the parturient. Typically, hemodynamics in the pt w/ AS are altered when the aortic valve area is reduced from one-third to one-fourth its original area. The normal aortic valve area is 3.0–4.0 cm^2. Physiologic perturbations often are apparent when the valve area is <1.0 cm^2. A reduced valve area increases the pressure gradient between the L ventricle & the ascending aorta. A significantly large pressure gradient increase for a given increase in flow occurs when the valve area is 0.75 cm^2 or less. Severe AS is associated w/ a mean pressure gradient of 50 mmHg or greater.

➤ The L ventricle must work harder to pump blood through a stenotic aortic valve. Increased pressure gradients across the stenotic valve present the L ventricle w/ an increased wall stress, or afterload. The L ventricle will hypertrophy to compensate for an increased afterload. Hypertrophy is often adequate to preserve ventricular performance as measured by the ejection fraction.

• As disease progresses, the stroke volume will eventually become fixed. The degree of hypertrophy will be insufficient to compensate for the increased intraventricular pressure & the contractile state of the ventricle may decrease.

➤ Coronary blood flow suffers as AS progresses. Coronary blood flow is dependent on the gradient that exists between the coronary ostia in the aortic root & the L ventricle during diastole. Coronary blood flow decreases when less time is spent in diastole, as occurs w/ an increased heart rate. Coronary blood flow decreases if the aortic diastolic pressure remains constant & L ventricular end-diastolic pressure increases. This is of concern to the pregnant pt, as systemic vascular resistance (SVR) decreases during pregnancy. With decreased SVR, the pressure head at the coronary ostia decreases to a greater extent, limiting the gradient that exists for coronary blood flow. Coronary blood flow decreases w/ increased L ventricular hypertrophy. There is reduced coronary blood per gram of muscle & there is limited reserve for coronary dilation. Coronary blood flow to the L ventricle occurs during diastole & flow to the R ventricle occurs during systole.

➤ Diastolic dysfunction ensues, w/ progressive L ventricular hypertrophy. L ventricular compliance increases w/ increased wall thickness. L ventricular end-diastolic pressure increases. Endocardial ischemia secondary to raised intracavitary pressures decreases ventricular relaxation. Ventricular relaxation is an active process requiring energy expenditure. Blood flow to the endocardium depends on the gradient between aortic pressure & L ventricular end-diastolic pressure. A coordinated atrial contraction becomes paramount for adequate ventricular filling in the setting of diastolic dysfunction. Loss of atrial contraction is not well tolerated by the pt w/ severe AS, usually leading to CHF.

  • The heart is less able to increase its output as AS progresses. Because stroke volume eventually becomes fixed, heart rate must increase to increase cardiac output. An increase in heart rate decreases coronary blood flow & increases myocardial oxygen demand. Less time is spent in diastole for coronary arterial flow. Myocardial oxygen demand increases w/ increased heart rate. Hypertrophied myocardium has an increased myocardial oxygen demand at baseline.

  • The parturient & fetus are at particular risk of heart failure w/ AS because cardiac output increases by up to 50% during pregnancy, w/ the greatest increase occurring during labor &

delivery. The heart may not be able to accommodate the parturient's need for an increased cardiac output. Placental blood flow, & thus the fetus, may suffer.

STUDIES

- Several sources of information or studies may be used to arrive at a diagnosis of AS.
  - ➤ A history of symptoms consistent w/ insufficient cardiac output may signal that the pt has significant AS. The pt may report syncope. There may be evidence of a non-reassuring fetal heart tracing. Placental blood flow is dependent on the systemic BP of the mother. Autoregulation does not govern blood flow in the placenta. Decreased blood flow results in fetal distress. The pt may report symptoms consistent w/ insufficient coronary blood flow: chest pain or an anginal equivalent, fatigue, palpitations secondary to premature ventricular contractions. A history of symptoms consistent w/ L atrial volume overload causing pulmonary edema suggests that the pt may have valvular disease. The pt may report dyspnea or orthopnea. The pt may report hemoptysis (occurs secondary to rupture of dilated bronchial veins), blood-tinged sputum secondary to pulmonary edema. The pt may have chest pain.
  - ➤ Auscultation may reveal evidence of AS. AS produces a systolic ejection murmur. The murmur may radiate to the carotid arteries & is heard best at the L upper sternal border. The murmur is in a crescendo-decrescendo pattern. The closure sequence of the pulmonic & aortic valve may be reversed. There may be a paradoxically split S_2 w/ expiration (pulmonic valve closes prior to aortic valve). There may be a single S_2 during inspiration (pulmonic & aortic valve close at the same time).
  - ➤ EKG may reveal evidence of dilated and/or hypertrophied L ventricle: L axis deviation, increased QRS voltage. Voltage criteria for L ventricular hypertrophy include R wave in AVL >12 mm; R wave in I >15 mm; sum of the S wave in V_1 or V_2 plus R wave in V_5 or V_6 equal to or greater than 35 mm.
  - ➤ Echocardiography is the best tool for evaluating & characterizing AS. The lesion can be examined in real-time. An anatomic assessment of the structure & function of the aortic valve can be made, including number of leaflets, extent of calcification, leaflet mobility & associated aortic insufficiency. Echocardiography is indicated when a diastolic murmur, a continuous murmur or a

loud systolic murmur is auscultated; when the murmur is associated w/ symptoms; & when the murmur is associated w/ an abnormal EKG.

- Echocardiography is a class I recommendation in the American College of Cardiology/American Heart Association guidelines for the clinical application of echocardiography for pts w/ known AS during pregnancy. Class I recommendations are supported by evidence and/or general agreement that the study is useful & effective. Echocardiography should be performed to assess changes in hemodynamic severity of the lesion. Echocardiography should be performed to assess ventricular function.

■ The following sources of information may be used to offer a prognosis for how the pregnant pt w/ AS will fare:

➤ The valve area associated w/ AS may provide prognostic information & as such should be determined via echocardiography.

- The American College of Cardiology & American Heart Association define the severity of AS according to valve area as determined by echocardiography: mild, valve area >1.5 cm^2; moderate, valve area 1.0–1.5 cm^2; severe, valve area <1.0 cm^2. Any degree of AS coupled w/ symptoms designates the lesion as severe.

➤ The American College of Cardiology & American Heart Association have classified maternal & fetal risk during pregnancy based on the type of valvular abnormality in conjunction w/ the New York Heart Association functional class.

- NYHA functional classification for congestive heart failure:
  - Class I: Pts have no limitation of activities, no symptoms from ordinary activities.
  - Class II: Pts have slight, mild limitation of activity; pts are comfortable w/ mild exertion.
  - Class III: Pts have marked limitation of activity & are asymptomatic only at rest.
  - Class IV: Any physical activity brings discomfort; symptoms occur at rest.
- Associated w/ a low maternal & fetal risk: asymptomatic AS w/ a transvalvular gradient <50 mmHg in the presence of normal systolic function
- Associated w/ a high maternal & fetal risk: severe AS w/ or w/o symptoms; aortic valve disease resulting in severe pulmonary hypertension (pulmonary pressure $>75\%$ of the sys-

temic pressure); aortic valve disease w/ L ventricular systolic dysfunction (ejection fraction <40%)
- The presence of a bicuspid aortic valve is associated w/ an abnormal aortic media, which may predispose to aortic dissection, esp. if there is enlargement of the aortic root.

MANAGEMENT/INTERVENTIONS

Medical mgt
■ Time course for evaluation by a cardiologist
  ➤ During pregnancy, women w/ valvular heart disease should be evaluated once each trimester for presence or worsening of symptoms & if there is a change in symptoms to assess for any deterioration in maternal cardiac status.
  ➤ The American College of Cardiology & the American Heart Association recommend that women w/ high-risk cardiac lesions undergo full evaluation prior to & during pregnancy (this includes AS).
■ During the antepartum period, medical therapy concentrates on prevention of endocarditis, avoidance of strenuous activity for the pt w/ severe AS & treatment of atrial fib.
  ➤ The American College of Cardiology/American Heart Association guidelines for the mgt of pts w/ valvular heart disease recommend that antibiotic prophylaxis be provided for the pt w/ AS to prevent endocarditis. Recommendations are that antibiotic prophylaxis be provided for dental procedures & certain respiratory, GI & GU procedures, as listed in the ACC/AHA guidelines. Antibiotic prophylaxis for endocarditis is not recommended for vaginal delivery or C-section.
  ➤ Pts w/ severe AS are advised to limit activity to low levels.
  ➤ Atrial fib w/ rapid ventricular rate should be aggressively treated; loss of a coordinated atrial contraction & ventricular tachycardia associated w/ atrial fib are not well tolerated by the pt w/ AS. Atrial fib w/ hemodynamic instability and/or pulmonary edema requires cardioversion. Atrial fib w/o hemodynamic instability should be rate-controlled pharmacologically.
    - Beta blockers have antiarrhythmic properties by their beta receptor-blocking action & direct membrane effects.
    - Prescribe w/ caution in the pt w/ symptoms of heart failure.
    - Digoxin has a cardioselective vagomimetic effect that depresses atrioventricular conduction & thus an excessively

high ventricular rate. It increases inotropy, which may improve symptoms of heart failure.

- Calcium channel blockers: verapamil & diltiazem have antiarrhythmic effects via their ability to block activated & inactivated calcium channels in the sinoatrial & atrioventricular node. Peripheral vasodilation is a side effect. Prescribe w/ caution in the pt w/ heart failure.
- Cardioversion often is performed when pharmacologic therapy fails to control the ventricular response to atrial fib.
- Meds that have a suppressive effect on atrial fib may be prescribed to the parturient in the antepartum period.
  - Procainamide, a sodium channel blocking drug (class I), may cause direct myocardial depression & reduced peripheral vascular resistance. It is listed as safe for use during pregnancy.
  - Quinidine, a sodium channel blocking drug (class I), decreases the pacemaker rate, decreases conduction & excitability & has alpha receptor-blocking properties. It may cause vasodilatation & a reflex increase in sinoatrial node rate. It is listed as safe for use during pregnancy.
  - Amiodarone, a blocker of sodium, potassium & calcium channels, suppresses supraventricular & ventricular arrhythmias. It may cause peripheral vascular dilation through alpha-blocking effects & may cause bradycardia. It is *not* listed as safe for use in pregnancy due to risk of hypothyroidism in the fetus as well as IUGR & prematurity.
  - Pts in atrial fib will need to be anticoagulated.
  - When the onset of atrial fib cannot be determined, the pt should not be cardioverted until she has been anticoagulated for a sufficient period of time as determined by her cardiologist (unless she is hemodynamically unstable).
- During the antepartum period, the pt may undergo surgical correction or palliation of her stenotic aortic valve.
  - Women w/ severe AS diagnosed prior to pregnancy should be evaluated by a cardiologist & a cardiac surgeon to determine if valvular surgery is appropriate.
  - Pts w/ symptoms of AS or a valve gradient >50 mm Hg should be advised to delay pregnancy until after valve correction.
  - The American College of Cardiology/American Heart Association guidelines recommend that women w/ severe AS diagnosed during pregnancy have a surgical intervention prior to labor &

delivery if syncope and/or heart failure has developed. Some pts may be a candidate for balloon valvotomy. Some pts may require aortic valve replacement. Surgery on the aortic valve in pregnant women is high risk for both mother & fetus. Women will have to be anticoagulated for the remainder of the pregnancy. Women who do not have an intervention are still at increased risk for morbidity & mortality; reviews have shown mortality rates as high as 17% for the mother.

- Obstetric concerns for the mgt of the pt w/ aortic valve disease
  - ➤ Women w/ severe AS or symptoms associated w/ AS should delay conception until their valvular disease is addressed.
  - ➤ Vaginal delivery should proceed w/ invasive hemodynamic monitoring if the pt has had symptomatic AS during pregnancy, or if her valvular lesion is classified as severe.
  - ➤ C-section is performed only when there are obstetrical indications for such a mode of delivery.
- The goals of the anesthetic mgt are the same as during the antepartum period: Avoid conditions that exacerbate AS & facilitate conditions that improve the symptoms of AS.
  - ➤ Maintain a normal to slow heart rate to increase diastolic time; this will facilitate L ventricular filling. Tachycardia will promote myocardial ischemia. A fast heart rate will increase myocardial oxygen consumption & will decrease time for myocardial perfusion.
  - ➤ Administer agents to decrease heart rate when indicated:
    - • Beta blockers: If the pt's symptom is angina concordant w/ an increased heart rate, a beta blocker may help. If the pt's symptoms are consistent w/ heart failure, a beta blocker will likely not help.
    - • Digoxin
    - • Calcium channel blockers
  - ➤ With respect to heart rate, administer agents that have a favorable side effect profile & avoid agents with an unfavorable side effect profile (phenylephrine instead of ephedrine; milrinone instead of dopamine or dobutamine; succinylcholine instead of pancuronium & high-dose mivacurium; opioids preferred to ketamine; avoid atropine, glycopyrrolate, meperidine). Some anesthesiologists choose not to include epinephrine in the test dose for epidural catheter position so as to avoid sudden-onset tachycardia if the catheter is intravenous.
  - ➤ Aggressively treat atrial fib (maintain normal sinus rhythm).

➤ Cardioversion is always indicated if new-onset atrial fib causes hemodynamic instability. Treat rapid ventricular rate: IV beta blockers, IV calcium channel blockers, IV digoxin.

■ Maintain cardiac output. Maintain normal to slow heart rate to optimize ventricular filling (see above). Avoid myocardial depression. During general anesthesia, avoid agents that are direct myocardial depressants. Thiopental for induction of anesthesia should be used w/ caution; etomidate is a better choice. Halothane is a direct myocardial depressant; this should not be the first choice of a volatile agent for general anesthesia. Use beta blockers w/ extreme caution in the pt w/ symptoms consistent w/ L ventricular failure secondary to AS.

➤ Maintain venous return. Avoid aortocaval compression by maintaining L uterine displacement. Maintain sufficient intravascular volume. For the parturient w/ severe AS, invasive hemodynamic monitoring will facilitate the mgt of intravascular volume. If a central venous catheter is in situ, maintain a high normal central venous pressure to allow for sufficient L ventricular filling. The L ventricle in the parturient w/ AS is less compliant if hypertrophy is present. L ventricular end-diastolic pressure will be higher for a given L ventricular end-diastolic volume for such pts. When guiding therapy w/ a central venous pressure only, one uses central venous pressure as a surrogate for L ventricular end-diastolic volume.

➤ If a pulmonary artery catheter is in situ, optimize pulmonary artery wedge pressure to maximize cardiac output while avoiding pulmonary edema. Hypovolemia is far more dangerous to the parturient w/ AS than is pulmonary edema. The pulmonary capillary wedge pressure should be maintained at the higher end of normal, roughly 18 mmHg. For a given pulmonary capillary wedge pressure, the L ventricular end-diastolic volume is likely to be less than it would be for a pt w/o AS: the L ventricle is less compliant in the pt w/ AS.

  • Avoid an increase in pulmonary vascular resistance. Avoid pain, hypoxia, hypercarbia, acidosis. Boluses of oxytocin, methylergonovine & 15 methyl prostaglandin F2-alpha may result in increased pulmonary vascular resistance. Nitrous oxide will increase pulmonary vascular resistance; bear this in mind during general anesthesia for C-section.

➤ Maintain adequate SVR for sufficient perfusion pressure. Insufficient perfusion pressure at the level of the coronary ostia will limit coronary flow. Decreased perfusion of the hypertrophic heart is not well tolerated by the parturient. The pt w/ AS has limited ability to increase cardiac output to maintain perfusion pressure if SVR decreases. Avoid spinal anesthesia, as it is associated w/ a precipitous drop in SVR. Dose epidural catheters carefully, paying close attention to the development of hypotension and/or signs & symptoms consistent w/ insufficient cardiac output. Consider weaker concentrations of local anesthetic for epidural analgesia. Consider the use of combined spinal-epidural technique. Prior intrathecal administration of an opioid may permit smaller doses of epidural local anesthetics. The presence of an epidural catheter facilitates the provision of perineal anesthesia during the second stage of labor. The presence of an epidural catheter also facilitates the provision of perineal anesthesia for episiotomy repair.

➤ During general anesthesia, be cognizant that propofol, isoflurane, sevoflurane & desflurane are associated w/ a decrease in SVR. Central access & an arterial line are mandatory. Phenylephrine should be ready prior to induction. An intra-arterial catheter should be placed to monitor for hypotension during labor & delivery; L ventricular dysfunction secondary to hypoperfusion of the myocardium from an insufficient SVR will be evident in real time.

CAVEATS & PEARLS

- Some anesthesiologists choose not to include epinephrine in the test dose for epidural catheter position so as to avoid sudden-onset tachycardia if the catheter is intravenous.
- For a general anesthetic, halothane should not be the first choice of volatile agent as it is a direct myocardial depressant & it sensitizes the myocardium to catecholamines.
- Hypovolemia is far more dangerous to the parturient w/ AS than is pulmonary edema.
- For the pt w/ AS who is likely to have a stiff L ventricle, L ventricular end-diastolic pressure will be much higher for a given L ventricular end-diastolic volume than for a pt who does not have L ventricular hypertrophy.
- Avoid spinal anesthesia, as it is associated w/ a precipitous drop in SVR.
- Use oxytocin, methylergonovine & prostaglandin F2-alpha w/ caution as these agents increase pulmonary vascular resistance.

■ A bicuspid aortic valve can be associated w/ aortic dissection in the third trimester.

CHECKLIST
■ Ascertain if the pt has had angina, syncope or symptoms of heart failure before and/or during pregnancy.
■ Obtain echocardiographic data to characterize the severity of AS if it has not been obtained during the pt's pregnancy.
■ The pt is high risk if she has severe AS w/ or without symptoms; she has aortic valve disease resulting in pulmonary hypertension; or she has aortic valve disease w/ L ventricular systolic dysfunction.
■ Review meds that the pt may be taking for rate control, atrial fib suppressive therapy, symptoms of heart failure & anticoagulation.
■ Women w/ severe AS or symptoms associated w/ AS should have invasive monitoring during labor & delivery, as this is the period w/ the greatest magnitude in change w/ regard to hemodynamics.
■ If GU procedures are to be performed other than routine vaginal delivery or C-section, administer prophylactic antibiotics to prevent endocarditis from bacteremia.
■ C-section is performed only when there are obstetrical indications for such a mode of delivery.
■ During anesthetic mgt, maintain a normal to slow heart rate, aggressively treat atrial fib, avoid myocardial depression & maintain venous return. Pts will require generous preload; maintain a high central venous pressure or pulmonary capillary wedge pressure. A sudden decrease in SVR and/or a sudden increase in venous capacitance as occurs w/ spinal anesthesia is unsafe. Avoid an increase in pulmonary vascular resistance. Treat pain, hypoxia, hypercarbia & acidosis. Use oxytocin, methylergonovine & prostaglandin F2-alpha w/ caution as these agents increase pulmonary vascular resistance.

ARDS

WILTON C. LEVINE, MD
TONG-YAN CHEN, MD

FUNDAMENTAL KNOWLEDGE
■ ARDS is a rare yet important endpoint of serious maternal pulmonary complications.
■ ARDS is defined as:
  ➤ Acute-onset bilateral infiltrate on chest x-ray

➤ Hypoxemia ($PaO_2/FIO_2 < 200$ mm Hg)
➤ No evidence of congestive heart failure, normal PCOP
■ Causes of ARDS in pregnancy
  ➤ Preeclampsia
  ➤ Sepsis
  ➤ Pyelonephritis
  ➤ Intrauterine infection
  ➤ Acute fatty liver of pregnancy
  ➤ Amniotic fluid embolism, pulmonary embolism, venous air embolism
  ➤ Aspiration

STUDIES
■ Chest x-ray, chest CT scan
■ Pulmonary artery catheterization & PAOP to help rule out congestive heart failure
■ Calculate PaO_2/FIO_2 ratio & consider intubation.

MANAGEMENT/INTERVENTIONS
See "*ICU Care of the Parturient.*"
■ Diagnosis of ARDS is critical to successful mgt.
■ Treatment is supportive.
■ Treatment is directed at preventing lung injury.
■ Maternal stabilization
  ➤ Intubation & ventilation when indicated
  ➤ The use of noninvasive positive-pressure ventilation is relatively contraindicated in the pregnant population given the risks related to full stomach.
  ➤ Ventilate pts following the ARDSnet guidelines.
  ➤ Fluid mgt should be based on hemodynamic monitoring.
■ Fetal monitoring
  ➤ May be difficult secondary to drugs used for maternal sedation
  ➤ Maternal hypoxia may precipitate preterm labor.
■ Treatment of underlying etiology
■ Avoid beta-agonists due to the increased risk of pulmonary edema. Use caution w/ magnesium sulfate as it may increase pulmonary capillary permeability.

CAVEATS/PEARLS
■ ARDS is a rare but important entity in the pregnant population.
■ Causes of ARDS during pregnancy are numerous.

- Workup & mgt involves diagnosis of underlying etiology & supportive medical care.
- Pts must be monitored & treated in an intensive care setting.
- Treatment requires treatment of the underlying etiology.
- Avoid beta-agonists.
- Use caution w/ magnesium sulfate.

CHECKLIST
- Determine if pt has ARDS or ARDS-like picture.
- Determine the underlying etiology of the ARDS.
- Transfer the pt to an ICU.
- Provide supportive care.
- Treat the underlying etiology.
- Provide adequate hemodynamic monitoring for the pt.

ARNOLD-CHIARI MALFORMATION

MEREDITH ALBRECHT, MD
MICHELE SZABO, MD

FUNDAMENTAL KNOWLEDGE

Definition
- Arnold-Chiari malformations (ACMs) are congenital anomalies characterized by descent of the cerebellar tonsils through the foramen magnum.
- There are four classes of ACM; the two most common are type I & II.
  Type I
- Characterized by elongation & caudal displacement of the cerebellar tonsils below the foramen magnum
  Type II
- Involves caudal displacement of cerebellar tonsils, inferior vermis, fourth ventricle, and & medulla oblongata. The remaining cerebellum is dysplastic and & the medulla is often elongated and & kinked
  Type III
  ➤ Involves caudal displacement of the cerebellum and & brain stem into a high cervical myelomeningocele
  Type IV
  ➤ Cerebellar hypoplasia w/o herniation

Epidemiology
- Type I

> Typically diagnosed in young adults
- Type II
  > Usually present in infancy or childhood

Pathophysiology
- Type I:
  > Rarely, obstruction of CSF flow occurs, resulting in non-communicating hydrocephalus.
  > Abnormalities of the cervical vertebrae (usually C1) occur roughly 5% of the time; very rarely, there is an associated myelomeningocele.
- Type II
  > Spina bifida, hydrocephalus & a syringohydromyelia generally present
  > Treatment consists of repair of the myelomeningocele, VP shunting to treat hydrocephalus.

Clinical Manifestations
Type 1
  > Valsalva-induced headache, neck/upper extremity pain & cerebellar symptoms (including ataxia, vertigo) are characteristic symptoms.
  > Extremity weakness & numbness may also be present.
- If tonsillar herniation is >5 mm, pts are more likely to be symptomatic.
Type II
  > Nystagmus, stridor, apnea & impaired gag reflex and upper extremity weakness

Effects of Pregnancy on ACM
- Valsalva w/ labor may produce significant neurologic impairment, including loss of consciousness.

Effects on Pregnancy/Fetus
- None unless parturient's well-being is compromised

STUDIES
- Diagnosis is made by neuroimaging (MRI is the preferred modality).

MANAGEMENT/INTERVENTIONS
- Treatment of the condition is often conservative, but it may include surgical decompression of the foramen magnum/cervical spine & or shunt insertion if hydrocephalus is present.

Surgical Management

- Asymptomatic pts are usually not treated surgically.
- Therapy for pts w/ progressive, severe symptoms includes suboccipital craniectomy w/ dural grafting.
  - ➤ If associated myelomeningocele (type II), surgical repair may be warranted.
  - ➤ If associated hydrocephalus (type II), pt may need VP shunting.

Anesthetic Implications

- Both regional anesthesia & general anesthesia have been used w/o complications in pts w/ ACMs w/ & w/o decompression surgery.
- If the pt has been treated w/ surgical decompression, then the risk of herniation is likely low. Consider regional anesthesia (spinal or epidural) or rapid sequence induction if general anesthesia is required.
- If intracerebral pressure above the level of the foramen magnum is high & the pt has not undergone surgical decompression, then dural puncture could result in further tonsillar herniation & neurologic deterioration.
  - ➤ There are case reports of initial diagnosis of ACM when pts developed neurologic symptoms (headache, auditory/visual changes) after dural puncture.
  - ➤ In addition, there are case reports & a small case series of pts w/ symptomatic Chiari malformations who have undergone successful spinal & epidural anesthetics.

CAVEATS/PEARLS

- ACMs are congenital anomalies characterized by descent of the cerebellum through the foramen magnum.
- There are four classes of ACM; the two most common are type I & II.
- Signs/symptoms (in decreasing order of frequency): include suboccipital headaches, ocular and & otoneurologic disturbances, ataxia/vertigo, and extremity weakness/numbness
- Diagnosis is made by neuroimaging (MRI is preferred modality).
- Both regional anesthesia & general anesthesia have been used without complications in pts w/ ACMs w/ & w/o decompression surgery.
- If the pt has been treated w/ surgical decompression, the risk of herniation is likely low.
- If intracerebral pressure above the level of the foramen magnum is high & the pt has not undergone surgical decompression, then dural puncture could result in further tonsillar herniation & neurologic deterioration.

CHECKLIST
- Neurosurgical consult
  - ➤ Gauge appropriateness of Valsalva during delivery (if not, consult w/ OB about non-Valsalva vaginal delivery w/ forceps or vacuum vs. C-section)
  - ➤ Evaluate whether dural puncture (either intentional during spinal anesthesia or unintentional during epidural placement) is likely to lead to herniation. Consider asking neurosurgeon whether s/he would be comfortable doing a lumbar puncture on this pt.
- Obtain MRI study to determine the presence & location of syringomyelia prior to attempting regional anesthesia.

ARRHYTHMIAS

JASMIN FIELD, MD
DWIGHT GEHA, MD

FUNDAMENTAL KNOWLEDGE
- Cardiovascular disease in pregnancy is rare, occurring in 1–5% of all deliveries.
- Arrhythmias represent 5% of all cardiac complications in pregnancy. Syndromes range from benign & asymptomatic to life threatening.
  - ➤ Arrhythmias are of critical importance: they may be the first sign of significant & previously undiagnosed disease.
  - ➤ Often fairly well tolerated during pregnancy when identified early & managed appropriately
- Normal physiologic changes associated w/ pregnancy can cause new arrhythmias or exacerbate preexisting issues, both previously active & quiescent.
  - ➤ Changes that may contribute directly to increased ectopy & arrhythmias:
    - Increased blood volume, heart rate, cardiac output
    - Increased atrial stretch & end-diastolic volume
    - Increased catecholamines & adrenergic receptor sensitivity
    - Hormonal, autonomic & emotional changes
- Benign EKG changes are associated w/ most normal pregnancies:
  - ➤ Increased heart rate shortens PR & QT intervals.
  - ➤ Axis deviation, R > L
  - ➤ Nonspecific changes of ST segments

> Inversion of T waves & presence of inferior Qs
> Premature beats (benign in previously normal hearts, but can initiate malignant arrhythmias in diseased hearts)
> 4-chamber enlargement leading to stretching of the conduction system

■ A handful of congenital & acquired rhythm disturbances are common to pregnant patients. These can be categorized in terms of bradycardias & tachycardias.

Bradycardias are disorders of AV conduction or sinus node function

■ Pacing function of the heart normally comes from sinoatrial node (SA), which lies at the junction of the SVC & RA.

■ Pacing impulse travels from the SA node to the AV node, located at the base of the intra-atrial septum.

> Normal delays in conduction through the AV node account for PR interval.
> Both SA & AV nodes are influenced by the autonomic nervous system.

■ The conduction system emerges from the AV node to become the bundle of His, R & L bundle branches & then the distal His-Purkinje system, which travels throughout both ventricles.

■ Activation of cardiac cells occurs through change in concentration of ions across cell membranes, creating a change in membrane potential & causing muscle cells to contract.

> The change in potential across the membrane occurs through movement of sodium, potassium & calcium ions.
> AH interval is the AV nodal conduction time.
> HV interval is the His-Purkinje conduction time.

■ Sinus node dysfunction can cause sinus bradycardia, tachycardia, sick sinus syndrome or tachy-brady syndrome.

■ AV conduction disturbances

> First-degree AV block: long PR
> Second-degree AV block: some atrial impulses fail to conduct to ventricles
  • Mobitz I or Wenckebach: progressively prolonged PR until atrial beat is dropped
  • Mobitz II: unpredictable dropping of atrial beat (conduction failure)
> Third-degree or complete heart block: no transmission of atrial signals to ventricles
  • Can be congenital or acquired

➤ AV dissociation
  • Present in complete heart block but can also be due to the presence of 2 independently functioning pacemakers
  • Can occur in the absence of conduction disturbance

Tachyarrhythmias are more common in women & are classified by dysfunction in impulse formation & impulse propagation:
■ Supraventricular tachycardias
  ➤ Characterized by HR > 120 bpm in pregnancy, w/ impulses originating or maintained in atrial or atrioventricular junctional tissue
  ➤ Atrial
    • Paroxysmal SVT begins & ends abruptly.
    • Exacerbated by pregnancy, tocolytics, oxytocics, sympathomimetics, anesthetics & cardiac events or lesions
    • Mortality is low, but morbidity may be significant in that emergency C-sections are often a consequence.
    • Treatments of choice are vagal maneuvers & adenosine.
  ➤ AV nodal reentrant (AVNRT)
    • Does not require accessory pathway for initiation or maintenance
  ➤ Atrioventricular reentrant (AVRT)
    • Also known as reciprocating tachycardia
    • Has 2 distinct pathways: normal & accessory
    • Pre-excitation occurs when bypass tract conducts to ventricles faster than via AV node
  ➤ Atrial fib/Atrial flutter
    • Less common in women of childbearing age but may occur as part of congenital pre-excitation syndromes such as WPW
    • Can occur when WPW tachyarrhythmias are treated w/ AV node blockers
■ Ventricular tachycardia
  ➤ Nonsustained VT
    • Benign if hemodynamically stable & not associated w/ structural heart disease or ischemia
  ➤ Sustained VT
    • Life-threatening
    • Treated w/ ICD

Congenital defects associated w/ arrhythmias in pregnancy
■ Neonatal lupus syndrome
  ➤ Causes 60–90% of congenital heart block

- ➤ Maternal IgG systemic lupus antibodies are transmitted transplacentally & damage fetal AV node.
- ➤ Most children born w/ CHB will require permanent pacemaker implantation & neonatal pacing.
- ➤ Third-trimester fetal mortality is high.
- ■ Ebstein's anomaly
  - ➤ Displacement of tricuspid valve into the RV due to abnormal tricuspid leaflets
  - ➤ Associated w/ paroxysmal atrial tachyarrhythmias
- ■ Transposition of the great arteries
  - ➤ Congenitally corrected transposition is associated w/ congenital heart block
- ■ WPW syndrome
  - ➤ Causes PSVT, atrial fib, atrial flutter
  - ➤ One example of a pre-excitation syndrome
  - ➤ AV node conduction occurs through an AV bypass tract called the bundle of Kent.
  - ➤ Results in earlier activation of ventricles than if signal had traveled through AV node
  - ➤ Short PR interval, & delta wave fuses w/ QRS complex on EKG
  - ➤ Treated w/ beta blockers, calcium channel blockers, digoxin, ablation of the bypass tract & cardioversion of unstable rhythms
    - In WPW w/ SVT & AF, blocking AV node (IV verapamil, digitalis & permanent pacing) can lead to acceleration through accessory tract, resulting in sustained tachyarrhythmias & VF.
- ■ Long QT syndrome
  - ➤ Often misdiagnosed as "vasovagal" or "hysterical" episodes
  - ➤ Can cause clinically significant hypoxia, though episodes usually resolve on their own
  - ➤ Strong family history often present
  - ➤ Can be triggered by stress or fever

Acquired conditions associated w/ arrhythmias in pregnancy

- ■ Normal physiology of pregnancy
- ■ Hyperthyroidism
- ■ Illicit drugs, caffeine, tobacco, alcohol
- ■ Coronary artery disease/ischemia
- ■ Underlying cardiomyopathy or valvular disease
- ■ Pheochromocytoma
- ■ Acquired long QT syndrome

➤ Caused by:
  • Drugs such as haloperidol, droperidol, benzodiazepines, antihistamines, antibiotics, cocaine, etc.
  • Electrolyte disturbances or other metabolic abnormalities
  • Bradyarrhythmias
  • Starvation or eating disorders
  • Nervous system disorders
■ Tocolytics, oxytocics

STUDIES

Standard workup for the parturient w/ arrhythmia
■ History & physical exam
  ➤ History of chest pain, palpitations, shortness of breath, syncope/presyncope
  ➤ History of seizures, esp. if present without postictal state
  ➤ Activity level, exercise tolerance
  ➤ Frequency, duration, severity, associated events
  ➤ Previous medical evaluation/treatment
■ Family history
  ➤ Syncope
  ➤ Sudden cardiac death
  ➤ Premature cardiac disease
  ➤ Familial hypercholesterolemia
■ EKG
■ Lab values
  ➤ Chem panel, electrolytes, CBC
  ➤ Urinary catecholamines
  ➤ Cardiac enzymes if clinically relevant
■ Holter monitor
■ Echo
  ➤ Uses deflections of ultrasound waves to give a 2-dimensional picture of the heart. Provides information on:
    • Valvular disease
    • Chamber size, wall motion abnormalities, wall thickness
    • Systolic, diastolic function & estimated ejection fraction
    • Pericardium & great vessels
  ➤ Doppler uses ultrasound deflected off RBCs to gather information about volume & flow.
■ Chest x-ray
  ➤ Heart size

➤ Pulmonary edema, effusions, etc.

If indicated, further relevant studies may include:

■ Exercise tolerance test/stress echo
  ➤ EKG & echo performed during exercise, or pharmacologically induced cardiac stress
    • Provides information on flow through coronary arteries & valves & on how heart responds to potential ischemia
    • Many pregnant women are not capable of nor encouraged to perform strenuous exercise, so pharmacologic induction is preferred.
    • Dobutamine 5–10 mcg/kg/min given to increase systolic myocardial contraction

■ Nuclear scans
  ➤ Radioactive isotopes that emit gamma rays during decay are injected into the bloodstream. Special cameras can then be used for imaging myocardium & vessels, along w/ size, function & perfusion of heart.
    • Commonly used isotopes: technetium 99m (or ^{99m}Tc sestamibi) & thallium 201
    • Multiple images are collected, under resting & stressed conditions, often over a 2-day protocol, allowing areas at risk for ischemia to be identified.
    • Sestamibi 99m scans tend to give better images but are more expensive.

■ Coronary angiogram & CT angiogram of coronary arteries
  ➤ Indicated for pregnant pts w/ signs & symptoms suggestive of unstable or progressive ischemia
  ➤ Potential cardiac risk factors such as advanced age, family history, smoking, obesity, diabetes, etc. may raise level of priority for imaging in the parturient.
  ➤ Risks of clinical picture must outweigh risk of invasive procedure w/ potential for serious complications & known radiation exposure.

MANAGEMENT/INTERVENTIONS

■ Risks & benefits of meds & interventions must be weighed carefully against severity of symptoms in the mother & potential harm to the fetus.

■ Few controlled trials have been done on meds during pregnancy, so much of the available information is observational or anecdotal.

Pharmacologic
- Drugs used to treat arrhythmias during pregnancy w/ reports of efficacy & few adverse events are listed in **bold**.
  - ➤ Prolong action potential duration (class IA)
    - **Quinidine**
    - **Procainamide**
    - **Disopyramide**
  - ➤ Shorten action potential duration (class IB)
    - **Lidocaine**
    - Mexiletine
    - Phenytoin
  - ➤ Slow conduction (class IC)
    - **Flecainide**
    - Propafenone
  - ➤ Beta blockers (class II)
    - **Propranolol**
    - **Metoprolol**
  - ➤ Potassium channel blockers (class III)
    - **Sotalol**
    - Amiodarone (FDA pregnancy risk classification D)
    - Ibutilide
  - ➤ Calcium channel blockers (class IV)
    - **Verapamil**
    - **Diltiazem**
  - ➤ **Adenosine**
    - Suppresses SA function
    - Slows atrioventricular conduction
    - Can cross placenta; reports of fetal bradycardia
    - 6–12 mg standard dosing in pregnancy
  - ➤ **Digoxin**
  - ➤ Replacement of electrolytes
    - Magnesium
    - Potassium
    - Calcium
  - ➤ Benzodiazepines
  - ➤ Anticoagulation
- Drugs used to treat arrhythmias during pregnancy for life-threatening emergencies only
  - ➤ Amiodarone
    - FDA pregnancy class D; multiple adverse fetal effects & teratogenicity have been reported

- Efficacious drug; has also been used safely in pregnant pts
- Risks to mother & fetus must be weighed in life-threatening emergencies.

Procedures

- Vagal maneuvers are effective in approx. 80% of pts w/ tachyarrhythmias who are not hemodynamically unstable or hypotensive.
  - Valsalva
  - Carotid massage
  - Facial cold water immersion
- Radiofrequency ablation
  - Performed via percutaneous catheter under fluoroscopy in EP lab
  - Arrhythmias are induced so that accessory tracts can be identified.
  - Eliminates supraventricular & ventricular arrhythmias such as:
    - AVNRT
    - AVRT
    - Atrial flutter
    - Idiopathic VT
- Temporary or permanent pacing
  - For symptomatic bradycardia, or cardiac disease w/ high risk of symptomatic bradycardia
  - Placed under fluoroscopy, but fetal shielding decreases risks (see "*Pacemakers*") to fetus from radiation exposure
- Cardioversion
  - Restores sinus rhythm
  - Direct current cardioversion safe at all stages of pregnancy
  - Amount of electrical current reaching fetus is insignificant.
  - Viable fetus should be monitored continuously as transient arrhythmias may occur.
- ICD (see "*Implantable Cardioverter Defibrillators*")
- Termination of pregnancy must be considered when interventions or treatments cannot resolve increased risks of continuing pregnancy.

CAVEATS & PEARLS

- Avoid all treatments of arrhythmias during first 8 weeks of pregnancy if able, as teratogenicity decreases after this period.
- Avoid maternal & fetal hypotension during unstable rhythms & during treatment of arrhythmias.
- Most anti-arrhythmic drugs are class C, meaning that there have been no controlled trials in pregnant women.

■ Though fluoroscopy is contraindicated during pregnancy because of radiation exposure, invasive procedures requiring fluoroscopy can be performed w/ fetal shielding when clinically indicated.

CHECKLIST
■ Basic suggestions for treatment of specific arrhythmias in pregnancy
  ➤ Stable VT: beta blockers, consider radiofrequency ablation
  ➤ Unstable VT: cardioversion, lidocaine, ICD
  ➤ Recurrent VT: quinidine, procainamide, sotalol, ICD
  ➤ SVT or acute AVNRT: vagal maneuvers, IV adenosine push, beta blockers, verapamil, digoxin, electrical cardioversion
  ➤ Chronic AVNRT: verapamil, digoxin, beta blockers, consider radiofrequency ablation prior to pregnancy
  ➤ Wide complex tachycardia: procainamide
  ➤ Atrial fib/atrial flutter:
    • Rate control w/ verapamil, digoxin, beta blockers
    • Chemical cardioversion w/ quinidine, procainamide short term
    • Electrical cardioversion
    • Consider radiofrequency ablation.
    • Anticoagulation w/ subcutaneous heparin based on risk factor criteria used in non-pregnant patients.
  ➤ Bradycardia: pacing
■ Plan on cardiac obstetric anesthetic mgt for labor & delivery in women w/ arrhythmias.
  ➤ C-section vs. cardiac vaginal delivery (see "*Ischemia & MI in Pregnancy*") Continuous invasive hemodynamic monitoring intra- & post-partum for parturients at high risk for symptomatic arrhythmias

ARTERIAL LINES

KRISTOPHER DAVIGNON, MD
HARISH LECAMWASAM, MD

FUNDAMENTAL KNOWLEDGE

Indications
■ Need for frequent lab analysis
■ Need for tight BP control
■ Expected large swings in BP over short time frames

Sites of cannulation

- Peripheral arteries w/ collateral circulation are preferred.
- Common sites for arterial cannulation are the radial & femoral arteries. Alternate sites of cannulation: ulnar artery, brachial artery, axillary artery, dorsalis pedis artery, posterior tibial artery
- The brachial, axillary & femoral arteries are "end arteries" & peripheral circulation must be monitored closely.
- Allen's test can be used to assess collateral circulation prior to cannulating the radial artery.
- Performed by occluding both the radial & ulnar arteries, observing blanching of the hand & then releasing the ulnar artery to document adequate flow

Transduction

- A disposable transducer is connected to a pressurized bag of saline or heparinized saline. This transducer will continuously flush at 2–3 mL/hr.
- Tubing should be rigid & as short as possible to avoid overdamping.
- The transducer must be zeroed to air & then leveled to the right atrium (4th intercostal space, midaxillary line).
- Meticulous care must be taken to avoid air in the transducer set.

STUDIES

- Blood gas determination will aid in confirming arterial placement.
- Transduction of a pressure waveform will confirm arterial placement.

MANAGEMENT & INTERVENTIONS

Technique

- Several techniques exist to cannulate arteries.
- After an appropriate-sized catheter is chosen (20- or 18-gauge, 1.25-inch catheter for radial, ulnar, dorsalis pedis, posterior tibial artery; 20 or 18-gauge, 4-inch catheter for femoral, brachial or axillary), the area is prepared in a sterile fashion.
- Next the pulse is palpated or located w/ ultrasound & the catheter is advanced at a 45- to 60-degree angle toward the artery.
- When the catheter enters the artery (as evidenced by a flash of bright red blood into the catheter hub), the catheter can be threaded directly into the artery or the catheter/needle combination can be used to transfix the artery.

- With the transfixation technique, the needle is removed & the catheter then withdrawn until pulsatile blood flows from the catheter.
- A small guidewire can then be inserted through the catheter into the artery to guide catheter placement. The wire is subsequently removed & the catheter connected to the transducer. Alternately, one may attempt to gently insert the catheter into the artery without wire-guided assistance.

CAVEATS & PEARLS
- Injection of 1% lidocaine in the area around the artery may prevent vasospasm.
- An arm board to maintain wrist extension may help w/ an arterial catheter that functions only when the wrist is extended.
- Longer 18- & 20-gauge catheters may be less prone to failure.
- Exsanguination can occur through a disconnected arterial line. Arterial lines should always be closely monitored & have an alarm system for disconnection.

CHECKLIST
- Confirm intra-arterial placement.
- Secure catheter appropriately w/ Tegaderm or suture.
- Monitor for adequate function; monitor insertion site for infection.

ASCITES

LAWRENCE WEINSTEIN, MD
DOUG RAINES, MD

FUNDAMENTAL KNOWLEDGE
- Ascites is a common result of many forms of cirrhosis. It consists of extravascular fluid in the abdominal cavity. This is due to increased portal hydrostatic pressures forcing fluid out of the portal circulation (portal hypertension), as well as decreased oncotic pressures (due to hypo-albuminemia), which would normally help keep fluid intravascular.
  - ➤ The presence of ascites is associated w/ higher operative risk & mortality, as well as an increased risk for bacterial peritonitis.
  - ➤ Ascites buildup in the abdominal compartment has important physiologic effects:
    - Increased portal venous pressure

- Increased intrathoracic pressure
- Decreased cardiac output
- Elevation of the diaphragm, causing atelectasis & V/Q mismatch in the lung

STUDIES

■ Diagnosis is made primarily by physical exam & appreciation of liver function compromise. Analysis of paracentesis fluid can support underlying etiology.

MANAGEMENT/INTERVENTIONS

■ Treatment of ascites includes preventing buildup & removing existing ascitic fluid:

> Salt-restricted diets & avoidance of sodium-rich IV fluids
> Avoid NSAIDs, which that enhance sodium retention.
> Use of spironolactone, a potassium-sparing diuretic
> Use furosemide cautiously, as aggressive use may cause enough sudden diuresis to diminish effective circulating plasma volume, which can compromise renal perfusion & exacerbate hepatorenal syndrome.
> Paracentesis of abdominal fluid is useful to quickly remove ascitic fluid & can improve respiratory dynamics & pt comfort.
- However, concurrent IV administration of a colloid such as albumin is essential to maintain effective circulating plasma volume.

■ Physiologic effects of ascites have implications for anesthesia.

■ Increased intrathoracic & intra-abdominal pressures make positive-pressure ventilation more difficult by decreasing thoracic compliance & leading to increased airway pressures and/or decreased tidal volumes.

■ In the setting of an already compromised cardiac output, be aware of further decreasing BP & organ perfusion w/ induction or inhalational agents.

■ If ascites is prominent & cardiovascular compromise present, then monitoring may include arterial & PA lines.

■ Ascites increases the volume of distribution for hydrophilic compounds & thus may alter the pharmacokinetics of certain drugs. Titrate meds w/ caution.

■ In the cirrhotic pt w/ ascites, replacement crystalloid fluids extravasate more easily, due to hypoalbuminemia & resulting low-oncotic pressure. Colloids & blood products may be more effective at restoring effective circulating volume in the setting of operative or peripartum hemorrhage.

CAVEATS/PEARLS
- Ascites can result from liver dysfunction of varying etiologies.
- Pressure differences (intrathoracic & intra-abdominal) can affect anesthetic course (ventilation more difficult & cardiac output can be impaired).
- Some drugs may have altered pharmacokinetics.

CHECKLIST
- Ascitic state optimized as much as possible
- Consider invasive hemodynamic monitoring if pt very compromised.
- Consider colloids.

ASPIRATION

WILTON C. LEVINE, MD
TONG-YAN CHEN, MD

FUNDAMENTAL KNOWLEDGE
- Aspiration is a leading cause of maternal morbidity & mortality.
- The risk of aspiration during C-section is estimated at 1/661 (as detailed in a single large American study) vs. 1/3,866 for elective surgery.
- Pregnancy
  - ➤ Increases intragastric pressure
  - ➤ Limits the ability of the lower esophageal sphincter to increase its tone & pushes the pylorus cephalad & anterior
  - ➤ Increases serum gastrin
  - ➤ Decreases serum motilin
  - ➤ Does not alter gastric emptying
- Progesterone
  - ➤ Relaxes smooth muscle
  - ➤ This may prevent the lower esophageal sphincter from increasing tone.
- Pregnancy is associated w/ increased serum gastrin & decreased serum motilin levels.

- Laboring women or women presenting for C-section should receive aspiration prophylaxis w/ a non-particulate antacid. In addition, some centers also recommend a promotility agent.
- Labor is associated w/ a decrease in gastric emptying.

STUDIES
- Chest x-ray evidence of aspiration may include a new opacity, most commonly in the right lower lobe but may occur in other areas of the lung.
- ABG may demonstrate hypoxemia.
- Rigid bronchoscopy may be necessary for removal of particulate material.
- Flexible bronchoscopy for evaluation of airways & suctioning of aspirated material
- Lavage is generally not recommended.

MANAGEMENT/INTERVENTIONS
- For pts in active labor or undergoing C-section
  - Give prophylaxis w/ a non-particulate antacid.
  - Consider metoclopramide; this increases lower esophageal sphincter tone & increases gastric motility.
- Pts for elective C-section should be NPO for at least 8 hours.
- Pts w/ uncomplicated labor may have "modest amounts of clear liquids" according to the ASA OB task force.
  - This must be avoided in pts w/ increased risk of aspiration:
    - Morbidly obese
    - Diabetic
    - Known or predicted difficult airway
- Solid foods must be avoided in laboring pts.
- The goal of antacid prophylaxis is to increase the gastric pH >2.5 and decrease gastric volume.
- Significant aspiration may lead to hypoxemia (secondary to increased shunt) & often bronchospasm.
- If a pt aspirates:
  - Suction the airways.
  - Consider rigid bronchoscopy, especially if particulate matter is involved.
  - Lung lavage will not remove acid & may actually worsen hypoxemia.
  - Steroid therapy has no effect on clinical course or outcome.
  - Airway mgt is supportive w/ FIO_2 as needed.

➤ Endotracheal intubation & mechanical ventilation w/ PEEP may become necessary.

➤ There is generally no immediate indication for antibiotics.

CAVEATS AND PEARLS

■ Aspiration is a leading cause of maternal morbidity & mortality.

■ The physiologic changes of pregnancy may predispose pts to aspiration.

■ Pts in active labor or scheduled for C-section should receive antacid prophylaxis w/ a non-particulate antacid.

■ Pts in active labor should remain NPO for solid foods but may have modest amounts of clear liquids, presuming there are no predictors of increased aspiration risk.

■ Pts scheduled for C-section should remain strictly NPO.

■ If aspiration occurs, there is no indication for lavage, steroids or antibiotics.

■ Endotracheal intubation & supportive care may be necessary.

CHECKLIST

■ Ensure aspiration prophylaxis.

■ Follow ASA OB guidelines for NPO status.

ASSISTED REPRODUCTIVE TECHNOLOGIES (ART)

YUMIKO ISHIZAWA, MD
LAWRENCE C. TSEN, MD

FUNDAMENTAL KNOWLEDGE

Background

■ Assisted reproductive technologies (ART) refer to all fertility treatments & procedures that involve the handling of oocytes & sperm. In general, ART involves hormonal stimulation, surgical removal of oocytes, the combination of oocytes & sperm in vitro & the transfer of embryos into the oocyte donor or a gestational carrier.

■ Approximately 1.2 million women (2% of the population of women of reproductive age) seek infertility-related treatments. Some of these individuals are seeking to preserve their fertility prior to undergoing other medical interventions, such as whole body radiation or chemotherapy. In addition, other individuals seek pre-genetic diagnosis of certain disease entities in the oocytes or embryos. In the

U.S., >100,000 cycles are performed each year, resulting in approx. 30,000 pregnancies & 40,000 infants.

- ■ Hormonal manipulation is performed to create oocytes for retrieval. This manipulation occurs in 3 stages:
  - ➤ **Down-regulation**: The ovaries are induced into a quiescent state to prevent a single dominant follicle (each follicle usually contains a single oocyte) from developing. This is usually accomplished via the pituitary w/ the administration of a gonadotropin-releasing hormone (GnRH) agonist (ie, leuprolide acetate). Down-regulation is usually achieved in 10–14 days when initiated in the mid-luteal phase of the menstrual cycle.
  - ➤ **Hyperstimulation**: The ovaries are stimulated by human menopausal gonadotropin (hMG) to produce multiple follicles. Follicular number & growth are followed by serial ultrasonographic exams & confirmation of progressive increases in serum estradiol levels.
  - ➤ **Ovulation**: The early processes associated w/ ovulation are initiated w/ the use of human chorionic gonadotropin (hCG). This induces the oocytes to move from the follicular wall into the follicular fluid. Oocyte retrieval (see below) occurs 34–36 hrs after the hCG but prior to the spontaneous rupture of the follicle (& subsequent loss of the follicular contents [ie, the oocyte]).
- ■ Hormonal stimulation is followed by the 3 procedures:
  - ➤ **Oocyte retrieval**: The extraction of oocytes is typically performed through a transvaginal ultrasound probe w/ a needle for puncture & aspiration. This is usually performed w/ the pt in the lithotomy position. On occasion, transabdominal needle puncture w/ ultrasound guidance or laparoscopic retrieval is performed. Laparoscopic retrieval is often reserved for immediate tubal transfer of the oocyte in a GIFT procedure (see below).
    - • **In Vitro Fertilization (IVF)**: The process by which oocytes & spermatozoa are combined in culture media. The term "IVF" is used frequently, but inappropriately, to mean all ART procedures.
    - • **Embryo Transfer (ET)**: The placement of embryos following IVF into the uterus via a transcervically placed catheter. In limited circumstances, this transfer can occur directly into the fallopian tubes (ZIFT). An ET usually occurs 3–5 days following the oocyte retrieval. Embryos not used may be cryopreserved until a later date. Special transfer protocols include:

- **Zygote Intrafallopian Transfer (ZIFT)** is the transfer of pronuclear-stage embryos into the distal portion of a fallopian tube approx. 16–20 hours after IVF.
- **Tubal Embryo Transfer (TET)** or **Tubal Embryo Stage Transfer (TEST)** occurs 48 hours after IVF.
- **Gamete Intrafallopian Transfer (GIFT)** is the injection of mature oocytes & washed sperm (gametes) into a distal fallopian tube via a catheter immediately after transabdominal or transvaginal collection of oocytes.

Complications of ART

➢ Increased coagulation & decreased fibrinolysis may result in thrombotic complications.

➢ Abdominal discomfort, exuberant ovarian enlargement & ascites may occur.

➢ Ovarian hyperstimulation syndrome is the most common complication associated w/ iatrogenic ovarian stimulation. Severe cases may result in follicular rupture & hemorrhage, pleural effusion, hemoconcentration, oliguria & thromboembolic events.

■ Hormonal stimulation may also result in ovarian cyst formation & rupture, or ovarian infarction from torsion.

■ Ectopic pregnancies occur more often w/ ART pregnancies, largely due to an increased prevalence of tubal disease in infertility pts.

■ Multiple gestation pregnancies, although often considered preferable by infertile couples, can result in poor outcomes. Maternal & perinatal morbidity & mortality for multiple gestation pregnancies is at least double that of singleton gestation pregnancies (see the chapter "*Multiple Gestations*").

■ Preterm delivery, low birth-weight babies & small-for-gestational-age babies are more common w/ IVF pregnancies.

Effects of Anesthesia on Reproduction

■ Although a number of studies suggest an effect of anesthetic agents on overall fertility success, the literature should be interpreted w/ caution for the following reasons: differences in the route, dose, timing & duration of drug exposure; differences in intraspecies & interspecies; differences in hormonal stimulation & reproductive lab techniques. Studies that incubate oocytes or embryos in anesthetic agents result in higher anesthetic concentrations than those occurring clinically; moreover, oocytes are washed & screened prior to fertilization & transfer.

➤ **Local anesthetics:** In animal models, subtle differences in fertilization & embryo development exist btwn oocytes incubated in various local anesthetics. However, in clinical studies, no trials have condemned the use of local anesthetics for oocyte retrieval, GIFT or ZIFT. Paracervical lidocaine blockade (vs. no anesthesia) for oocyte retrieval & epidural lidocaine (vs. general anesthesia) for GIFT showed similar, favorable pregnancy rates.

• **Opioids, Benzodiazepines, & Ketamine:** Fentanyl, alfentanil, remifentanil, or meperidine does not appear to interfere w/ either fertilization or embryo development in animal & human trials. Opioids given IV in clinically relevant doses are detected in the follicular fluid within 15 minutes, but exist in extremely low to nonexistent levels. Midazolam given in doses up to 500× those used clinically does not impair fertilization or embryo development in vivo or in vitro. Diazepam, given as an intraperitoneal dose of 35 mg/kg in mice, has been noted to produce more offspring w/ cleft lip/palate anomalies. Ketamine w/ midazolam has been observed, in a small study, to produce no differences in reproductive outcome when used as an alternative to general anesthesia w/ isoflurane.

• **Propofol & Thiopental:** Propofol accumulates in follicular fluid in a dose- & duration-dependent manner. High concentrations of propofol in animal studies suggest limited effects. When compared clinically to volatile agents or paracervical blocks, most studies suggest no differences in fertilization, embryo cleavage or implantation rates. Thiopental & thiamylal used for induction of anesthesia are detected in follicular fluid within 11 minutes & have been associated w/ no adverse reproductive effects compared to propofol.

• **Nitrous Oxide:** Although nitrous oxide is known to reduce methionine synthetase activity, animal studies suggest limited cell cleavage effects that resolve by later stages of embryo development. Clinical studies during laparoscopic ART procedures suggest no adverse effects on fertilization or pregnancy.

• **Volatile anesthetics:** Volatile agents have been observed to depress DNA synthesis & mitosis in cell cultures. The adverse effects of halothane are more significant than isoflurane. Sevoflurane & desflurane have not been adequately studied, but compound A & fluorine have been noted to have adverse effects on rapidly dividing cells. High prolactin levels

& spindle cell dysfunction may be the mechanisms involved in the adverse reproductive effects of volatile agents.

- **Antiemetic agents:** Droperidol & metoclopramide induce hyperprolactinemia w/ potential impairment of ovarian follicle maturation & corpus luteum function. Serotonin 5-HT3 antagonists (ie, ondansetron) have not been evaluated.

STUDIES

■ In general, the pts are relatively young & otherwise healthy & do not require pre-op lab studies, ECG or chest x-ray. However, as a growing percentage of pts desiring ART have significant comorbidities, including morbid obesity, diabetes, cancer, heart & pulmonary anomalies, the pre-op evaluation of each pt should be addressed individually.

MANAGEMENT/INTERVENTIONS

General considerations

■ ART involves ambulatory procedures. Anesthesia goals are effective pain relief w/ rapid recovery & minimal post-op nausea, sedation, pain & psychomotor impairment.

■ Standard fasting guidelines should apply & aspiration precautions should be applied to those pts at risk. If NPO guidelines are not followed, the decision to cancel or delay the case should be made weighing the risks & benefits. A spinal anesthetic is advocated if NPO guidelines are not followed.

■ If the window (34–36 hrs after hCG administration) for oocyte retrieval is missed, spontaneous ovulation & oocyte loss can occur. In addition, ovarian hyperstimulation syndrome may occur if follicle aspiration is not performed.

Transvaginal ultrasound-guided oocyte retrieval

■ Oocyte retrieval usually takes 10–15 minutes from the vaginal probe placement to the last follicular aspiration.

■ Conscious sedation & total intravenous anesthesia (TIVA) are the most commonly used techniques, but paracervical block, spinal, epidural or general inhalational anesthesia can be used. Pts need to be immobile at the time of retrieval.

■ Additional analgesia is often required w/ paracervical blocks as it does not adequately block vaginal & ovarian sensory fibers.

■ Spinal anesthesia, including low-dose spinal bupivacaine, can be a good option, although the times to urination, ambulation & discharge are usually longer in comparison to other techniques.

Laparoscopic ART procedures

■ Local, regional & general anesthesia can be used. General anesthesia may be induced just before the skin incision to minimize unnecessary exposure to anesthetic agents.

■ Commonly used for pneumoperitoneum, carbon dioxide may acidify follicular fluid & decrease fertilization rates. Venous gas embolism is an omnipresent risk w/ laparoscopy; if it occurs, resuscitation efforts including oxygen, IV fluid, hemodynamic support & aspiration of gas should be performed promptly.

■ Trendelenburg position is often used to facilitate visualization of the fallopian tubes & other pelvis structures & can produce physiologic changes, especially when used in the presence of a pneumoperitoneum.

Embryo transfer

■ When performed transcervically, this procedure is typically performed w/o anesthesia. On rare occasions, analgesia or anesthesia is requested, particularly for difficult cervical anatomy. Transabdominal gamete or embryo transfer (ie, GIFT, ZIFT) is usually performed via laparoscopy under local, regional or general anesthesia.

Post-op mgt

■ The incidence of unplanned hospital admission after ART procedures is <0.2%. Reasons include syncope, hemoperitoneum & ovarian hematoma.

■ Post-op pain can be treated w/ small doses of fentanyl, meperidine or oral acetaminophen w/ codeine. Avoid NSAIDs, as changes in the prostaglandin milieu can affect embryo implantation.

■ Post-op nausea & vomiting may occur; consider non-dopaminergic agents.

■ Pts undergoing anesthesia for ART should be followed in 24–48 hours after the procedure.

CAVEATS & PEARLS

■ ART is being applied to an increasingly diverse population of pts w/ a wide range of comorbid conditions. The total number of ART procedures is increasing dramatically.

■ Hormonal stimulation creates multiple oocytes for retrieval, but other mild to severe physiologic sequelae may occur, including ovarian hyperstimulation syndrome.

■ If NPO guidelines prior to oocyte retrieval have not been followed, consider the risks & benefits of proceeding. Delaying or canceling the case may result in oocyte loss & ovarian hyperstimulation syndrome. Review the "stimulation sheet" immediately prior to the oocyte retrieval. This indicates the number of follicles available for retrieval, which appears related to both the duration of the procedure & the degree of discomfort experienced.

■ Conscious sedation, regional anesthesia & general anesthesia have all been used successfully to anesthetize women for ART procedures. Lab studies have suggested that local anesthetic agents, nitrous oxide & the volatile halogenated agents interfere w/ some aspect of reproductive physiology in vitro. Clinical data suggest that brief administration of most anesthetic agents (except halothane) has limited to no adverse effects on live-birth rates; however, as a principle, agents should be minimized.

■ Avoid anti-dopaminergic agents (ie, metoclopramide, droperidol) prior to oocyte retrieval & NSAIDs due to the potential for adversely affecting the fertility outcome.

Updated information may be obtained at the websites of the American Society of Reproductive Medicine (http://www.asrm.org/) & Society for Assisted Reproductive Technology (http://sart.org/).

CHECKLIST

■ Review the medical history of pts in advance of procedures requiring analgesia or anesthesia. As more individuals have significant comorbid conditions, additional information or evaluative studies may be necessary.

■ Communicate w/ pts that most anesthetic agents (of those listed above) in clinically used doses have limited or no known adverse effects on fertility outcome.

■ Review the "stimulation sheet" to determine the number of follicles & the location of the ovaries; this may assist in determining the most appropriate type & amount of anesthesia & post-op analgesia.

■ As ART procedures may result in perforation of vessels or vital organs, be prepared for adverse events or emergencies. Backup airway equipment & emergency resuscitation meds should be immediately available.

■ Communicate w/ the reproductive endocrinologist involved w/ the procedures to assess the timing of critical moments & the duration of the procedures.

■ Determine if there are any additional concerns, including ovarian hyperstimulation syndrome.

ASTHMA

WILTON C. LEVINE, MD
TONG-YAN CHEN, MD

FUNDAMENTAL KNOWLEDGE

- Asthma is a disease characterized by hyperactive airways leading to episodic bronchoconstriction.
- Asthma is associated w/
  - ➤ Reversible airway obstruction
  - ➤ Airway inflammation
  - ➤ Airway hyperresponsiveness
- Asthma is the most common medical condition occurring during pregnancy & can lead to an increase in maternal & fetal morbidity & mortality if not well controlled.
- Studies in the literature note that asthma severity during pregnancy improves, stays the same or worsens in equal proportions.
  - ➤ Unfortunately, the course of asthma in an individual parturient is difficult to predict.
  - ➤ Women w/ mild disease are unlikely to develop significant asthma-related morbidity, while women w/ severe disease are at greater risk for asthma-related morbidity.
  - ➤ Increased levels of progesterone during pregnancy lead to bronchodilation.
  - ➤ Increased levels of serum cortisol during pregnancy may be beneficial to the parturient.
  - ➤ Increased gastroesophageal reflux may lead some parturients to experience worsening asthma and asthma-like symptoms.
  - ➤ Decreased sensitivity to beta-adrenergic agonists may worsen asthma during pregnancy
  - ➤ The effects of asthma on pregnancy are unclear; there are no clear data in the literature on rates of preterm labor, pre-eclampsia, C-section or congenital abnormalities.
- Severe & poorly controlled asthma may lead to adverse fetal outcomes as a result of chronic or intermittent maternal hypoxemia.
- Severe attacks are rare during labor & delivery.

STUDIES

- A history must be taken to determine symptoms of wheezing, cough, dyspnea, chest tightness, pattern & severity of symptoms & triggers.

- Determine if the pt has ever been hospitalized, taken oral steroids (including date and dose of most recent steroid course) or been intubated secondary to her asthma.
- Determine if the pt is currently taking oral steroids.
- Determine if the pt is medically optimized.
- Do a physical exam focusing on lung auscultation, presence or absence of wheezing & ratio of inspiratory/expiratory phase.
- Pts should monitor peak flow rates throughout pregnancy.
- PFTs are useful to document the severity of asthma. With asthma, PFTs may show a reduction of FEV_1, FVC & FEV_1/FVC.
- Chest x-ray can help differentiate symptoms & physical exam findings from pneumonia, pneumothorax & heart failure.

MANAGEMENT/INTERVENTIONS
- Avoid things that trigger the pt's asthma.
- Pts need to be managed w/ both rapidly acting & chronic meds.
  - ➤ Chronic meds help prevent symptoms; rapidly acting meds can help treat acute symptoms.
  - ➤ Short- & long-acting beta-2 agonists, inhaled corticosteroids & methylxanthines are safe for use during pregnancy.
  - ➤ Oral corticosteroids are generally safe for use during pregnancy w/o increased risk of abortion, stillbirth, congenital malformation, adverse fetal effect or neonatal death attributable to the steroids.
  - ➤ Leukotriene antagonists should be continued in pts w/ resistant asthma who have previously responded well to these drugs.
- Treatment of acute severe asthma during pregnancy is no different from treatment outside of pregnancy:
  - ➤ Oxygen
  - ➤ Nebulized beta-2 agonists & ipratropium
  - ➤ Oral & IV steroids
  - ➤ IV beta-2 agonists
  - ➤ Occasionally IV aminophylline
  - ➤ Chest x-ray & ABG needed
- Pts taking oral steroids should receive hydrocortisone 100 mg IV q8h at the onset of labor.
- PGE2 is safe, as it is a bronchodilator
- PGF2a (Hemabate) should be used w/ caution as it may cause bronchospasm.
- Goals of labor analgesia
  - ➤ Pain relief

> Reduction of stimulus to hyperpnea
  • This is especially important for pts w/ asthma triggered by exercise or stress.
> Prevention or relief of maternal stress

CAVEATS AND PEARLS

■ Asthma is a disease of hyperactive airways & airway inflammation.
■ Asthma is the most common medical condition encountered during pregnancy.
■ Asthma may improve, worsen or stay the same during pregnancy.
■ Severe or poorly controlled asthma may lead to adverse fetal outcomes.
■ Pts need optimal mgt & treatment for their asthma.
■ PGF2a should be used w/ caution as it may cause bronchospasm.

CHECKLIST

■ Perform a focused history & physical exam.
■ Check PFTs or peak flow if clinically indicated.
■ Provide stress-dose steroids if clinically indicated.
■ Continue all asthma meds.
■ Avoid triggers of the pt's asthma.

AUTOIMMUNE HEPATITIS

LAWRENCE WEINSTEIN, MD
DOUG RAINES, MD

FUNDAMENTAL KNOWLEDGE

■ Autoimmune hepatitis is a chronic hepatitis of unknown etiology most prevalent in young women.
■ Onset is usually insidious, but about 25% of cases present as an acute hepatitis.
  > May follow a viral illness such as Hep A, Epstein-Barr or measles.
■ Many pts are asymptomatic. Those w/ symptoms may present w/ malaise, anorexia, nausea, abdominal pain, lethargy or itching.
■ Autoimmune hepatitis is often co-existent w/ other autoimmune diseases, such as rheumatoid arthritis, Sjögren syndrome, ulcerative colitis & Coombs-positive hemolytic anemia.
■ Physical exam usually reveals a normal-appearing young woman w/ spider nevi, cutaneous striae, acne, hirsutism & hepatomegaly.
■ Amenorrhea may be present, even in the non-pregnant pt.

STUDIES

- Elevated aminotransferases
- Bilirubin is often elevated, but pts may be anicteric.
- Elevated serum autoantibody titers, including anti-nuclear (ANA), anti-smooth muscle & anti-mitochondrial antibodies
- Serum gamma globulin levels are typically elevated.
- Pts often positive for HLA-B8, HLA DR3 or HLA-DR4
- Frequently, diagnosis is made by detecting elevated aminotransferases in an otherwise asymptomatic woman.

MANAGEMENT/INTERVENTIONS

- Unlike chronic Hep C, autoimmune hepatitis usually responds very well to treatment w/ prednisone & azathioprine.
  - ➤ With this regimen, CBCs should be checked weekly for the first 2 months because of a small risk of bone marrow suppression.
  - ➤ This drug combination improves symptoms in 80–90% of pts.
- Symptoms improve rapidly following drug treatment, but biochemical improvement of aminotransferases levels may take up to several months, & histologic resolution of hepatic inflammation can take up to 2 years.
  - ➤ Failure of aminotransferase elevation to normalize predicts a lack of histologic resolution of inflammation & fibrosis.
- Pre-existent cirrhotic liver changes will not reverse, even following successful therapy w/ normalization of aminotransferase levels.
- Non-responders to treatment may be considered for cyclosporine, tacrolimus or methotrexate.
- Liver transplant is an option of last resort for treatment failures.
- As w/ all liver disease pts, anesthetic decisions should be guided by the symptoms & manifestations of the liver process. Various manifestations will have differing effects on physiology & choice of anesthetic technique for labor or delivery.
  - ➤ If pt is coagulopathic, see the section on *"General Concepts."*
  - ➤ If pt is cirrhotic, see sections on *"General Concepts," "Cirrhosis," "Portal Hypertension," "Ascites," "Hepatic Encephalopathy."*
    - For general discussion of regional & general anesthesia considerations, see the section on *"General Concepts."*

CAVEATS/PEARLS

- Autoimmune hepatitis is a chronic hepatitis of unknown etiology most prevalent in young women, making parturients susceptible.

- Lab abnormalities include elevated transaminases, bilirubin & auto-antibodies.
- Treatment is most often prednisone plus azathioprine.

CHECKLIST
- Check for other autoimmune processes: comorbid illnesses may have an impact on anesthesia (eg, airway, metabolic derangements).
- Consider stress-dose steroids if appropriate given recent administration.

BASICS OF REGIONAL ANESTHESIA

KRISTEN STADTLANDER, MD; MAY PIAN-SMITH, MD; AND LISA LEFFERT, MD

FUNDAMENTAL KNOWLEDGE

Stages of labor
- First stage of labor
  - Begins w/ uterine contractions & ends w/ full cervical dilation. Marked by crampy, abdominal, visceral pain carried by the spinal nerves in the T10-L1 dermatomes.
  - The pain of first stage worsens as cervix dilates & w/ the use of oxytocin to augment contractions.
- Second stage of labor
  - Begins w/ a fully dilated cervix & ends w/ delivery of the infant
  - Marked by somatic sharp pain caused by fetal head compressing perineal structures (via the pudendal nerve, S2-S4 dermatomes)
- Third stage of labor
  - Begins w/ delivery of the infant & ends w/ delivery of the placenta
  - Generally associated w/ little pain compared to the first two stages

Anatomy of the subarachnoid, subdural & epidural spaces
- Subarachnoid space
  - The spinal canal begins at the foramen magnum cranially & extends to the sacral hiatus caudally.
  - The spinal cord has three successive coverings or meninges: pia, dura & arachnoid mater.
  - The subarachnoid space is a space btwn the pia & arachnoid mater.
  - It extends from the cerebral ventricles down to S2.

➤ The spinal space contains CSF, spinal cord & its exiting nerve roots & blood vessels supplying the cord.

➤ The volume of CSF in the spinal canal below the foramen magnum is 25–40 mL; the total volume of CSF is 100–150 mL.

➤ CSF is continuously made (about 450 mL/day) by the choroid plexuses in the cerebral ventricles & reabsorbed at the arachnoid granulations.

➤ The spinal cord extends to L3 at birth & slowly moves cephalad to reach its adult position of L1–2 by the age of 2.

➤ For this reason, obstetric spinal anesthesia is usually administered at the L2–3 or L3–4 interspace to minimize possible spinal cord injury w/ the spinal needle. To ensure proper positioning, Tuffier's line is used.

➤ Tuffier's line is the theoretical line drawn horizontally from one iliac crest to the other & corresponds to the L4 spinous process (although considerable variation has been found in studies). Thus, by directing the needle to the interspace 1 or 2 spaces above Tuffier's line, a safe margin for the passage of the spinal needle is obtained.

■ Epidural space

➤ The epidural space is a potential space that has a triangular shape w/ the apex of the triangle facing posteriorly.

➤ It is bordered superiorly by the foramen magnum, inferiorly by the sacrococcygeal ligament at S2–3, anteriorly by the posterior longitudinal ligament, posteriorly by the ligamentum flavum & laterally by dura, lamina & pedicles. The epidural space contains fat, nerve roots, arteries that supply the cord & vertebral veins.

➤ The distance from skin to epidural space is 3–9 cm; for 80% of the population, the distance from skin to epidural space is 4–6 cm.

➤ To reach the epidural space, the order of structures the needle must pass through is skin, subcutaneous tissue, supraspinous ligament, interspinous ligament, ligamentum flavum, epidural space.

■ Subdural space

➤ The subdural space is a potential space between the dura & the arachnoid mater. Inadvertent injection of local anesthetic into the subdural space can be the cause of failed spinal or epidural.

■ Bony landmarks

➤ The bony landmarks are made of vertebrae (7 cervical, 12 thoracic, 5 lumbar, 4 coccygeal).

➤ The lumbar vertebrae encountered in obstetric anesthesia contain a vertebral body, two pedicles & two laminae.

➤ The vertebral bodies border the spinal canal anteriorly, the pedicles laterally & the laminae posteriorly.

➤ Each vertebra has a spinous process, which in the lumbar territory projects more horizontally but in the thoracic levels projects more caudally.

➤ The spinous processes can obstruct the space between vertebrae & make it more difficult to access the epidural or intrathecal spaces at a thoracic level.

➤ For this reason, at the thoracic level, a paramedian approach to the epidural space is sometimes employed.

■ Vertebral ligaments

➤ There are 3 ligaments that are encountered when performing neuraxial anesthesia.

➤ Supraspinous ligaments connect the spinous processes at their apices.

➤ Interspinous ligaments connect the spinous processes at their horizontal edges.

➤ Ligamentum flavum connects the caudal edge of the vertebra above to the cephalad edge of the lamina below.

➤ Ligamentum flavum is the ligament that gives the characteristic feel when the "loss of resistance" technique is employed to locate the epidural space. This ligament is made up of 80% elastin & provides significant resistance to passage of the epidural needle. In contrast, the interspinous ligament has less elastin & therefore usually provides less resistance to the passage of the epidural needle.

Physiology of Regional Anesthesia

■ Local anesthesia affects nerve conduction via inhibition of sodium channels.

■ The termination of local anesthetic action is due to reabsorption of the agent into the systemic circulation.

■ When spinal anesthesia is performed, the sequence of neural blockade is as follows: sympathetic block w/ vasodilation of the affected area, loss of pain & temperature sensation, loss of proprioception, loss of pressure sensation & finally motor block.

■ This sequence occurs because the smaller autonomic fibers are blocked more easily than the larger sensory fibers. The largest motor fibers are most resistant.

- The level of sympathetic blockade in a spinal anesthetic will extend approximately 2 segments higher than the sensory block, & the motor block will be approximately 2 segments lower than the sensory blockade.
- During epidural anesthesia, this neural block differential is not as apparent. With dilute epidural medication mixes, the pt may even ambulate while sensory blockade is present.

Organ System Effects of Regional Anesthesia
- Cardiovascular
  - ➤ Regional anesthesia blocks sympathetic nerve fibers & results in vasodilation.
  - ➤ This decreased systemic vascular resistance can result in marked hypotension, which can be accompanied by increased heart rate (reflex tachycardia) or decreased heart rate (due to the Bezold Jarisch & analogous reflexes).
  - ➤ If a regional block is high enough to block the cardiac accelerator fibers at T1–T5, the heart cannot mount a tachycardic response to decreased SVR & cardiovascular collapse can ensue.
  - ➤ The hypotensive effects of regional anesthesia can be attenuated by volume loading the pt w/ 10–20 mL/kg (avg. dose 1L LR or NS) before placing the spinal or epidural. Hypotension is less common during labor analgesia than it is w/ surgical anesthesia.
  - ➤ Maintaining L uterine displacement immediately after placement also helps to prevent obstruction of venous return.
  - ➤ IV pressors such as ephedrine & phenylephrine should be immediately available if hypotension ensues.
- Pulmonary system
  - ➤ The block obtained by a lumbar spinal or epidural anesthetic should not affect ventilatory function.
  - ➤ Even at thoracic levels, tidal volume is usually not diminished. A small decrease in vital capacity can occur due to loss of abdominal & intercostal muscle function.
  - ➤ For pts w/ severe lung disease who rely on accessory muscles for respiration, a high thoracic spinal can result in respiratory impairment necessitating intubation.
  - ➤ For the majority of the population, fully functioning phrenic nerves (innervated by C3/4/5) provide ample oxygenation & ventilation.
  - ➤ If high spinal anesthesia occurs, the airway may need to be quickly secured until phrenic nerve function is regained.

- GI system
  - ➤ Neuraxial block causes a sympathectomy, which can affect the GI organs.
  - ➤ Sympathetic outflow to the gut originates at T5-L1 levels.
  - ➤ Abolishing sympathetic outflow results in unopposed parasympathetic tone, which can lead to increased peristalsis.
- Urinary system
  - ➤ Neuraxial anesthesia results in loss of autonomic bladder control & urinary retention.
  - ➤ If extended periods of analgesia are planned, the bladder should be emptied w/ a urinary catheter.
- Endocrine system
  - ➤ Neuraxial anesthesia can at least partially block the release of catecholamines, cortisol & ADH.

STUDIES
MANAGEMENT/INTERVENTIONS
CAVEATS/PEARLS
CHECKLIST
N/A

BELL'S PALSY

MEREDITH ALBRECHT, MD; LISA LEFFERT, MD; AND MICHELE SZABO, MD

FUNDAMENTAL KNOWLEDGE

Definition
- Syndrome of acute onset involving the facial nerve

Epidemiology
- Incidence is 188 per 100,000 during pregnancy (especially 3rd trimester & post-partum).
- Incidence is $10\times$ higher in pregnant than in non-pregnant pts (11–40 per 100,000).

Pathophysiology
- Idiopathic
- Associated w/ herpes simplex virus type I, Lyme disease

Clinical Manifestations
- Facial paralysis
- Abrupt onset; maximal weakness by 48 hours
- May be preceded by pain behind the ear

- Taste sensation may be lost unilaterally.
- 80% recover within a few weeks or months.
- Incomplete paralysis at 1 week is a favorable prognostic sign.
- Bilateral paralysis is a poor prognostic sign.
- Can be associated w/ hypertensive disorders or pregnancy/pre-eclampsia

Effect of Pregnancy on Bell's Palsy
- Pregnancy may worsen the course of the disease.

Effect of Bell's Palsy on Pregnancy & the Fetus
- Associated w/ pre-eclampsia
- Neonatal outcome unaffected

STUDIES

History & Physical
- Acute onset of facial paralysis
- Look for lesions of herpes zoster, especially in the ear canal or tympanic membrane (Ramsey-Hunt syndrome).
- Normal neurologic exam except the facial nerve

Laboratory
- CSF shows mild lymphocytosis.
- Check Lyme titer.

Imaging
- MRI shows swelling & uniform enhancement of the facial nerve & possible entrapment of the nerve.
- Other
- EMG: denervation after 10 days: long delay (>3 months) prior to regeneration

MANAGEMENT/INTERVENTIONS

Medical Treatment
- Antibiotics for CSF-positive Lyme titers
- Symptomatic
  - ➤ Tape & Lacri-Lube ointment to protect cornea during sleep
  - ➤ Massage of weakened muscles
- Prednisone (60–80 mg over 5 days, then taper over 5 days)
- Possible advantage of acyclovir (avoid during pregnancy)

Anesthesia
- Spinal anesthesia or inadvertent dural puncture has been associated w/ Bell's palsy, but a retrospective study showed no increase in

incidence of Bell's palsy in groups w/ no anesthesia vs. spinal anesthesia vs. epidural anesthesia.

CAVEATS & PEARLS
- Facial paralysis
- Generally presents in 3rd trimester or post-partum
- Increased incidence in pregnancy
- All types of anesthesia acceptable
- No increased incidence w/ spinal anesthesia
- Can be associated w/ preeclampsia

CHECKLIST
- Careful physical exam to document facial paralysis & other neurologic findings
- Observe for signs of preeclampsia.

BENIGN INTRACRANIAL HYPERTENSION (BIH)

MEREDITH ALBRECHT, MD
MICHELE SZABO, MD

FUNDAMENTAL KNOWLEDGE

Definition
- Syndrome of increased ICP w/o hydrocephalus or mass lesion w/ elevated CSF pressure but otherwise normal CSF composition

Epidemiology
- Most prevalent in obese female pts of child-bearing age
- 8–19 per 100,000 obstetric pts

Pathophysiology
- Etiology unknown
- Presumed due to altered CSF reabsorption by arachnoid villi

Clinical Manifestations
- Headaches
  - Worse in morning
  - Aggravated by Valsalva maneuvers such as coughing
- Papilledema
  - Visual disturbances can occur secondary to optic nerve edema.
  - Visual field deficits or altered visual acuity
  - Blindness in severe cases; optic nerve atrophy w/ sustained edema

Effect of Pregnancy on BIH
- Unclear whether pregnancy worsens BIH
- Visual outcome same as for non-pregnant pts w/ BIH

Effect of BIH on Pregnancy
- No evidence that BIH has adverse effect on fetus
- No increased rate of spontaneous abortion

STUDIES

History & Physical
- Determine course & extent of disease.
- Presence/extent of visual symptoms
  - ➤ Examine for papilledema.
- Obtain a history of previous treatment: meds, need for CSF drainage.
- Obtain surgical record if treatment has included a lumbar-peritoneal shunt.
  - ➤ Document shunt location.
- If indwelling lumbar-peritoneal shunt, examine back to confirm level of placement.

Imaging
- Lumbar spine radiograph to determine level of shunt should history of shunt placement be unavailable & regional anesthesia planned
  - ➤ Consider PA rather than AP x-rays to decrease fetal radiation dose.

MANAGEMENT/INTERVENTIONS
- Treatment goals
  - ➤ Preserve vision
  - ➤ Improve symptoms
- Weight loss
  - ➤ 7–10% weight loss (non-ketotic) improves symptoms.
- Analgesics
- Diuretics: acetazolamide
  - ➤ Carbonic anhydrase inhibitor
  - ➤ Decreases CSF production
  - ➤ Can cause a metabolic acidosis
  - ➤ Increases risk of reduced intravascular volume
- Steroids: less effective
- Repeated lumbar puncture: fenestrates dura & drains CSF

- Lumbo-peritoneal (LP) shunt: for continuous CSF drainage in serious cases
- Optic nerve sheath fenestration if vision is threatened

Anesthesia
General
- Avoid maneuvers that produce sustained increases in ICP (eg, coughing).
- Control BP.
- Consider hyperventilation following delivery of fetus.
- Induction w/ thiopental or propofol plus succinylcholine; reported safe
- Sometimes chosen for pts w/ indwelling lumbo-peritoneal shunt
  - When surgical history is unknown
  - Avoids radiographic exposure to determine shunt location
- Back-up for ineffective regional anesthesia
  - Scarring from LP shunt placement may impair successful epidural analgesia.
  - Spinal analgesia: possibly short-lived due to rapid removal of drug via LP shunt
- Most are obese pts, therefore potential difficult airway

Regional
- Often preferred
- Reduces BP & ICP response to pain
- Avoids systemic maternal sedation & hypercarbia
- Abolishes Valsalva maneuver, which increases CVP & ICP
- "Wet tap": does not cause herniation
  - Increased ICP evenly distributed w/ no focal lesion
  - Spinal or lumbar puncture therapeutic
- Theoretical risk of puncturing indwelling shunt
- Rapid injection of volume into the epidural space could increase ICP, so inject slowly.

CAVEATS & PEARLS
- Anesthetic decision making is based on the presence of papilledema.
  - If papilledema +/− visual symptoms present, take measures to control ICP to prevent visual loss.
  - No papilledema: standard anesthetic mgt
- Presence of a functioning LP shunt
  - Decreases the likelihood of symptoms

➤ Risk of catheter disruption w/ regional anesthesia
➤ Risk of catheter disruption is decreased if location of the shunt is well documented

CHECKLIST

■ Document preexisting visual disturbances prior to administering general or regional anesthesia.
■ Identify & inform the pt's neurosurgeon of your anesthetic plans. Determine most efficient mode of contact in case of emergency.
■ Consider stress-dose steroids during labor & delivery for pts on chronic steroid therapy.
■ Antibiotic prophylaxis for pts w/ indwelling LP shunt

BILATERAL RENAL CORTICAL NECROSIS

JOSHUA WEBER, MD
PETER DUNN, MD

FUNDAMENTAL KNOWLEDGE

■ Bilateral renal cortical necrosis (BRCN) is rare in non-pregnant pts.
■ BRCN causes 10–38% of ARF in pregnancy.
■ Placental abruption is the most common cause of BRCN. Other causes include:
➤ Placenta previa
➤ Intrauterine fetal death
➤ Amniotic fluid embolism
■ Pathophysiology unclear but may involve renal ischemia or endotoxin release
■ Presentation
➤ Oliguria/anuria
➤ Flank pain
➤ Gross hematuria
➤ Hypotension

STUDIES

■ Lab tests commonly ordered to evaluate renal function in pregnancy, including:
➤ Creatinine
➤ BUN
➤ Electrolytes
➤ Creatinine clearance

- ➤ CBC
- ➤ Urinalysis
- ■ In addition:
  - ➤ Renal ultrasound or CT: shows hypodensities in renal cortex
  - ➤ Renal arteriography: shows absent or patchy renal cortex
  - ➤ Renal biopsy: shows extensive microthrombi in renal arterioles & glomeruli

MANAGEMENT & INTERVENTIONS

Medical/OB mgt of BRCN

- ■ No therapy has been shown to be effective for BRCN.
- ■ Many pts will need hemodialysis.
- ■ For decreased renal function
  - ➤ Increased frequency of prenatal visits (q2 wks in 1st & 2nd trimesters, then q1 week)
  - ➤ Monitoring: monthly measurements of serum creatinine, creatinine clearance, fetal development, BP
  - ➤ Erythropoietin may be used for maternal anemia.
  - ➤ Preterm delivery is considered for worsening renal function, fetal compromise or pre-eclampsia.
  - ➤ Renal biopsy is considered if rapid deterioration in renal function occurs prior to 32 weeks gestation.
  - ➤ See "*Parturients on Dialysis*" for dialysis mgt.
- ■ Anesthetic mgt for pts w/ significant renal dysfunction

Pre-op

- ■ Evaluate degree of renal dysfunction & hypertension.
- ■ Evaluate for anemia & electrolyte abnormalities.

Intraoperative mgt

- ■ Monitors: standard monitoring + fetal HR +/– arterial line +/– CVP
- ■ Limit fluids in pts w/ marginal renal function to prevent volume overload.
- ■ Use strict aseptic technique, as uremic pts are more prone to infection.
- ■ Careful padding/protection of dialysis access is important.
- ■ Consider promotility agents, as uremic pts may have impaired GI motility.

Regional anesthesia

- ■ Uremia-induced platelet dysfunction leads to increased bleeding time.

- Pts may have thrombocytopenia from peripheral destruction of platelets.
- Increased toxicity from local anesthetics has been reported in pts w/ renal disease, but amides & esters can be used safely.
- Contraindications to regional technique: pt refusal, bacteremia, hypovolemia, hemorrhage, coagulopathy, neuropathy

General anesthesia
- Uremic pts may have hypersensitivity to CNS drugs due to increased permeability of blood-brain barrier.
- Uremia causes delayed gastric emptying & increased acidity, leading to increased risk of aspiration pneumonitis (consider sodium citrate, H2-receptor blocker, metoclopramide).
- Hypoalbuminemia leads to increased free drug concentration of drugs that are bound to albumin (ie, thiopental).
- Succinylcholine is relatively contraindicated, as it causes approx. 1-mEq/L increase in serum potassium, which may precipitate cardiac dysrhythmias.
- Use caution w/ drugs dependent on renal excretion (gallamine, vecuronium, pancuronium) & clearance (mivacurium, rocuronium).

CAVEATS & PEARLS
- Triad of BRCN: anuria, gross hematuria & flank pain
- Increased toxicity from local anesthetics has been reported in pts w/ renal disease, but amides & esters can be used safely.
- Succinylcholine is relatively contraindicated, as it causes approx. 1 mEq/L increase in serum potassium, which may precipitate cardiac dysrhythmias.
- Use caution w/ drugs dependent on renal excretion (gallamine, vecuronium, pancuronium) & clearance (mivacurium, rocuronium).

CHECKLIST
- Check OB plan.
- Correct underlying hemodynamic abnormalities, especially volume status.
- Be prepared to treat hypertension.
- Use meds & dosages adjusted to reflect degree of renal dysfunction.

BONE MARROW MALIGNANCIES AND BONE MARROW TRANSPLANT PATIENTS

JEANNA VIOLA, MD
JANE BALLANTYNE, MD

FUNDAMENTAL KNOWLEDGE

■ Myeloproliferative disorders: the most common in pregnancy are:
  ➤ Essential thrombocytopenia
   • Asymptomatic thrombocytosis
   • 50% have splenomegaly + elevated plt count >1,000,000 at presentation.
   • Morbidity is due to arterial & venous thrombosis as well as hemorrhage. Immediately post-partum, pts may have severe thrombocytosis to 1,500,000 w/ essential thrombocytopenia.
  ➤ Polycythemia rubra vera
   • Occasionally seen in pregnancy
   • Symptoms are related to increased blood volume & viscosity.
   • Pts are at risk of bleeding.
■ Leukemias: classified as either acute or chronic; myelogenous or lymphocytic
  ➤ Myelogenous leukemia: myeloblasts proliferate in the bone marrow & spread to extramedullary organs.
   • 80% of acute myelogenous leukemia (AML) cases occur in adults.
   • AML pts may develop renal failure from the precipitation of uric acid, a breakdown product from nucleic acids, in the renal tubules.
   • Chronic myelogenous leukemia (CML) accounts for 20–30% of leukemias & is most prevalent in middle-aged adults. CML may transform into AML or ALL.
   • CML pts experience a 40% increase in metabolic requirements due to the production of excessive white cells.
  ➤ Lymphoblastic leukemia: lymphoblasts proliferate in the lymph nodes:
   • Acute lymphocytic leukemia (ALL) is mainly a disease of children; long-term survival rate in adults is poor.
   • Chronic lymphocytic leukemia (CLL) usually occurs at age 60 or older & accounts for 25% of adult leukemias. A hemolytic anemia may be associated with CLL. CLL-induced lymph node proliferation around ureters results in renal failure.

> Pregnancy does not alter the incidence or prognosis of leukemia.
- Bone marrow transplant pts
  > May be from a histocompatible donor or be the pt's own "post-remission" marrow
  > Infusion of the bone marrow transplant follows total body irradiation and/or intensive chemotherapy.
  > Autologous transplants avoid the possibility of graft-versus-host disease.
- Hodgkin's lymphoma
  > Most common lymphoproliferative disease in young people
  > Fourth most common cancer diagnosis in parturients
  > Pregnancy does not alter the prognosis of lymphoma; however, treatment during pregnancy is often required.

STUDIES
- Essential thrombocytopenia
  > Symptoms: sensation of burning in the fingertips, headaches, easy bruising & mucous membrane hemorrhages
  > No specific lab tests predict this disease; elevated platelet count on CBC.
  > Reduced responsiveness to epinephrine, or spontaneous in vitro platelet aggregation
- Leukemia
  > Clinical manifestations include fatigue, pallor (from anemia), infection (from neutropenia) & hemorrhage (thrombocytopenia).
  > Pts may exhibit splenomegaly, hepatomegaly.
  > Bone marrow biopsy confirms the diagnosis of leukemia.
- Hodgkin's lymphoma
  > Usually asymptomatic lymphadenopathy (painless neck mass) or a mediastinal mass on chest x-ray on presentation
  > Systemic symptoms include fever, pruritus, severe pain after ingestion of alcohol.
  > Diagnosis made by lymph node biopsy
  > PA chest x-ray w/ adequate abdominal shielding
  > CBC, ESR, serum creatinine concentration, serum liver enzymes
  > Bone marrow biopsy

MANAGEMENT/INTERVENTIONS
- Essential thrombocytopenia
  > Pts do well with low-dose ASA.

➤ Avoid hydroxyurea & busulfan in pregnancy if possible.
➤ Regional anesthesia is safe unless there is ongoing hemorrhage.
◼ Polycythemia rubra vera
  ➤ Treated w/ recurrent phlebotomy.
  ➤ Careful iron supplementation may be necessary.
  ➤ Maintain Hct <45 through phlebotomy.
  ➤ Take care w/ positioning to prevent venous stasis.
◼ Leukemia
  ➤ Standard chemotherapy used to treat leukemia can be safely administered during the second & third trimesters.
  ➤ Anthracycline antibiotics (daunorubicin, doxorubicin) & cytosine arabinoside are used in treating AML; remission rate is 60–80%.
    • These drugs can impair ventricular dysfunction & cause ventricular tachydysrhythmias, heart block & sudden death.
  ➤ Post-remission, pts receive bone marrow transplant, which sustains remission for >2 yrs in 40% of AML pts.
  ➤ CML treatment includes busulfan (an alkylating agent), steroids, radiation of the spleen & radioactive phosphorus treatment.
    • Hypoadrenalism may occur due to suppression of the pituitary axis by busulfan.
    • Busulfan can produce pulmonary fibrosis; assess pulmonary function.
  ➤ Treatment of CLL involves administration of alkylating agents such as chlorambucil & cyclophosphamide.
    • Cyclophosphamide can prolong the effect of succinylcholine.
  ➤ Leukophoresis or rapid reduction of white count w/ chemotherapy may be needed to decrease risk of labor or surgery.
  ➤ Vigorous hydration is important.
  ➤ In general, no contraindications to regional anesthesia
◼ Hodgkin's lymphoma
  ➤ Most parturients diagnosed w/ Hodgkin's during pregnancy undergo therapy. Delaying treatment until second trimester is safest for the fetus.
  ➤ Irradiation (second or third trimester)
    • The whole-body fetal dose should be limited to 0.10 Gy or less.
    • Aim for partial therapy until delivery.
  ➤ Both MOPP & ABVD have been administered to pregnant women w/ Hodgkin's.
    • Avoid administration of chemo close to delivery: the neonate's ability to metabolize & excrete these drugs is low.

- Monitor CBC of mother & infant for cytopenia if chemo given prior to delivery.

CAVEATS AND PEARLS
- Strict aseptic technique is important in pts w/ neutropenia.
- These pts have received multiple blood transfusions & are at increased risk for a transfusion reaction due to allo-immunization.

CHECKLIST
- Pts w/ AML should have Hct, Hgb measured, serum electrolytes, BUN, liver enzymes.
- Determine blast cell count in untreated leukemic pts at delivery; consider plasmapheresis to reduce the hyperviscosity of the blood.
- Consider CXR to rule out anterior mediastinal mass if Hodgkin's pt may require GETA.
- Early & frequent consultation w/ pt's oncologist
- Determine what chemotherapy has been administered & where irradiation has been given.

BRAIN TUMOR

MEREDITH ALBRECHT, MD
MICHELE SZABO, MD

FUNDAMENTAL KNOWLEDGE

Definition
- Any growth of abnormal cells or uncontrolled proliferation of cells in the brain

Epidemiology
- 14 per 100,000 general population
- Most studies suggest incidence is slightly lower in pregnant women than age-matched non-pregnant women; suggested contributing factors are brain tumor-induced decreased libido, infertility
- Third leading cause of death in pts age 20–29

Pathophysiology
- Etiology is likely complex & as yet unknown.
- Tumor type is diverse.
- Distribution of histologic type in pregnant women is similar to that of non-pregnant women.
  - ➤ Glial tumors: most common, constituting 35% of all intracranial tumors

- Meningiomas: 18% of intracranial tumors, 2:1 female to male ratio
- Pituitary adenoma: 7% of tumors, peak incidence in young women of child-bearing age
- Hemangioblastoma: usually occurs in posterior fossa
- Acoustic neuroma: 7% of brain tumors
- Ependymoma
- Primary brain lymphoma: incidence increased w/ AIDS
- Metastatic tumor: melanoma, breast, lung cancer & choriocarcinoma are tumors most likely to metastasize to the brain

Clinical Manifestations
- Symptoms vary & depend on size & location, rate of tumor growth & amount of edema formation. Usually present w/ any of 3 syndromes:
  - Focal neurologic deficit: resulting from compression of the neurons from an expanding lesion
  - Seizures: brain tumors involving the cerebral cortex more likely associated w/ seizures
    - 20% of brain tumor pts present w/ new-onset seizure.
  - Nonfocal neurologic disorder: usually related to increased ICP
    - Headaches: worse in morning
      - Headaches are presenting symptom in 36–90% of pts.
    - Vomiting
    - Visual changes
    - Dementia
    - Personality change
    - Gait disorder

Effect of pregnancy on brain tumor
- Two primary brain tumors are well documented to grow w/ pregnancy.
  Effect attributed to presence of tumor hormone growth receptors.
  - Meningioma
    - Benign tumor
    - Well-documented hormone growth receptors
    - Possible regression following delivery
  - Pituitary adenoma
    - 5–20% of macroadenomas will enlarge during pregnancy.
    - Most pronounced effect in 2nd & 3rd trimester
    - Pituitary gland size normally increases by 45% during pregnancy & lactation.
    - Effect of tumor growth + pituitary enlargement may combine to make pt more symptomatic.

- Metastatic tumors
  - Breast & melanoma: well-described tumor hormonal growth receptors
  - Choriocarcinoma: result of pregnancy
- Physiologic changes of pregnancy also have the potential to exacerbate the symptoms of any brain tumor.
  - Pregnancy causes increase in brain water content.
  - Pregnancy causes intracranial venous distention.
  - Glial tumors (malignant tumor) are example where physiologic changes worsen the tumor.
    - More extensive perineoplastic brain edema develops.
    - Leads to more severe symptoms

Effect of brain tumor on pregnancy
- Increased risk of spontaneous abortion
- Increased risk of fetal mortality
- Possible teratogenic & carcinogenic effects of radiation during diagnostic testing & treatment
- Possible teratogenic effects of drug therapy
- Pituitary adenoma or insufficiency
  - Increased rate of infertility, spontaneous abortion
  - GH antagonizes insulin action in acromegalics & leads to increased risk of diabetes.
- Increased risk of DVT

STUDIES

History & Physical
- History
  - Ascertain tumor onset, presenting symptoms & type.
  - Determine course of the neurologic disease.
  - Determine seizure history.
  - Determine what treatment, if any, the pt has received.
  - If pt is acromegalic, determine if symptoms of sleep apnea or voice changes are present.
- Physical
  - Airway
    - Acromegalic: examine for a potentially difficult airway
      - Enlarged tongue
      - Enlarged jaw
      - Coarse voice: associated w/ enlarged supraglottic folds
    - Others
      - Meticulous airway evaluation

- May require emergency GA for C-section
> Neurologic
  - Mental status exam
  - Examine for focal neurologic deficits.
  - For pts w/ pituitary tumors, document visual field testing.
  - Repeat mental status & neurologic exam as often as needed during & following labor & delivery.
> Ophthalmologic
  - Perform funduscopic exam looking for evidence of papilledema.

Imaging
- MRI or CT scan: examine most recent films, looking for evidence of increased ICP or potential for herniation
  > Size & location of tumor
  > Supratentorial or infratentorial lesion
  > Presence of non-communicating hydrocephalus or pre-existing VP shunt
  > Are the ventricles midline, or are they compressed?
  > Examine for evidence of brain herniation.
- CT scan
  > Usually initial diagnostic procedure of choice for pregnant pt
  > Appropriately shielded fetus, safe radiation exposure
- MRI
  > No long-term data on fetal outcome
  > MRI generally avoided during first trimester
  > MRI contrast agent, gadolinium, crosses the placenta.
  > No reported adverse effects of fetal exposure to gadolinium
  > Nevertheless, most advise against contrast use during pregnancy unless clinically necessary.
- Echocardiogram: consider if pt previously treated w/ doxorubicin

Other
- CBC: consider if pt has received chemotherapy
- Free drug level of anticonvulsant at onset of labor
- Glucose: consider for the acromegalic or pt on dexamethasone

MANAGEMENT / INTERVENTIONS
- Mgt of these complex pts varies & depends on:
  > Type of tumor (benign or malignant, potential responsiveness to Rx)
  > Location of tumor
    - Infratentorial vs. supratentorial

- Surgical accessibility
- ➤ Size of tumor
  - Growth rate
- ➤ Presence of increased ICP (eg, non-communicating hydrocephalus)
- ➤ Symptoms of tumor
  - Progression of symptoms
  - Responsiveness to pharmacologic therapy
- ➤ Gestational age of fetus
  - Fetal pulmonary maturity
- ➤ Pt's wishes
- ■ Multidisciplinary team meeting should be held once a pregnant pt is diagnosed w/ a brain tumor.
  - ➤ Treatment plan should be discussed & established.
  - ➤ Backup emergency plan should be established.
- ■ Some possible treatment plans
  1) Defer surgery until after pregnancy:
     - Benign tumors
     - Controlled symptoms
     - Follow w/ serial neurologic exams & imaging
  2) Neurosurgical resection of tumor in 2nd or beginning 3rd trimester
     - Symptomatic benign tumor or low-grade astrocytoma
     - Diagnosed in 1st, 2nd or beginning of 3rd trimester
     - Neurosurgical resection
     - Followed by normal gestation
  3) Concurrent C-section & neurosurgical resection in 3rd trimester
     - Malignant but treatable brain tumor or benign tumor that has become symptomatic
     - Plan C-section at time of established fetal maturity.
     - C-section, then craniotomy
  4) Stereotactic biopsy & no surgical treatment
     - Suspected high-grade glioblastoma for which there is no neurosurgical treatment
  5) C-section
     - Planned at fetal maturity for pt w/ high-grade tumor
     - Earlier if mother becomes neurologically unstable
  6) Termination of pregnancy

Medical Treatment
- ■ Dexamethasone

➤ Significantly reduces perineoplastic brain edema
➤ No evidence of teratogenicity, not systematically studied
➤ Not recommended during 1st trimester
➤ May precipitate gestational diabetes & hypertension
➤ May induce neonatal hypoadrenalism
■ Antiemetics
■ Bromocriptine
➤ Used to treat prolactinoma
➤ Usually discontinued during pregnancy
➤ Hypertension, stroke & seizures reported to occur in pts in puerperium after suppression of lactation w/ bromocriptine
■ Octreotide
➤ Used to treat acromegaly
➤ Usually discontinued during pregnancy
➤ Unknown fetal effects
■ Anticonvulsants
➤ Phenytoin, carbamazepine, valproate, phenobarbital
➤ All associated w/ teratogenic effects
➤ During first trimester, many use only for motor seizures or those that would endanger mother or fetus
➤ Alter folate absorption, requires replacement
➤ Induce vitamin K deficiency in newborn
  • At risk for hemorrhagic disease of newborn
  • Treat all pts on anticonvulsants w/ vitamin K supplementation.
➤ Free drug levels dramatically change throughout pregnancy.
  • Assess free drug level every week in last month of pregnancy & at onset of labor or prior to C section.
■ Chemotherapy
➤ During last two trimesters
➤ Often indicated for high-grade, inoperable tumor
■ Radiation therapy
➤ Safe for fetus w/ appropriate shielding
➤ Often indicated for high-grade, inoperable tumor or metastasis

Anesthesia
■ There are insufficient data and no conclusive evidence for the safest anesthetics in these complex pts, so the selection of anesthetic technique remains controversial.
■ Brain tumors are diverse & their complexity is multiplied by pregnancy; anesthetic mgt should be individually tailored.

- Anesthetic plan should be discussed & approved by a multidisciplinary care team.
- The following are examples of mgt for various clinical scenarios.
  1) Neurologically stable parturient at term w/ unresected brain tumor (eg, supratentorial meningioma, small acoustic neuroma)
     - Regional (epidural)
       - Reasonable, if pt not at risk for herniation w/ an inadvertent dural puncture
         - For example, supratentorial meningioma w/o mass effect, frontal glioma w/o mass effect, pituitary adenoma or small acoustic neuroma
       - Consult neurosurgery & neurology
         - Establish whether there is a risk for herniation w/ CSF leak.
         - Litmus test: ask both neurologist & neurosurgeon whether they would perform a lumbar puncture in the pt.
       - Advantage: pt has clear sensorium & ability to follow serial neurologic exams
       - Attenuates increases in ICP that occur w/ uterine contractions
       - Prevents Valsalva if dense block
       - Can titrate local anesthetics to effect
     - General
       - Preferred if epidural is contraindicated because of risk for herniation from inadvertent dural puncture & CSF leak
       - Manage ICP
         - Avoid hypoventilation.
         - Avoid hypoxia (preoxygenate well!).
         - Blunt or treat hypertensive response to noxious stimuli (avoid coughing).
         - Avoid & aggressively treat hypotension.
         - Pentothal & succinylcholine well tolerated & well described for use in this setting
         - Succinylcholine causes only a transient rise in ICP, which is blunted by prior administration of pentothal.
         - Isoflurane or sevoflurane w/ nitrous oxide well tolerated until delivery
         - Consider adding short-acting narcotic such as fentanyl following delivery of fetus to blunt response to noxious stimuli.
         - Prompt emergence is important so that serial neurologic exams can be performed; plan accordingly.

2) Craniotomy during 2nd or early 3rd trimester
   - ➤ Often planned for low-grade glioma, for tumor in "risky" location such as near motor cortex where tumor expansion could lead to significant neurologic deficit, when imaging shows significant tumor growth or presence of progressive neurologic deficit
   - ➤ General anesthesia
   - ➤ Direct arterial BP measurement w/ A-line
   - ➤ Consider CVP.
   - ➤ Controlled, "modified" rapid sequence induction
   - ➤ Goal: ensure hemodynamic stability & adequate cerebral perfusion pressure & control ICP
     - Cricoid pressure
     - Graded doses of pentothal or propofol: assess hemodynamic effect
     - Titrated doses of narcotic to prevent hypertensive response to intubation
     - Rocuronium: monitor w/ TOF to ensure twitch suppression to prevent Valsalva response to intubation
   - ➤ Brain "relaxation"
     - Lumbar CSF drainage: preferred if there is not risk for herniation (eg, no evidence of non-communicating hydrocephalus) as it helps avoid use & potential risks of mannitol or furosemide
     - Mannitol
       - Potential to cause temporary fetal dehydration
       - Fetal outcome data are limited.
       - Anecdotal case reports suggest it is safe for these circumstances.
   - ➤ Choice of maintenance anesthetic agent should include need for rapid emergence.
   - ➤ If pt is on anticonvulsants
     - Shorter duration of neuromuscular blockade
     - Decreased sensitivity to narcotics
     - Avoid drugs that lower seizure threshold (meperidine & sevoflurane).
3) Concurrent C-section & craniotomy at term
   - ➤ Often planned when tumor is diagnosed in middle of 3rd trimester & pt is neurologically stable but would benefit from earlier resection (eg, metastatic tumor, low-grade glioma)
   - ➤ C-section should precede craniotomy.
   - ➤ General anesthesia

➤ Direct arterial BP measurement w/ A-line
➤ Consider CVP.
➤ Controlled, "modified" rapid sequence induction
  - Cricoid pressure
  - Graded doses of pentothal or propofol: assess hemodynamic effect
  - Titrated doses of narcotic to prevent hypertensive response to intubation in pts w/ increased ICP
  - Rocuronium: monitor w/ TOF to ensure twitch suppression to prevent Valsalva response to intubation
➤ Brain "relaxation"
  - Lumbar CSF drainage: preferred if there is not risk for herniation (eg, no evidence of non-communicating hydrocephalus), as it helps avoid use & potential risks of mannitol or furosemide
  - Mannitol
    - Potential to cause temporary fetal dehydration
    - Fetal outcome data are limited.
    - Anecdotal case reports suggest it is safe for these circumstances.
➤ Choice of maintenance anesthetic agent should include need for rapid emergence.
➤ If pt is on anticonvulsants
  - Shorter duration of neuromuscular blockade
  - Decreased sensitivity to narcotics
  - Avoid drugs that lower seizure threshold (meperidine & sevoflurane).
➤ Administer prophylactic antibiotics.
➤ Administer dexamethasone to treat tumor edema.
➤ Oxytocin
  - Effect in pts w/ intracranial vascular lesions is unclear; likely it causes cerebral vasoconstriction.
  - Can cause maternal hypertension; vigilant attention to BP
  - Has been used clinically in these circumstances w/o adverse effect
  - Check for uterine bleeding at regular intervals throughout the craniotomy.
4) Urgent or emergent craniotomy w/ or w/o concurrent C-section
➤ General anesthesia is the only feasible choice.
➤ Mother is at great health risk & preventing her morbidity & mortality is a top priority.

➤ Goals: manage ICP, prevent maternal aspiration & avoid harm to the fetus

➤ If feasible & time permits, insert arterial line for BP monitoring.

➤ Rapid sequence induction
- Pentothal or propofol, succinylcholine (unless pt has paresis >48 hrs), narcotic or IV lidocaine to blunt BP response to intubation
- Effects of succinylcholine on ICP are short-lived & attenuated w/ prior administration of pentothal (advantage of rapid onset outweighs the potential transient adverse effect on ICP)

➤ Hypotension &/or hypoxia will dramatically worsen neurologic injury; treat aggressively.

➤ Hyperventilation is indicated in life-threatening intracranial emergency; cease once brain is decompressed
- Reliably reduces ICP
- Marked hyperventilation causes uteroplacental vasoconstriction, resulting in fetal hypoxia & acidosis.
- Reduction in cardiac output caused by positive-pressure ventilation is likely cause of decreased uterine blood flow & not alkalosis per se.

➤ Mannitol is indicated to treat life-threatening emergency.
- Potential to cause temporary fetal dehydration
- Fetal outcome data are limited.
- Anecdotal case reports suggest it is safe for these circumstances.

➤ Choice of maintenance anesthetic agent should include need for rapid emergence.
- For the emergent craniotomy w/ significantly increased ICP: recommend TIVA prior to decompression w/ dural incision, to minimize increase in ICP
- Low-dose volatile w/ nitrous oxide following decompression

➤ Administer dexamethasone to decrease tumor edema.

➤ Administer prophylactic antibiotics.

➤ If pt is on anticonvulsants
- Shorter duration of neuromuscular blockade
- Decreased sensitivity to narcotics
- Avoid drugs that lower seizure threshold (meperidine & sevoflurane)

➤ If a concurrent C-section is planned
- If urgent, perform craniotomy first.
- Follow same recommendations as above & be prepared to treat the mannitol-induced fetal dehydration & narcotic-induced respiratory depression.
- Fetal monitoring as per OB consult
- If labor begins during craniotomy & delivery is imminent
  - Suspend intracranial procedure.
  - Deliver infant as indicated obstetrically.
- Oxytocin
  - Effect in pts w/ intracranial vascular lesions is unclear; likely to cause cerebral vasoconstriction
  - Can cause maternal hypotension; vigilant attention to BP
  - Has been used clinically in these circumstances w/o adverse effect
- After delivery of the infant, anesthesia may be modified as required for the neurosurgical procedure.

5) Stereotactic biopsy
➤ Performed when high-grade brain glioma is suspected to obtain a diagnosis
➤ Performed under local anesthesia

CAVEATS & PEARLS
- Diagnosis of brain tumor during pregnancy is devastating, creates obstacles for diagnostic procedures & affects the nature & timing of treatment.
- Team approach is critical for successful mgt of these pts.
- Timing of the delivery &/or neurosurgical procedure is based on the course of the neurologic disease as well as obstetrical considerations.
- Tumors are diverse, so each pt's mgt must be individualized & flexible.
- Always have a well-published emergency plan.
- Brain tumor symptoms of headache, nausea, vomiting & seizures are similar to those of eclampsia; examine pt for focal neurologic deficits & papilledema to help distinguish the cause.

CHECKLIST
- Make certain you know how to contact the neurosurgeon emergently.
- Administer prophylactic antibiotics if performing a concurrent neurosurgical procedure.

- Check serum anticonvulsant levels.
- Perform serial neurologic exams whenever feasible before, during & after delivery.
- Fetal monitoring as per obstetric consult

BREECH IN LABOR

SUSANNE PAREKH, MD
ANDREA TORRI, MD

FUNDAMENTAL KNOWLEDGE

- Most singleton breech presentations at mid-term convert to vertex presentation by the time they reach term. Breech presentation is observed in about 2–4% of singleton term pregnancies but is more common in pregnancies with premature labor: 7% when the duration of the pregnancy is <32 weeks, 25–40% when <28 weeks.
- In obstetrics, *presentation* of the infant denotes the fetal anatomic part that overlies the inlet of the mother's pelvis. The breech infant is oriented along the longitudinal axis (ie, longitudinal *lie*) & the cephalic pole lies in the uterine fundus. The presenting part of the breech infant is the buttocks &/or the fetal lower extremities. The relationship between them (ie, the *attitude*) describes the 3 possible breech presentations & influences both the obstetrical conduct of labor & the anesthetic plan.
  - ➤ The 3 varieties of breech presentation are frank breech, complete breech & incomplete (or footling) breech.

Frank breech
- Most common variety
- Infant w/ flexed hips & extension of both knees
- Fetus typically remains in this position throughout labor & the fetal aggregate is regularly shaped & completely fills the pelvic outlet.
- These characteristics are considered favorable for progressive, regular & complete dilatation of the birth canal & for the possibility of a successful vaginal delivery.

Complete breech
- Infant w/ flexed hips & flexed knees
- Least common of the 3 varieties
- The fetal aggregate is less regular & hip & knee flexion might decrease any time during labor, causing sudden modification of the presentation into an incomplete or footling breech.

Incomplete or footling breech

- Infant w/ incomplete flexion of 1 hip & knee
- More common variety of breech presentation in preterm gestations
- Fetal aggregate is irregular & incompletely fills the pelvic outlet.
- This is the variety of breech associated w/ the highest rate of umbilical cord prolapse & entrapment of the after-coming head.

STUDIES

- OBs will use physical exam &/or ultrasonography to determine fetal presentation.
- Obtain standard pre-op lab studies (blood type & screen, hematocrit, platelet count) if time permits.

MANAGEMENT AND INTERVENTIONS

External Cephalic Version (ECV)

- An obstetrical maneuver that by external palpation & manipulation of the fetus converts a breech (or transverse) presentation into a vertex one
- Overall success of ECV is higher when an adequate amount of amniotic fluid is present, the fetal spine is not lying against the posterior uterine wall & the presenting fetal part has not yet engaged the pelvic inlet.
- Most OBs choose to perform ECV after 37 weeks gestation because there is a 5–10% risk of bradycardia & may require urgent delivery. This is most likely due to transient cord compression.
- Other risks include cord entanglement, bleeding from an abruption & labor.
- Most pts are monitored throughout the version & for a period of time after the procedure.
- The use of epidural analgesia for ECV is controversial because it might increase the likelihood of maternal & fetal injury by allowing more forceful manipulations because of the analgesia present. However, some authors have shown that epidural analgesia for ECV increases the success rate of the procedure. According to the ACOG bulletin of July 1997, there is not enough current evidence to recommend the use of epidural analgesia before attempting ECV. Many OBs do not ask for epidural analgesia before performing external cephalic rotation, but it seems wise to alert the anesthesiologist before attempting ECV.

■ When choosing how to dose an epidural for ECV, remember that using a concentrated local anesthetic can mask pain associated w/ maternal or fetal injury. However, w/ the use of ultrasound monitoring during the procedure, changes in FHR can be immediately recognized. Given the potential for fetal intolerance, it is prudent to achieve a dense enough block to allow the obstetrician to do an urgent cesarean delivery.

■ Some obstetricians electively plan a C-section for all cases of breech presentation. The largest randomized breech trial showed that cesarean delivery was less traumatic for the singleton breech than vaginal delivery.

■ If a vaginal breech birth of a singleton fetus is planned, then a functional epidural is extremely important. This requires epidural analgesia of the sacral roots S2 to S4 to block transmission of the pudendal nerves. On the other hand, the level of analgesia should never be so intense as to prevent adequate pushing during the 2nd stage. The delivery of the head may be accomplished by maternal expulsive efforts or use of forceps. Since entrapment of the fetal head is always a possibility in the vaginal breech delivery, the anesthesiologist should formulate a plan to quickly provide skeletal & smooth muscle relaxation. A small dose of IV nitroglycerin (100–500 mcg) provides immediate & brief cervical smooth muscle relaxation. When time permits, epidural reinforcement by 5 mL of 3% chloroprocaine helps to achieve more intense perineal muscle relaxation. Immediate rapid sequence induction of general anesthesia offers the advantage of uterine and cervical smooth muscle relaxation from the halogenated agent combined w/ skeletal muscle relaxation from the succinylcholine, but it carries the risk of emergency general anesthesia in the parturient & requires intubation of the trachea.

■ The possibility of head entrapment in the birth canal during fetal extraction & the higher incidence of umbilical cord prolapse in breech presentation may suddenly convert an elective vaginal breech delivery into a dire emergency in a significant proportion of cases.

CAVEATS AND PEARLS
■ Due to urgency of delivery, there may not be time to wait for lab results or for the patient to be NPO for at least 8 hours.

■ Planning a safe anesthetic relies heavily on careful history (including a history of bleeding problems) & physical exam (w/ a focus on the airway).

CHECKLIST
- Airway assessment
- Aspiration prophylaxis, including sodium citrate (Bicitra) and metoclopramide (Reglan)
- Operative/anesthetic plan discussed w/ OBs & nurses

CARDIAC ARREST

JASMIN FIELD, MD
DWIGHT GEHA, MD

FUNDAMENTAL KNOWLEDGE
Cardiac arrest in late pregnancy is rare:
- Approx. 1 in 30,000 pregnancies
- Most often due to medical conditions common to pregnancy & comorbidities exacerbated by pregnancy; more rarely due to underlying cardiac disease (not due to normal stresses of pregnancy alone)

  Although most cardiac arrests in the parturient occur in acute care settings, successful resuscitation is exceedingly rare due to obstacles created by the normal physiologic changes of pregnancy:
  - ➤ Increased oxygen consumption
  - ➤ Decreased functional residual capacity & oxygen-carrying capacity result in rapid desaturation.
  - ➤ Aortocaval compression by gravid uterus in supine position can obstruct venous return.
  - ➤ Low fetal tolerance of hypotension
  - ➤ Potential airway swelling
  - ➤ Full stomach of pregnancy, w/ increased risk of aspiration
  - ➤ Decreased sternal area & compliance secondary to breast hypertrophy & elevation of diaphragm w/ flaring of ribs due to fetal displacement
- ASSISTED VENTILATION & AIRWAY MGT MUST START IMMEDIATELY!

Causes of cardiac arrest in the parturient
- Thromboembolism
  - ➤ Coagulation enhanced during pregnancy & for 4–6 weeks postpartum via 3 mechanisms:
    - Elevated coagulation factors 2, 7, 8, 10
    - Elevated fibrinogen
    - Augmented platelet adhesion

- Amniotic fluid embolism
- Sepsis
- DIC
- Arrhythmia (see "*Arrhythmias*")
- Trauma
  - ➤ The leading cause of non-obstetric maternal death is trauma during pregnancy.
  - ➤ Maternal death is the leading cause of fetal death.
- Postpartum hemorrhage
- Anesthetic-related meds
  - ➤ Spinal anesthesia
    - Epidural anesthesia
    - Vagal
    - Seizures
    - Arrhythmias
    - Other meds
  - ➤ IV magnesium sulfate therapy for eclampsia
  - ➤ Reports of intraoperative asystolic cardiac arrest occurring w/ injection of 0.2 mg IV methylergonovine during C-section under spinal bupivacaine/fentanyl/morphine, also following IV bolus of 10 IU oxytocin
    - One pt was found via subsequent cardiac catheterization to have subtotal LAD occlusion due to coronary vasospasm, with post-MI LVEF of 15% requiring several days of vasopressor support, w/ intra-aortic balloon pump, & multiple doses of intracoronary nitroglycerin
    - Sublingual nitroglycerin may be useful as immediate intervention if pts experience symptoms of intra-op coronary vasospasm after ergot derivatives.

STUDIES
- All interventions must occur simultaneously & immediately.
- Staff on labor & delivery floor should be prepared for the specific nuances of CPR in the pregnant pt.
- Pt should be immediately placed on full monitors & 100% O_2 w/ reservoir bag.
- Establish large-bore IV access.
- Once CPR has been initiated, send stat electrolytes, CBC, cardiac enzymes, w/ 12-lead EKG, chest x-ray as time allows.
- Cardiac catheterization & echo as indicated

MANAGEMENT/INTERVENTIONS

ACLS for the parturient

- Anticipate potential airway edema/difficult airway.
  - ➤ Short-handled blade
  - ➤ LMA, gum-elastic bougie, fiberoptic scope readily available
- Full stomach of pregnancy requires rapid sequence intubation w/ cricoid pressure & cuffed endotracheal tube.
  - ➤ Increased intra-abdominal pressure
  - ➤ Decreased lower esophageal sphincter tone due to negative pressure of intrathoracic migration & hormonal changes
  - ➤ Delayed gastric emptying during labor
  - ➤ Proceed quickly w/ difficult airway algorithm, as desaturation is rapid & not tolerated by fetus.
  - ➤ Maintain cricoid pressure w/ bag-mask ventilation & LMA.
- Compressions & ventilations done in standard ratio
  - ➤ Hand position for compressions is more cephalad.
- Left uterine displacement required throughout resuscitation
  - ➤ Roll to 15–30 degrees
  - ➤ Premade wedge available
  - ➤ Can be supported/displaced on caregiver's knees
  - ➤ May need manual displacement of abdomen using multiple assistants for positioning while chest is turned more supine for compressions
  - ➤ Raising pt's legs can improve venous return.
- Meds & defibrillation are otherwise unchanged from standard ACLS.

Emergency C-section

- If efforts at resuscitation are unsuccessful *after only 4–5 minutes*, emergency bedside C-section should occur w/o delay for sterile prep or anesthesia.
  - ➤ Removal of fetus is often a necessary component of restoring maternal & fetal circulation, not just a last-ditch effort.
  - ➤ CPR must be maintained during surgical evacuation of fetus.
  - ➤ Transabdominal and/or open chest cardiac massage via thoracotomy may be necessary or beneficial.
  - ➤ Resuscitations taking >15 minutes *rarely* produce viable pts (mother or fetus).

CAVEATS AND PEARLS

- Expect rapid deoxygenation & challenging airways.

- Maintain cricoid pressure until cuffed endotracheal tube can be placed.
- Have multiple rescuers who are trained in specifics of gravid resuscitation, who can move as quickly & efficiently as possible.
- Simultaneously establish 100% O_2, monitors, large-bore IV access.
- Positioning w/ wedge under right side for left uterine displacement
- Recommendations for drugs & defibrillation are unchanged, w/ the following caveats in mind:
  - Application of defibrillator electrodes may be difficult & limited by body habitus & pt positioning.
  - Adhesive defibrillator pads may be easier to apply & more effective than hand-held paddles.
  - Pre-eclamptic & eclamptic pts can have arrest due to cardiotoxicity of magnesium sulfate treatment & will need correction of hypermagnesemia w/ calcium chloride
  - Cardiotoxicity from local anesthetics: may need emergent cardiopulmonary bypass
- Vasopressors likely will not increase uteroplacental flow after arrest w/o delivery of fetus.
- Sublingual nitroglycerin may be useful as immediate intervention for signs & symptoms suggestive of acute coronary vasospasm after ergot derivatives.
  - IV ergot administration causes immediate symptoms, but IM administration (more common) can be delayed up to 20 minutes.
- If efforts at resuscitation are unsuccessful *after 4–5 minutes*, emergency bedside C-section should occur w/o delay for sterile prep or anesthesia.
- Transabdominal and/or open chest cardiac massage via thoracotomy may be necessary.
- Resuscitations taking > 15 minutes rarely produce viable pts (mother or fetus).

CHECKLIST
- RAPID RESPONSE!
- Difficult airway mgt tools readily available & accessible
- Rapid sequence intubation/immediate control of airway
- Left uterine displacement crucial in resuscitation
- Standard code cart, meds & defibrillator
- Correct underlying cause of arrest while performing CPR, monitoring, getting access, etc.

- Surgical removal of fetus after 4–5 minutes of CPR
- Consider early cardiac massage transabdominally or via thoracotomy.

CARDIOMYOPATHY

MATTHEW CIRIGLIANA, MD
DWIGHT G. GEHA, MD

FUNDAMENTAL KNOWLEDGE

- Peripartum cardiomyopathy is a serious condition that may develop during or after pregnancy. It is associated w/ high morbidity & mortality for the parturient.
- Maternal mortality approaches 60%. Estimates are that 50% of women w/ peripartum cardiomyopathy have persistent ventricular dysfunction.
- Figures for the incidence of peripartum cardiomyopathy are not based on the current definition of peripartum cardiomyopathy & as such are probably inaccurate. Cunningham et al. published a rate of 1 in 15,000 in 1986. Ventura et al. published a rate of 1 per 300 to 4,000 live births in the U.S. Estimates are 1,000 to 1,300 women will be affected each year. The figures reported are all larger than the figures reported for the incidence of idiopathic cardiomyopathy, suggesting that peripartum cardiomyopathy is a separate entity.
- Proposed causes of peripartum cardiomyopathy
  - ➤ Evidence obtained via endomyocardial biopsy suggests that peripartum cardiomyopathy may be secondary to viral infection of the myocyte. A depressed immune system during pregnancy may allow for increased viral replication. The post-viral response against the infected myocyte leads to ventricular dysfunction.
  - ➤ Chimeric cells of the hematopoietic system from the fetus may take residence in maternal myocardium. This is facilitated by pregnancy-associated immunosuppression. Later immune response may lead to ventricular dysfunction.
  - ➤ Other sources suggest that peripartum cardiomyopathy may be a maladaptive response to the hemodynamic stress of pregnancy.
  - ➤ Peripartum cardiomyopathy may be in fact be familial dilated cardiomyopathy unmasked by pregnancy.
- The parturient is faced w/ numerous hemodynamic changes during pregnancy.

➤ Systemic vascular resistance (SVR) decreases during pregnancy. Prostacyclin, estrogen & progesterone plasma concentrations increase, resulting in decreased vascular resistance. The vascular beds of the uterus & kidneys display this change.

➤ To maintain the same cardiac output in the face of decreased vascular resistance, there is a compensatory increase in heart rate, on the order of 15–25%.

➤ To maintain the same pre-gravid cardiac output would be insufficient for the growing fetus. Metabolic demands of the growing fetus require adaptation on the part of the maternal cardiovascular system. Oxygen consumption increases, up to 20% by term, so more oxygen must be delivered. Cardiac output must increase during pregnancy, upwards of 50%.

➤ Heart rate alone does not produce the increase in cardiac output associated w/ pregnancy. To compensate for decreased SVR, the maternal blood volume increases by 25–40% by term. Plasma volume increases by upwards of 50% by term due to sodium retention from increased mineralocorticoid activity during pregnancy. RBC volume increases by 20%, which is less than the increase in plasma volume, resulting in a decreased hematocrit. The increased blood volume allows for increased venous return, which in turn increases cardiac output via increased stroke volume. The increase in intravascular volume has been shown to result in gradual dilatation of all four cardiac chambers.
 • Compensation occurs via L ventricular remodeling, which peaks by the third trimester. There is an increase is L ventricular wall thickness & an increase in contractility.

➤ During labor, stress on the cardiovascular system increases further. Cardiac output may increase by 60% over pre-pregnancy values during labor. During the immediate post-partum period, the uterus contracts, providing an autotransfusion of blood. This increased blood volume allows for a further increase in cardiac output.

■ The parturient w/ ventricular dysfunction due to dilated cardiomyopathy is faced w/ the above physiologic demands, but little if any physiologic reserve to meet them. The myocyte in such pts docs not contract efficiently. For a given amount of oxygen consumption, the myocyte contracts less. The increase in heart rate associated w/ pregnancy increases oxygen & metabolic demands for an already overtaxed myocyte. As L ventricular function deteriorates, forward flow will decrease. There may be insufficient cardiac output to satisfy the metabolic demands of the parturient & the fetus. Pulmonary congestion may occur & arrhythmias may be present. Atrial fibrillation & atrial flutter may occur from a dilated L atrium. Ventricular ectopy may be noted. Renal insufficiency may develop from insufficient renal perfusion. Cardiogenic shock may ensue. The pt may become lethargic or lose consciousness.

STUDIES
- Peripartum cardiomyopathy is a poorly understood condition, and as such, its definition & diagnosis is based on consensus.
  - In 1972, Demakis et al. provided diagnostic criteria for peripartum cardiomyopathy. Criteria were used in recruitment of subjects for a study examining the natural course of peripartum cardiomyopathy. The criteria were development of cardiac failure w/ no identifiable cause; onset of cardiac failure within the last month of pregnancy, or within 5 months of delivery; & absence of heart disease before the last month of pregnancy.
  - The definition of peripartum cardiomyopathy was formalized by the National Heart Lung & Blood Institute of the National Institutes of Health in 1997 & then revised in 2000. Peripartum cardiomyopathy is defined as the condition that satisfies the following criteria:
    - Development of cardiac failure in the last month of pregnancy or within 5 months of delivery
    - Absence of an identifiable cause for the cardiac failure
    - Absence of recognizable heart disease prior to the last month of pregnancy
    - L ventricular systolic dysfunction demonstrated by classic echocardiographic criteria such as depressed shortening fraction or ejection fraction
- Risk factors for peripartum cardiomyopathy to be noted in the pt's history include advanced maternal age, multiparity, black race, multiple fetuses, history of preeclampsia, and prior history of peripartum cardiomyopathy.
  - Elkayam et al. published a study in the *New England Journal of Medicine* in 2001 surveying the outcomes of pregnancies occurring after a diagnosis of peripartum cardiomyopathy during a previous pregnancy. 60 pregnancies in 44 women were identified & the cohort was divided into two groups.
  - The first group comprised 28 pregnancies in parturients for whom L ventricular function returned to normal. Subsequent pregnancies were associated w/ a reduction in L ventricular

function. Ejection fraction decreased from $56 +/- 75\%$ to $49 +/- 10\%$. One fifth of the pregnancies in this group was associated w/ symptoms of heart failure. The mortality rate in this group was 0%.

➤ The second group comprised 16 pregnancies in parturients for whom L ventricular function dysfunction persisted. Subsequent pregnancies were associated w/ a further reduction in L ventricular function. Ejection fraction decreased from $36 +/- 9\%$ to $32 +/- 11\%$. 44% of these pregnancies were associated w/ heart failure. The mortality rate in this group was 19%.

➤ This study demonstrates that outcomes of pregnancies in women who had peripartum cardiomyopathy in a prior pregnancy are poor. The same holds true both for women whose L ventricular dysfunction persists or returns to normal.

➤ In an earlier study, Sutton et al. suggested that pregnancy was safe so long as L ventricular dysfunction returned to normal. Four pts who had peripartum cardiomyopathy during prior pregnancies were studied. Echocardiographic data of L ventricular dysfunction were obtained prior to pregnancy, during the third trimester & a mean of 6 weeks postpartum. L ventricular mean diameters at end-diastole & end-systole did not change during pregnancy, nor did ventricular fractional shortening. The authors concluded that women w/ a history of peripartum cardiomyopathy should not be discouraged from attempting pregnancy so long as their L ventricular function returns to normal.

■ Obtaining a list of symptoms may aid in the diagnosis of peripartum cardiomyopathy:
➤ Orthopnea
➤ Paroxysmal nocturnal dyspnea
➤ Lower extremity edema
➤ Fatigue
➤ Shortness of breath
➤ Hemoptysis secondary to pulmonary congestion

■ The exam may provide evidence that the parturient is suffering from heart failure & perhaps peripartum cardiomyopathy:
➤ Rales
➤ S3 gallop
➤ Elevated jugular venous pulse
➤ Hepatojugular reflex
➤ Pitting edema in the lower extremities

■ An echocardiographic exam is essential for the diagnosis of peripartum cardiomyopathy.

➤ The exam will show evidence of impaired ventricular function. The ECHO exam will also rule out evidence of valvular disease or other cardiomyopathies that may be the etiology of heart failure.

➤ Hibbard et al. published a modified definition for peripartum cardiomyopathy based on echocardiography: ejection fraction <45%; fractional shortening <30% on an M-mode echocardiographic scan; L ventricular end-diastolic dimension >2.7 cm per square meter of body surface area.

■ EKG may provide evidence of cardiomyopathy
  ➤ Left atrial dilatation
  ➤ Widened QRS complexes
■ Chest x-ray
  ➤ Enlarged heart
  ➤ Pulmonary congestion

MANAGEMENT/INTERVENTIONS
■ Anesthetic goals for management of the parturient w/ peripartum cardiomyopathy during labor & vaginal delivery are as follows:
  ➤ Vaginal delivery should proceed w/ invasive hemodynamic monitoring. An arterial line should be placed for monitoring arterial pressure & arterial blood gas sampling. Central venous pressures at the least should be followed. A pulmonary artery catheter offers the advantage of following serial cardiac outputs so that intravascular volume may be optimized. Additional volume may be necessary if labor analgesia is initiated w/ epidural local anesthetics. Vasodilation w/ nitroglycerin & diuresis may be necessary immediately after delivery when autotransfusion from the uterus abruptly increases intravascular volume.
  ➤ Stage II & III should take place in an ICU setting if sufficient monitoring equipment is not available on the labor & delivery floor.
  ➤ During the second stage of labor, the obstetric goal is to avoid maneuvers that worsen symptoms of heart failure. The Valsalva maneuver may result in a sudden increase in SVR & should be avoided. The obstetrician may discourage maternal expulsive efforts during the second stage of labor to avoid Valsalva. Uterine contraction will facilitate fetal descent. The parturient should avoid pushing. Low forceps & vacuum extraction are techniques used to facilitate delivery after fetal descent.
  ➤ Several case reports have described successful administration of a labor epidural during labor. The decrease in SVR associated

w/ epidural local anesthetics may unload the heart & increase cardiac output. The pulmonary capillary wedge pressure or central venous pressure should be followed as the epidural local anesthetics are administered, as additional fluid may be necessary to maintain cardiac output if the decrease in SVR is precipitous.

- There is no consensus on which type of anesthesia is most appropriate for the pt w/ peripartum cardiomyopathy who is to undergo C-section.
  - General anesthesia has several advantages over epidural anesthesia for C-section. The airway is secured prior to the autotransfusion from uterine contraction following delivery. The acute increase in intravascular volume may result in flash pulmonary edema w/ hypoxia. Cardiogenic shock during the C-section may lead to syncope & aspiration. Ventilation can be controlled if a high-dose narcotic technique is chosen to induce & maintain anesthesia.
  - General anesthesia has several pitfalls, however. Because the parturient is considered to have a full stomach, one must perform a rapid sequence induction or secure the airway w/ an awake fiberoptic intubation. Bolus doses of induction agents may result in severe myocardial depression: thiopental is cardiodepressant; propofol is cardiodepressant & a vasodilator; high-dose narcotics may avoid myocardial depression. Ventilatory depression in the newborn can occur, however. Remifentanil for induction may be considered for its short half-life in the parturient & the fetus, but bolus doses are often associated w/ hypotension. Etomidate is associated w/ hemodynamic stability & may be the best choice for a rapid sequence induction. Ketamine will increase SVR & heart rate, which may precipitate heart failure.
    - The possibility remains that the airway may not be secured.
    - Inhalational agents used for maintenance are associated w/ myocardial depression.
  - Epidural anesthesia is a viable option for the parturient w/ peripartum cardiomyopathy who must undergo delivery via C-section. One can titrate in a controlled manner the decrease in SVR that accompanies the onset of surgical anesthesia. The decrease in SVR occurs without concomitant myocardial depression. A decrease in SVR will decrease afterload & may improve myocardial function. The slow onset affords time to replace intravascular volume to maintain sufficient preload. As w/

general anesthesia, hemodynamics should be monitored & managed w/ the aid of invasive monitoring.

- If the epidural works well, the pt may avoid a rapid sequence induction, which can be associated w/ severe hypotension & myocardial depression.
- One main disadvantage of epidural anesthesia is that the airway remains unsecured, & the need for intubation may arise during the operation. The pt may develop cardiogenic shock & become lethargic or unresponsive. The pt may develop pulmonary edema when intravascular volume increases abruptly w/ uterine contraction after delivery.

■ Vasoactive drugs should be readily available when a pt w/ peripartum cardiomyopathy is laboring on the floor.

Ephedrine has been used safely in the parturient for augmentation of BP. Pts w/ severe heart failure may not respond to ephedrine, as part of its efficacy is dependent on release of endogenous catecholamines. Pts w/ heart failure have increased release of endogenous catecholamines at baseline. Pts may develop tachyphylaxis to ephedrine w/ repeated doses.

Phenylephrine, a pure alpha agonist, may be used safely in the parturient to treat hypotension. Phenylephrine will increase aortic root pressure & thus increase myocardial perfusion. Phenylephrine will increase work for the L ventricle as it increases afterload; this may decrease cardiac output.

Norepinephrine is an alpha agonist that may be used to increase SVR when necessary. Unlike phenylephrine, norepinephrine has beta-agonist activity, which may increase contractility as well as SVR. Norepinephrine may constrict the vascular supply of the uterus & precipitate fetal distress. It must be administered via a central line.

Milrinone may be infused to increase contractility in a failing heart. Milrinone is a phosphodiesterase inhibitor. A side effect of milrinone is vasodilation. Milrinone is often infused w/ norepinephrine to treat the concomitant vasodilation.

Dopamine may be infused to increase cardiac output in the parturient w/ heart failure. This drug is a beta, alpha & dopamine receptor agonist & is associated w/ tachycardia & arrhythmias.

Hydralazine is a safe drug for the parturient who requires afterload reduction.

ACE inhibitors should be avoided in the parturient. ACE inhibitors are associated w/ renal damage in the fetus in all trimesters. An ACE inhibitor should be prescribed for the parturient post-partum.

Diuretics may also be necessary to remove excess intravascular volume if the pt develops pulmonary edema.

Management of the parturient w/ peripartum cardiomyopathy will require the assistance of a cardiologist. Refractory heart failure may require an intraoperative balloon pump. The pt may require a ventricular assist device or, ultimately, a heart transplant.

CAVEATS, PEARLS

- An echocardiographic exam will provide the best assessment of how the pt's heart is functioning & is recommended by the National Institutes of Health for the diagnosis of peripartum cardiomyopathy.
- Invasive hemodynamic monitoring should be instituted prior to delivery. The heart will experience a volume load immediately after delivery as the uterus contracts.
- Consider transferring the pt to an ICU setting for labor & delivery if appropriate monitoring is not available in the labor & delivery suite.
- Slow titration of an epidural catheter has been used successfully to provide labor analgesia & surgical anesthesia for pts w/ peripartum cardiomyopathy.
- Emergency airway equipment should be available, as the pt w/ peri partum cardiomyopathy is at higher risk for needing intubation.
- Do not administer ACE inhibitors until after the pt has delivered.

CHECKLIST

- Call cardiologist for echocardiographic exam.
- Place invasive lines early.
- Inquire about ICU beds early & consider transferring pt for labor & delivery.
- Vasoactive meds must be immediately available.
- Emergency airway equipment must be stocked, checked & immediately available.
- Have plan for placement of ventricular assist device should pt's condition deteriorate rapidly.

CARPAL TUNNEL SYNDROME

MEREDITH ALBRECHT, MD; LISA LEFFERT, MD; AND MICHELE SZABO, MD

FUNDAMENTAL KNOWLEDGE

Definition

- Entrapment of the median nerve in the carpal tunnel

Epidemiology
- Can be as high as 62% of pregnant women in the later stages of pregnancy

Pathophysiology
- The median nerve & 9 tendons lie in close proximity in the carpal tunnel.
- Entrapment of the nerve can easily occur w/ overuse or swelling (due to fluid retention).

Clinical Manifestations
- Paresthesias & weakness in a median nerve distribution
- Nocturnal paresthesias of thumb, index & middle fingers
- Severe cases result in weakness & atrophy of the thenar eminence.
- Generally resolves within 2 months post-partum
- Can be associated w/ hypothyroidism, rheumatoid arthritis, diabetes

Effect of Pregnancy on Carpal Tunnel Syndrome
- Can increase the severity of & induce carpel tunnel syndrome

Effect of Carpal Tunnel Syndrome on Pregnancy & the Fetus
- No effect

STUDIES

History & Physical
- Paresthesias & weakness in the median nerve distribution
- Possible weakness
- Atrophy of the thenar eminence
- Symptoms elicited w/ hyperextension of the wrist

Laboratory
- EMG/nerve conduction studies to confirm diagnosis

Imaging
- None

MANAGEMENT/INTERVENTIONS

Medical Treatment
- Supportive: splinting
- Glucocorticoid injections
- Severe symptoms require surgery.

Anesthesia
- No type is contraindicated.
- Avoid radial arterial line placement on involved side

CAVEATS/PEARLS
- Due to entrapment of the median nerve in the carpal tunnel
- Weakness & paresthesias in the median nerve distribution
- Pregnancy can increase the severity of & induce carpel tunnel syndrome
- Avoid radial arterial line placement on involved side.

CHECKLIST
- Careful physical exam to document other neurologic deficits

---

CAUSES OF ACUTE RENAL FAILURE IN PREGNANCY

JOSHUA WEBER, MD
PETER DUNN, MD

FUNDAMENTAL KNOWLEDGE
Prerenal
- Hyperemesis gravidarum
- Uterine hemorrhage
- Heart failure

Postrenal
- Urolithiasis
- Obstruction of ureters by gravid uterus

Intrarenal
- Acute pyelonephritis
- Septic abortion
- Acute tubular necrosis (ATN)
- Amniotic fluid embolism
- Drug-induced interstitial nephritis
- Bilateral renal cortical necrosis
- Acute glomerulonephritis
- Preeclampsia/eclampsia
- HELLP syndrome
- Acute fatty liver of pregnancy
- Idiopathic postpartum renal failure

STUDIES, MANAGEMENT/INTERVENTIONS, CAVEATS/ PEARLS, CHECKLIST
N/A

CENTRAL VENOUS LINES

KRISTOPHER DAVIGNON, MD
HARISH LECAMWASAM, MD

FUNDAMENTAL KNOWLEDGE

Indications

- For delivery of certain drugs (potent vasoactive medications: norepinephrine, epinephrine, dobutamine, milrinone, others) & TPN
- For assessment of central venous pressure (CVP)
- CVP in the normal parturient is 0–5 cm H20 (as in the non-parturient).

Sites of cannulation

- Most common sites for central venous access: internal jugular veins, external jugular veins, subclavian veins, femoral veins
- Alternately, central venous access can be obtained via cannulation of peripheral veins, most commonly the basilic.

Normal values

- CVP should be measured at end-expiration in the respiratory cycle & end-diastole in the cardiac cycle.
- Normal CVP: 0–5 mm Hg

Waveforms

- A normal CVP waveform consists of a, c & waves w/ x & y descents. These waves correspond to atrial contraction, ventricular contraction, atrial relaxation, atrial filling & atrial emptying, respectively.
- If abnormal waveforms are noted, be sure the catheter is appropriately situated in a central vein.
- Commonly seen abnormal waveforms
  - ➤ Cannon a waves: represent atrial contraction against a closed atrioventricular valve due to atrioventricular dissociation
  - ➤ Large waves: most often represent incompetent atrioventricular valve w/ tricuspid regurgitation. Large waves may also be seen w/ volume loading & diminished atrial compliance.

STUDIES

- Evaluate chest x-ray for line position & complications (pneumothorax, hemothorax) following any central venous line placement using a jugular or subclavian venous approach.
- Pressure transduction allows an operator to confirm venous access even prior to vessel dilation for catheter placement. The pressure

waveform may also give an indication regarding catheter location (an abnormal trace often means the catheter is not in a central vein).

MANAGEMENT & INTERVENTIONS

Technique
- "Blind" Seldinger technique
- Ultrasound-assisted Seldinger technique

Interpretation of data
- CVP must be combined w/ some assessment or assumptions about the cardiac status to be interpreted. A trend in CVP associated w/ interventions can also be helpful in assessing a pt's volume status.

    Decreasing CVP: represents an improvement in cardiac performance or a decrease in venous return (either due to increased impedance to venous return or decrease in relative volume status). The clinical context must be used to decide on the appropriate diagnosis.

    Increasing CVP: represents either a decrease in cardiac performance or an increase in venous return (either from a decrease in impedance or a relative increase in volume status). Again, the clinical context must be used to interpret the CVP.

CAVEATS & PEARLS
- To aid placement, use Trendelenburg position to increase CVP & jugular filling.
- To aid in differentiating between arterial & venous cannulation, compare the blood's color w/ a sample from the arterial line or use pressure manometry. Attaching a fluid-filled extension set & raising it 15–20 cm above the pt should result in a falling column of fluid if the cannulation is venous. These tests should be done prior to cannulation w/ larger-bore catheters.
- Ultrasound may also aid in difficult placement. Ultrasound can display anatomical aberrations & venous thrombus.
- Dysrhythmias can occur, most commonly from wire placement during Seldinger-guided placement.
- Pneumothorax, air embolus, hemothorax & hemopericardium are common complications to be aware of in the post-line period.
- Arterial puncture (subclavian, carotid, femoral or radial) may occur. This may be an issue in the anticoagulated pt or if the artery is cannulated w/ a large-diameter catheter.

CHECKLIST
- Confirm intra-arterial placement.

- Secure catheter appropriately w/ Tegaderm or suture.
- Monitor for adequate function; monitor insertion site for infection.

CEREBRAL VENOUS SINUS THROMBOSIS

MEREDITH ALBRECHT, MD
MICHELE SZABO, MD

FUNDAMENTAL KNOWLEDGE

Definition
- Thrombosis of intracranial cortical veins

Epidemiology
- 1–4 per 10,000 deliveries
- Accounts for 20–40% of ischemic strokes during pregnancy
- Often affects young to middle-aged pts, more commonly women

Pathophysiology
- More than 100 cases reported in literature; categorized as:
  - Local factors such as meningitis, sinusitis, tumor
  - Inherited pro-thrombotic tendencies such as factor V Leiden mutations
  - Drugs such as BCP or HRT
  - Systemic factors such as pregnancy, malignancy
  - Blood dyscrasias

Clinical Manifestations
- Clinical presentation can be extremely variable.
- Evolves over hours to weeks
- Venous absorption of CSF is blocked.
- If collateral venous drainage is insufficient, ICP will increase.
- Venous infarction & focal hemorrhage may occur.
- Headache, 95%
- Focal seizures w/ or w/o generalization, 47%
- Paresis, 43%
- Papilledema, 41%
- Impairment of consciousness, 39%
- Coma, 15%

Effect of pregnancy on cerebral venous thrombosis
- Pregnancy & particularly post-partum period are times of increased susceptibility.
- Risk increased further w/:

> Cesarean delivery
> Increasing maternal age
> Presence of co-morbid conditions, including hypertension, intercurrent infection & hyperemesis

■ Most occur post-partum, usually 2–3 weeks following delivery.
■ Contributing factors are thought to be:
> Traumatic damage to venous endothelium during 2nd stage of labor
> Hypercoagulable state

Effect on pregnancy & fetus
■ Related to effects of diagnostic studies
■ Related to treatment w/ anticoagulants & anticonvulsants

STUDIES

History & physical
■ Neurologic
> Document mental status exam.
> Document neurologic deficits.
> Determine presence & characteristics of seizures.
> Look for evidence of increased ICP; funduscopic exam: papilledema

Imaging
■ MRI venography
> Gold standard for diagnosis
> Used in puerperium & following 1st trimester
■ CT venography
> Alternative test for pregnant pt in 1st trimester
> Appropriately shielded fetus, radiation exposure considered safe

Other
■ LP may be performed to exclude diagnosis of meningitis.
■ Screen for hypercoagulable disorders.
■ PTT or PT for anticoagulated pt
■ Platelet count in pts on heparin; HIT antibody if heparin-induced thrombocytopenia
■ Serum anticonvulsant level where appropriate
■ Creatinine if given contrast dye for CT

MANAGEMENT / INTERVENTIONS
■ Goals
> Prevent clot propagation.
> Possible clot disruption

- ➤ Mgt of seizures
- ➤ Mgt of increased ICP
- ■ Anticoagulation
  - ➤ Unfractionated heparin
    - Gold standard treatment for prevention of clot propagation; well-documented improved outcome
    - Titrated to target a therapeutic PTT
    - Increased risk of osteoporosis after long-term (>1 month) administration
    - Can produce heparin-induced thrombocytopenia
    - No teratogenic effects have been reported, but no direct studies have been performed.
    - Not excreted in breast milk
    - Given safely to pts w/ preexisting intracerebral hemorrhagic infarction
  - ➤ Low-molecular-weight heparin
    - Uncertainty of its efficacy compared to unfractionated heparin
  - ➤ Coumadin
    - Safe for post-partum pt
      - Typically given for 3–6 months following presentation of thrombosis
      - Does appear in breast milk
    - For the pregnant pt
      - Readily crosses placenta
      - Potential to cause bleeding in fetus
      - Established teratogenicity
      - Not recommended for use
    - Monitor anticoagulant activity w/ INR.
- ■ Thrombolysis
  - ➤ Transvenous catheter thrombolysis
    - Generally accepted to be beneficial to pt
    - Clinical outcome during pregnancy limited to anecdotal case reports
    - Use reported to have no adverse maternal complications
    - No teratogenic effects have been observed, though not systematically studied.
- ■ Anticonvulsants are indicated for some pts.
  - ➤ All are established teratogens, w/ greatest risk during 1st trimester.
  - ➤ Risk of maternal & fetal hypoxia & acidosis associated w/ seizure justifies their use in pt at risk for seizure.

> Drug pharmacokinetics are altered during pregnancy, so check serum anticonvulsant levels.
> Interfere w/ folic acid & vitamin K metabolism; give supplementation
■ Treat elevated ICP.
> Promote venous drainage w/ head-up position.
> Keep pt well oxygenated; manage hypoxia aggressively.
> Ensure adequate ventilation; hypercarbia will exacerbate elevations in ICP.
> Aggressively treat hypotension.
> Hyperventilate only as a temporizing measure during emergency in which other definitive treatment modalities are being instituted.
  • Marked hyperventilation causes uteroplacental vasoconstriction, resulting in fetal hypoxia & acidosis.
  • Reduction in cardiac output caused by positive-pressure ventilation likely cause of decreased uterine blood flow
  • Used when there is evidence of increased ICP; effects on fetus minimized w/ normovolemia & low airway pressures
> Mannitol
  • Osmotic diuretic
  • Effective in treating intracranial hypertension
  • Can increase fetal plasma osmolality & cause fetal dehydration; effect likely temporary
  • Fetal outcome data are limited.
  • Limited use for life-threatening elevated ICP
> Furosemide
  • Not as effective as mannitol
  • Causes less fetal dehydration than mannitol
> Prevent or treat maneuvers that increase ICP
  • Coughing or straining
  • Vomiting
  • Fever
  • Seizure

Anesthesia
■ Most likely the pt will be anticoagulated w/ heparin at the time of delivery.
■ Discontinue heparin on the morning of planned labor induction or C-section.
■ Regional anesthesia

➤ Preferred if pt is not coagulopathic & symptoms of increased ICP have resolved

➤ Permits continuous neurologic monitoring

➤ Prevents maneuvers that might cause further venous injury or increases in ICP

■ General anesthesia

➤ Preferred if ICP is elevated

➤ Goal is to control ventilation, prevent hypoxia, aggressively treat hypotension, prevent maneuvers that would increase cerebral venous pressure (eg, coughing).

➤ Directly measure arterial pressure w/ a-line.

➤ Hydrate pt prior to induction.

➤ Avoid succinylcholine if pt is paretic >48 hours.

➤ "Modified" rapid sequence induction w/ rocuronium or succinylcholine if appropriate, pentothal or propofol narcotic, titrated to minimize hypotension & blunt response to noxious stimulation of intubation

➤ Treat narcotic-induced fetal respiratory depression w/ naloxone or respiratory support.

➤ Hyperventilate only if ICP elevation is life-threatening.
  • Adverse fetal effects can be minimized w/ adequate maternal hydration & minimizing Valsalva.

➤ Mannitol
  • Indicated if ICP elevation is severe
  • Effective for mother; can cause fetal hypovolemia
  • Be prepared for fluid resuscitation of the newborn.

➤ Plan anesthetic for a prompt emergence that would permit early neurologic exam

CAVEATS & PEARLS

■ Usual presentation will be a postpartum headache.

➤ Important to differentiate it from other causes of post-partum headache: post-dural puncture headache (PDPH), migraine, tension headache, pre-eclampsia, meningitis, brain tumor, SAH

■ Presence or absence of intracranial hypertension will be main determinant of anesthetic mgt.

■ Check for normalization of coagulation status prior to regional technique.

■ Identify & inform the pt's neurologist of your anesthetic plans. Determine most efficient means of emergency contact.

CHECKLIST

■ Identify pt's neurologist & mechanism of contact.

■ Hold anticoagulants & check for normalization of coagulation studies prior to regional technique or C-section.

■ Perform frequent neurologic exams for detection of worsening neurologic status.

CERVICAL CERCLAGE

JAMES WILLIAMS, MD
RODGER WHITE, MD

FUNDAMENTAL KNOWLEDGE

■ Incompetent cervix cannot sustain pregnancy to full term.

   ➤ Causes are both structural & functional & can include trauma (from previous pregnancy), anatomic disorders, hormonal abnormalities

   ➤ Clinical diagnosis

■ Typically procedures are done transvaginally.

■ Prophylactic procedure (before & during pregnancy) as well as urgent

   ➤ Greatest risk during emergency is rupture of membranes, so uterine relaxation is essential.

   ➤ Preterm labor can be induced by procedure.

■ Cerclage removed at 37 or 38 weeks gestation, but depending on type placed alternative is elective cesarean delivery.

   ➤ Once cerclage is removed, labor may begin in few hours or days.

STUDIES

■ FHR monitoring at least before & after procedure; often done continuously if >20 weeks gestation

■ Other studies are dictated by clinical scenario & comorbidities.

MANAGEMENT/INTERVENTIONS

Spinal

■ T8–10 level

■ Bupivacaine 10mg +/− intrathecal opioid (fentanyl 10–25 mcg)

■ Lidocaine is used less commonly because of the relatively high incidence of transient radicular irritation (TRI).

■ Mepivacaine 45 mg (hyperbaric) is another option.

■ Alternative is "low-dose" bupivacaine (hyperbaric 5.25 mg) + fentanyl 20 mcg.

Epidural
- Lumbar placement for T8–T10 level
- Incremental dosing w/ 15–18 mL 2% lidocaine +/− neuraxial opoid (fentanyl 50–100 mcg)
- Alternative is "low-dose" 0.125% bupivacaine 15–20 mL

General anesthesia
- May be preferred if dilated cervix & herniation of fetal membranes, since volatile anesthetics cause uterine relaxation

Uterine relaxation
- Volatile anesthetics
- Tocolytics (terbutaline, ritodrine)
- Nitroglycerin

CAVEATS AND PEARLS
- Single IV catheter & standard monitors are typically sufficient.
- Increased rate of cesarean delivery following cerclage
- Avoid causing increased intrauterine pressure if cervix is dilated (ie, urgent cerclage).
  - ➤ Coughing on induction of general anesthesia
  - ➤ Dorsiflexion during placement of regional anesthetic (controversial)
- Intrathecal lidocaine is being used less frequently due to concern for transient neurologic symptoms.

CHECKLIST
- Full pre-op evaluation
- Prepare to provide uterine relaxation, especially if preterm labor is precipitated.

CHEST COMPRESSIONS

RICHARD ARCHULETA, MD
SANDRA WEINREB, MD

FUNDAMENTAL KNOWLEDGE
- Chest compressions are a necessary part of neonatal resuscitation if effective PPV is insufficient to maintain the heart rate >60 bpm.
- The neonate is fragile, & chest compressions should be administered such that the depth of compression is one-third the anterior-posterior diameter of the neonate's chest.

- The location of compression is the lower third of the sternum.
  - ➤ This point can be located by palpating the sternum just below an imaginary line connecting the nipples.
  - ➤ Carefully avoid applying pressure on the xiphoid process, which could cause internal damage.

STUDIES
- Continue to evaluate neonate's respiration, heart rate & color at least every 30 seconds until neonate's cardiopulmonary status has stabilized.

MANAGEMENT/INTERVENTIONS
- Neonate should be intubated for PPV during chest compressions.
- Pressure for chest compressions is applied w/ 1 of 2 techniques:
  - ➤ Technique 1: both hands are wrapped around the chest w/ the thumbs placed on the lower third of the sternum
    - • This is the preferred technique because it provides a higher cardiac output, higher systolic BP & higher coronary perfusion pressure.
    - • Requires 2 trained personnel (other rescuer is providing PPV)
  - ➤ Technique 2: two fingers (second & third digits) are applied to the lower third of the sternum
    - • The other hand is supporting the neonate's back.
    - • Use this technique when there is only 1 qualified rescuer, or if the hands of the rescuer applying chest compressions are too small for the 2-handed technique.
- Depth of chest compressions
  - ➤ Depress the sternum 1–1.5 cm (approx. one third of the anterior-posterior diameter of the neonate).
  - ➤ The duration of compression & release should be equal.
- Rate of chest compressions
  - ➤ Apply 3 chest compressions for every positive-pressure breath delivered.
  - ➤ Ideally, 90 chest compressions & 30 breaths should be delivered per minute in a 3:1 ratio.
- Re-evaluate spontaneous heart rate periodically
  - ➤ Discontinue chest compressions when spontaneous heart rate >60 bpm.

CAVEATS & PEARLS
- Ensure there is a good pulse w/ each compression.
  - ➤ Palpate pulse at base of umbilical cord.

➤ If there is no reliable pulse detected w/ chest compressions
  • Deepen the compressions beyond one third of the anterior-posterior diameter of the chest until a pulse is detected.
  • Consider IV fluids.
■ Avoid lifting fingers off sternum w/ each compression.
■ Apply pressure smoothly while performing compressions; avoid jerky movements that can cause trauma to the neonate's chest.

CHECKLIST
■ Ensure neonate is intubated.
■ Apply pressure to lower third of sternum for chest compression.
■ Depress sternum approximately one third of the anterior-posterior diameter.
■ Apply 3 chest compressions & PPV breaths in a 3:1 ratio.
  ➤ Deliver 90 chest compressions & 30 PPV breaths per minute.

CHRONIC LOW BACK PAIN/HISTORY OF PREVIOUS SPINE SURGERY

STEPHEN PANARO, MD
EDWARD MICHNA, MD

FUNDAMENTAL KNOWLEDGE
■ 50% of women w/ chronic back pain experience an exacerbation of their symptoms w/ pregnancy.
■ Regional anesthesia is statistically less successful in women w/ chronic low back pain or a history of previous spine surgery, but is most often successful.
  ➤ Higher failure rate may be due to distortion of surface anatomy & to a tethering of the dura to the ligamentum flavum, a supposition supported by animal models.
  ➤ Back surgeries that disrupt the epidural space are more likely to result in failed epidural blocks than those that do not.
  ➤ There is a higher risk of dural puncture during attempted epidural placement due to the scarring & distortion of the epidural space.
■ Effect of regional anesthesia may be incomplete or delayed in onset in these pts:
  ➤ For instance, pts w/ sciatica or nerve root compression may experience delay in the onset of block because the local anesthetic may have difficulty in diffusing to the affected root.

➤ Pts w/ disc disease may have poor or delayed blocks because of the compromised ability of local anesthetic to diffuse beyond the affected disc space.

STUDIES
- Plain films may be helpful in pts w/ previous surgery (w/ or w/o skin markers on scar) to define the precise location of previous surgery.
- MRI may be useful to assess likelihood of scarring in & around the epidural space.

MANAGEMENT/INTERVENTION
- Neuraxial anesthesia can be successful after back surgery; one study cites a 91.2% success rate.
- Informed consent must include the increased risk of patchy block or inadvertent dural puncture.
- If available, consider neurologic/neurosurgical consultation to help delineate the anatomic implications of the surgical intervention.
- If feasible, perform the neuraxial block at 1 or 2 interspaces above the previous surgical site or site of disc disease to minimize the risk of distorted landmarks, spinal stenosis immediately above a fusion & tethering of the dura to the ligamentum flavum.
  - ➤ From a practical standpoint, this can be difficult to accomplish if there is no surgical scar, since the anesthesiologist's ability to identify a particular interspace can be limited w/o the use of fluoroscopy.
  - ➤ The surgical scar may extend beyond the level of the surgery.
  - ➤ Despite these limitations, there is support in the literature for attempting neuraxial anesthesia in pts w/ history of back surgery.
  - ➤ It is reasonable to consider "early" epidural placement in these pts in anticipation of difficulty w/ placement.

CAVEATS/PEARLS
- Regional anesthesia is statistically less successful in women w/ chronic low back pain or a history of previous spine surgery, but it is most often successful.
- If feasible, perform the neuraxial block at 1 or 2 interspaces above the affected level or previous surgical site to minimize the risk of distorted landmarks, spinal stenosis immediately above a fusion & tethering of the dura to the ligamentum flavum.
- Should an inadvertent dural puncture occur, continuous spinal analgesia is an effective anesthetic option.

- Continuous spinal analgesia can also be an initial anesthetic option for both labor analgesia & surgical anesthesia, although the risk of post-dural puncture headache in this population is significant.

CHECKLIST
- Check available scans if pt has had back surgery.
- Consider neurologic/neurosurgical consult if feasible.
- Initiate informed consent documenting potential increased risk of inadequate regional anesthetic or inadvertent dural puncture.

CHRONIC PAIN

HUMAYON KHAN, MD
JYOTSNA NAGDA, MD

FUNDAMENTAL KNOWLEDGE
- Managing chronic pain pts during pregnancy & labor can be quite challenging.
- Concern about the fetal well-being & fear of fetal malformations force most physicians to take a least invasive & most conservative path for managing these pts whenever possible.
- Sometimes the use of meds & other invasive modalities is necessary to attenuate the suffering of pregnant pts; choosing the right medication & invasive treatment is of utmost importance.
- The aim of this chapter is to review the common chronic pain conditions encountered by OBs & obstetric anesthesiologists during pregnancy & parturition & their correct mgt, citing literature.

FDA Pregnancy Categories

Category A: Adequate, well-controlled studies in pregnant women have not shown an increased risk of fetal abnormalities to the fetus in any trimester of pregnancy.

Category B: Animal studies have revealed no evidence of harm to the fetus; however, there are no adequate & well-controlled studies in pregnant women. OR Animal studies have shown an adverse effect, but adequate & well-controlled studies in pregnant women have failed to demonstrate a risk to the fetus in any trimester.

Category C: Animal studies have shown an adverse effect & there are no adequate & well-controlled studies in pregnant women. OR No animal studies have been conducted & there are no adequate & well-controlled studies in pregnant women.

Category D: Adequate well-controlled or observational studies in pregnant women have demonstrated a risk to the fetus. However, the benefits of therapy may outweigh the potential risk. For example, the drug may be acceptable if needed in a life-threatening situation or serious disease for which safer drugs cannot be used or are ineffective.

Category X: Adequate well-controlled or observational studies in animals or pregnant women have demonstrated positive evidence of fetal abnormalities or risks. The use of the product is contraindicated in women who are or may become pregnant.

NR = Not rated

Commonly used medications & their categories during pregnancy

Simple analgesics
Acetaminophen	B
Caffeine	B

NSAIDs
Naproxen	B
Diclofenac sodium	B
Indomethacin	NR
Ibuprofen	D
Aspirin	D (only for 3rd trimester)
Etodolac	C
Meloxicam	C
Rofecoxib	C
Salicylates	C

Anti-epileptic drugs
Gabapentin	C
Topiramate	C
Carbamazepine	D
Valproate	D
Levetiracetam	C
Zonegran	C
Tiagabine	C

Antidepressants
Venlafaxine	C
Citalopram	C
Escitalopram	C
Amitriptyline	D
Imipramine	D
Nortriptyline	D
Desipramine	C
Fluoxetine	B
Paroxetine	B
Doxepin	C

Opioids
Oxycodone	B
Codeine	B
Morphine	C
Hydromorphone	C
Remifentanil	C
Propoxyphene	NR
Meperidine	C
Nubain	B

Muscle relaxants
Tizanidine	C
Cyclobenzaprine	B
Metaxalone	NR
Baclofen	C
Orphenadrine	C
Carisoprodol	NR

Triptans
Almotriptan	C
Eletriptan	C
Frovatriptan	C
Naratriptan	C

Rizatriptan	C		Promethazine	C
Sumatriptan	C			
Zolmitriptan	C		**Beta-blockers**	
			Atenolol	D
Ergots			Metoprolol	C
Ergotamine	D		Nadolol	C
			Propranolol	C
Corticosteroids			Timolol	C
Dexamethasone	C		Labetalol	C
Prednisone	B			
Barbiturates			**Others**	
Butalbital	C (D if used during the 3rd trimester or near delivery)		Hydralazine	C
			Verapamil	C
			Magnesium sulfate	B
			Promethazine	C
			Hydroxyzine	C
Antiemetics			Ketamine	NR
Granisetron	B		Prednisone	B
Metoclopramide	B		Mexiletine	C
Ondansetron	B		Clonazepam	D
Prochlorperazine	C		Botulinum toxin	A C

Acetaminophen

- Acetaminophen is widely used during pregnancy. Although there is no known association w/ teratogenicity, few clinical data are available to support the lack of association. Hence, acetaminophen is currently considered the pain reliever of choice during pregnancy. It is extremely important to rule out fatty liver of pregnancy, HELLP syndrome or any concomitant liver disease before starting a pt on acetaminophen because fulminant liver failure has been reported w/ acetaminophen (treated w/ orthotopic liver transplantation) in pts w/ preexisting fatty liver of pregnancy. There is also a case report of exanthematous pustulosis in a pregnant woman using acetaminophen.

NSAIDs

- Prostaglandins play an important role in human ovulation & implantation through their own effect and w/ interaction w/ platelet activating factors & cytokines, both in the uterus & in the embryo. Hence, there is increasing concern of miscarriage w/ NSAID use. This risk is highest w/ NSAID use around the time of conception & increases w/ its use for >1 week.

Salicylates: Chronic ingestion of salicylates during pregnancy has been associated w/ an increased incidence of postmaturity, significant prolongation of labor, decrease in birthweight & increased incidence of spontaneous abortion & stillbirth. Salicylates are not recommended for analgesia in pregnant women.

Aspirin: Has been used during pregnancy for a long time. It is not associated w/ any teratogenic effects in fetus. Aspirin should be avoided in 3rd trimester because of the risk of intracranial hemorrhage, prolonged gestation & protracted labor.

Indomethacin, which had shown promise in the treatment of preterm labor, should not be used because of concern over antenatal narrowing & closure of fetal ductus arteriosus. It has also been associated w/ persistent pulmonary hypertension, renal failure, necrotizing enterocolitis & neonatal death.

Ibuprofen, which is category D, is associated w/ reversible oligohydramnios & diameter narrowing of PDA.

Ketorolac, which has been associated w/ dystocia in rodents, has not been found to be harmful during pregnancy. It is not recommended during egg retrieval for IVF because it might affect the implantation of zygote.

Goals of NSAID therapy

- Use non-pharmacologic therapy or acetaminophen first.
- Continue aspirin or other NSAID, especially naproxen, diclofenac (category B), if symptoms are not controlled w/ acetaminophen.
- Avoid using NSAIDs during embryogenesis (15–55 days) & 3rd trimester.
- Restrict use of NSAIDs to 48 hours if possible.
- If prolonged use of NSAID is required, close fetal monitoring, including ultrasound & echocardiography, is recommended to monitor amniotic fluid volume & patency of PDA.
- Avoid the use of NSAIDs after 32 weeks of pregnancy to reduce the risk of neonatal hemorrhage, peripartum bleeding & early closure of PDA.

Opioids

- **Methadone** maintenance is safe for opioid & heroin addicts. It is a category B drug & only in rare instances has been associated w/ increased birthweight, prolonged gestation & neonatal withdrawal syndrome. Pregnancy affects methadone metabolism & elimination: bioavailability & half-life are lower & its clearance is greater. For mothers who are breast-feeding, infants are exposed to 2.79% of the maternal dose.

■ Other opioids, including morphine, hydromorphone, oxycodone & fentanyl, have been used during pregnancy w/o any untoward events. They do increase the risk of neonatal opioid withdrawal syndrome if taken regularly & in high doses.

Goals of opioid therapy

■ Use acetaminophen first; can combine w/ hydrocodone if pain is severe.

■ Oxycodone can be used if pain is not controlled w/ acetaminophen or codeine.

■ Morphine, hydromorphone, fentanyl are next in the ladder; can be used in the IV form if above measures are not helpful.

■ Meperidine has also been used safely during pregnancy & labor but should be avoided during breast-feeding because normeperidine has a long half-life in newborns.

■ Remifentanil pt-controlled analgesia has been used w/ success for labor analgesia in those who refuse neuroaxial anesthesia or in whom it is contraindicated.

Steroids

■ Most steroids cross the placenta, although prednisone & prednisolone are inactivated by the placenta. Prednisone use during the 1st trimester has been associated w/ increased risk of oral clefts. Use of steroids during pregnancy poses a minimal risk to the developing fetus.

■ Epidural steroids are given in many pain clinics for treatment of lumbar radiculopathy. These procedures are usually done w/o any x-ray guidance.

■ Breast-feeding is safe during steroid administration.

Anticonvulsants

■ Anticonvulsants are increasingly being used for neuropathic pain, chronic daily headaches & migraine headache prophylaxis. Newer anticonvulsants including Neurontin, lamotrigine & topiramate are category C; older anticonvulsants, including carbamazepine, phenytoin & valproic sodium, are category D. The first generation of antiepileptic drugs, phenobarbital & phenytoin, are mainly associated w/ heart defects & facial clefts. Among women w/ epilepsy treated w/ phenytoin, approximately 7% develop 1 or more features of fetal hydantoin syndrome, which comprises microcephaly, mental deficiency & craniofacial abnormalities. The second-generation AEDs, valproate & carbamazepine, are associated w/ spina bifida aperta, neural tube defects, hypospadias, radial aplasia & probably autism-like disorder. Several factors have been identified to account for the increased risk, including the direct teratogenic effects of the AEDs, indirect effects of these drugs interfering w/ folate metabolism & possible arrhythmogenic effect of maternal drug therapy on the embryonic heart, leading to ischemia in developing tissues.

- All anticonvulsants should be discontinued during pregnancy, especially during the 1st trimester; even newer anticonvulsants should be avoided during the 1st trimester.
- Consultation w/ a perinatologist is recommended if continued use of anticonvulsants during pregnancy is being considered.

Antidepressants

- Most antidepressants are classified as FDA category C. One concern regarding the use of TCAs is the small risk of a neonatal withdrawal syndrome, which may include tachypnea, tachycardia, irritability & seizures of the newborn. MAO inhibitors should be avoided during pregnancy in part because of greater hepatic toxicity, the need of low-tyramine diet & toxic interactions w/ other meds. Several studies involving SSRIs have been unable to show a significant incidence of teratogenicity, although one study of fluoxetine did report an increase in minor physical anomalies of no cosmetic or functional significance & a decline in birthweight.

Common chronic pain conditions seen during pregnancy

Low Back Pain

- Low back pain is seen in almost 50% of pregnant pts. There is accentuation of lumbar lordosis during pregnancy, which may be partly responsible for back pain. Though uncommon, osteoporosis leading to vertebral or hip pain & fracture can occur during pregnancy & breast-feeding. Pts w/ chronic back pain secondary to trauma or surgery may be managed w/ a combination of narcotic & non-narcotic meds. Injection therapies, including epidural steroids & sacroiliac injections, are also relatively safe. Fluoroscopy should be avoided during pregnancy, especially during organogenesis.
- Nonpharmacologic measures including biofeedback, relaxation training, massage therapy, aquatic therapy, aerobic body conditioning, acupuncture, acupressure, TENS & application of heat or cold should be used as a first treatment option to minimize the use of

medication; medication should be used only if symptoms are not controlled by nonpharmacologic measures.

Sacroiliac Joint Pain

■ The hormonal changes during pregnancy, including production of relaxin by the corpus luteum, lead to widening & increasing mobility of the sacroiliac & symphysis pubis joints. This pain can radiate to the posterior thigh & groin respectively. Sometimes sacroiliac joint pain mimics sciatica; in these circumstances a focused exam of the sacroiliac joint may help in reaching the diagnosis. Nonpharmacologic measures & physical therapy may be sufficient, but in some pts the use of acetaminophen w/ or w/o narcotics &/or limited use of NSAIDs becomes necessary to control symptoms. Sacroiliac steroid injections may provide 4–8 weeks of good pain relief. Fluoroscopy should be avoided if possible. Pts w/ sacroiliac joint hardware or sacroiliac joint fusion may be very difficult to manage & usually require high doses of narcotic meds. Use of a trochanteric belt is suitable to stabilize painful pelvic joints & decrease back pain on the recommendation of a physical therapist.

Migraine

■ Migraine improves during pregnancy in 50–80% of pts, & attacks typically diminish by the end of the 1st trimester. It is thought to be due to 50x–100x increase in estrogen concentration. In some rare instances headaches begin during pregnancy. It is of utmost importance to make a thorough search for the potentially serious causes, including preeclampsia, pseudotumor cerebri & intracranial/SAH. MRI, serum toxicology screens & coagulation studies may be necessary. Rarely, migraine may appear for the first time in pregnancy or more commonly during the postpartum period w/ a rapid fall in the estrogen level.

■ Inadequately treated migraine can lead to poor nutritional intake, dehydration, sleep deprivation, increased stress, poor marital relations & depression, w/ the associated adverse sequelae on maternal & fetal well-being.

■ Symptomatic nonpharmacologic treatment including ice, relaxation, massage, biofeedback, stress mgt & cognitive-behavior therapy should always be recommended. Prophylactic treatment during pregnancy is indicated for women w/ intractable & frequent migraines, particularly when prolonged vomiting results in dehydration. When possible, these pts should be managed jointly by the obstetrician & a headache specialist. Beta-blockers may be used earlier during pregnancy. However, when used later in pregnancy, IUGR & bradycardia can occur.

■ First-line abortive treatment consists of acetaminophen, NSAIDs & caffeine-containing analgesics. Opioids may be used in selected cases. Antiemetics such as prochlorperazine & promethazine can provide useful adjunctive therapy. Use of triptans should be reserved for migraines that do not respond to other treatment options, as they are category C drugs.

■ For protracted migraine attacks, treatment options include IV hydration & parenteral prochlorperazine, diphenhydramine hydrochloride, metoclopramide or magnesium sulfate. In refractory cases these drugs may be supplemented w/ parenteral opioids or corticosteroids.

■ Use of Botox for chronic headaches & migraine mgt is also controversial. Botox is a category C drug. There are no adequate & well-controlled studies of Botox in pregnant women. It should be administered in pregnancy only if the potential benefits justify the risk to the fetus.

Sickle cell crises

■ Sickle cell disease is the most common hemoglobinopathy in the U.S., w/ 8% of African-American subjects carrying the sickle hemoglobin gene. Modern technology & scientific advances have revolutionized sickle cell mgt & obstetric & perinatal care, allowing more aggressive intervention & subsequent improvement in the outcome.

■ Pregnant pts are prone to develop vaso-occlusive crises, especially in the 3rd trimester & the postpartum period. These crises manifest as abdominal, joint, chest or back pain. These pts are usually managed by hydration, oxygen & opioid analgesics. Sometimes it is important to decrease the polymerized Hgb S level by partial exchange transfusions. During labor it is of utmost importance to give these pts oxygen & hydrate them judiciously & prevent hypoxia. Epidural or spinal anesthesia can be safely placed in these pts. Many maternal & fetal complications of pregnancy are more common in pts w/ sickle cell disease, including preeclampsia, premature labor & IUGR.

Pts w/ Complex regional pain syndrome

■ Pts w/ complex regional pain syndrome are seen quite uncommonly during pregnancy or labor. There are isolated case reports of pts w/ complex regional syndrome becoming pregnant. There is some indication that the symptoms may worsen during pregnancy, w/

patchy reduction in the bone density in the area involved. These pts have severe neuropathic pain & are on multiple meds, including high-dose opioids & AEDs, so they avoid pregnancy. If they become pregnant it is highly advisable to stop the AEDs & if possible narcotics during the period of organogenesis (15–55 days). If continuation of medication is necessary, close fetal monitoring w/ ultrasound, serum markers & echocardiography may be necessary to avoid any fetal abnormalities, & early therapeutic abortion may be considered. During labor these pts should have an early epidural placement. It is also important not to touch the areas that have tactile allodynia & hyperalgesia (features of complex regional pain syndrome) because this can result in extreme pain of varying duration.

■ A disorder involving lower extremity & hip pain w/ arthropathy & locoregional trophic disturbance can develop during pregnancy; it has been labeled reflex sympathetic dystrophy, also algodystrophy in some cases. It is a poorly understood disorder & is associated w/ patchy demineralization. MRI is helpful in the diagnosis, w/ regional low signal intensity on T1-weighted images & regional high signal intensity on T2-weighted images. This disorder resolves over several weeks or months after delivery but can recur during subsequent pregnancies.

Fibromyalgia

■ Fibromyalgia is a complex syndrome characterized by widespread musculoskeletal pain accompanied by multiple areas of tender points at many locations. Fibromyalgia syndrome has no adverse effects on the outcome of the pregnancy or the health of neonate. Many pts experience worsening of their fibromyalgia symptoms during pregnancy, especially in the 3rd trimester. There is increased incidence of postpartum depression & anxiety in these pts.

Pts w/ Intrathecal infusion pumps

■ Intrathecal infusion therapies are increasingly being used for malignant & non-malignant pain. There are limited data on the safety of the various intrathecal agents in pregnancy, but there is an isolated case report of a mother who continued her intrathecal morphine infusion through a pump w/ an unremarkable antenatal & postnatal course. Minimal maternal serum & breast milk levels of morphine were found in the first 7 weeks postpartum.

■ Although these pts are seen uncommonly during pregnancy, they can present many challenges to OBs & obstetric anesthesiologists.

Guidelines for taking care of these pts during the antenatal period & labor are as follows:

➤ Anesthesia consults in the antenatal period, detailed information on intrathecal meds & their dosages. Get a computer printout after the pump interrogation. Talk directly to the pain specialist or neurosurgeon who placed the pump.

➤ The pain specialist might be able to give the pt a small bolus of medication on top of the baseline requirement to control the labor pain. Common meds used in intrathecal pumps are baclofen, morphine, hydromorphone, clonidine & bupivacaine.

➤ If an epidural has to be placed, it can be placed below the incision. Dural puncture should be avoided at all costs because it can lead to headaches and also result in increasing pain & loss of intrathecal medication once the catheter is removed.

➤ An epidural blood patch might be technically difficult if the infusion pump was placed for failed back surgery or post-laminectomy syndrome, as post-op scarring may result in difficult placement & spread of blood in the epidural space may not result in improvement of symptoms.

➤ If the infusion pump has only an opioid analgesic, an epidural w/ bupivacaine only may be adequate for labor analgesia.

➤ A lumbar spine x-ray may be recommended to see integral parts of the system & location of the pump. Pumps are usually implanted in the anterior lower abdominal wall. The integrity of the intrathecal system can be confirmed w/ a dye study, which is not recommended.

➤ A neonatologist should be readily available to treat any neonatal opioid withdrawal symptoms.

Patients w/ Spinal cord stimulators

■ As w/ intrathecal pumps, spinal cord stimulator pts are not commonly seen during pregnancy & labor. FDA recommends that spinal cord stimulators should be turned off during pregnancy because the effect of stimulation on the fetus is not known. However, there is an isolated case report of a pt w/ complex regional pain syndrome who continued to use the spinal cord stimulator for analgesia during pregnancy w/o any untoward effect on the fetus.

■ Animal studies regarding spinal cord stimulation & pregnancy revealed that milk ejection was obtained by electrical stimulation of the anterolateral spinal cord in lactating rats. This was attributed to the release of oxytocin. Although the functional significance of this reflex may be relevant in pregnancy, it is unlikely that the ventral spinal cord pathways responsible would be stimulated during the epidural stimulation of the dorsal spinal cord.

- Common indications for spinal cord stimulators are complex regional pain syndrome & post-laminectomy syndrome. These pts can present a host of challenges to the anesthesiologist, including a difficult epidural placement, failed epidural analgesia, dural puncture, damage to stimulator leads, potential intrathecal catheter & post-dural puncture headaches. Obtain a lumbar spine x-ray before placing the epidural catheter to determine the location of the implantable pulse generator & leads.
- The opioid requirement may be slightly higher in these pts because of cross-tolerance.

STUDIES
- **MRI**

  If a pregnant pt presents w/ new headache or any sensory or motor deficit, an MRI of the involved region becomes necessary to prevent any future disability. MRI is relatively safe during pregnancy. Pts w/ spinal cord stimulators cannot undergo MRI, but they should have a CT scan instead. Pts w/ intrathecal infusion pumps can safely undergo MRI, but their pump should be interrogated after the procedure is completed.

- **EMG & NCS**

  Nerve conduction studies & electromyography are rarely performed during pregnancy. They are indicated only if the pt has developed a new sensory deficit that cannot be explained in the setting of the pregnancy

- **X-Rays**

  Lumbar spine x-rays should be performed in pts w/ spinal cord stimulators undergoing epidural placement to avoid any damage to the stimulator leads.

- **Pump interrogation**

  It should be done by a pain specialist as soon as the pt comes to the triage room or should be available from the antenatal consult.

- **Urine toxicology**

  Many pain pts abuse other illicit substances, including cocaine & marijuana. These pts should be routinely screened for the presence of illicit substances.

MANAGEMENT/INTERVENTIONS
- Mgt is discussed in the individual section of chronic pain problems encountered by the obstetric anesthesiologist.
- Early placement of the epidural remains the key in managing these pts.

CAVEATS/PEARLS
- Identify the chronic pain problem that the pt is suffering from.
- Establish a rapport w/ the pt.
- If the pt is seen in the pre-op clinic, get the phone number of the primary care physician & pain mgt physician & talk to them personally.
- Be aware of comorbidities.
- If the pt has an implantable device, determine the exact location of the catheter (in case of an intrathecal pump) or leads (in case of a spinal cord stimulator).
- MRI cannot be performed in pts who have spinal cord stimulators but is safe in pts w/ intrathecal pumps. Pumps should be interrogated after the MRI is complete.

CHECKLIST
- Avoid use of drugs during organogenesis.
- Incorporate conservative, nonpharmacologic & alternative medicine in your practice when dealing w/ chronic pain pts during pregnancy.
- Once you establish a rapport w/ your pt, ask about any substance abuse during pregnancy. These pts think it is legitimate to use substances such as marijuana if pain is not adequately controlled by other measures.
- Preplan the anesthetic & anticipate the complications if the pt is seen pre-op.
- Have the printout of the last pump interrogation & any drug or dosage change.
- Avoid a wet tap at all costs in these pts during epidural placement, because this complication can open the doors for new chronic pain problems.
- If the pt has an intrathecal pump, determine the location of the reservoir by palpation or x-ray & outline the catheter (which is tunneled under the skin on the pt's back) while performing the epidural, to avoid damage to the catheter.

CIRRHOSIS

LAWRENCE WEINSTEIN, MD
DOUG RAINES, MD

FUNDAMENTAL KNOWLEDGE

Cirrhosis is an irreversible chronic liver disease in which parenchymal injury results in fibrosis. Since it is a sign of advanced liver disease & a poor overall health state, cirrhosis is uncommon in pregnant pts.

- Causes of cirrhosis include alcoholism, chronic viral hepatitis, biliary cirrhosis.
- Signs & symptoms include weakness, spider angiomata, palmar erythema, caput medusa, icterus, ascites, GI bleeding, varices, right upper quadrant pain, encephalopathy.
- Important consequences for the anesthesiologist include esophageal varices, coagulopathy, portal hypertension, ascites, circulatory alterations & the effect of hepatic failure on drug pharmacokinetics.
- Cirrhosis is associated w/ hyperdynamic circulation w/ elevated cardiac output.
  - ➤ Secondary to generalized peripheral vasodilation, increased intravascular volume, decreased blood viscosity & arteriovenous communications in the lungs
  - ➤ Because of this, an apparently *normal* cardiac output value in a cirrhotic pt may actually represent a low cardiac output state & require further evaluation of cardiac function.
- Despite increased overall cardiac output, perfusion to organs such as liver & kidneys may be inadequate secondary to shunting.
- If pt has concomitant heart failure secondary to alcoholic cardiomyopathy, then increased blood volume can result in congestive heart failure.
- Some people w/ liver failure have a downregulation of alpha adrenoreceptors, attenuating their response to norepinephrine & making intractable hypotension a concern for the anesthesiologist.
- Cirrhotic pts tend to have baseline hyperventilation w/ a resultant respiratory alkalosis.
- Chronic hypoxemia can result from several causes.

STUDIES

- Lab abnormalities can relate to underlying etiology of liver disease.

- Pathologic findings include fibrosis, regenerative nodules; special stains may be helpful.
- Special tests include liver biopsy, cholangiography, Doppler ultrasound evaluation of portal & hepatic veins, ultrasound evaluation of bile duct & space-occupying lesions.

MANAGEMENT/INTERVENTIONS

- Hemodynamic changes are important for the anesthesiologist.
- In an already vasodilated cirrhotic pt, BP swings are poorly tolerated & induction of neuraxial or general anesthesia may be associated w/ sudden profound hypotension.
  - BP monitoring is vital, & an arterial line is indicated before induction of any anesthesia in pts w/ cirrhotic liver disease.
  - Monitor urine output to assess effective circulation & volume status.
  - Because of hyperdynamic circulation & systemic vasodilation, central venous monitoring & PA catheters may not reflect fluid status accurately, although PA catheters do become useful in the setting of co-existent pulmonary hypertension or oliguric renal failure.
- Due to the associated pulmonary effects, the cirrhotic pt under general anesthesia may require higher FIO2 &/or PEEP to maintain adequate oxygen saturation & tissue delivery.
  - Pre-oxygenation for general anesthesia becomes even more important than usual, as V/Q mismatching will result in more rapid desaturation w/ apnea.
- Higher inspiratory pressures may be necessary to maintain adequate tidal volumes in the setting of increased abdominal & thoracic pressures secondary to ascites.
  - Muscle paralysis may be useful in decreasing the muscular component of chest wall resistance to positive-pressure ventilation.

Ventilation strategies should aim for normocapnia, as alkalosis shifts ammonium ions to a less ionized equilibrium, facilitating diffusion across the blood brain barrier & potentially exacerbating hepatic encephalopathy.

CAVEATS/PEARLS

It is rare for pts w/ true cirrhosis to be able to carry a pregnancy to term. As w/ most liver disease, it is useful to understand the etiology of the cirrhosis so that associated abnormalities can be appropriately managed.

CHECKLIST
See details in sections below, related to specific causes of cirrhosis.

CNS INFECTION (BACTERIAL MENINGITIS & VIRAL ENCEPHALITIS)

MEREDITH ALBRECHT, MD; LISA LEFFERT, MD; AND MICHELE SZABO, MD

FUNDAMENTAL KNOWLEDGE
See also chapters on "*HIV & AIDS*," "*Fever*," "*Increased ICP*" (with brain abscess).

Definition
- Infection of CNS, either bacterial or viral

Epidemiology
- Possible CNS infections during pregnancy
  - Bacterial meningitis
  - Herpes simplex encephalitis
  - Tuberculosis meningitis
  - Leprosy
  - Cryptococcal meningitis
  - Listeriosis
  - Tetanus
  - Syphilis
  - Lyme disease
  - Cytomegalovirus
  - HIV

Pathophysiology
- Pregnancy is associated w/ decreased immune function.
- Infection can be spread by contiguous infection or via hematogenous seeding.

Clinical Manifestations
- Signs of infection such as fever & fatigue
- Signs of neurologic involvement such as headache, focal neurologic deficits, mental status changes, seizures
- Due to mass effect in the case of abscess

Effect of Pregnancy on CNS Infection
- Pregnancy is associated w/ decreased immune function & can worsen disease course.

Effect of CNS Infection on Pregnancy & the Fetus
■ Increased incidence of perinatal & maternal morbidity

STUDIES
History & Physical
■ Fever
■ Headache
■ Mental status changes
■ Focal neurologic findings
■ Personality changes
■ Amnesia
■ Aphasia
■ Seizures
■ Nuchal rigidity in case of bacterial meningitis

Laboratory
■ CSF chemistries
  ➤ Viral: mononuclear pleocytosis, normal glucose, increased protein
  ➤ Bacterial: elevated neutrophils, decreased glucose, elevated protein
■ Gram stain
■ Culture
■ Lumbar puncture if abscess not present
■ Brain biopsy

Imaging
■ CT
■ MRI
■ EEG: diffuse slowing or periodic complexes

MANAGEMENT/INTERVENTIONS
Medical Treatment
■ Antibiotic or antiviral therapy for the specific organism
■ Abscesses >2.5–3 cm in diameter require surgical aspiration & drainage.
■ If mass effect is present, dexamethasone is recommended.
■ Anticonvulsants if seizures are present

Anesthesia
■ Physical exam documenting extent of existing deficit
■ Look for signs of possible sepsis.

- In the case of brain abscess or global cerebral edema, if increased ICP is present, institute ICP precautions.
  - ➤ No regional anesthesia (possibility of herniation w/ dural puncture)
  - ➤ Hyperventilation (after delivery)
  - ➤ Limit fluid resuscitation.
  - ➤ Mannitol
  - ➤ Steroids
- Avoid regional anesthesia due to concern about neuraxial spread of disease.

CAVEATS & PEARLS
- Multiple different causative organisms
- Investigate for signs of ICP or sepsis.
- Avoid regional anesthesia.

CHECKLIST
- Use universal precautions.
- Complete physical exam documenting extent of existing neural deficits
- Look for signs of possible sepsis.
- General anesthesia recommended due to concern about possible neuraxial spread
- In the case of a brain abscess or global cerebral edema, assess the degree of ICP & institute ICP precautions.

COMBINED SPINAL/EPIDURAL ANESTHESIA-ANALGESIA

KRISTEN STADTLANDER, MD; MAY PIAN-SMITH, MD; AND LISA LEFFERT, MD

FUNDAMENTAL KNOWLEDGE
- The combined spinal/epidural (CSE) technique has become popular in the past decade. The main benefit of this technique is the profound & immediate analgesic relief the spinal delivers, followed by the ability to provide extended relief when the epidural catheter is activated. It is often used when a pt arrives in late-stage labor & there is not enough time to establish an epidural block.
- There are three main techniques of CSE: the spinal needle-through-needle technique, the "backeye" technique (using a specially designed epidural needle w/ ports for both the spinal needle & epidural

catheter) & the separate needle technique, in which the epidural is placed after the spinal placement is completed.

- A fourth technique is a separate needle technique that allows the epidural catheter to be placed first & test-dosed, which is not possible w/ the needle-through-needle technique. However, this introduces the possibility of damaging the epidural catheter when introducing the spinal needle. It is also more time- & labor-intensive, as two different interspaces must be navigated. Because of these reasons, it is rarely used.
- The "backeye" technique is essentially the same as the needle-through-needle technique & will be described in the Management /Interventions section.
- The needle-through-needle technique involves placing an epidural needle in the epidural space (through the "loss of resistance" or "hanging drop" method) & then placing a long spinal needle through the epidural needle. When CSF is obtained, a spinal dose is given & the spinal needle is removed. The epidural catheter is then threaded but usually not immediately tested.

STUDIES

- CBC: The literature is insufficient to assess the predictive value of a platelet count for anesthesia complications in parturients without comorbid illness, or in those w/ pregnancy-induced hypertension.
- ACOG 1999 Practice Bulletin states, "Although limited, data support the safety of epidural anesthesia in patients with platelet counts greater than 100K. In women with gestational thrombocytopenia with platelet counts less than 99K but greater than 50K, epidural anesthesia also may be safe, but its use in such patients will require a consensus among the obstetrician, anesthesiologist, and patients. When platelet counts are less than 50K, epidural anesthesia should not be given."
- Normal coagulation profile
- Examination of the area where the epidural will be administered
- Informed consent w/ full explanation of the procedure & possible complications (headache 1–2%; rarely bleeding, infection, nerve/neck/back injury) & the risk of failed block
- Detailed history & physical highlighting bleeding abnormalities or pre-anesthetic neurologic deficits
- Access to fetal monitoring

MANAGEMENT/INTERVENTIONS

Technique

- Find epidural space w/ an epidural needle in usual manner (see "*Epidural Analgesia*"). Many experts recommend obtaining "loss of resistance" w/ saline instead of air to decrease the chance of pneumocephalus & patchy block. Once in the epidural space, place long spinal needle through epidural needle & advance until "pop" is felt and/or CSF is obtained.
- It is crucial to stabilize the spinal needle prior to injection. To stabilize the spinal needle, rest the back of your nondominant hand on the back of the pt w/ the fingers locking the epidural & spinal needle hubs together. The dominant hand delivers the spinal dose.
- There are many combinations of medicines for spinal labor analgesia. A common practice is to deliver 2.5 mg bupivacaine (0.25%) w/ or w/out 10–25 mcg fentanyl.
- After the spinal is dosed, remove the spinal needle & quickly thread the epidural catheter. The resulting spinal block can mask the symptoms of a paresthesia. Therefore, it is critical to advance the epidural catheter only if no resistance is encountered.
- "Test dose" in CSE is controversial. Giving a test dose through the epidural right after the spinal has taken effect can precipitate hypotension.
- Once the procedure is completed, the epidural infusion (w/o a loading dose) can be initiated, or alternatively, once the spinal begins to wear off, the epidural catheter can be test dosed & bolused as needed.

CAVEATS & PEARLS

1. The main advantage of the CSE technique is rapid onset of pain relief.
2. The main drawback of the CSE technique is the possibility of masking a potentially ineffective catheter & the small additional risk of postdural puncture headache from the dural puncture.
3. Be vigilant for signs of intravascular or intrathecal epidural placement, particularly if no test dose is given.
4. When using the CSE in labor, hypotension can be encountered immediately after administering the spinal. Make sure the pt has received adequate hydration before placement & make sure that a pressor such as ephedrine is readily available.
5. Use fetal monitoring.

CHECKLIST

1. Before placing an epidural, review the contraindications to regional anesthesia, w/ special attention to bleeding disorders/coagulopathies & pre-existing neurologic deficits.
2. Make sure the parturient has full monitoring, including fetal monitoring (if applicable) & a working IV.
3. Make sure the pt is prehydrated, pressors are readily available & emergency airway & cardiovascular supplies are accessible.
4. Always aspirate before injecting local anesthetic.
5. Obtain informed consent, including all possible complications of an epidural anesthetic & the possibility of a failed block/epidural replacement.

Monitor closely for hypotension & intravascular or intrathecal placement. Catheter removal & prompt treatment w/ pressors, hydration & ventilatory support can prevent disastrous complications (see "*Troubleshooting/Managing Inadequate Regional Anesthesia*").

CONGENITAL FIBRINOGEN DISORDERS

JEANNA VIOLA, MD
JANE BALLANTYNE, MD

FUNDAMENTAL KNOWLEDGE

- Divided into subgroups of afibrinogenemia, dysfibrinogenemia & hypofibrinogenemia, all of which predispose the pt to hemorrhage.
- Severe bleeding in pregnancy is rare & usually occurs post-partum.
- Approx. 20% of pts w/ this disorder develop a thrombophilia.
  - ➤ Likely due to the defective binding of thrombin to the abnormal fibrin
  - ➤ Thrombin levels are increased.
  - ➤ Stimulation of abnormal fibrin during fibrinolysis is ineffective.

STUDIES

N/A

MANAGEMENT/INTERVENTIONS

- Periodic transfusions of thrombin may be necessary to prevent miscarriage in pts prone to hemorrhage.
- Thrombophilic pts may require low-dose heparin & aspirin prophylaxis.
- Regional anesthesia is usually contraindicated in these pts.

CAVEATS AND PEARLS

- Congenital fibrinogen disorders are rare but serious diseases.

■ Pts may be prone to miscarriage.
■ Pts may be prone to either excessive bleeding or clotting.
■ Avoid regional anesthesia & IM injections in most cases.

CHECKLIST
■ Categorize the pt's status as either coagulopathic or thrombophilic, as mgt will differ.
■ Obtain consult w/ hematologist.
  Careful airway exam, as most pts will require GETA for C-section

CYSTIC FIBROSIS

WILTON C. LEVINE, MD
TONG-YAN CHEN, MD

FUNDAMENTAL KNOWLEDGE
■ Cystic fibrosis (CF) is an autosomal recessive disease of the exocrine glands causing production of excess secretions w/ abnormal electrolyte concentrations, leading to glandular obstruction.
■ Pregnancy in women w/ CF is no longer rare.
■ The overall rate of spontaneous abortion in pts w/ CF is 4.6%.
■ Maternal death during pregnancy in pts w/ CF is directly related to pulmonary status.
■ Pregnant CF pts often deteriorate with pregnancy due to:
  ➤ Increased airway responsiveness & obstruction
  ➤ Increased work of breathing
  ➤ Cardiovascular changes such as CHF & pulmonary hypertension that may result from increased blood volume
■ Pre-pregnancy pulmonary function correlates w/ pulmonary function during pregnancy (better pre-pregnancy function leads to better function while pregnant).

STUDIES
■ Evaluate pt for clinical status, nutritional status, chest x-ray abnormalities, pulmonary function.
■ Pts w/ prepregnancy FVC < 50% predicted or w/ cor pulmonale may be discouraged from becoming pregnant as they are at significant risk for morbidity & mortality.
■ Pregnancy is associated w/ a 13% decrease in FEV_1 & an 11% decrease in FVC. These decreases are typically regained post-partum.

- $FEV_1 < 60\%$ predicted is associated w/ preterm infants & increased loss of pulmonary function during pregnancy.
- Monitor pregnancy w/ serial PFTs, pulse oximetry & ABG monitoring when needed.

MANAGEMENT/INTERVENTIONS

- Given the risk of hypoxia w/ CF, pts should have continuous monitoring of oxygen saturation during labor & delivery.
- Anesthetic goals
  - ➤ Pain relief or prevention
  - ➤ Avoid high thoracic motor block
  - ➤ Avoid respiratory depression & hypoxia
  - ➤ Avoid maternal hyperventilation
    - Hyperventilation causes increased work of breathing & may lead to respiratory decompensation in pts w/ severe pulmonary dysfunction.
  - ➤ Use opioids w/ caution to avoid respiratory depression.

CAVEATS AND PEARLS

- Pregnancy in a pt w/ CF is no longer rare.
- Pts w/ prepregnancy FVC < 50% predicted or cor pulmonale should be discouraged from pregnancy.
- Pregnancy should be followed w/ serial PFTs, pulse oximetry & ABG monitoring as needed.
- In labor, CF pts should have continuous pulse oximetry.
- Avoid a high thoracic motor block when placing an epidural.
- Avoid narcotic-related hypoventilation & respiratory depression.

CHECKLIST

- Assess pt's pre-pregnant & current pulmonary status.
- Provide continuous monitoring w/ pulse oximetry.

DEPRESSION

LATA POTTURI, MD
ADELE VIGUERA, MD

FUNDAMENTAL KNOWLEDGE

DSM IV diagnostic criteria

At least 5 of the following symptoms must have been present during the same 2-week period & represent a change from previous functioning;

at least one of the symptoms is either (1) "depressed mood" or (2) "loss of interest or pleasure" (Do not include symptoms that are clearly due to a general medical condition, or mood-incongruent delusions or hallucinations)

(1) Depressed mood most of the day, nearly every day, as indicated by either subjective report (e.g., feels sad or empty) or observation made by others (e.g., appears tearful)

(2) Markedly diminished interest or pleasure in all, or almost all, activities most of the day, nearly every day (as indicated either by subjective account or observation by others)

(3) Significant weight loss when not dieting or weight gain (e.g., a change of >5% of body weight in a month), decrease in appetite, or increase in appetite, nearly every day

(4) Insomnia or hypersomnia, nearly every day

(5) Psychomotor agitation or retardation, nearly every day (observable by others, not merely subjective feelings of restlessness or being slowed down)

(6) Fatigue or loss of energy nearly every day

(7) Feelings of worthlessness or excessive or inappropriate guilt (which may be delusional) nearly every day (not merely self-reproach or guilt about being sick)

(8) Diminished ability to think or concentrate or indecisiveness, nearly every day (either by subjective account or as observed by others)

(9) Recurrent thoughts of death (not just fear of dying), recurrent suicidal ideation w/o a specific plan, or a suicide attempt or a specific plan for committing suicide

The symptoms cause clinically significant distress or impairment in social, occupational, or other important areas of functioning.

The symptoms are not due to the direct physiological effects of a substance (e.g., a drug of abuse, a medication) or a general medical condition (e.g., hypothyroidism).

The symptoms are not better accounted for by bereavement, i.e., after the loss of a loved one, the symptoms persist for >2 months or are characterized by marked functional impairment, morbid preoccupation w/ worthlessness, suicidal ideation, psychotic symptoms, or psychomotor retardation.

Course during pregnancy/postpartum

Up to 70% of women report negative mood symptoms during their pregnancy; however, the prevalence among pregnant women who fulfill the diagnostic criteria for major depression is 10–20%.

Depression is difficult to recognize during pregnancy since symptoms can often be challenging to distinguish from normal pregnancy-related discomforts. The course varies throughout pregnancy. Most data indicate that symptoms peak during the 1st trimester, improve during the 2nd trimester & increase again during the 3rd trimester.

In general, pregnancy represents a time of increased vulnerability for the onset of depression. Risk factors that have been found to contribute to depression in pregnancy include history of depression prior to pregnancy, history of antepartum or postpartum depression & a family history of depression, particularly during pregnancy or postpartum. Other risk factors for depression during pregnancy include poor social support, adverse life events, marital discord, unplanned pregnancy & ambivalence toward the pregnancy.

Relapses during the postpartum period are common. Women who are depressed in pregnancy will usually go on to develop postpartum depression. If they are stable during pregnancy but have a prior history of major depression, 30% will go on to develop postpartum depression. In women who have a history of antepartum or postpartum depression, 50–60% will develop postpartum depression.

Meds commonly used in treatment
- SSRIs
- TCAs

Fetal issues & medications
The risks of treating a pregnant pt w/ psychotropic meds must be weighed against potentially harmful effects to the fetus. All psychotropic meds cross the placenta. Studies have not consistently reported an increased risk of fetal malformations or miscarriages in women taking SSRIs or TCAs. Reproductive safety data for SSRIs or TCAs do not demonstrate an elevated risk for major malformations w/ 1st-trimester exposure above the baseline risk for major malformations of 2–4%.

STUDIES
- History & physical
  - In addition to a thorough history & physical, ask pt about all prenatal psychiatric diagnoses. How has her illness been managed prior to pregnancy & during pregnancy? Ask about psychological counseling, psychiatric treatment & all meds she has taken during pregnancy.
  - Also ask the pt regarding the course of her depression during pregnancy, symptoms encountered & last dose of medication.

- Lab tests
  - When applicable, check serum medication level & a full electrolyte panel.

EKG

A number of conduction abnormalities have been noted in pts on TCAs. It may be worthwhile to check an EKG or analyze the pt's rhythm on a cardiac monitor. Barring another indication, pts w/ a history of depression taking other psychotropic meds do not need a baseline EKG.

MANAGEMENT & INTERVENTIONS

- Psychosocial approach to the pt: Depressed pts can benefit from reassurance & a thorough explanation of the events surrounding labor. Social supports & family members should be involved as deemed appropriate.
- Tailoring anesthetic plan: Pts w/ a history of depression who are able to give informed consent for anesthesia can safely undergo both general & regional anesthesia. Awareness of potential drug interactions will aid in developing a safe anesthetic plan.
- Informed consent: Determine the pt's ability to give informed consent.

CAVEATS & PEARLS

- Depression can be difficult to diagnose during pregnancy since normal pregnancy-related discomforts can mimic symptoms of depression. Screen pts carefully.

CHECKLIST

- Be familiar w/ the diagnostic criteria for depression.
- Know what meds the pt is taking & when her last dose was.
- Consider checking an EKG or analyzing cardiac rhythm in pts taking TCAs.

DIABETES INSIPIDUS

GRACE C. CHANG, MD, MBA; ROBERT A. PETERFREUND, MD, PhD; AND STEPHANIE L. LEE, MD, PhD

FUNDAMENTAL KNOWLEDGE

Definition

- Absence of antidiuretic hormone (ADH) secondary to destruction of posterior pituitary (neurogenic diabetes insipidus)

- Lack of response to ADH by renal tubules (nephrogenic diabetes insipidus)

Epidemiology
- Rarely complicates pregnancy
- Very few cases have been reported.

Signs/Symptoms
- Polydipsia
- High output of poorly concentrated urine
- Increased serum osmolarity

Etiology
- Indirect head injury
- Direct injury to posterior pituitary during surgery
- Meningitis
- Infectious disease of pituitary & hypothalamus (Langerhans histiocytosis)

Changes w/ Pregnancy
- Subclinical DI, either nephrogenic or neurogenic, can become symptomatic in pregnancy due to breakdown of ADH by placental vasopressinase.
- Pt may have associated abnormal labor due to insufficient levels of oxytocin.

STUDIES
- Desmopressin (L-deamino-8-D arginine vasopressin) response test
  - ➤ If neurogenic DI, will have concentration of urine after challenge w/ 1 mcg desmopressin (DDAVP), subcutaneous or IV, or 20 mcg DDAVP, intranasal
  - ➤ Nephrogenic DI will not respond to vasopressin or DDAVP.

MANAGEMENT/INTERVENTIONS
- Desmopressin (DDAVP) if neurogenic DI
  - ➤ 0.1–0.2 mL bid or tid by rhinal tube (100 mcg/mL) or nasal spray pump, 1–2 sprays bid-tid (10 mcg/spray)
  - ➤ 0.5–1.0 mL IV or subcutaneous bid (4 mcg/mL)
  - ➤ 0.5–4 tabs po bid-tid (0.1 mg /tablet) for partial DI only
  - ➤ Dose is greater in pregnant pts because of breakdown of DDAVP by placental vasopressinase.
- Chlorpropamide if partial neurogenic to increase renal tubule sensitivity to ADH

- Diuretics (hydrochlorothiazide) to reduce volume delivered to proximal tubule if nephrogenic DI
- Aggressive fluid replacement
- Weigh pt daily.

Anesthetic management
- Assess volume status.
- Aggressive fluid replacement
- Ensure adequate treatment w/ DDAVP.
  - Partial deficiency of ADH needs replacement only if plasma osmolality >290 mOsm/L.
- Monitor electrolytes & replete as necessary.
- Monitor urine output.
- Regional anesthesia & general anesthesia are equally safe.

CAVEATS/PEARLS
- Monitor fluid & electrolyte status carefully.

CHECKLIST
- Aggressive fluid hydration
- Monitor electrolytes & plasma osmolality or urine specific gravity.
- Monitor urine output, keep input/output balanced & weigh pt daily.

DIABETES MELLITUS

GRACE C. CHANG, MD, MBA; STEPHANIE L. LEE, MD, PhD; AND ROBERT A. PETERFREUND, MD, PhD

FUNDAMENTAL KNOWLEDGE

Definition

Chronic, systemic metabolic disease characterized by absolute or relative deficiency of insulin action, resulting in hyperglycemia. Insulin increases transport of glucose into fat & muscle & potassium across cell membranes, inhibits lipolysis, increases glycolysis in fat & muscle & stimulates glycogen synthesis & inhibits both glycogenolysis & gluconeogenesis in all tissues.

- DM type 1
  - Characterized by autoimmune process that destroys insulin-producing pancreatic beta cells
  - Pts usually diagnosed early in life, typically not susceptible to obesity

➤ Must be treated w/ insulin replacement
➤ Pts susceptible to diabetic ketoacidosis

■ DM type 2
  ➤ Characterized by relative insulin deficiency & peripheral resistance to insulin
  ➤ Onset later in life; obesity; resistance to ketosis
  ➤ Can be treated w/ oral hypoglycemics, oral insulin sensitizers, insulin or both oral agent(s) & insulin

■ Gestational diabetes mellitus (GDM)
  ➤ Glucose intolerance of variable severity; onset or first detection during pregnancy
  ➤ Characterized by postprandial hyperglycemia, resulting from impaired insulin release & exaggeration of insulin resistance seen in normal pregnancies
  ➤ This definition applies regardless of use of insulin as therapy or if the disease persists after pregnancy.

Epidemiology

■ DM: 2–5% of all pregnancies; GDM: 90% of all cases of diabetes complicating pregnancy, remaining cases divided between two types of pregestational DM
■ About 135,000 cases of GDM diagnosed annually in United States
■ More than half who develop GDM will go on to develop DM type 2 later in life.
■ Risk factors for GDM: older maternal age, family history of diabetes, increased pregravid body mass index
■ More common in populations w/ higher rate of DM type 2: African Americans, Asians, Hispanics, Native Americans (prevalence is 3.3–6.1%; in low-risk populations prevalence is 1.4–2.8%)

Pathophysiology

■ Normal changes in carbohydrate metabolism associated w/ pregnancy include increased insulin resistance due to production of human placental lactogen & progesterone; also prolactin, cortisol & chorionic somatomammotropin levels increase; this promotes higher circulating glucose & amino acid levels.
■ Hormone levels increase linearly during 2nd & 3rd trimesters.
■ Glucose crosses placenta via facilitated diffusion; maternal blood glucose level determines fetal concentration.
■ Insulin does not cross placenta.
■ In normal pregnancy maternal fasting glucose is lower than in non-pregnant state due to fetal glucose uptake.

- Postprandial glucose levels are maintained at normal levels at cost of maternal hyperinsulinemia.
- 1st trimester: relatively higher levels of estrogen enhance insulin sensitivity; in combination w/ nausea & vomiting, increased risk of maternal hypoglycemia. Pts w/ poorly controlled DM type 1 at conception & early weeks of gestation have a higher incidence of spontaneous abortion & major congenital malformations.
- 2nd trimester: maternal hyperglycemia produces fetal hyperglycemia, stimulating fetal pancreatic beta cells & fetal hyperinsulinemia. Since insulin is major fetal growth hormone, hyperinsulinemia can produce macrosomia (doubles risk for shoulder dystocia at vaginal delivery). Fetal growth restriction can also result during this time from maternal nephropathy & hypertension.
- 3rd trimester: insulin resistance most marked; GDM most often occurs at this time; risk of ketoacidosis greatest, diabetogenic hormone levels plateau during last few weeks of pregnancy

Classification
Modified White Classification
- Criteria related to severity of disease in terms of duration since diagnosis & presence of end organ effects
- Class C, D, F, H, or R diabetics have increased risk of poor pregnancy outcome compared w/ women in classes A or B.
- Class A: any age of onset, any duration of pregestational DM, no vascular disease, therapy is diet only
- Class A1 (GDM): fasting glucose level <105 mg/dL & postprandial glucose level <120 mg/dL; therapy is diet only
- Class A2 (GDM): fasting glucose level ≥105 mg/dL &/or postprandial glucose level ≥120 mg/dL; therapy is insulin
- Class B: >20 years age of onset, <10 years duration of pregestational DM, no vascular disease, therapy is insulin
- Class C: onset at 10–19 years of age, 10–19 years duration of pregestational DM, no vascular disease, on insulin
- Class D: onset <10 years of age or 20 years or greater duration of pregestational DM, benign retinopathy, on insulin
- Class F: onset at any age, any duration of pregestational DM, nephropathy, on insulin
- Class R: onset at any age, any duration of pregestational DM, proliferative retinopathy, on insulin
- Class H: onset at any age, any duration of pregestational DM, heart disease, on insulin

Maternal Complications
- Dependent on woman's condition at conception
- Infection: increased frequency of pyelonephritis & vaginitis
- Pregnancy-induced hypertension: risk directly related to severity of diabetes
- Retinopathy: tends to progress during pregnancy
  - Pts w/ minimal or no retinopathy, 10% chance of progression
  - Pts w/ proliferative retinopathy or severe preproliferative retinopathy: 50% chance of further progression of eye disease
  - Likely etiology: growth factors associated w/ pregnancy & increased retinal blood flow
  - Rapid institution of strict glycemic control during pregnancy has been associated w/ short-term progression of retinopathy.
- Nephropathy: if normal renal function, usually no significant deterioration seen other than mild proteinuria, which returns to normal after pregnancy
  - If microalbuminuria is present prepregnancy, 1/3 progress to nephrotic-range proteinuria by end of pregnancy.
  - If macroproteinuria (24-hour urine protein >190 mg/day) is present prepregnancy, 30% chance of developing pre-eclampsia by term
  - If creatinine clearance reduced to <80 mL/min or urine protein is >2 g/day, net loss of renal function is evident postpartum in up to 50% of women. Birthweight is proportional to creatinine clearance. Risk of fetal growth restriction is increased, especially in pts who also are hypertensive.
- Neuropathy: no major changes expected in any neuropathy during pregnancy, but greater incidence of entrapment neuropathies (ie, carpal tunnel syndrome)
  - Autonomic neuropathy is stable; gastroparesis can contribute to worsening of nausea/vomiting.
- Cardiovascular disease
  - MI during pregnancy in the diabetic pt can result in maternal mortality >60%.
  - Hemodynamic changes associated w/ pregnancy increase myocardial stress. Epinephrine released in response to hypoglycemia may exacerbate risk of myocardial injury.
  - May need cardiac evaluation, especially in higher-risk women (diabetes >20 years, signs/symptoms of vascular disease, presence of cardiovascular autonomic neuropathy)

Fetal & Neonatal Complications

■ Intrauterine fetal death: increased risk associated w/ fasting maternal glucose level >105 mg/dL during last 4–8 weeks of gestation

■ Congenital malformations: caudal regression & renal, cardiac & CNS abnormalities
  ➤ All occur by 8 weeks gestation, so important for women to have well-controlled DM (HgbA$_{1C}$<7%) prior to conception; HgbA$_{1C}$ level is directly related to risk of malformation of fetus.

■ IUGR: seen in pregnancies complicated by nephropathy & vascular disease, related to poor placental vasculature

■ Macrosomia
  ➤ In pts w/ DM type 1, risk is 25%.
  ➤ Also increased risk w/ DM type 2

■ Respiratory distress syndrome: risk used to be 20% but has dropped to 1.6%, which is similar to pregnancies not complicated by DM

■ Neonatal hypoglycemia: in pts w/ DM type 1, risk is 8%; risk also increased w/ DM type 2

■ Shoulder dystocia: rate as high as 20–50% in fetuses >4,500 g

■ Brachial plexus injury: due to macrosomia, occurs at time of vaginal delivery
  ➤ In pts w/ GDM treated for severe hyperglycemia, risk 4–8% w/ fetuses >4,500 g
  ➤ Studies show 80–90% of these injuries resolve by 1 year of life.

■ Clavicular fracture: also due to macrosomia at time of delivery
  ➤ In pts who were treated for severe hyperglycemia, there is 6% increased risk of development in their fetuses compared w/ pts w/ well-controlled diabetes.
  ➤ >95% of clavicular fractures heal within several months without residual effects.

■ Neonatal hyperbilirubinemia, polycythemia, hypocalcemia: evidence unclear & limited about increased risk

■ Long-term consequences in children of mothers w/ DM
  ➤ Increased risk of impaired glucose tolerance, childhood obesity & neuropsychological disturbances; however, no large studies have clearly shown this

STUDIES

■ Screening for GDM controversial
  ➤ Unclear evidence of correlation between screening & improved outcome

➤ Current practice is to screen most pts despite absence of data-driven justification.

■ American Diabetes Association recommends glucose testing as soon as possible in pts at high risk for GDM (marked obesity, history of GDM, glycosuria or strong family history of diabetes).

➤ If negative at initial screening, pts should be retested at 24–28 weeks gestation.

➤ Women of average risk should be tested at 24–28 weeks gestation.

■ Glucose screening: conducted at 24–28 weeks gestation w/ use of 50-g oral glucose load; no regard to time of day or time of last meal; plasma glucose measured 1 hour later

➤ Value ≥130 mg/dL considered abnormal & requires full glucose tolerance test (GTT)

■ GTT performed after overnight fast, fasting plasma level drawn, followed by samples at 1, 2 & 3 hours.

➤ If 2 or more threshold values met, pt diagnosed w/ GDM

➤ Women w/ 1 abnormal result show insulin resistance & are more likely to deliver macrosomic infants; recommended that they be treated as having GDM & repeat GTT in 4 weeks

➤ 3 organizations have slightly different criteria for positive GTT:

- National Diabetes Data Group (NDDG): most often used in North America
  - 100 g oral glucose load
  - Fasting: abnormal if ≥105 mg/dL
  - 1 hour: abnormal if ≥190 mg/dL
  - 2 hour: abnormal if ≥165 mg/dL
  - 3 hour: abnormal if ≥145 mg/dL
- American Diabetes Association: also used in North America
  - 100-g oral glucose load
  - Fasting: abnormal if ≥95 mg/dL
  - 1 hour: abnormal if ≥180 mg/dL
  - 2 hour: abnormal if ≥155 mg/dL
  - 3 hour: abnormal if ≥140 mg/dL
- World Health Organization: most often used in rest of world
  - 75-g oral glucose load
  - Fasting: abnormal if ≥126 mg/dL
  - 2 hour: abnormal if ≥140 mg/dL

MANAGEMENT/INTERVENTIONS

- Diet
  - ➤ For those diagnosed w/ GDM, diet is most important factor for controlling blood glucose
    - Consists of 2,000–2,200 calories/day; focuses on complex, high-fiber carbohydrates w/ exclusion of concentrated sweets
    - Calorie target based on pt's ideal prepregnancy weight; 30 kcal/kg for average pt, 35 kcal/kg for underweight pt, 25 kcal/kg for obese women
    - If more restricted diet is used (1,600–1,800 calories/day) for obese pt, she should monitor morning urine for ketones.
- Exercise
  - ➤ Pts encouraged to exercise 3 or 4 times/week for 20–30 minutes
  - ➤ Brisk walking ideal
  - ➤ Studies show better glucose control w/ combination of diet & exercise compared w/ diet alone.
- Oral hypoglycemics
  - ➤ First-generation sulfonylurea drugs (tolbutamide & chlorpropamide)
    - Teratogenic in animals
    - Possibly teratogenic in humans
    - Shown to cross placenta
    - Drug levels detected in umbilical cord blood in concentrations similar to maternal blood
    - Generally avoided in pregnant pts
  - ➤ Second-generation sulfonylurea drugs (glyburide)
    - Do not cross placenta
    - Generally not recommended during pregnancy but in randomized uncontrolled study showed similar fetal outcome w/ either insulin or glyburide when administered after 1st trimester
    - Glyburide not FDA approved for treatment of GDM
    - No difference in maternal complications or neonatal outcomes, but rate of maternal hypoglycemia significantly lower than in pts on insulin
  - ➤ Biguanides (metformin)
    - Insulin-sensitizing agents should not be used during pregnancy.
- Insulin
  - ➤ Human insulin is mainstay in pts w/ pregestational DM.

➤ Insulin requirements rise throughout pregnancy (especially btwn 28–32 weeks gestation).

➤ Recommended dose during 1st trimester 0.8 U/kg/day; 2nd trimester 1.0 U/kg/day; 3rd trimester 1.2 U/kg/day

➤ Insulin-resistant DM type 2 pts may require much higher doses of insulin, while insulin-dependent DM type 1 pts may require much less insulin.

➤ Total dose divided w/ 2/3 administered in fasting state as 2/3 NPH & 1/3 rapid-acting insulin & remaining 1/3 of total dose given as 1/2 rapid-acting insulin at evening meal & 1/2 at bedtime as NPH

➤ Rapid-acting insulin (regular & lispro)
  • Regular insulin should be given 30 minutes before eating & insulin lispro should be given 10–15 minutes before eating because of rapid onset of action.
  • Insulin lispro improves compliance but can lead to severe hypoglycemia if pt is unprepared.
  • Studies have shown pts treated w/ insulin lispro had lower $HgbA_{1C}$ & higher satisfaction.

➤ Intermediate-acting insulin (NPH & lente)
  • Usually given before breakfast w/ short-acting insulin & before evening meal or at bedtime
  • Bedtime dosing may be preferable since decreases risk of nocturnal hypoglycemia that can occur when given prior to evening meal

➤ Long-acting insulin (ultralente & glargine)
  • Administered 1 or 2 times daily
  • Long duration of action makes it difficult to determine timing.
  • Glargine is a recently developed insulin analog produced w/ recombinant DNA technology.
  • Experience w/ glargine in pregnancy is limited; many diabetologists prefer glargine because of smooth absorption rate, providing for basal insulin requirements.

➤ Regular U-500 insulin (500 U/mL)
  • Pts who are highly insulin-resistant can use this concentrated insulin.
  • Usually recommended for pts who require >200 U/day

➤ Insulin pumps
  • Usually 50–60% of total daily dose is administered as continuous basal rate, while boluses before meals & snacks account for 20–50% of daily dose.

- Requires pt who is highly motivated & compliant
- Pump associated w/ more flexible lifestyle, improved satisfaction, decrease in severe hypoglycemia & better control of early-morning hyperglycemia

■ Monitoring
  ➤ Pt should check fasting glucose level preprandial, 1 hour or 2 hours after each meal & at bedtime for a total of 7 checks each day.
  ➤ If fasting capillary glucose is $\geq$95 mg/dL, the 1-hour is $\geq$130–140 mg/dL or the 2-hour is $\geq$120 mg/dL, then additional intervention is required (diet & exercise compliance should be reviewed, then insulin can be instituted).
  ➤ During the night, the blood glucose should not be $\leq$60 mg/dL.
  ➤ Mean capillary glucose levels should be maintained at 100 mg/dL & HgbA$_{1C}$ $\leq$6%.
  ➤ Pts w/ diet-controlled GDM should be seen every 1–2 weeks until 36 weeks gestation, weekly thereafter.
  ➤ At 40 weeks gestation, pts get twice-weekly nonstress tests.
  ➤ Pts w/ GDM who have had a history of stillborn fetus or hypertension are started on twice-weekly nonstress tests at 32 weeks gestation.
  ➤ If estimated fetal weight $\geq$4,500 g, then C-section is considered to reduce risk of shoulder dystocia.
  ➤ Poorly controlled pts may require elective delivery at 38–39 weeks gestation; if delivery is before 39 weeks, amniocentesis may be used to assess fetal lung maturity.
  ➤ While in labor, pts who require insulin or glyburide should have blood glucose checked every 1–2 hours; goal glucose level is $\leq$110 mg/dL.
  ➤ After birth, neonate should be monitored for hypoglycemia, hypocalcemia, hyperbilirubinemia.

■ Diabetic ketoacidosis (DKA)
  ➤ Occurs in 1–3% of all pregnancies complicated by DM type 1
  ➤ Can be seen at glucose levels exceeding 200 mg/dL
  ➤ Associated w/ infections or poor compliance w/ treatment, also seen in previously undiagnosed, new-onset GDM
    - DKA & hyperglycemia can lead to decreased intravascular volume, decreased serum sodium & potassium levels & acidosis, all of which can lead to cardiovascular collapse & shock.
    - Treatment focused on volume replacement & insulin therapy

- Start normal saline at rate of 1,000 mL/hr & IV insulin given initially as a bolus dose of 5–10 U, followed by insulin infusion of 1–5 U/hr.
- When glucose levels are ≤250 mg/dL, D5 1/2 NS should be used while continuing insulin infusion.
- If glucose levels fall <25% over 2 hours, double insulin infusion rate.
- Potassium should be measured frequently; if normal or reduced, start infusion rate of 15–20 mEq/hr; if elevated, wait until level is in normal range & normal kidney function confirmation w/ urine output & normal creatinine before considering repletion.
- Use bicarbonate only if severe acidosis (pH < 7.1), since rapid normalization of maternal pH & pCO_2 can increase fetal pCO_2 & reduce oxygen delivery to fetal tissues; use 1.5 ampules in 1 L of 1/2 normal saline if needed.

■ Hyperosmolar hyperglycemic nonketotic coma (HONK): occurs predominantly in pts w/ DM type 2
  ➤ Hyperglycemia (often >600 mg/dL), hyperosmolarity (>310 mOsm) & moderate azotemia (BUN 70–90 mg/dL) w/o ketonemia or significant acidosis
  ➤ Absence of significant ketosis may indicate inhibition of lipolysis by hyperosmolarity or low levels of insulin.
  ➤ Fluid administration is important.
   - If initial serum osmolarity is <320 mOsm/L, give 2–3 L of NS.
   - If serum osmolarity >320 mOsm/L, may need to use hypotonic crystalloid initially & change to isotonic crystalloid when serum osmolarity <320 mOsm/L
   - Use hypotonic crystalloid w/ caution as rapid decrease of serum osmolarity can lead to cerebral edema.
   - If pt is hypotensive but cannot tolerate aggressive fluid administration, colloids or vasopressors may be used.
   - Administer D5 when plasma glucose is <250 mg/dL.
  ➤ Give bolus of regular insulin & begin at a low-dose continuous infusion; if no decrease in glucose level occurs over the first 2–4 hours, increase the insulin infusion rate every hour until a response occurs.
  ➤ Pts w/ DM type 2 are highly insulin-resistant & will require high doses of insulin.
  ➤ Potassium chloride can be given as part of fluid regimen; monitor levels closely because levels will drop w/ hydration & as acidosis is corrected.

➤ Do not give bicarbonate unless lactic acidosis leads to pH < 7.0 (acidosis in this setting is not from ketoacidosis, but poor perfusion).

Anesthetic Management
- Obtain thorough preanesthetic evaluation, history & physical, looking for acute & chronic complications of DM.
- Labor mgt for GDM pts controlled on diet alone or <0.5 units/kg/day of insulin
  ➤ Monitor glucose every 1–2 hours; goal to titrate IV insulin & glucose so that maternal blood glucose concentration is 70–100 mg/dL.
  ➤ If pt is on insulin drip, check glucose level every hour.
- Maternal insulin requirements decrease w/ onset of labor, increase during 2nd stage of labor & decrease markedly during early postpartum period.
- IV insulin therapy is the most flexible method of treatment during labor; subcutaneous insulin therapy may increase risk of maternal hypoglycemia.
- Other systemic mgt
  ➤ If pt has complications from DM (coronary, cerebral, peripheral vascular, renal, GI or autonomic system), these must also be managed during delivery or surgery.
- Pain has been demonstrated to impair insulin sensitivity by affecting non-oxidative glucose metabolism.
  ➤ Data suggest glucose regulation can be improved w/ better control of pain.
    • In a study comparing epidural & general anesthesia, attenuation of the hyperglycemic response to abdominal surgery was observed through modification of glucose production w/o affecting glucose utilization.
    • Protein metabolism was not influenced by epidural blockade.
    • Neuraxial analgesia may be beneficial to parturients w/ DM.
- Regional anesthesia
  ➤ Neuraxial blockade may lead to decreased uteroplacental blood flow, which is accompanied by possibility of cardiovascular pathology & autonomic instability; must prevent hypotension
  ➤ A study showed that w/ strict observation & reaction to maternal BP, volume expansion w/ a non-dextrose-containing solution & maternal glucose control, spinal or epidural was not associated w/ fetal acidosis & is safe for pts w/ DM.

➤ Pts w/ evidence of autonomic dysfunction may benefit from more frequent BP determinations & more vigorous IV hydration before & during regional anesthesia.

■ General anesthesia
➤ No studies have compared relative maternal safety of general vs. regional anesthesia in pregnant diabetic pts.
➤ Consider impaired counterregulatory hormone responses to hypoglycemia, limited atlanto-occipital joint extension & gastroparesis.
➤ Pre-op evidence of autonomic cardiovascular dysfunction is predictive of need for vasopressor support during general anesthesia.

CAVEATS & PEARLS
■ Determine whether pt has GDM or DM type 1 or 2.
■ Preanesthetic evaluation w/ focus on identification of acute & chronic complications of DM, especially DKA, HONK & cardiovascular & renal complications
■ DM is associated w/ increased incidence of polyhydramnios, preterm labor, preeclampsia, fetal macrosomia, C-section.
■ Pts w/ autonomic dysfunction should have more aggressive IV hydration & frequent BP monitoring before & during labor when regional anesthesia is used.
■ Closely monitor maternal blood glucose levels.
■ Insulin requirements decrease during 1st stage of labor, increase during 2nd stage & decrease after delivery.
■ Use IV glucose & insulin to titrate maternal blood glucose to 70–90 mg/dL.
■ Avoiding maternal hyperglycemia intrapartum will prevent fetal hyperglycemia & reduce likelihood of neonatal hypoglycemia.

CHECKLIST
N/A

DILATION & CURETTAGE/EVACUATION (D&C, D&E)

JAMES WILLIAMS, MD
RODGER WHITE, MD

FUNDAMENTAL KNOWLEDGE
Clinical scenarios include abortion/miscarriage, retained products of conception (POC), intrauterine fetal demise (IUFD).

Types of spontaneous abortion/miscarriage

- Threatened = uterine bleeding w/o cervical dilation before 20 weeks gestation
- Inevitable = cervical dilation or rupture of membranes w/o expulsion of the fetus
- Complete = spontaneous expulsion of fetus & placenta
- Incomplete = partial expulsion of uterine contents
- Missed = fetal death goes unrecognized for several weeks

STUDIES

Dictated by clinical scenario; can include type & screen/cross, CBC, coagulation studies

MANAGEMENT/INTERVENTIONS

General considerations

- Ensure adequate intravascular volume & consider IV hydration w/ 1–2 L crystalloid prior to regional anesthesia.
- Standard monitors unless clinical scenario dictates invasive monitoring.
- Single IV catheter typically sufficient, but consider large-bore IV access if pt has had or is at risk for substantial blood loss.

MAC

- Paracervical block (especially if cervix not dilated)
- IV sedation/anxiolysis typically w/ benzodiazepines, short-acting opioids, possibly propofol

Spinal

- T8–10 level
- Bupivacaine 10 mg +/– intrathecal opoid (fentanyl 10–25 mcg)
- Lidocaine not currently used by most practitioners because of high incidence of transient radicular irritation.
- Mepivacaine 45–60 mg (hyperbaric) is another option.
- "Saddle block"

Epidural

- Lumbar placement for T8–T10 level
- Incremental dosing w/ 15–18 mL 2% lidocaine

General anesthesia

- Rapid sequence induction if full stomach
- Typical induction agents are propofol & thiopental, but consider ketamine or etomidate if hemodynamically unstable.
- Mask/LMA if no contraindications

■ Avoid high concentrations of volatile anesthetic (>0.5 MAC) to prevent bleeding & uterine atony.

Anesthetic adjuncts
■ Oxytocin
■ Ergots

CAVEATS AND PEARLS
■ Sepsis may complicate retained POC or spontaneous abortion.
■ Coagulation defects including DIC can accompany retained POC & IUFD.
■ If cervix dilated &/or early gestation, procedure can be well tolerated w/ MAC.
■ 2nd trimester D&Es have increased risk of bleeding/uterine perforation.
■ Avoid regional anesthesia if concern for decreased intravascular volume, sepsis or coagulopathy.
■ Rhogam for Rh-negative pts
■ Intrathecal lidocaine is being used less frequently due to concern for transient neurologic symptoms.

CHECKLIST
■ Full pre-op evaluation
■ Awareness of serious perioperative complications, including uterine perforation, sepsis & DIC

DISSEMINATED INTRAVASCULAR COAGULATION (DIC)

JEANNA VIOLA, MD
JANE BALLANTYNE, MD

FUNDAMENTAL KNOWLEDGE
■ Platelets & procoagulant proteins are consumed following a systemic insult.
■ Homeostasis of clotting becomes dysregulated: either thrombosis or bleeding may result.
■ There are many inciting factors for DIC, but the common thread is thrombin formation:
  ➤ Caused by injury of either endothelium or tissues
  ➤ Kinin & complement cascades are activated, leading to vascular permeability & vasodilation.

- ➤ Fibrin deposited within the microvasculature is thought to cause end-organ damage.
- ■ Pregnancy itself is a state of low-grade, self-limited DIC; levels of all of the factors in the clotting cascade increase & levels of antithrombin III decrease.
- ■ Most common triggers of DIC in pregnancy:
  - ➤ Placental abruption: most common cause of DIC
    - Coagulopathy results from local extravascular clotting protein consumption & systemic activation of fibrin.
    - Severity of hemodynamic instability correlates w/ amount of abruption.
    - DIC is usually self-limited, but pts are at greater risk of post-partum hemorrhage.
  - ➤ Pre-eclampsia/eclampsia syndrome: chronic, subclinical coagulopathy
    - Increased fibrin deposits in glomerular, hepatic & placental microvessels
    - Increased levels of fibrin degradation products & decreased AT III activity
    - Thrombocytopenia may be the only clinical manifestation.
  - ➤ Amniotic fluid embolism: likely to result in hemodynamic collapse
    - Amniotic fluid stimulates conversion of fibrinogen & activates platelets.
    - Maternal mortality is extremely high, usually within hours.
    - Most patients go on to develop DIC if they survive the initial CV insult.
  - ➤ Gram-negative sepsis
    - Triggered by circulating endotoxins, enhanced in pregnancy
    - Coagulopathy can worsen the state of shock as kinins, histamine, serotonin & prostaglandins are released.
    - Fibrinogen production initially increases, but consumptive coagulopathy (due to hypofibrinogenemia) ensues & thrombocytopenia may be marked.

STUDIES

- ■ Clinical observation of bleeding from operative & venipuncture sites, associated w/ hypotension & renal failure
- ■ Chronic low-grade DIC may manifest as easy bruising, gingival bleeding or epistaxis.

- Thrombocytopenia: 50% of pts will have a plt count <50,000.
- BT, PT, PTT are all elevated due to inadequate levels of coagulation proteins, especially factor V.
- Thrombin time is prolonged due to hypofibrinogenemia & fibrin degradation products (FDPs).
- FDPs are normally increased (D-dimer).
- Other tests include measurement of the concentration of fibrinopeptides & plasmin-antiplasmin complexes & TEG (thromboelastogram).

MANAGEMENT/INTERVENTIONS
- Eliminate the cause.
- Replenish consumed factors, such as platelets & fibrinogen:
  - Each unit of platelets raises plt count 5–10,000.
  - FFP (fibrinogen levels should rise 10–20 mg/dL per unit transfused)
  - Cryoprecipitate
    - Same amount of fibrinogen as FFP in 1/3 amount of volume
    - Used when close mgt of volume control is required.
- Frequent (hourly) measurements of plt counts & fibrinogen levels
  - Goal: plt >50,000, fibrinogen >100 mg/dL
- Transfuse PRBCs if hemorrhage occurs (goal Hct >30).
- Maintain hemodynamic stability w/ volume; avoid hypovolemia.
- Left uterine displacement is the preferred pt position.
- Normothermia is also important, as hypothermia exacerbates coagulopathy.
- Administration of heparin blocks the formation of thrombin & may slow consumption enough to establish sufficient concentrations of platelets, fibrinogen & other hemostatic factors.
- Consider adjunct therapies:
  - Replacement of activated protein C (anticoagulant, protects against endotoxin shock)
  - Antifibrinolytic agents such as aminocaproic acid or tranexamic acid, aprotinin (inactivates plasmin)
  - Use these agents w/ care as fibrinolysis may be the only mechanism maintaining patency of vessels, and stopping fibrinolysis may lead to microvascular occlusion.
- In potential for DIC (pre-eclampsia, infection, retained dead fetus, etc.), early epidural placement is appropriate prior to the deterioration of coagulation, provided that the plt count is >75,000.

- If the pt develops significant coagulopathy, the epidural catheter is then left in place until coagulation studies normalize & the plt count is >75,000.
- Regional anesthesia is contraindicated w/ a documented coagulopathy.
- Perform C-section only when blood products are in the room; general anesthesia w/ RSI required.
- Careful intubation is necessary to avoid airway hematoma.
- With hypovolemia, reduce dose of barbiturate or ketamine induction is suggested w/ a minimal amount of volatile as maintenance to preserve hemodynamic stability.
- Be aware of DIC-induced renal or hepatic insufficiency; dose drugs accordingly.
- Keep temp above 34C to avoid further coagulopathy from hypothermia.
- An arterial line is helpful as serial blood samples will be needed. PA line is also sometimes needed to monitor hemodynamic status.

CAVEATS AND PEARLS
- Transfuse carefully, as components may facilitate the consumptive process.
- Fibrinogen is an acute phase reactant; this test alone is not an accurate diagnostic test.
- DIC is usually brought on in pregnancy by fetal pathology. The fetus will be affected by the hemodynamic compromise & coagulopathy or thrombosis that occurs in the mother.

CHECKLIST
- Are precipitating causes being treated?
- Prepare for adequate level of invasive monitoring relative to the severity of the case.
- Obtain adequate IV access.
- Careful exam of airway to prepare for GETA
- Warm OR

EATING DISORDERS

LATA POTTURI, MD
ADELE VIGUERA, MD

FUNDAMENTAL KNOWLEDGE
- *DSM IV Diagnostic criteria*

Diagnostic criteria for anorexia nervosa

A. Refusal to maintain body weight at or above a minimally normal weight for age & height (e.g., weight loss leading to maintenance of body weight <85% of that expected or a BMI of <17.5); or failure to make expected weight gain during periods of growth, leading to body weight <85% of that expected)

B. Intense fear of gaining weight or becoming fat, even though underweight

C. Disturbance in the way in which one's body weight or shape is experienced, undue influence of body weight or shape on self-evaluation, or denial of the seriousness of the current low body weight

D. In postmenarchal females, amenorrhea, i.e., the absence of at least three consecutive menstrual cycles. (A woman is considered to have amenorrhea if her periods occur only following hormone, e.g., estrogen, administration. Obviously, this is not applicable during pregnancy.)

Diagnostic criteria for bulimia nervosa

A. Recurrent episodes of binge eating. An episode of binge eating is characterized by both of the following:
   (1) eating, in a discrete period of time (e.g., within any 2-hour period), an amount of food that is definitely larger than most people would eat during a similar period of time & under similar circumstances.
   (2) a sense of lack of control over eating during the episode (i.e., a feeling that one cannot stop eating or control what or how much one is eating)

B. Recurrent inappropriate compensatory behavior in order to prevent weight gain, such as self-induced vomiting, misuse of laxatives, diuretics, enemas, or other medications, fasting, or excessive exercise

C. The binge eating & inappropriate compensatory behaviors both occur, on average, at least twice a week for 3 months.

D. Self-evaluation is unduly influenced by body shape & weight.

E. The disturbance does not occur exclusively during episodes of Anorexia Nervosa.

Diagnostic criteria for binge eating disorder

A. Recurrent episodes of binge eating. An episode of binge eating is characterized by both of the following:
   (1) eating, in a discrete period of time (e.g., within any 2-hour period), an amount of food that is definitely larger than most

people would eat in a similar period of time under similar circumstances.

(2) a sense of lack of control over eating during the episode (i.e., feeling that one cannot stop eating or control what or how much one is eating)

B. The binge-eating episodes are associated w/ 3 (or more) of the following:

   (1) eating much more rapidly than normal
   (2) eating until feeling uncomfortably full
   (3) eating large amounts of food when not feeling physically hungry
   (4) eating alone because of being embarrassed by how much one is eating
   (5) feeling disgusted w/ oneself, depressed, or very guilty after overeating

C. Marked distress regarding binge eating is present.

D. The binge eating occurs, on average, at least 2 days a week for 6 months.

E. The binge eating is not associated w/ the regular use of inappropriate compensatory behaviors (e.g., purging, fasting, excessive exercise) & does not occur exclusively during the course of Anorexia Nervosa or Bulimia Nervosa.

Course during pregnancy/postpartum

Many pregnant women express concerns about gaining weight & maintaining their figure. When there has been a history of an eating disorder, the weight gain & body shape changes accompanying pregnancy can provoke extreme distress. Very little is known about the impact of pregnancy on women w/ anorexia nervosa or bulimia nervosa. The evidence that is available suggests that serious eating disorders are rarely precipitated during pregnancy. Bulimic symptoms frequently improve temporarily during pregnancy, while the course of anorexia is less vulnerable to change. There is an association btwn eating disorders & a variety of complications of pregnancy, including fetal growth restriction, malnutrition & increased rates of hyperemesis gravidarum, miscarriage, preterm birth, C-sections & postpartum depression. However, most pregnancies in women w/ eating disorders yield healthy term babies.

Meds commonly used in treatment

Meds are used in conjunction w/ psychotherapy to help treat the depression, anxiety &/or obsessions associated w/ disordered eating habits.

■ SSRIs

- TCAs
- Antipsychotics

Fetal issues & medications

All psychotropic meds cross the placenta. The risks of treating a pregnant pt w/ psychotropic meds must be weighed against potentially harmful effects to the fetus. However, the best risk/benefit assessment should be made on an individual basis depending on the pt's history & illness severity & potential risks associated w/ no treatment. Potential risks of no treatment include the pt not following up w/ prenatal care or the pt engaging in high-risk behaviors such as substance abuse, smoking & other reckless behaviors. Studies have also shown that untreated anxiety or depression in pregnancy is associated w/ a high risk for neonatal complications, including low birthweight & preterm delivery.

Studies consistently report no increased risk of fetal malformations in women taking SSRIs or TCAs. Studies have shown no increased risk for major malformations w/ conventional antipsychotics. However, reproductive safety data on the newer atypical antipsychotics remain too limited to make any definitive conclusions. Neonates exposed to antipsychotics have been reported to have transient effects such as hypotension, extrapyramidal symptoms, sedation, tachycardia, restlessness, dystonic & parkinsonian movements.

STUDIES

- History & physical

In addition to a routine history & physical, ask specific questions regarding the history of the pt's eating disorder. Ask about body image, weight gain, eating habits & "compensatory behaviors" such as purging or laxative use during pregnancy. Find out if the pt has been receiving counseling or has been taking psychiatric medications for her illness. Note the duration of medication therapy & timing of the pt's last dose.

- Lab tests

The pt w/ an eating disorder is at high risk for malnutrition & electrolyte derangement. Along w/ routine peripartum lab studies, a full chemistry panel w/ liver function tests, coagulation profile, & an albumin level should be checked.

> EKG

A baseline EKG should be checked in any pt w/ an eating disorder w/ electrolyte abnormalities or a history of cardiac conduction abnormalities (ie, palpitations or arrhythmias). Additionally, a number of conduction abnormalities have been noted in pts on TCAs. It may be worthwhile to check an EKG or analyze the pt's rhythm on a cardiac monitor.

MANAGEMENT & INTERVENTIONS

■ Psychosocial approach to the pt: The pt w/ an eating disorder may feel depressed about weight gain or change in body image during pregnancy. Conversely, she may feel guilty about her behaviors & possible adverse effects on her fetus. Approach the pt in a reassuring manner free of judgment. Social supports & family members should be involved as deemed appropriate.

➤ Tailoring anesthetic plan: Take care when administering regional or general anesthesia to the pt w/ an eating disorder. Chronic malnutrition can cause electrolyte & coagulation abnormalities. Awareness of potential drug interactions will aid in developing a safe anesthetic plan.

➤ Informed consent: Determine the pt's ability to give informed consent.

CAVEATS & PEARLS

■ Eating disorders during pregnancy increase the risk for complications during pregnancy, but most women w/ eating disorders have healthy term babies.

■ Pts w/ eating disorders are at high risk for malnutrition & electrolyte derangements.

CHECKLIST

■ Be familiar w/ the diagnostic criteria for eating disorders.

■ Know what med the pt is taking & when her last dose was.

■ Consider checking an EKG or analyzing cardiac rhythm in pts taking TCAs.

ECT DURING PREGNANCY

LATA POTTURI, MD
ADELE VIGUERA, MD

FUNDAMENTAL KNOWLEDGE

■ Common psychiatric diagnoses

ECT can be used for treating the pregnant pt w/ depression, mania, catatonia or schizophrenia.

➤ Basics of ECT

ECT acts via an induced seizure. This is thought to release norepinephrine, serotonin & dopamine in the brain stem. The pt is given a short-acting sedative-hypnotic, usually propofol or thiopental, &

succinylcholine for muscle relaxation. Paralysis suppresses the peripheral manifestations of the seizure, protecting the pt from potential injury caused by muscular contractions & other injuries induced by the seizure. The pt is ventilated w/ 100% oxygen through an Ambu bag & hyperventilated before the electrical stimulus.

Physiologic changes that can occur during ECT include hypotension & bradycardia, followed by sympathetic hyperactivity, tachycardia & a rise in BP. These changes are transient & usually resolve quickly. Side effects include confusion, headache, nausea, myalgias & anterograde amnesia following the treatment. These side effects in general clear over several weeks but can take up to 6 months to resolve. The mortality rate associated w/ ECT is approximately 4 per 100,000 treatments & is usually cardiac in origin.

■ Special considerations during pregnancy/postpartum
  ➤ Safety: ECT has few side effects in pregnancy & may actually be safer than untreated psychiatric illness or treatment w/ a medication that can potentially be teratogenic.
  ➤ Potential risks to fetus & mother: The complications of ECT were evaluated in a retrospective study by Miller (1994), who reviewed the literature from 1942 to 1991. The most common complication found was fetal cardiac arrhythmia. In each case, the arrhythmias were self-limited & a healthy baby was ultimately delivered. Five cases of vaginal bleeding, 2 cases of uterine contraction, 3 cases of abdominal pain, 4 cases of premature labor, 5 miscarriages & 3 cases of stillbirth were found. However, the author noted that ECT was likely not the causative factor in these cases, & in the cases not involving miscarriage or stillbirth, a healthy infant was born. Currently, there is no definitive evidence that ECT is harmful to the fetus in utero.

The anesthetic agents commonly used during ECT have been studied w/ regard to potential complications. Succinylcholine is the paralytic most commonly used during ECT. It does not cross the placenta in appreciable amounts. Pseudocholinesterase, the enzyme that deactivates succinylcholine, is present in lower levels during pregnancy. Additionally, 4% of the general population is pseudocholinesterase deficient. Studies have shown prolonged apnea & the need for continuous ventilation among mothers undergoing C-section & exposed to succinylcholine in the 3rd trimester. The neonates in these cases had low Apgar scores & respiratory depression.

To control excessive pharyngeal secretions & bradycardia, anticholinergic agents, usually atropine or glycopyrrolate, are often used.

Studies have shown that women receiving atropine had more congenital malformations than women receiving glycopyrrolate. However, women who received atropine had no higher incidence of malformations than women in the general public. Use of these drugs during C-section also did not result in an increased rate of complications.

With regard to neonatal complications, studies have not proven that ECT confers a teratogenic risk or has a long-term effect on childhood development.

In general, complications of ECT are infrequent & self-limited. Clinicians should be aware of medication side effects. Atropine can cause tachycardia in the fetus & decrease variability in fetal heart rate. Thiopental can also decrease fetal heart rate beat-to-beat variability. To decrease the risk of fetal arrhythmias, avoid atropine, maximize oxygenation, avoid extreme hyperventilation & elevate the right hip for uterine displacement. Fetal monitoring during ECT can also be considered.

➤ Potential benefits: Along w/ a psychiatrist, if an obstetrician & an anesthesiologist are part of the team caring for the pt & all safety guidelines are followed, ECT appears to be a very safe & effective treatment for refractory psychiatric disorders in pregnant women.

STUDIES

■ History & physical: In addition to a thorough history & physical, ask pt about all prenatal psychiatric diagnoses. How has her illness been managed prior to pregnancy & during pregnancy? Ask about psychological counseling, psychiatric treatment & all meds she has taken during pregnancy. Ask about the pt's prior experience w/ ECT & any problems she may have encountered.

➤ Lab tests: When applicable, check serum medication level & a full electrolyte panel. Since pts receiving ECT are usually given succinylcholine, it may be useful to check serum potassium levels & serum creatinine if abnormalities in these levels are suspected.

➤ EKG: A number of conduction abnormalities have been noted in pts on TCAs. It may be worthwhile to check an EKG or analyze the pt's rhythm on a cardiac monitor. Barring another indication, pts taking other psychotropic medications do not need a baseline EKG.

MANAGEMENT & INTERVENTIONS

■ Anesthetic plan: Propofol or thiopental is used to put the pt to sleep & succinylcholine is used for paralysis. Atropine or glycopyrrolate is used to control secretions & minimize bradycardia. The pt is ventilated w/ 100% oxygen & hyperventilated before the electrical stimulus is administered. Seizure threshold can be decreased by estrogen & increased by progesterone. Changes in the ratio of hormone levels during pregnancy can affect seizure threshold, thereby altering the optimal stimulus needed for administering ECT. The first treatment should be initiated w/ standard stimulus parameters & subsequent treatments should be adjusted accordingly.

➤ Full stomach/RSI considerations: Prolonged gastric emptying time during pregnancy increases the risk for aspiration during anesthesia. Intubation is an option to prevent this; however, in general, pregnant women can be difficult to intubate secondary to weight gain, edema of the airway & hypervascularity. A nonparticulate antacid such as sodium citrate can be administered prior to ECT to raise gastric pH & decrease the risk of aspiration pneumonitis.

➤ Informed consent: Determine the pt's ability to give informed consent.

CAVEATS & PEARLS

■ ECT acts via an induced seizure that is thought to release various neurotransmitters.

■ Side effects include confusion, headache, nausea, myalgias & anterograde amnesia. These can take several weeks to 6 months to resolve.

■ ECT may be safer than untreated psychiatric illness or treatment w/ a potentially teratogenic medication during pregnancy.

■ The most common fetal complication is cardiac arrhythmia. To decrease the risk of arrhythmias, avoid atropine, maximize oxygenation, avoid extreme hyperventilation & elevate the right hip for uterine displacement.

■ Increased progesterone levels found during pregnancy can increase the seizure threshold.

■ Pregnant women have delayed gastric emptying times, which can increase the risk for aspiration during anesthesia.

CHECKLIST

■ Be aware of pt's psychiatric disorder.

■ Know possible physiologic changes that can occur during ECT.

■ Inform pt of potential maternal & fetal complications of ECT.

■ Use succinylcholine carefully in pregnant pts, as pseudocholinesterase levels are decreased.

- Atropine increases the risk of fetal cardiac arrhythmias & causes more birth defects than glycopyrrolate. Use w/ caution.
- Consider fetal cardiac monitoring during ECT.
- Know what meds the pt is taking & when her last dose was.
- Consider checking an EKG or analyzing cardiac rhythm in pts taking TCAs.
- The seizure threshold may be increased in pregnant women & a higher-than-usual stimulus may be needed to induce a seizure.
- Consider giving a non-particulate antacid to decrease the risk of aspiration pneumonitis during anesthesia.

EPIDURAL ABSCESS

SISSELA PARK, MD
LAURA RILEY, MD

FUNDAMENTAL KNOWLEDGE

- Rare
- Diagnosis is difficult because of low frequency.
- Symptoms
  - Back pain
    - Seen first
    - Most important symptom
    - Severe
    - May appear suddenly or progressively
  - Tenderness w/ percussion of spine
  - Within a week of onset of a back pain
    - Root pain
    - Weakness
    - Paralysis
  - Neurologic problems may appear suddenly or gradually & are often irreversible.
  - Pt may also have:
    - Headache
    - Fever & chills
    - Leukocytosis
- Reports suggest that epidural infections are usually secondary to trauma, surgical procedures or hematogenous spread rather than from regional anesthesia.
- No documented connection btwn epidural vein puncture in a febrile pt & the development of an epidural abscess

■ DDx is extensive since there are many causes of back pain. Consider:
  ➤ Disc disease
  ➤ Bony disease
  ➤ Metastatic tumors
  ➤ Meningitis
  ➤ Vertebral diskitis
  ➤ Osteomyelitis
  ➤ Herpes zoster

Complications
■ Abscess can expand longitudinally in the epidural space, causing damage to the spinal cord by:
  ➤ Direct compression
  ➤ Interruption of arterial blood supply
  ➤ Focal vasculitis
  ➤ Thrombosis & thrombophlebitis of nearby veins
  ➤ Bacterial toxins
  ➤ Mediators of inflammation
  ➤ These factors can act at the same time.

STUDIES
■ MRI is the method of choice for diagnosis.
  ➤ Positive early in the course of infection
  ➤ Offers the best imaging of inflammatory signs
■ CT scan w/ gadolinium contrast is also useful.
■ Routine blood tests are rarely beneficial.
■ X-rays of the spine are seldom helpful.
■ Once epidural abscess is suspected, attempt to culture causative organism from blood, abscess or CSF.

MANAGEMENT/INTERVENTIONS
■ Two goals of therapy
  ➤ Decrease size of, then eliminate, the inflammatory mass.
  ➤ Eliminate causative organism.
■ Therapy consists of aspiration, drainage & antibiotics.
■ Early (within 24 hours of admission) surgical decompression & drainage is crucial to improve overall prognosis.
■ If causative organism is known, target antibiotic therapy.
■ If organism is not known, use antibiotics that cover staphylococci, streptococci & gram-negative bacilli.
  ➤ Nafcillin 1.5 g IV q4h w/ cefotaxime 2 g IV q6h plus metronidazole 500 mg IV q6h

> Substitute vancomycin 1 g IV q12h for nafcillin if pt has a penicillin allergy.
> Can also use ticarcillin-clavulanate 3.1 g IV q6h
- Antibiotics should be continued for 4–6 weeks.

CAVEATS & PEARLS
- Postpartum infection = temp > 100.4 degrees F, 24 hours after delivery
- Epidural abscess
  > Initial symptom is back pain followed by root pain, weakness & paralysis.
  > MRI is the best method of diagnosis.
  > Treatment consists of aspiration, drainage & antibiotics.

CHECKLIST
- With postpartum fever, determine & treat cause.
- Epidural abscess can expand longitudinally in epidural space, damaging the spinal cord.

EPIDURAL ANALGESIA

KRISTEN STADLANDER, MD; MAY PIAN-SMITH, MD; AND LISA LEFFERT, MD

FUNDAMENTAL KNOWLEDGE
See "*Basics of Regional Anesthesia.*"
- Lumbar epidurals for labor are usually placed at the L2–3, L3–4 or L4–5 interspaces.
- Epidurals can be single-shot or continuous infusion through a catheter (most common modality).
- Epidural anesthesia can be slower in onset & may not cause as dense a block as spinal anesthesia, but this is highly dependent on the type & concentration of local anesthetic and/or opiates administered.
- There is controversy over the appropriate time to administer epidural anesthesia in a laboring pt. Take into account the pt's discomfort & the availability of the necessary personnel. The literature has shown that epidural analgesia may prolong labor by roughly 1 hour & may be associated w/ a decrease in the rate of spontaneous vaginal delivery. That being said, it has not been proven that the epidural itself causes a parturient to need a cesarean delivery or assisted vaginal birth. A more lengthy discussion of this topic is beyond the scope of this chapter, but several meta-analyses have been conducted to examine the issue.

Some of the beneficial effects of epidural anesthesia are as follows:

- By alleviating pain, epidurals decrease catecholamine levels, which can have a negative impact on uteroplacental blood flow.
- The mother can more actively participate & be aware during the birthing process w/ an epidural in place (as opposed to under general anesthesia).
- By alleviating pain, epidural anesthesia decreases respiratory alkalosis & maternal hypocarbia. Maternal hypocarbia can have a detrimental effect by shifting the oxyhemoglobin curve to the left, resulting in increased maternal oxygen affinity & reduced fetal oxygen delivery.
- Epidurals can have a beneficial effect in pre-eclamptic pts by decreasing systemic vascular resistance & decreasing BP.
- A well-functioning epidural can be a potentially safer alternative to a general anesthetic in pts who are at a high risk of cesarean section & who may be difficult to intubate. Due to the hyperemia & the edematous state of laboring pts & the often emergent nature of obstetric cesarean deliveries, an otherwise benign airway can become more difficult to secure.

Determinants of the spread of epidural anesthesia

- Pregnancy: A 20–30% reduction in overall dose of local anesthetic is seen in pregnant pts. The proposed explanations for this observation include:
  - ➤ Increased progesterone levels
  - ➤ Pregnancy-related changes in diffusion barriers
  - ➤ Endogenous analgesic systems
- Gravity: Much less important than in spinal anesthesia. However, lateral decubitus & Trendelenburg positions are sometimes used to extend a low or one-sided epidural block.
- Onset of an epidural block is usually faster in the cephalad direction due to the smaller size of the nerve roots. The larger sacral nerve roots are often the last to be blocked & can be sometimes be spared entirely. Injection w/ the pt in the sitting position sometimes facilitates delivery of more anesthetic to the lower lumbar & sacral nerve roots.
- Obesity: Epidural fat as well as engorged epidural veins can displace volume in the epidural space & potentiate spread of block.

Determinants of the duration & onset of epidural anesthesia

- The order of onset of local anesthetic block from fastest onset to slowest is: 3% 2-chloroprocaine, lidocaine, bupivacaine (onset of action of chloroprocaine is related to its high concentration, not pKa).

- The time to 2 dermatome regression (the time for the local anesthetic to wear off by 2 dermatomal levels) is agent-specific. The times are chloroprocaine, 60 minutes; lidocaine, 90–120 minutes, mepivacaine, 120–160 minutes; bupivacaine, 200–240 minutes.

- The speed of onset, duration of block & quality of block are increased by adding 1:200,000 (5 mcg/mL) epinephrine to the local anesthetic. This effect is more apparent w/ lidocaine & chloroprocaine & less w/ bupivacaine & ropivacaine. Phenylephrine is less effective in this capacity. The mechanism of this effect is that the epinephrine constricts blood vessels, preventing the local anesthetic from being taken away from the nerve roots where it exerts its action.

- Adding an opiate (e.g., 50–100 mcg fentanyl) also increases speed of onset, duration & block quality. There is some evidence that chloroprocaine interferes w/ the subsequent effects of epidural opiates, especially morphine.

- Adding sodium bicarbonate to chloroprocaine or lidocaine (in the ratio of 1 mL of 8.4% sodium bicarbonate per 9 mL local anesthetic) decreases the onset time of the block. This effect is a result of an increase in the pH of the local anesthetic mixture, which increases the non-ionized fraction of the drug. It is this un-ionized fraction that can cross the axonal membrane. (Ultimately, the ionized form binds to intracellular receptors.)

- Bupivacaine should not be routinely mixed w/ sodium bicarbonate at doses greater than 0.5 mEq/10 cc (if used at all) as it readily precipitates at a pH > 6.8.

STUDIES
- CBC: The literature is insufficient to assess the predictive value of a platelet count for anesthesia complications in parturients without comorbid illness, or in those w/ pregnancy-induced hypertension.

- ACOG 1999 Practice Bulletin states, "Although limited, data support the safety of epidural anesthesia in patients with platelet counts greater than 100K. In women with gestational thrombocytopenia with platelet counts less than 99K but greater than 50K, epidural anesthesia also may be safe, but its use in such patients will require a consensus among the obstetrician, anesthesiologist, and patients. When platelet counts are less than 50K, epidural anesthesia should not be given."

- Normal coagulation profile
- Exam of the area where the epidural will be administered
- Informed consent w/ full explanation of the procedure & possible complications (headache 1–2%; rarely bleeding, infection, nerve/neck/back injury) & the risk of failed block
- Detailed history & physical highlighting bleeding abnormalities or pre-anesthetic neurologic deficits
- Access to fetal monitoring

MANAGEMENT/INTERVENTIONS

Minimum equipment to perform an epidural anesthetic includes:

- Monitoring equipment, including BP, pulse oximetry, EKG
- A functioning IV to facilitate administration of IV fluids & resuscitative medications
- Airway equipment including a face mask, Ambu bag, oxygen source & emergency intubation equipment & medications
- Suction device.
- A bed capable of Trendelenburg position
- A commercial sterile epidural kit & sterile gloves
- A code cart should be located within reach.

Types of needles & catheters

- Usually a 17-gauge Tuohy or Weiss needle is used. These needles are typically blunted at the end w/ a bevel to allow passage of the epidural catheter. The blunted end lowers the risk of accidental dural puncture should the needle contact the dura. Catheters can be made of stiffer plastic or softer materials that are wire-reinforced. The softer catheters are often preferred as they are less likely to enter an epidural vessel or to cause paresthesias.

Technique for placing an epidural catheter

- Check w/ nurse & OB staff to ensure readiness.
- Infuse 250–500 cc-1 L NS/LR through functioning IV.
- Have ephedrine or phenylephrine prepared in the event of hypotension.
- Make sure BP, EKG & pulse oximeter are functioning & emergency equipment is ready.
- Administer 30 cc sodium citrate (Bicitra) orally to the pt.
- Have pt assume lateral or sitting position.
- Palpate the pt's back to find optimal interspace.
- Prep/drape w/ sterile technique, assemble epidural tray, & numb the area w/ the smaller-gauge, local anesthetic needle.

- Enter epidural space by either the "loss of resistance" technique or "hanging drop" method.
- Thread catheter. If a paresthesia occurs & is transient, proceed w/ threading the catheter. Consider injecting 2–3 cc of preservative-free NS through the catheter to confirm that the paresthesia does not recur. If a paresthesia is persistent or particularly painful, withdraw the needle & the catheter at the same time. Before proceeding w/ another attempt, document that the paresthesia has completely resolved.
- Thread 4–5 cm of the catheter into the epidural space to minimize the chance that the block will be one-sided & to maximize the chance that a sufficient length of catheter will remain in the pt's back. Remove the needle w/ the catheter left in place.
- Aspirate catheter, looking for blood or CSF, & then administer test dose.
- If test dose is negative, use a sterile dressing & tape to affix catheter securely to the pt's back; laboring pts are active. Label catheter to avoid epidural administration of IV medications. Administer loading dose of epidural anesthesia in small, incremental doses.
- Monitor BP every 2–3 minutes in the first 10 minutes & then every 5–15 minutes thereafter.
- Maintain pt w/ uterine displacement, switching sides to enhance the even distribution of local anesthetic.
- Treat hypotension as needed w/ pressors (ephedrine, phenylephrine), IV fluids & changes in position.

Ways to access the epidural space

- Loss of resistance: In this method, the epidural needle w/ stylet is advanced between 2 vertebrae (usually midline) until either the interspinous ligament or the ligamentum flavum is encountered (signaled by increased tissue resistance). At this point the stylet is removed & a plastic or glass "loss of resistance" syringe filled w/ 2–8 mL sterile saline or air is attached to the needle. As the needle is slowly advanced through the ligament w/ the nondominant hand, the dominant hand is either continuously or intermittently placing pressure on the syringe, attempting to inject the saline/air. While the needle is in the ligamentum flavum, a resistant or "bouncy" feeling is encountered as the air/saline is compressed. As the tip of the needle enters the epidural space, there is a loss of resistance & the air or saline from the syringe should inject easily. There is some evidence that injecting more than a very small volume of air can lead to a patchy block.

- Hanging drop: This method relies on the fact that negative pressure exists in the epidural space. When the needle is engaged in the interspinous ligament or ligamentum flavum, the stylet is removed & the hub of the needle is filled w/ saline until a drop of liquid remains hanging from the hub. When the needle is advanced & the tip of the needle enters the epidural space, the drop is sucked up into the needle. The epidural catheter is then threaded. This technique can fail if the needle becomes plugged w/ tissue or if the negative pressure is minimized, as is often the case in pregnancy. As a result, the loss of resistance technique is more reliable & more often used in pregnancy.

Use of epidural test dose: The purpose of the test dose is to determine if an intravascular or intrathecal catheter placement has occurred. Always have monitors, emergency airway equipment & pressors available as described above.

- Detecting intravascular placement
  - ➤ Due to the engorgement of epidural blood vessels in late pregnancy, an intravascular epidural placement is more common in the pregnant population. Even when a test dose is negative, the epidural should always be dosed incrementally to minimize the chance of large intravascular injection, which can lead to cardiovascular & respiratory collapse. An intravascular catheter placement may have occurred even when blood cannot be aspirated through the catheter. The low pressure in the epidural space can cause the epidural vein to collapse upon the catheter tip when the anesthesiologist aspirates. Holding the end of the catheter below the level of the pt can be useful to see if blood flows through it under the force of gravity.
  - ➤ One method for employing a test dose is to inject 3 cc of 1.5% lidocaine w/ 1:200,000 (15 mcg) epinephrine through the epidural catheter. If the catheter is intravascular, the pt will typically have an increase in heart rate of 20 bpm or an increase in systolic BP of at least 15 mm Hg within 60 seconds due to the epinephrine. The pt may also report symptoms such as tinnitus, hearing changes or palpitations.
  - ➤ If the pt is on beta-blocker therapy, the heart rate increase may not occur, but the BP increase may still be evident.
  - ➤ Increases in BP & heart rate may be especially difficult to detect in the laboring pt because contractions can cause transient increases in heart rate & BP that can mimic a positive test dose.

Because of this, the test dose is ideally administered immediately following a contraction.

➤ It can be dangerous to administer the epinephrine contained in a standard test dose to a pre-eclamptic pt w/ an already dangerously high systolic BP. Because of this, some practitioners omit the epinephrine from the test dose & rely on the subjective symptoms of intravascular dose of local anesthetic (e.g., metallic taste, perioral numbness, tinnitus, dizziness or sense of impending doom).

■ Detecting intrathecal placement

➤ First the catheter is aspirated to see if CSF is obtained. If no fluid is aspirated, then a test dose (3 cc of 1.5% lidocaine w/ 1:200,000 epinephrine) is administered. If the catheter is intrathecal, the pt should report a loss of sacral motor function (tested by the ability to perform a straight leg raise) 3–4 minutes after administration. Studies have shown that in a few cases, a standard test dose inadvertently administered intrathecally has resulted in a dangerously high spinal level. If the test dose is administered into the epidural space, little or no motor block ensues.

■ If the catheter is determined to be intrathecal (either because of aspiration of CSF or because of a positive test dose), then follow the steps outlined in continuous spinal anesthesia (CSA) section. Alternatively, remove the intrathecal catheter & attempt to place an epidural catheter.

■ Alternative test dose options

➤ 60 mg lidocaine w/ or without epinephrine

➤ 7.5–12.5 mg bupivacaine

➤ 15 mcg epinephrine w/o local anesthetic

➤ 1–2 mL air injected intravascularly may be heard as it goes through the heart w/ a Doppler ultrasound. It is important not to use this option in a patient w/ a known atrial septal defect or patent foramen ovale.

Medications that can be used for epidural analgesia

■ Epidurals can be dosed intermittently or continuously.

■ Epidurals require frequent monitoring of vital signs & motor function.

■ Pt-controlled epidural anesthesia (PCEA) can be used to allow the pt to administer a bolus dose of epidural anesthesia when necessary. Studies have shown that PCEA often results in lower overall local anesthetic requirements & increased satisfaction among parturients.

With careful dosing parameters & an educated pt, undesirable side effects can be avoided.

■ Dosing schedules include:
  ➤ Intermittent lidocaine: 5–10 mL of 0.75–1.5% every 60–90 minutes or bupivacaine 5–10 mL of 0.125–0.375% q1–2h
  ➤ Continuous lidocaine: 8–15 mL/hr of 0.5–1.0%, or bupivacaine: 8–15 mL/hr of 0.0625%-0.25%
  ➤ PCEA = bupivacaine: 0.125% basal rate 4 mL/hr, bolus 4 mL, lockout 20 minutes, maximum hourly dose 16 mL, or bupivacaine 0.125% w/ 2 mcg/mL fentanyl basal rate 6 mL/hr, bolus 3 mL, lockout 10 minutes, maximum hourly dose 24 mL
    • Adding narcotics (fentanyl 1–2 mcg/mL or sufentanil 0.1–0.2 mcg/mL) to the epidural:
    • Results in less motor block
    • Decreases the concentration of local anesthetic needed for adequate analgesia
    • An additional bolus dose of 50 mcg epidural fentanyl (diluted in preservative-free normal saline) can be used to alleviate rectal or back pain caused by the descent of the fetal head
    • The narcotics act on mu receptors in the substantia gelatinosa of the spinal cord. The more lipophilic narcotics such as fentanyl & sufentanil have a fast onset & short duration, while the more hydrophilic narcotics such as morphine have a longer onset & duration.

CAVEATS & PEARLS

■ Contraindications to regional anesthesia
  ➤ Absolute: Pt refusal, uncorrected coagulation disorder, localized infection at proposed injection site, generalized sepsis, increased intracranial pressure, extreme hypovolemia
  ➤ Relative: Demyelinating disease, chronic back pain or lumbar surgery, skin infection close to proposed site, mild hypovolemia, severe aortic or mitral stenosis. Spinals & epidurals have been used safely in some pts w/ demyelinating disease (e.g., multiple sclerosis) & some pts who have undergone back surgery (e.g., laminectomy).
■ Aspirate before injecting medication through an epidural catheter.
■ Monitor carefully for signs of intravascular/intrathecal injection.
■ Maximize pt positioning.
■ If bone is encountered when placing an epidural, withdraw the needle & use the small local needle to "feel" the bony landmarks.

- If the midline approach is used, make sure the epidural needle is engaged firmly in the ligament. If the needle is angled to one direction, there is an increased chance that the epidural catheter may exit the space laterally & deliver the local to only one side.
- An intravascular catheter may have a negative blood aspiration test. For this reason, use a test dose & always dose incrementally.
- Always label & tape the epidural carefully.
- Be vigilant for complications.
- Consider placing an epidural early in labor (an "early epidural") if pt is at particular risk for needing a cesarean section or if pt appears to have a difficult airway.

CHECKLIST

1. Before placing an epidural, review contraindications to regional anesthesia, w/ special attention to bleeding disorders/coagulopathies & pre-existing neurologic deficits.
2. Make sure the parturient has full monitoring, including fetal monitoring (if applicable) & a working IV.
3. Make sure the patient is prehydrated, pressors are readily available & emergency airway & cardiovascular supplies are accessible.
4. Always aspirate before injecting local anesthetic.
5. Obtain informed consent, including all possible complications of an epidural anesthetic & the possibility of a failed block/epidural replacement.

Monitor closely for hypotension & intravascular or intrathecal placement. Catheter removal & prompt treatment w/ pressors, hydration & ventilatory support can prevent disastrous complications (see "*Troubleshooting/Managing Inadequate Regional Anesthesia*").

EPILEPSY

MEREDITH ALBRECHT, MD
MICHELE SZABO, MD

FUNDAMENTAL KNOWLEDGE

Definition

- Group of disorders characterized by chronic, recurrent, paroxysmal changes in neurologic function caused by abnormalities in the electrical activity of the brain

- Seizures are convulsive when accompanied by motor manifestations.
- Seizures can also produce paroxysmal changes in sensory, cognitive or emotional neurologic function.
- Seizures can be generalized, partial or focal.

Epidemiology
- Incidence: 3–5/1,000 births
- Most common neurologic disorder in pregnant women
- Pre-eclampsia is likely not more common in epileptic women.

Pathophysiology
- The pathophysiology is complex & linked to a variety of mechanisms
  - ➤ Diminution of neuronal inhibitory mechanisms
  - ➤ Enhancement of excitatory synaptic mechanisms
  - ➤ Enhancement of endogenous neuronal burst firing
  - ➤ Metabolic abnormalities & anatomic brain lesions
- Results in the hallmark rhythmical & repetitive hypersynchronous discharge of many neurons

Clinical manifestations
- A motor seizure produces either a focal or generalized tonic clonic movement
- Other types of seizures can be manifest by absence spells, paroxysmal change in emotional behavior, abnormal senses.

Effect of pregnancy on epilepsy
- Seizure incidence increases in 25% of pts.
- Highest risk in pts w/ pre-existing poor seizure control
- Status epilepticus incidence: thought not to increase in pregnancy
- Bioavailability of anticonvulsants changed during pregnancy
  - ➤ Alterations in drug protein binding
  - ➤ Clearance & absorption changes
  - ➤ Results in dramatic decreases in free unbound drug & sub-therapeutic drug levels
- Sleep deprivation, stress & alkalosis may contribute to seizure recurrence.

Effect on pregnancy & fetus
- More than 90% of pregnancies among women w/ epilepsy have a favorable outcome.

- Major fetal malformations ("fetal anticonvulsant syndrome") occur in 4–8% of pregnancies; neural tube defects & congenital heart disease are most frequent.
- Minor fetal anomalies occur in 6–20% of pregnancies & include cleft lip & palate, facial dysmorphisms.
- Described w/ all anticonvulsants
- Risk increased w/ polytherapy
- Goal of anticonvulsant therapy is to taper medications to a minimal effective dose & monotherapy.
- Fetus at risk for preterm delivery & IUGR
- Anticonvulsants impair folate absorption.
- Anticonvulsants induce vitamin K deficiency in fetus.
  - Vitamin K deficiency causes hemorrhagic disease of newborn.
  - Prevalence 10% if untreated
- Seizures pose risk to fetus.
  - Persistent generalized tonic-clonic seizure causes fetal hypoxia & acidosis.
  - After single seizure, fetal intracranial hemorrhages, miscarriages & stillbirths have been reported, although self-limited seizures can be well tolerated.
  - Complex partial seizures reported to affect fetal heart rate during labor.
  - Maternal status epilepticus associated w/ 50% fetal mortality
- Maternal mortality is increased in women w/ epilepsy.

STUDIES

Imaging

- None indicated for mother if well-established diagnosis
- New-onset seizures require full neurologic evaluation.
- High-resolution ultrasound evaluation to detect major fetal malformations

Other

- Assess free drug levels of anticonvulsants
  - Monthly during pregnancy
  - Every week during the last month of pregnancy
  - At the onset of labor
- Alpha-fetoprotein to rule out neural tube defect in fetus

MANAGEMENT/INTERVENTIONS

- 1–2% of epileptic pts have generalized seizures during labor.

- During prolonged labor, oral absorption of anticonvulsants is erratic.
  - ➤ Give fosphenytoin, pentobarbital or valproic acid IV rather than PO at same maintenance dose.
- A self-limited seizure (convulsions lasting <5 minutes) does not necessarily require treatment to abort the seizure.
  - ➤ Maintain a patent airway; limit potential for aspiration.
  - ➤ Monitor fetal heart rate (if no inherent uteroplacental insufficiency exists, then most fetal bradycardias that occur during self-limited seizures are transient).
- Status epilepticus (continuous convulsions) is a medical emergency.
  - ➤ Requires abortive seizure therapy
  - ➤ If seizures cannot be controlled, perform prompt C-section.
  - ➤ Fetal loss reported to be 50%
  - ➤ Call for help; administer oxygen & immediately establish an airway.
  - ➤ Maintain left uterine displacement.
  - ➤ Obtain continuous EEG recording while treating seizures.
  - ➤ Immediately attempt to terminate seizure w/ IV benzodiazepine.
    - Lorazepam 0.075 mg/kg at 2 mg/min is recommended because it results in less respiratory depression.
    - Diazepam is an acceptable alternative.
  - ➤ If seizures are not controlled w/ benzodiazepine, then administer:
    - Fosphenytoin 5–10 mg/kg IV at 150 mg/min
    - If seizures continue, add phenobarbital 20 mg/kg IV at 65 mg/min.
    - If seizures persist >60 min, begin midazolam, propofol, or barbiturate infusion to induce burst suppression.

Anesthesia
- General
  - ➤ Avoid drugs that lower seizure threshold:
    - Ketamine
    - Meperidine
    - Sevoflurane
  - ➤ Anticonvulsants alter drug pharmacokinetics & dynamics.
    - Increase metabolism of nondepolarizing relaxants
    - Increase narcotic threshold (require more narcotics)
  - ➤ Avoid complete neuromuscular paralysis; obscures ability to detect a motor seizure.

■ Regional
  ➤ Preferred as it facilitates neurologic monitoring

CAVEATS & PEARLS
■ Identify & inform pt's neurologist of seizure treatment & anesthetic plan.
■ A self-limited seizure (convulsions lasting <5 minutes) does not necessarily require treatment to abort the seizure.
  ➤ Maintain a patent airway; limit potential for aspiration.
  ➤ Monitor fetal heart rate (if no inherent uteroplacental insufficiency exists, then most fetal bradycardias that occur during self-limited seizures are transient).
■ Prolonged seizures are potentially harmful to mother & fetus. Decrease risk by:
  ➤ Ensuring adequate anticonvulsant levels w/ IV supplementation during labor
  ➤ Immediately & aggressively treating continuous generalized convulsions lasting >5 min
  ➤ Instituting seizure abortive therapy as described above for pts w/ status epilepticus

CHECKLIST
■ Know the pt's seizure history/seizure presentation.
■ Ensure well-secured IV access.
■ Check pt's most recent therapeutic anticonvulsant drug level.
■ Have oxygen, Ambu bag & bite block immediately available for use.
■ If seizures are not well controlled, have IV benzodiazepine available.

FACTOR DEFCIENCIES

JEANNA VIOLA, MD
JANE BALLANTYNE, MD

FUNDAMENTAL KNOWLEDGE
■ Hemophilia A
  ➤ Pts have normal levels of factor VIII but experience a reduction in the coagulation activity of this factor (<1–30% of normal coagulation activity) & therefore are prone to bleeding.
  ➤ Variable penetrance: some pts exhibit mild disease; others have severe hemorrhage.
  ➤ This trait is inherited in an X-linked recessive pattern; therefore, females who are affected by this disease are very rare.

➤ Levels of factor VIIIc rise in pregnancy, so many pts will experience a remission.
■ Hemophilia B
  ➤ AKA Christmas disease, factor IX deficiency
  ➤ Follows an X-linked recessive inheritance pattern & is clinically indistinguishable from Hemophilia A
  ➤ Unlike factor VIIIc, levels of factor IX do not rise during pregnancy.
■ Platelets maintain normal function in hemophiliacs.
■ Deficiency of either factor VIII or factor IX impairs factor X, the first coagulation factor in the common pathway.
■ Factor X deficiency
  ➤ Very rare disease, inherited in an autosomal recessive fashion
  ➤ In pregnancy, levels of factor X rise to >150% of normal, causing a remission of the disease.
■ Factor deficiency
  ➤ Transmitted as an autosomal recessive trait; most common in pts of Ashkenazi Jewish, Italian, and German descent
  ➤ In contrast to the other factor deficiency disorders, the level of factor does not correlate well w/ the amount of bleeding.
  ➤ Factor levels normally decrease during pregnancy.

STUDIES
■ Diagnosis & prediction of the severity of hemophilia A are based on the level of factor VIII.
■ Diagnosis & prediction of the severity of hemophilia B are based on factor IX levels.
■ Factor X deficiency is diagnosed by measurement of factor X levels.
■ Pts w/ factor present w/ prolonged PTT, normal PT.
■ Prothrombin deficiency results in prolongation of PT, PTT.

MANAGEMENT/INTERVENTIONS
■ An assessment of factor levels & the response to pregnancy helps guide mgt during labor & delivery.
■ Supplementation of the deficient factor, either via FFP or by direct administration of the factor, will limit the symptoms of the disease.
■ Hemophilia A
  ➤ Pts w/ mild-moderate disease respond to desmopressin, which increases factor VIII coagulation activity by 2–4×.
  ➤ Factor VIII is administered as a concentrate or in cryoprecipitate. The replacement amount is calculated by determining the percentage of the pt's deficiency.

- Each unit/ kg infused raises the pt's factor VIII coagulation activity by 2%.
  - Levels >30% required for labor & post-op, >80% for surgery
- Hemophilia B
  ➤ Replacement therapy for factor IX deficiency can be accomplished by administration of FFP.
    - 1 unit/kg will increase factor IX activity by 1%.
    - 20–40% for post-op, 60% level needed for surgery
- Factor deficiency
  ➤ Pt may also develop an inhibitor to factor activity; must be supplemented w/ an anti-inhibitor complex to correct the coagulopathy.
  ➤ Goal for factor level is 20% activity prior to surgery.
- In the case of an overt coagulopathy, regional anesthesia is contraindicated. GETA is the most appropriate anesthetic for C-section.

CAVEATS AND PEARLS
- Pts need an antepartum consultation w/ a hematologist & anesthesiologist.
- Factor levels should be normalized by supplementation or transfusion of FFP prior to labor or C-section.
- Hemophilia A pts often respond well to DDAVP; it may normalize the factor VIIIc level, making regional anesthesia safe.
- Most pts will require GETA for C-section.

CHECKLIST
- Obtain consult w/ hematologist as early in pregnancy as possible.
- Check factor levels prior to delivery & administer appropriate repletion therapy.
- Careful assessment of airway, as GETA likely needed for C-section.

FAMILIAL DYSAUTONOMIA (RILEY-DAY SYNDROME)

MEREDITH ALBRECHT, MD; LISA LEFFERT, MD; AND MICHELE SZABO, MD

FUNDAMENTAL KNOWLEDGE
Definition
- Reduced number of cells in the autonomic ganglia & fewer nerve fibers

Epidemiology
- Five known subtypes
- Type I: autosomal dominant
- Type III
  - Autosomal recessive
  - Ashkenazi Jewish population
  - Very rare

Pathophysiology
- Loss of small nerve fibers, myelinated & unmyelinated
- Unknown
  - Possible decrease in an enzyme triggers apoptosis
  - Possible abnormal transcription of molecules during development
- Possible depletion of catecholamines
- Both sensory & autonomic dysfunctions are present.

Clinical Manifestations
- Dysphagia
- Vomiting
- Intravascular volume depletion
- Prerenal azotemia
- Extreme cardiovascular instability (secondary to decreased autonomic innervation of blood vessels & organs)
- Increased risk of aspiration/gastroesophageal reflex
- Recurrent pneumonias
- Localized sensory anesthesia
- Impaired thermoregulation
- Decreased peripheral pain perception
- Normal visceral pain sensation
- Areflexia
- Insensitivity to pain
- Poor temperature control
- Possible self-mutilation
- Emotional lability & fits
- Dysautonomic crises triggered by stress
  - Intractable vomiting
  - Tachycardia
  - Hypertension
  - Flushing
  - Diaphoresis

Effect of Pregnancy on Familial Dysautonomia
- Unknown

Effect of Familial Dysautonomia on Pregnancy & the Fetus
- Decreased fertility
- Can deliver normal children

STUDIES

History & Physical
- History of numbness or shooting pain in the lower extremities
- Loss of pain & temperature sensation in the lower extremities
- Anhydrosis
- Trophic ulcers
- Poor temperature control
- Poor coordination
- Scoliosis

Laboratory
- Intradermal injection of histamine fails to elicit a normal "Schwarzman" reaction in affected areas.
- Sural nerve biopsy

Imaging
- None

Other
- Nerve conduction studies: reduced velocities (motor & sensory)

MANAGEMENT/INTERVENTIONS

Medical Treatment
- Supportive treatment
- Physical & occupational therapy

Anesthesia
- Initial assessment
  - Evaluate respiratory, neurologic function.
  - Assess whether pt can cooperate w/ regional anesthesia
- General anesthesia
  - May be necessary if respiratory status is affected
  - May be necessary if pt is too emotionally labile
  - Pretreat w/ H2 antagonist & metoclopramide due to increased risk of aspiration.
  - Pretreat w/ anxiolytic (diazepam is a good choice).

➤ Baseline SVR is low. Cardiac output is very dependent on preload, so intravascular volume repletion is recommended prior to induction.
➤ Increased sensitivity to direct-acting amines
➤ Unpredictable response to indirect-acting agents
➤ Invasive pressure monitoring recommended
➤ Recommend rapid sequence induction: the literature contains case reports of succinylcholine being used w/o untoward event.
➤ Response to muscle-relaxant reversal agents is unpredictable.
➤ Dysautonomic pts require lower doses of anesthetics.
➤ Post-op pain control difficult but necessary to prevent dysautonomic crisis
➤ May require post-op ventilation
➤ Requires vigorous pulmonary toilet & prophylactic antibiotics
■ Regional anesthesia
➤ Fluid prehydration is key.
➤ Can be technically difficult due to scolosis
➤ Improved post-op pain control & potentially decreased autonomic instability
➤ Local anesthetic boluses can cause increased drop in BP.
➤ If decreased BP unresponsive to fluid boluses, try small doses of direct-acting alpha-adrenergic agents.

CAVEATS & PEARLS
■ Due to reduced number of cells in autonomic ganglia leading to autonomic instability
■ Goals of care are to reduce pt anxiety, optimize respiratory function, maximize pain control & attain euvolemia.
■ Increased risk of aspiration; recommend pretreatment.
■ Enhanced response to direct-acting amines
■ Unpredictable response to indirect-acting agents
■ Careful control of pain reduces the incidence of dysautonomic crisis.

CHECKLIST
■ Careful history & physical exam to assess pulmonary function & autonomic instability & preexisting neurologic dysfunction
■ Pretreat w/ H2-antagonists, sodium citrate & metoclopramide due to increased risk of aspiration
■ Rapid sequence induction recommended
■ Hydrate pts, as chronic dehydration is common
■ Invasive pressure monitoring recommended

- Control of pain important to prevent dysautonomic crisis
- Maximize pulmonary status, as pulmonary complications & need for post-op ventilation common

FETAL CIRCULATION AND PLACENTAL TRANSFER OF DRUGS

MARK STONEY, MD
LISA LEFFERT, MD

FUNDAMENTAL KNOWLEDGE

- Adequate blood flow to the fetus is essential. This is made possible through the complex structure of the placenta. A nongravid uterus receives approx. 50 cc of blood/min. However, the gravid uterus can receive up to 600–700 cc/min. 80% of the blood flow to the uterus (approx. 500 cc/min) is directed to the placenta through an estimated 200 spiral arteries. At the placenta, the transfer of important nutrients, respiratory gases & waste occurs.

Basic Anatomy

- The placenta is often thought of as a simple structure that drugs and nutrients must cross from the mother to the fetus. However, it is very complex & a better understanding of its many functions can be gained from a basic understanding of the anatomy.
- The placenta is formed from both maternal & fetal tissues after the blastocyst erodes into the maternal decidua. This process results in a blastocyst surrounded by maternal blood. This is the origin of the intervillous space (described below). The placenta receives blood from the mother as well as the fetus. This is essential for transfer across the placental membrane, which is approximately 1.8 m^2.
- The anatomy of the placenta is best understood by considering the path that a drug or other molecule will follow when traveling from the mother to the fetus.
- Maternal blood travels to the uterus via the uterine artery. At this point a portion of the blood supply supports the myometrium, but a majority of the flow travels to the placenta. Blood travels through the spiral arteries to the maternal arterioles that direct flow into the intervillous space of the placenta. Maternal blood fills this space that surrounds the villi. The villi are of fetal origin. This is the location of the uteroplacental membrane. All fetal transfer occurs at this point. After crossing the membrane, the nutrients or drugs enter the fetal capillaries, which are inside the tertiary or terminal villi. At this point

flow is directed back toward the fetus, leaving the placenta via the umbilical vein.

■ Respiratory gases & waste leaving the fetus travel to the placenta by the two umbilical arteries. The site of transfer to the mother is once again a fetal capillary in the tertiary villi. Here transfer occurs across the uteroplacental membrane back into the intervillous space w/ maternal blood. Blood then travels back into the maternal venous circulation.

Fetal Circulation

■ The fetal circulation is completely different from the adult. It involves two separate systems w/ one supplying primarily the upper body through the L side of the heart. Circulation from the R side of the heart bypasses the lungs & supplies the lower body. The R ventricle has a cardiac output almost twice that of the L. This is in contrast to one continuous circulation in the adult. As noted, all gas, nutrient & drug exchange occurs in the placenta. Only half of the fetal cardiac output travels to the placenta. This occurs because of a system of shunts that result in mixing of oxygenated & deoxygenated blood.

Review of the fetal circulation:

■ Blood leaving the placenta in the umbilical vein is oxygenated w/ an oxygen saturation of approx. 80%. Once at the liver, blood flow is split to two different locations. Half of the flow mixes w/ blood in the portal vein & passes through the liver for detoxification before returning to the heart. The other 50% of blood in the umbilical vein bypasses the liver, through the ductus venosus, & mixes w/ deoxygenated blood from the lower extremities in the IVC. Blood from the IVC returns to the R atrium w/ a saturation of 67% secondary to mixing in the IVC. Once in the R atrium, blood from the IVC is shunted to the L atrium via the foramen ovale. L atrial flow is directed into the L ventricle & then primarily to the brain & heart.

■ Blood from the upper torso & brain returns to the R atrium via the SVC. Once in the R atrium it mixes w/ blood that returned to the heart from the IVC. At this point it is directed into the R ventricle. From here flow is directed into the pulmonary artery, where (secondary to high pulmonary vascular resistance) flow is preferentially directed through a patent ductus arteriosus. This blood has a saturation of approx. 55–60% & supplies the lower body via the descending aorta. Blood then exits the fetus through the 2 umbilical arteries into the placenta.

■ Once the baby is born, the fetal circulation changes rapidly to the adult form. These rapid adjustments in circulation are made possible by several processes. First, w/ several breaths the neonatal lungs fill with air & rapidly expand, leading to decreased PVR. In addition, the increase in pO_2 results in decreased PVR & dilation of the pulmonary arteries. This change results in flow being preferentially directed through the lungs instead of the ductus arteriosus & subsequently returning to the L heart. Increasing pressures in the L atrium result in the functional closing of the foramen ovale. The ductus arteriosus also closes w/ increasing pO_2, so blood flow leaves the L ventricle supplying the entire body. Hypoxia or acidosis results in persistent fetal circulation secondary to failure of closure of shunts because of the absence of the normal triggers for closure described above.

Basic Principles of Transfer Across the Placenta

■ Transfer from the intervillous space to the fetal capillaries within the tertiary villi occurs across several cell membranes. The cell layers consist of a syncytiotrophoblast & fetal capillary endothelium. Transfer across these cell layers is based on several methods of transport. The primary modes of transport include passive diffusion, facilitated diffusion, active transport & endocytosis/exocytosis.

■ Various factors unique to each solute affect the transfer across the cell membranes. The characteristics that affect a substance's transfer include molecular size, lipid solubility, ionic charge & maternal plasma protein binding. Smaller size, increased lipid solubility, uncharged form & less maternal plasma protein binding lead to increased transfer across the cell membrane.

STUDIES
MANAGEMENT/INTERVENTIONS
CAVEATS/PEARLS
CHECKLIST
N/A

FEVER DURING PREGNANCY

SISSELA PARK, MD
LAURA RILEY, MD

FUNDAMENTAL KNOWLEDGE

Temperature regulation

■ Normal temp range in healthy adults: 36–37.5 degrees Celsius

- Human body has a critical or "set-point" temp.
- Temp control mechanisms constantly adjust to keep body temp at the set-point.
- Body temp is regulated by hypothalamic integration of signals from receptors in the skin & CNS.
  - Hypothermia
    - Causes vasoconstriction in peripheral tissues to:
      - Limit blood flow to the skin
      - Reduce heat loss
      - Keep heat in the core compartment
    - When vasoconstriction is not enough, shivering is initiated to increase heat production. Shivering is controlled by the CNS.
  - Hyperthermia/fever
    - Vasodilation occurs secondary to the inhibition of sympathetic tone.
      - Raises the rate of heat transfer to the periphery as much as $8\times$
    - If vasodilation is not enough, sweating occurs.
      - Heat loss occurs by evaporation.
      - Can eliminate up to 10x the basal rate of heat production
    - Inhibition of heat-producing processes such as shivering
- Endothelial cell production of prostaglandins causes resetting of the hypothalamic set-point.

Fever

- Temp >38 degrees Celsius
- Causes
  - Drugs
  - Diseases
  - Elevated temps have been seen in laboring women w/ epidurals.
- Pyrogens
  - Substances that trigger fever (pyrexia)
  - Exogenous or endogenous
    - Exogenous pyrogens are elements of many microorganisms.
    - Endogenous pyrogens are cytokines produced by certain drugs or released from cells of the immune system.
    - Cytokines bind to receptors on the vascular endothelium in certain areas of the hypothalamus, causing:
      - Elevation of the "set-point" temp
      - Activation of the mechanisms of increased heat production

Changes during pregnancy
- Increased heat production due to increased basal metabolic rate caused by:
  - Fetal metabolism
  - Maternal adjustment to pregnancy
  - Inability to dissipate heat due to alterations in sweating mechanism
  - Physiologic changes during pregnancy confound the diagnosis of infection in a febrile pt.
    - Production of prostaglandins
      - Cause a resetting of the set-point temp
      - Key aspect of the start of labor
    - Since uterine perfusion is not autoregulated, peripheral vasodilation & increased blood flow to an infection site could theoretically decrease uterine & fetal perfusion.
    - Elevated leukocyte counts are common in labor.

Fetal complications
- One study has suggested that there is increased perinatal morbidity.
- Mild maternal fever (about 1 degree Celsius above normal) may be associated w/:
  - Hypotonia
  - 1-minute Apgar scores <7
  - Need for manual ventilation by bag-&-mask in delivery room
  - Increased need for supplemental oxygen in the nursery
  - Neonatal seizures
  - Cerebral palsy
  - Neonatal encephalopathy

Maternal complications
- Tachycardia
- Increased cardiac output
- Augmented oxygen consumption
- Elevated catecholamine production
- Increased incidence of cesarean delivery or operative vaginal delivery w/ instruments

STUDIES
- Temp measurement
- Leukocyte count may not be useful since leukocytosis is common in labor.

MANAGEMENT/INTERVENTIONS

General management

■ Issues to consider
- ➤ Possible causes:
  - • Infection
    - • Determine the source.
    - • Differentiate between infections that could spread to the fetus & those unlikely to affect the fetus directly.
  - • Neoplastic disease
  - • Connective tissue disease
  - • Pulmonary emboli
- ➤ Risks to mother & baby
  - • If well-being of the two are in conflict, consider the thoughts of the mother & her family.
- ➤ Some treatments may not be an option.
  - • Be aware of teratogenic potential of meds.
- ➤ Premature labor may occur secondary to fever.
  - • Assess febrile pts for the occurrence of uterine contractions.
  - • Perform cervical exam if not contraindicated.

■ Treatment as needed for the cause of the fever

■ May need to adjust drug dosages due to physiologic changes of pregnancy
- ➤ Glomerular filtration rate increases by about 50%, increasing clearance of renally excreted meds.

Regional anesthesia in the febrile pt

■ Concerns of a connection between dural puncture in a bacteremic pt & the subsequent development of meningitis
- ➤ Lumbar puncture may disrupt the venous plexus around the spinal cord, causing direct seeding of infected blood into the CNS by the needle.

■ Such concerns also apply to epidurals & the possible development of epidural abscesses.
- ➤ Epidural placement frequently disrupts blood vessels.
- ➤ Introduction of a foreign body, which could serve as a nidus for infection

■ Some clinicians hypothesize that disruption of the dura may allow hematogenous spread of infection into the CNS w/o direct vessel disturbance.

- No epidemiologic study has conclusively shown a causal relationship btwn dural puncture in a bacteremic pt & the subsequent diagnosis of meningitis or epidural abscess.
- Several epidemiologic studies have found an extremely low frequency of CNS infection after regional anesthesia (one study showed 0 episodes in 10,098 spinal anesthetics; another showed 0 incidents in 10,440 spinal anesthetics).
- Multiple retrospective studies have shown no evidence of meningitis or epidural abscess after epidural or spinal anesthesia in women w/ intra-amniotic infection.
  - ➤ These studies were small.
  - ➤ CNS infection is relatively rare after regional anesthesia in healthy pts, so these studies are not big enough to rule out the possibility that intra-amniotic infection could increase the risk of meningitis or epidural abscess
- Generally accepted that regional anesthesia can be performed in healthy pts at risk for bacteremia
- Most clinicians feel that regional anesthesia is acceptable in the pt w/ intra-amniotic infection in the setting of systemic antibiotics.
- It is thought that appropriate antibiotics decrease the risk of CNS infections.

CAVEATS & PEARLS
- Fever = temp >38 degrees Celsius
- In pregnancy, elevated temps can be seen in setting of:
  - ➤ Infection
  - ➤ Response to some drugs
  - ➤ Laboring women w/ epidurals
- It is generally accepted that regional anesthesia can be performed in:
  - ➤ Healthy pts at risk of bacteremia
  - ➤ Pts w/ intra-amniotic infection in the setting of systemic antibiotics
- Maternal fever may be associated w/ increased perinatal morbidity.

CHECKLIST
- Consider likely causes of infection.
- Be prepared for fetal resuscitation if there is maternal fever during labor.

GALLSTONES

LAWRENCE WEINSTEIN, MD
DOUG RAINES, MD

FUNDAMENTAL KNOWLEDGE

- Gallstones are more common in women than men.
- Risk factors include obesity, advancing age, female gender, diabetes mellitus, elevated serum triglycerides, cirrhosis & pregnancy.
- Gallstones alone are often asymptomatic. However, pts may have biliary colic, RUQ intermittent pain, often associated w/ meals.
- Complications of gallstone disease
  - ➤ Biliary colic: RUQ intermittent pain, often associated w/ meals
  - ➤ Acute cholecystitis: marked by RUQ pain, fever & nausea. Physical exam will elicit a positive Murphy sign in many instances
  - ➤ Pancreatitis
  - ➤ Choledocholithiasis (gallstones in the common bile duct): when obstructive, these stones can result on colicky RUQ pain & jaundice. If fever & chills are also present, may represent the more serious condition of ascending cholangitis.

STUDIES

Labs

- Asymptomatic gallstones confined to the gallbladder are often associated w/ normal lab values.
- Acute cholecystitis
  - ➤ Elevated WBC count
  - ➤ Elevated aminotransferases & alkaline phosphatase
  - ➤ Possibly elevated amylase & total bilirubin
- Choledocholithiasis (common duct obstruction)
  - ➤ Serum bilirubin & alkaline phosphatase are elevated.
  - ➤ Acute obstruction of the duct can raise aminotransferases dramatically.
  - ➤ WBC count can be normal, but will be markedly elevated w/ progression to cholangitis.

Imaging

- Abdominal ultrasound is excellent for the detection of gallstones but is not specific for demonstrating acute cholecystitis or common duct obstruction.

➤ Advantages of ultrasound include speed, lack of invasiveness, lack of pt discomfort.

■ CT scan can demonstrate stones & is also good for showing hepatic ductal dilation secondary to obstructive disease, or gallbladder inflammation in the setting of acute cholecystitis.

■ HIDA scan is very sensitive for showing cystic duct obstruction, which is often the cause of acute cholecystitis.

■ Endoscopic retrograde cholangiopancreatography (ERCP) provides a direct means of determining the cause, location & extent of a common bile duct obstruction.

➤ An advantage of ERCP is that it allows treatment of ductal obstruction at the time of the study via papillotomy w/ stone extraction or stent placement.

MANAGEMENT/INTERVENTIONS

■ Asymptomatic gallstones can be left alone & do not need urgent treatment.

■ When gallstones are symptomatic, treatment of choice is a cholecystectomy.

➤ It is preferable to perform this laparoscopically because of considerably less post-op pain & hospital stay.

➤ In the pregnant population, the risks of general anesthesia & abdominal surgery for the pt & fetus must be weighed against the severity of the gallstone-related symptoms.

■ In a pt w/ acute cholecystitis, treatment consists of IV antibiotics, NPO status & analgesia.

➤ Acute disease will generally subside within a couple of days, at which point cholecystectomy is recommended because there is a high rate of recurrence.

➤ If there is evidence of gallbladder gangrene or perforation, then surgery is needed as soon as feasible.

➤ Choledocholithiasis can be managed by ERCP w/ stone extraction, followed by eventual cholecystectomy.

➤ In the case of ascending cholangitis, treatment must be done urgently, as the biliary system needs to be decompressed for recovery to occur. Antibiotics are used in conjunction w/ ERCP or surgical decompression.

■ ERCP is not an easily tolerated procedure w/o considerable sedation or anesthesia. This becomes important in the case of the parturient w/ common duct gallstone disease.

CAVEATS/PEARLS

- Gallstone disease is more common in women than men, & both pregnancy & liver disease are additional risk factors.
- Gallstones are clinically important only when they are symptomatic (biliary colic) or when they cause processes such as acute cholecystitis or choledocholithiasis w/ cholangitis.
- Useful imaging modalities include ultrasound, CT scan, HIDA scan & ERCP.
- Surgical treatment during pregnancy should be reserved for those who are very symptomatic or have a pressing indication for surgery (see chapter "*Non-Obstetric Surgery in Pregnancy*").

CHECKLIST

- Abnormal lab values may be nonspecific.
- See chapter "*Non-obstetric Surgery in Pregnancy.*"
- Beware of signs of infection & treat accordingly.

GENERAL ANESTHESIA AND THE DIFFICULT AIRWAY

TODD JEN, MD
WARD R. MAIER, MD

FUNDAMENTAL KNOWLEDGE

Delivery by caesarean section (C-section) continues to increase worldwide, with rates of 20–25% in the U.S. between 1998–2000, 26.1% in 2001.

- Most common indications for C-section
  - ➤ Previous C-section
  - ➤ Dystocia
  - ➤ Cephalopelvic disproportion
  - ➤ Non-reassuring fetal stress (acute continuous bradycardia <60–80 bpm or severe decelerations)
  - ➤ Hemorrhage

The choice of anesthetic technique depends on multiple factors; the chosen technique should be the safest for the mother & should minimize neonatal depression while still providing optimal surgical conditions. Most C-sections are performed under regional anesthesia (see "*Anesthesia for Cesarean Delivery*" chapter). General anesthesia (GA), however, can, in some instances, enable a more reliable & rapid induction, more hemodynamic stability & a more secure airway w/ better control of ventilation.

- Common indications for GA
  - ➤ Non-reassuring fetal stress w/o preexisting epidural
  - ➤ Acute maternal hypovolemia
  - ➤ Significant coagulopathy
  - ➤ Inadequate regional anesthesia
  - ➤ Some forms of preexisting neurologic, lumbar spine/disc disease
  - ➤ Maternal refusal of regional anesthesia

Anesthesia-related deaths are the 6th leading cause of pregnancy-related mortality in the U.S. Airway mgt problems, specifically maternal aspiration & failed intubation, are the most common cause of GA-related morbidity & mortality.

- **Aspiration**
  - ➤ Obstetric pts are theoretically at higher risk than the general population for aspiration of gastric contents.
  - ➤ All pts in the second half of pregnancy should be considered to have "full stomachs."
  - ➤ Risk factors
    - • Delayed gastric emptying during labor
    - • Increased intra-abdominal contents
    - • Increased gastric volume
    - • Increased gastric acidity
    - • Decreased lower esophageal sphincter (LES) tone
  - ➤ Studies have suggested that both volume & pH of gastric contents are important in the severity of aspiration pneumonitis, w/ an increased incidence of morbidity & mortality when pH < 2.5 & volume > 0.4 mL/kg.
  - ➤ NPO guidelines
    - • Clear liquids
      - • Uncomplicated labor: modest amounts of PO water, fruit juice (no pulp), carbonated beverages, clear tea, black coffee
      - • High risk (obesity, difficult airway, high C-section risk): further PO restrictions, case-by-case. NPO 2 hours before elective C-section.
    - • Solids
      - • NPO 6–8 hours before elective C-section
      - • NPO in laboring pts

- **Difficult airway**
  - ➤ The pregnant pt has been thought to be at higher risk than the general population for airway difficulties & failed intubation.

Large population studies outside of the U.S. have shown that failed intubation at the time of C-section is correlated w/ inadequate pt preparation, less skilled anesthesia personnel & airway characteristics (eg, protruding incisors, foreshortened chin). Pregnancy-related factors include both anatomic & physiologic:

- Weight gain
- Increased Mallampati scores
- Capillary engorgement & mucosal edema
- Decreased functional residual capacity (FRC)
- Increased O_2 consumption (by 20%)
- Increased risk of hypoxia during apnea
- Increased risk of aspiration
- Preexisting obesity
- Preexisting airway abnormalities

■ **Maintenance of GA**
➤ Obstetric pts have reduced anesthetic requirements, so induction is more rapid & lower MAC values are required for maintenance of GA. Awareness is virtually abolished when a combination of 50% N_2O, 50% O_2 & 0.5 MAC volatile agent is used.
  - N_2O at 50% does not produce significant uterine relaxation or neonatal depression.
  - 0.5 MAC of isoflurane (0.75%), sevoflurane (1.0%), desflurane (2–4%), enflurane (1.0%) & halothane (0.5%) contributes to maintenance of GA by:
    - Allowing the use of decreased N_2O%
    - Allowing increased FiO_2
    - Decreasing awareness/recall
    - Minimizing decreased uterine tone
    - Minimizing neonatal depression

STUDIES
■ The choice of preop lab studies will depend on individual maternal/fetal indications (see "*Anesthesia for Cesarean Delivery*" chapter).
■ Monitoring during GA should include BP, O_2 saturation, ECG, $ETCO_2$, temperature, FHR, neuromuscular conduction.

MANAGEMENT/INTERVENTIONS
Preanesthetic Mgt
■ Prevention of maternal aspiration

➤ Follow NPO guidelines (see "Fundamental Knowledge" in this chapter).
➤ Administer nonparticulate PO antacid within 1 hour of induction.
  • 0.3 M sodium citrate 30 ml PO
    • Neutralizes 255 mL of HCl with pH 1.0 for 40–60 minutes
➤ Consider H2-blocker, proton pump inhibitor & metoclopramide.
  • Cimetidine 300 mg or ranitidine 50 mg IV at least 30 minutes prior to induction
  • Omeprazole 20–40 mg PO at least 30 minutes prior to induction
  • Metoclopramide 10 mg IV given 3–5 minutes prior to induction
■ Placement of large-bore IV catheter
■ Apply monitors: BP, O_2 saturation, ECG, $ETCO_2$, temperature, FHR, nerve stimulator.
■ Left uterine displacement (LUD) to avoid aortocaval compression

Induction
■ Pt prepped and draped; obstetrician ready to begin
■ Preoxygenation w/ FiO_2 1.00:
  ➤ 3–5 minutes or 8 vital capacity (VC) breaths
■ Rapid sequence induction (RSI) w/ cricoid pressure (see "Intubation and the difficult airway" below)
■ Do not release cricoid pressure until tracheal placement of ETT is confirmed (positive $ETCO_2$, fogging of ETT during expiration, symmetrical chest movement, auscultation of breath sounds) & cuff inflated.
■ Induction agents
  ➤ Thiopental: 4–5 mg/kg IV
  ➤ Propofol: 2–2.5 mg/kg IV
  ➤ Ketamine: 1 mg/kg IV
  ➤ Etomidate: 0.2–0.3 mg/kg IV
■ Muscle relaxants/neuromuscular blocking drugs (NMBDs)
  ➤ Succinylcholine: 1–1.5 mg/kg IV (onset 45 secs)
  ➤ Rocuronium: 0.6 mg/kg IV (onset 98 secs)
  ➤ Vecuronium: 0.2 mg/kg IV (onset 175 secs)
  ➤ Cis-atracurium: 0.2 mg/kg IV (onset 2–8 mins)

Intubation and the difficult airway
■ Airway exam
  ➤ Examine mouth opening (MO), thyromental distance (TMD), Mallampati class (MP), neck flexion/extension, dentition, body habitus.

- ➤ Predictors of difficult intubation
  - MO < 4 cm
  - TMD < 6.5 cm
  - Atlanto-occipital extension < 10° (normal extension approx. 35°)
  - Short, bull neck
  - Large tongue
  - Prominent upper teeth
  - Microagnathia
  - Large chest
- ■ Equipment
  - ➤ Suction device
  - ➤ Masks: 3 sizes
  - ➤ Oral, nasal airways: 3 sizes of each
  - ➤ Laryngoscopes: curved and straight blades, short handle
  - ➤ ETTs: 5–7 mm
  - ➤ Bougie: gum elastic, Eschmann intubating stylet
  - ➤ LMA/FasTrach LMA: #3, 4
  - ➤ Combitube
  - ➤ Magill forceps
  - ➤ Fiberoptic bronchoscope (FOB)
  - ➤ Transtracheal jet ventilator (TTJV)
  - ➤ Percutaneous cricothyrotomy kit
    - Our institution has 24-hour on-call surgical team available.
- ■ Positioning
  - ➤ LUD
  - ➤ Elevation of head, shoulders & thorax to achieve "sniffing" position
    - Use folded blankets to "ramp" up thorax, shoulders & head.
    - Consider reverse Trendelenburg to off-load breasts & abdominal contents.
  - ➤ Cricoid pressure
  - ➤ BURP maneuver: external pressure on cricoid cartilage in a Backward, Upward & Rightward Position to assist in obtaining view of larynx
- ■ Recognized vs. unrecognized difficult airway
  - ➤ Recognized
    - Attempt regional anesthesia if conditions permissible.
      - Non-urgent, coagulation studies acceptable
    - Awake fiberoptic intubation (FOI)
      - Consider anticholinergic drying agent.
      - Consider sedation, by titrating small amounts.

- Consider topical anesthetics, nerve blocks (e.g., nebulized lidocaine, superior laryngeal nerve block, transtracheal topicalization).
- To avoid aspiration, avoid oversedation.
- LMA-facilitated intubation, using FasTrach LMA.
- Unrecognized
  - Call for help.
  - Ventilate w/ FiO$_2$ 1.00, using face mask vs. LMA & applying cricoid pressure.
  - Adequate ventilation/oxygenation
    - Fetal distress?
      - **No:** allow drugs to wear off & wake pt.
      - Regional vs. awake FOI/LMA facilitated intubation
      - **Yes:** maintain cricoid pressure.
      - Continue FiO$_2$ 1.00.
      - Add volatile agent.
      - Allow spontaneous ventilation if possible.
      - If pt apneic, continue mask ventilation vs. placing LMA.
      - Inform OB to expedite delivery.
  - Inadequate ventilation/oxygenation
    - Before proceeding w/ surgery:
      - Maintain cricoid pressure.
      - Consider non-surgical airway.
        - LMA, Combitube, TTJV
      - Consider surgical airway.

Maintenance of anesthesia
- After induction & intubation, maintain GA w/ 50% N$_2$O, 50% O$_2$ at high flow rates & 0.5 MAC volatile agent.
- Avoid hyperventilation, hypotension.

Postdelivery
- Consider increasing N$_2$0% & decreasing volatile agent.
- Administer oxytocin IV, 10–40 U diluted in 500 mL lactated Ringer's solution.
  - Consider methylergonovine 0.2 mg IM or prostaglandin-F2a 0.25 mg IM for persistent uterine atony (see "*Postpartum Hemorrhage*" chapter).
- Titrate opioid.

Extubation
- Reverse any NMBDs.

■ Suction oropharynx.
■ Extubate only after pt is fully awake w/ airway reflexes intact.

CAVEATS AND PEARLS
■ Aspiration & difficult intubation are the most common causes of GA-related morbidity & mortality in the obstetric pt.
■ Most difficult airways are unrecognized in the pregnant pt.
■ If the pt has a potentially difficult airway or is at high risk (morbidly obese), early consultation w/ an anesthesiologist is recommended.
■ High-risk pts, who are also at high risk for C-section, should be considered for an epidural placed early in labor (see "*Anesthesia for Cesarean Delivery*" chapter).
■ In an emergency, if a choice has to be made btwn the survival of the fetus vs. the mother, the mother should be protected over the fetus.
■ Whenever GA is being given for non-reassuring FHR tracing, FHR should be rechecked in the OR. A normalized FHR pattern may signal an opportunity to administer a regional anesthetic instead of GA.

CHECKLIST
■ Prevention of maternal aspiration
■ Recheck FHR in OR
■ Plan of action ready for difficult airway/failed intubation
■ Prevention of hypotension
■ Maintenance of adequate maternal ventilation & oxygenation
■ Minimize duration of GA

GENERAL CONCEPTS: LIVER DISEASE

LAWRENCE WEINSTEIN, MD
DOUG RAINES, MD

FUNDAMENTAL KNOWLEDGE

Introduction
The liver is the largest solid organ in the human body & is responsible for regulating many metabolic & homeostatic functions. Functions of the liver include:
■ Production of bile
■ Carbohydrate storage & release (in the form of glycogen)
■ Formation of urea from nitrogenous waste products
■ Cholesterol metabolism
■ Manufacture of plasma proteins, such as albumin

- Many roles in fat metabolism
- Metabolism of certain polypeptide hormones
- Reduction & conjugation of adrenocortical & gonadal steroid hormones
- Detoxification of many drugs & toxins

Because of its many important roles, problems w/ the liver can be very detrimental to one's overall health, w/ many physiologic consequences

Pregnancy & Liver Disease: An Overview

- Severe liver disease involving cirrhosis & severely impaired hepatocyte function is rare in pregnancy.
- Women of child-bearing age w/ severe liver dysfunction are unlikely to be able to sustain a pregnancy, w/ its associated increases in nutritional & metabolic demands.
- Anesthetic decisions for the mgt of vaginal & cesarean delivery must take into account alterations in hepatic function, maternal physiology & coagulation derangements.
- Pregnant women have an increase in plasma volume of about 50% from the 6th to 36th weeks of gestation.
- There is a concurrent, but smaller, increase in RBC mass (about 20%) & thus a resultant decrease in hematocrit (hemodilution) during pregnancy.

Hepatic Blood Flow

- Cardiac output increases until the 2nd trimester, then plateaus until delivery.
- Despite these hemodynamic changes, absolute hepatic blood flow remains constant, a result of a decrease in the percentage of cardiac output directed toward the liver.
- The liver receives a dual blood supply:
  - ➤ The oxygen-rich hepatic artery (about 25% of blood supply, but roughly half of oxygen supply)
  - ➤ The relatively oxygen-poor portal vein
- Normally, there is autoregulation of hepatic arterial flow, such that when portal vein delivery decreases, hepatic arterioles dilate to maintain blood flow to the liver.
- Hepatic blood flow is determined by:
  - ➤ *Perfusion pressure*, which is equal to mean arterial or portal vein pressure minus hepatic vein pressure
  - ➤ *Splanchnic vascular resistance*: The splanchnic vascular bed is innervated by sympathetic vasoconstricting fibers, which

will increase activity in the settings of hypoxia, hypercarbia & increased catecholamines.

Pulmonary Effects of Liver Disease

➤ Intrapulmonary arteriovenous shunting can represent 10–40% of the cardiac output. These are right-to-left shunts & result in decreased arterial oxygen saturation.

➤ *Ascites* causes upward pressure on the diaphragm w/ atelectasis & V/Q mismatch.

• This reduces overall lung volumes & FRC & can lead to a restrictive lung disease pattern on spirometry.

➤ Hypoalbuminemia leads to pleural effusion, which exacerbates atelectasis as well.

■ Liver disease pts have increased 2,3-DPG levels & a subsequent right shift of the hemoglobin-oxygen dissociation curve, w/ a reduced hemoglobin affinity for oxygen.

➤ This will increase oxygen delivery to the peripheral tissues but hinder oxygen pickup & carrying capacity. Anemia in this setting further compromises oxygen-carrying capacity.

Renal effects of Liver Disease

■ Pts w/ cirrhosis & ascites have decreased renal perfusion & an increased risk of hyponatremia & hypokalemia.

➤ Decreased perfusion is due to relative hypovolemia; although cirrhotic pts have increased total body water & intravascular volume, portal-systemic shunting results in decreased effective plasma volume & renal blood flow. This decreased flow causes renin, angiotensin & aldosterone levels to be elevated.

➤ In cirrhosis there is a decrease in sodium excretion due to active reabsorption of sodium secondary to high levels of renin & angiotensin.

• Consequently, total body sodium is increased & any exogenous sodium can further exacerbate ascites & edema. Plasma hyponatremia is thus dilutional owing to decreased free water clearance, often a result of inappropriate ADH secretion.

➤ Hypokalemia is secondary to increased renal losses, as a result of high angiotensin & aldosterone.

• This can be exacerbated when diuretics are used to treat ascites.

• Because of the association of hypokalemia w/ cardiac arrhythmias (flat, broadened T waves, PVCs, ST-segment depression), careful EKG monitoring is essential peri-operatively, & potassium should be replaced to maintain normal plasma concentrations.

■ **Hepatorenal syndrome** is a functional defect in cirrhotic pts marked by oliguria, sodium retention, azotemia, intractable ascites & high mortality.

➤ Usually precipitated by GI bleeding, rapid diuresis, surgical blood losses or sepsis

➤ Once hepatorenal syndrome has developed, operative mortality is close to 100%, w/ the exception of a liver transplantation.

Metabolic Effects of Liver Disease

■ Liver failure pts are often hypoglycemic due to decreased hepatic gluconeogenesis & glycogenolysis. Frequent glucose monitoring is necessary to prevent dangerously low blood sugar levels, which can manifest as seizures or coma when severe.

STUDIES

■ Hemodilution of pregnancy causes serum albumin levels to decrease during pregnancy, w/ mean values of about 3 g/dL.

■ Serum alkaline phosphatase levels are elevated ($2-4\times$ normal) in the 3rd trimester, secondary to presence of placental alkaline phosphatase.

■ Serum ALT levels can be slightly elevated in the 2nd trimester but tend to be within normal limits during pregnancy.

■ AST levels remain fairly constant & normal in pregnancy.

■ Total & free bilirubin concentrations are lower in pregnancy. Conjugated bilirubin is decreased in the 2nd & 3rd trimesters.

■ Prothrombin time (PT) is normal & unchanged during pregnancy.

■ The majority of hepatic studies are normal or near normal during pregnancy (with the exception of alkaline phosphatase & albumin). Thus, intra-pregnancy increases in ALT, AST, bilirubin or PT should prompt a workup to investigate the presence of co-existent pathology.

MANAGEMENT/INTERVENTIONS

Hepatic Blood Flow

■ Both general & regional anesthesia reduce hepatic blood flow, an important consequence in the setting of already impaired hepatic function.

■ General anesthesia can decrease hepatic blood flow through a number of mechanisms.

➤ Volatile agents decrease hepatic blood flow secondary to reduction of systemic BP & cardiac output. This effect is exacerbated by reflex sympathetic activation, which constricts the splanchnic vasculature & increases resistance to hepatic blood flow.

➤ Volatile agents can decrease the ability of the hepatic artery to autoregulate blood flow in the setting of decreased portal vein delivery.
  • This effect is less severe w/ isoflurane & sevoflurane compared w/ halothane. Thus, isoflurane & sevoflurane are better choices for the anesthesiologist concerned w/ preserving hepatic blood supply.
  • Halothane has the additional drawback of generating hepatotoxic reductive metabolites in the setting of hypoxia.

➤ The reduction in hepatic flow associated w/ volatile agents can be lessened by using lower concentrations of volatile agents in conjunction w/ nitrous oxide, as hypotension increases w/ higher levels of volatile agent.

➤ Use of vasopressors to offset hypotension during anesthesia can increase splanchnic vascular resistance through activity at alpha-adrenergic receptors, thereby potentially reducing hepatic blood flow.
  • Decreases in blood flow are also seen w/ beta-blockers & vasopressin, whereas low-dose dopamine may *increase* hepatic blood flow.

➤ Mechanical ventilation can decrease hepatic blood flow.
  • Positive-pressure ventilation increases intrathoracic pressure, decreasing venous return & cardiac output, which in turn results in less hepatic blood delivery.
  • PEEP can worsen this effect.
  • Consequently, spontaneous ventilation may be a better alternative for maintenance of hepatic blood flow.

➤ Avoid hypoxemia because it causes splanchnic constriction & reduced blood flow. Inspired oxygen content should be adjusted to maintain good oxygen saturation & arterial oxygen partial pressure.

➤ Maintenance of adequate intravascular volume via IV fluids, colloids &/or blood products can help to attenuate some of these effects & maintain perfusion.

➤ Regional neuraxial anesthesia reduces hepatic blood flow predominantly via reduced systemic BP secondary to sympathectomy w/ deceased venous return & cardiac output.

- Reduction of hepatic blood flow can be minimized w/ good volume resuscitation & slow titration of epidural dosing.
- Spinal anesthesia has a rapid onset & often more precipitous changes in BP & cardiac output. For this reason, it is potentially less safe than epidural anesthesia when preservation of hepatic blood flow is paramount.

Pulmonary Effects of Hepatic Disease

- Due to the associated pulmonary effects, the cirrhotic pt under general anesthesia may require higher FIO2 &/or PEEP to maintain adequate oxygen saturation & tissue delivery.
  - ➤ Preoxygenation for general anesthesia becomes even more important than usual, as V/Q mismatching will result in more rapid desaturation w/ apnea.
- Higher inspiratory pressures may be necessary to maintain adequate tidal volumes in the setting of increased abdominal & thoracic pressures secondary to ascites.
  - ➤ Muscle paralysis may be useful in decreasing the muscular component of chest wall resistance to positive-pressure ventilation.
- Ventilation strategies should aim for normocapnia, as alkalosis shifts ammonium ions to a less ionized equilibrium, facilitating diffusion across the blood-brain barrier & potentially exacerbating hepatic encephalopathy.

Renal Effects of Hepatic Disease

- Severe hyponatremia (<120 mEq/L) is associated w/ mental status changes & possibly seizures, & efforts should be made to maintain sodium >130 mEq/L. Strategies to this end include:
  - ➤ Free water restriction
  - ➤ Administration of albumin w/ a loop diuretic
  - ➤ Normal saline will elevate plasma sodium but can have the negative effect of worsening total body sodium & ascites.
- Hypoglycemia is treated w/ exogenous dextrose via IV fluids.
  - ➤ Frequent monitoring of glucose & potassium is recommended, as administration of sugar shifts potassium intracellularly & can exacerbate hypokalemia.
    - To this end, an arterial line is useful for frequent blood sampling.
- The anesthesiologist can play a role in preventing post-op renal failure by paying careful attention to operative fluid losses & replacing intravascular volume w/ colloids.
  - ➤ A Foley catheter to track urine output & an arterial line would be standard monitors in this setting.

- Central venous lines may be useful for the administration of vasoactive drugs, but pressure values will likely NOT reflect effective plasma volumes in the setting of ascites & portal hypertension.

Monitors & Lines
- Monitoring is of vital importance given that parturients w/ liver disease tolerate hypotension & hypoxemia poorly.
  - ➤ Standard monitoring includes a 5-lead EKG, pulse oximetry & non-invasive BP monitors.
  - ➤ An arterial line is often the best choice, as it allows more precise BP monitoring & easy access for drawing blood for gas analysis, electrolytes & glucose levels.
  - ➤ As discussed above, central venous access &/or PA catheters may be of value in the setting of pulmonary hypertension
- Large-bore IV access should be available, & the operating environment should be equipped w/ fluid warmers & a rapid infusion system.

Cross-matched blood products should be available, if time permits, because many women w/ liver disease or the HELLP syndrome are coagulopathic & have the potential for significant peri-operative hemorrhage.

Coagulopathy & Anesthetic Considerations
Coagulopathy is a major concern for the anesthesiologist in the pregnant population. Regional neuraxial anesthesia is usually preferred for the term parturient, especially in the setting of severe liver disease & its associated pulmonary & circulatory consequences, which make general anesthesia less desirable. However, neuraxial anesthesia is contraindicated in the setting of clinically significant coagulopathy because of the risk of potentially devastating epidural hematoma.
- The parturient w/ cirrhosis or acute liver disease may have an elevated PT as a result of decreased hepatic synthesis of clotting factors.
- If PT is elevated as a result of severe hepatic disease, vitamin K supplementation will not be effective in reversing coagulopathy, since the hepatocytes themselves are not working properly.
- Thrombocytopenia may be present as a result of congestive splenomegaly (secondary to portal hypertension) & bone marrow suppression in the cirrhotic parturient.
- Coagulation studies & platelet number should be carefully reviewed before undertaking spinal or epidural anesthesia.
  - ➤ If INR is >1.5 or if platelets are <50K, consider replacing factors or platelets prior to proceeding w/ neuraxial anesthesia.

- In the case of elevated INR, 10–15 mL/kg of FFP is sufficient to replace clotting factors in most pts.

Post-partum bleeding secondary to thrombocytopenia at levels above 50K is rare, & transfusion of platelets should be based on clinical bleeding.

- Regardless of anesthetic type, large-bore IV access should be obtained & cross-matched blood should be available in the event of hemorrhage during either vaginal or cesarean delivery.
- For additional discussion, see "*Hematologic Disorders.*"

Regional/Neuraxial Anesthesia in Liver Disease

- For the majority of pregnant women at term (including those w/ hepatic disease), regional anesthesia is preferred to general in the absence of contraindications. Advantages include:
  - ➤ Awake pt: this avoids induction & muscle relaxation & the associated risk of aspiration w/ a diminished gag reflex. It also allows avoidance of systemic sedatives & opiates, which can have effects on the newborn.
  - ➤ Spontaneous ventilation: by avoiding positive-pressure ventilation & volatile anesthetic gases, there is better preservation of hepatic blood flow
  - ➤ Airway mgt is more difficult in the term parturient than in the non-pregnant pt because of increased airway edema & abdominal girth. As a result, mask ventilation & intubation can present challenges that may be avoided by opting for a regional anesthetic.
- Spinals & epidurals may safely be administered to parturients w/ co-existing liver disease, so long as there are no contraindications.
- Prior to administration of epidural or spinal anesthesia, a thorough workup for coagulopathy should be done, including evaluation of platelet count, PT, INR & fibrinogen.
  - ➤ Coagulation disorders are common in the setting of acute fatty liver of pregnancy & pre-eclampsia.
  - ➤ Any coagulopathy should be corrected via administration of FFP, platelets or cryoprecipitate prior to epidural or spinal placement.
- As discussed above, neuraxial blockade causes a sympathectomy that decreases cardiac output, BP, hepatic blood flow & sometimes heart rate.
  - ➤ Maintenance of intravascular volume is essential when planning a regional anesthetic, & large-bore IV access should be obtained prior to placement.
  - ➤ Vasopressors such as ephedrine should be immediately available to treat hypotension & bradycardia.

➤ When liver disease is severe, an arterial catheter may be invaluable for BP monitoring.

■ Because of its slower onset, epidural anesthesia may be less likely to cause hypotension & bradycardia than spinal anesthesia & is the best choice for non-urgent delivery in the parturient w/ liver dysfunction.

■ Amide local anesthetics (lidocaine, bupivacaine, mepivacaine) undergo hepatic biotransformation & have increased half-lives in pts w/ compromised liver function.

➤ Potential toxicity is somewhat offset by an increased volume of distribution in cirrhotic pts.

■ Systemic toxicity is a particular concern in the pregnant pt w/ liver disease.

➤ Both pregnancy & portal hypertension can cause engorgement of epidural veins, increasing the chance of intravascular injection of local anesthetic.

➤ Test dosing is mandatory in this setting, & it is prudent to dose epidurals slowly, titrating to effect, in non-emergent situations.

➤ Addition of epinephrine to all local anesthetics used can alert the anesthesiologist to intravascular migration of the catheter, which can occur even after an initially negative test dose.

■ For a planned cesarean delivery, the issue of local anesthetic toxicity can be mitigated by opting for spinal anesthesia, which requires a much lower dose of local anesthetic.

➤ However, as mentioned, spinals can cause more adverse hemodynamic shifts. Carefully titrated epidural anesthesia is overall the more preferred option.

■ 2-Chloroprocaine, an ester local anesthetic, is often used for emergent cesarean delivery in parturients w/ an indwelling epidural catheter. It is preferred in these situations because it is broken down rapidly by plasma pseudocholinesterase & thus has very little potential for systemic or neonatal toxicity.

➤ With liver disease, pseudocholinesterase levels may be low, though the clinical significance of this as relates to metabolism of 2-chloroprocaine use is uncertain.

■ Coagulation status should be re-checked & if necessary corrected prior to removal of an epidural catheter.

General Anesthesia in Liver Disease

Airway Mgt

■ Airway mgt is particularly challenging in the parturient owing to increased pharyngeal edema & higher risk of aspiration compared w/ the non-pregnant pt.

- Pts should be positioned to optimize direct laryngoscopy.
- Backup airway measures such as fiberoptic scopes, elastic gum bougies & LMA should be available.
- Pre-oxygenation via spontaneous ventilation should be thorough, if time permits.
- Inductions should be planned as rapid sequence to minimize aspiration risk. Continuous cricoid pressure is applied until tube placement is confirmed w/ end-tidal carbon dioxide & bilateral chest auscultation.
- Endotracheal intubation is absolutely indicated, as the LMA & mask ventilation cannot protect against aspiration & are often not as effective for positive-pressure ventilation.
  - ➤ Higher inspiratory pressures may be necessary to counteract the decreased respiratory compliance that results from the gravid uterus & possible presence of ascites.
- Do not extubate the pt until it is well demonstrated that she is awake & strong enough to protect the airway.
  - ➤ Certain non-depolarizing muscle relaxants have prolonged effects in the setting of liver disease & reversal should be double-checked prior to extubation.

Maintenance of Anesthesia & Anesthetic Drugs
- **Induction**
- Induction can be obtained w/ propofol, thiopental or etomidate. Both propofol & thiopental cause hypotension & should be used w/ caution & close hemodynamic monitoring. Etomidate is a good choice when hypovolemia is suspected but has the disadvantage of slower onset.
  - ➤ Thiopental has unaltered metabolism, since redistribution is the primary means of termination.
  - ➤ Propofol has unaltered pharmacokinetics but prolonged duration of action in liver disease.
  - ➤ Etomidate has prolonged half-life in liver disease.
- As above, general anesthetic agents & positive-pressure ventilation act to decrease hepatic blood flow.
  - ➤ Volatile agent doses can be decreased by co-administering nitrous oxide (which has very little effect on hepatic blood flow), so long as the pt's oxygen saturation can tolerate a lower inspired oxygen fraction.
  - ➤ Avoid halothane, as it decreases hepatic blood flow to a greater extent than the other volatile agents (isoflurane, sevoflurane, desflurane).

- Paralysis is often necessary for an easy rapid sequence induction & for abdominal relaxation to facilitate surgical cesarean delivery.
  - Succinylcholine may have a prolonged duration of action since plasma cholinesterase is often decreased w/ hepatic disease.
    - Clinically, this is not very important, & the rapid onset of paralysis still makes succinylcholine the agent of choice for rapid sequence induction.
  - Atracurium & cis-atracurium are the non-depolarizing muscle relaxants of choice owing to their non-hepatic metabolism.
    - Atracurium is a less attractive choice because of the side effect of histamine release.
  - Non-depolarizing agents vecuronium, rocuronium & pancuronium have increased recovery times in the setting of hepatic insufficiency & should not be used if cis-atracurium is available.
    - Also, these agents have an increased volume of distribution & require larger loading doses in pts w/ hepatic dysfunction.
  - Reversal of paralysis is safely accomplished w/ neostigmine, which is excreted renally.
    - Reversal should be documented w/ a nerve stimulator because of the high risk of aspiration in the parturient & cirrhotic populations.
- **Pain Management & Sedation**
  - Systemic administration of narcotics & sedatives is generally limited prior to delivery of the neonate, as they can cross the placenta & result in respiratory depression of the newborn.
  - After delivery, it is reasonable to give IV narcotics to treat surgical pain.
    - In the setting of hepatic insufficiency, morphine & meperidine have prolonged durations of action & should be carefully titrated so that respiratory depression does not complicate wake-up & extubation.
  - At low clinical doses, fentanyl metabolism is unaltered by liver disease because of binding to muscle & fat (increased volume of distribution).
  - Always titrate narcotic usage to pt demands & respiratory status.
    - Naloxone should be available in the case of overdose or respiratory depression.
  - Benzodiazepines, such as midazolam, have increased half-lives in liver disease & may exacerbate hepatic encephalopathy in a cirrhotic pt. They should be used sparingly.

■ **Emergence**
■ Emergence from anesthesia is a critical moment & a time at which a pt is at increased risk for aspiration & airway compromise
  ➤ Neuromuscular blockade should be fully reversed & muscle strength demonstrated prior to extubation.
  ➤ The pt should be awake & following commands.
  ➤ If a pt has received massive volume resuscitation w/ crystalloid &/or blood products, airway edema may be a concern.
    • There should be a low threshold for leaving pts intubated & transferring them to an ICU setting for airway observation.
  ➤ Any parturient w/ liver disease should probably go to a closely monitored recovery unit for vital sign & airway observation after emergence.

CAVEATS/PEARLS
■ In most cases, regional anesthesia is preferred over general for the parturient w/ co-existing liver disease.
■ Important considerations when planning a neuraxial anesthetic are coagulation status & urgency of the clinical situation.
■ When time or comorbidity precludes the use of regional anesthesia, general anesthesia is performed w/ careful attention to airway mgt, hemodynamic monitoring & fluid resuscitation.
■ Be aware of the physiologic & pharmacokinetic consequences of hepatic disease & plan to deal w/ them in a cautious manner.

CHECKLIST
See details for specific syndromes.

GESTATIONAL BACK PAIN

STEPHEN PANARO, MD
EDWARD MICHNA, MD

FUNDAMENTAL KNOWLEDGE
■ **Prevalence:** Nearly 50% of pregnancies
■ **Risk factors:** Antecedent history, multiparity (in most but not all studies), young age, low socioeconomic class, excessive weight gain, spondylolisthesis
■ **Impact:** It is estimated that almost one third of women report that back pain of pregnancy limits their ability to work, perform normal daily activities & sleep.

■ **Etiology:** Although multifactorial, it is widely attributed to mechanical & hormonal factors:
  ➤ Relaxin (produced by the corpus luteum) is the hormone that induces ligamentous softening & pelvic joint laxity, promoting instability of the SI joints & symphysis pubis. These changes tend to be responsible for back pain as early as the 1st trimester.
  ➤ Mechanical factors associated w/ back pain play a larger role in the final trimesters. Uterine enlargement rotates the sacrum forward & increases the lumbar lordosis by closing the lumbar interlaminar space. These effects increase the burden on the facets & the posterior aspect of the intervertebral discs, effects that can compromise the nerve root foramina & precipitate sciatica (present in 1% of pregnant women). Sciatica must be distinguished from the more common posterior pelvic pain, which may radiate to the posterior thighs & sometimes below the knees. This pain should not extend to the foot or involve neurologic change.
  ➤ Disc herniation, although rare in pregnancy, can be associated w/ bladder or bowel dysfunction.

STUDIES
■ MRI may be useful if neurologic deficit is present. It is important to distinguish between incidental findings & those that relate to symptoms & will change clinical mgt.

MANAGEMENT/INTERVENTIONS
■ **Medical Treatment**
  ➤ Conservative w/ exercise, acetaminophen, heat/ice
  ➤ TENS
  ➤ In cases of sciatica, consider epidural steroid injection after consultation w/ OB.
■ **Anesthesia**
  ➤ Document a complete history & physical exam w/ special attention to any neurologic findings prior to performing a regional anesthetic.
  ➤ Spinal or epidural anesthesia is rarely contraindicated in these pts.
  ➤ Discontinue epidural anesthesia (or at least the local anesthetic administration) & obtain a neurology consult for any pt who reports new or worsening neurologic symptoms.
  ➤ After performing a regional anesthetic, the pt should be placed in a position that was comfortable for her prior to anesthesia,

since the associated sensory block makes her less likely to protect herself from the effects of potentially harmful positions.

➤ Rotational movements & the lithotomy position should be minimized.

CAVEATS / PEARLS

■ Gestational back pain is highly prevalent.

■ Inform pts that back pain prior to delivery is a significant risk factor for post-partum back pain, regardless of whether regional anesthesia is used.

■ Hormonal factors contribute to gestational back pain early, mechanical factors later.

■ Regional anesthesia is not contraindicated.

■ Take care not to put the pt into a position that was uncomfortable for her prior to induction of regional anesthesia.

CHECKLIST

■ Pre-procedure documentation of neurologic exam

■ Neurology consultation & assistance in selected cases

GESTATIONAL THROMBOCYTOPENIA

JEANNA VIOLA, MD
JANE BALLANTYNE, MD

FUNDAMENTAL KNOWLEDGE

■ Common; occurs in 8% of parturients

■ Usually appears late in third trimester

■ New-onset mild thrombocytopenia w/o platelet dysfunction

■ Not associated w/ history of thrombocytopenia or bleeding

■ Usually recurs in subsequent pregnancies

■ No increased bleeding risk to mother or neonate

■ Normalizes 3–5 days post-partum

STUDIES

■ Mild platelet drop: $>90 \times 10^9$/L

■ Platelets may appear larger.

■ No other cytopenias

■ Normal coagulation indices

■ Normal urinalysis, liver function tests (no clinical evidence of pre-eclampsia)

■ Document platelet count in neonates.

MANAGEMENT/INTERVENTIONS
■ No particular intervention necessary in the absence of true coagulopathy
■ No contraindications to regional anesthesia

CAVEATS AND PEARLS
■ Diagnosis of exclusion; causes of significant bleeding abnormalities must be ruled out by history, exam & repeat studies of coagulation & platelet count
■ First-trimester thrombocytopenia is more likely to be idiopathic thrombocytopenia (ITP).

CHECKLIST
■ Recheck labs to rule out other coagulopathies.
■ Rule out pre-eclampsia or HELLP syndrome.

GLOMERULONEPHROPATHIES

JOSHUA WEBER, MD
PETER DUNN, MD

FUNDAMENTAL KNOWLEDGE
■ Glomerulonephropathies are characterized by glomerular dysfunction.
■ The glomerulonephropathies can be divided into 2 categories:
  ➤ *Nephritic syndromes* (inflammatory or necrotizing lesions of the glomeruli)
  ➤ *Nephrotic syndromes* (abnormal permeability of the glomeruli to proteins)
■ Glomerulonephropathies account for 2/3 of pts w/ chronic renal failure.
■ Pts w/ parenchymal disease may be asymptomatic for years or may have progressive renal insufficiency & hypertension.
Severe renal dysfunction before pregnancy is associated w/:
■ Higher likelihood of worsened renal function during pregnancy. The pathophysiology of how pregnancy worsens renal disease is unknown.
■ Higher incidence of obstetric complications (prematurity, fetal death)

STUDIES

Lab tests commonly ordered to evaluate renal function in pregnancy include:

- Creatinine (Cr > 0.8 is abnormal in pregnancy)
- BUN
- Electrolytes
- Creatinine clearance
- CBC
- Urinalysis

In addition to labs commonly used to evaluate renal function in pregnancy, the following tests may be performed:

- Serial BP monitoring
- Fetal ultrasound at 20 weeks to monitor growth
- Renal biopsy: generally not performed after 32 weeks gestation

MANAGEMENT & INTERVENTIONS

Medical/OB mgt of pts w/ pre-existing renal dysfunction

- Increased frequency of prenatal visits (q2 wks in 1st & 2nd trimesters, then q1 week)
- Monitoring: monthly measurements of serum creatinine, creatinine clearance, fetal development, maternal BP
- Erythropoietin may be used for maternal anemia.
- Preterm delivery considered for worsening renal function, fetal compromise or pre-eclampsia.
- Renal biopsy considered if rapid deterioration in renal function prior to 32 weeks gestation
- If glomerulonephropathy is responsive to steroids, these should be continued during pregnancy.
- See "*Parturients on Dialysis*" for dialysis mgt.

Anesthetic management for pts w/ pre-existing renal dysfunction

Pre-op

- Evaluate degree of renal dysfunction & hypertension.
- Evaluate for anemia & electrolyte abnormalities.
- Pre-existing peripheral neuropathy may confound recovery from regional anesthetic techniques (if regional anesthesia is used, carefully document baseline deficits). Intraoperative mgt
- Monitors: standard monitoring + fetal heart rate (FHR) +/− arterial line +/− CVP
- Limit fluids in pts w/ marginal renal function to prevent volume overload.

- Use strict aseptic technique, as uremic pts are more prone to infection.
- Careful padding/protection of dialysis access is important.
- Consider promotility agents, as uremic pts may have impaired GI motility.

Regional anesthesia
- Uremia-induced platelet dysfunction leads to increased bleeding time.
- Pts may have thrombocytopenia from peripheral destruction of platelets.
- Increased toxicity from local anesthetics has been reported in pts w/ renal disease, but ester & amide local anesthetics can be used.
- Contraindications to regional technique: pt refusal, bacteremia, significant hypovolemia, severe hemorrhage, coagulopathy, potentially pre-existing neuropathy

General anesthesia
- Uremic pts may have hypersensitivity to CNS drugs due to increased permeability of blood-brain barrier.
- Uremia causes delayed gastric emptying & increased acidity, leading to increased risk of aspiration pneumonitis (consider sodium citrate, H2-receptor blocker, metoclopramide).
- Hypoalbuminemia leads to increased free drug concentration of drugs that are bound to albumin (ie, thiopental).
- Succinylcholine is relatively contraindicated, as it causes approx. 1-mEq/L increase in serum potassium, which may precipitate cardiac dysrhythmias.
- Use caution w/ drugs dependent on renal excretion (gallamine, vecuronium, pancuronium) & clearance (mivacurium, rocuronium).

CAVEATS & PEARLS
- Serum Cr of 2.0 or greater prior to pregnancy implies a 33% chance of developing dialysis-dependent end-stage renal disease during or shortly after pregnancy.
- Cisatracurium is a good muscle relaxant for pts w/ renal dysfunction, as its clearance is independent of renal function (Hoffman degradation).
- Standard doses of anticholinesterases are used for reversal of neuromuscular blockade.

- Consider whether pt is likely to have platelet dysfunction (secondary to uremia) or significant peripheral neuropathy before doing regional anesthetic.

CHECKLIST
- Check OB plan for pt.
- Document degree of renal dysfunction.
- Be prepared to manage hypertension.
- Consider effects of uremia, hypoalbuminemia, impaired renal excretion when choosing meds.

HELLP SYNDROME

LAWRENCE WEINSTEIN, MD
DOUG RAINES, MD

FUNDAMENTAL KNOWLEDGE
- HELLP syndrome is a pathophysiologic state of pregnancy that is marked by hemolysis, elevated liver enzymes & low platelet counts.
- Occurs in 10–20% of women w/ pre-eclampsia
- Occasionally occurs w/o pre-existing pre-eclampsia
- For a detailed discussion of HELLP, see chapters on "*Severe Preeclampsia*" & "*Hematologic Disorders.*"

STUDIES
- Hemolytic anemia w/ schistocytes on blood smear
- Platelet count <100,000 cells/uL
- Serum lactate dehydrogenase >600 IU/L
- Elevated total bilirubin
- Serum AST >70 IU/L

MANAGEMENT/INTERVENTIONS
- Treatment for HELLP is maternal stabilization & correction of coagulopathy if needed
- In the case of co-existing pre-eclampsia, treatment consists of fetal delivery as soon as safely possible.
- As w/ all liver disease pts, anesthetic decisions should be guided by the symptoms & manifestations of the liver process. Various manifestations will have differing effects on physiology & choice of anesthetic technique for labor or delivery. In the case of HELLP syndrome, special attention should be paid to coagulation status & platelet count.
    - ➤ If pt is coagulopathic, see the section on "*General Concepts.*"

> If pt is cirrhotic, see sections on "*General Concepts*," "*Cirrhosis*," "*Portal Hypertension*," "*Ascites*," "*Hepatic Encephalopathy*."
> For general discussion of regional & general anesthesia considerations, see the section on "*General Concepts*."

CAVEATS/PEARLS

- HELLP syndrome is a pathophysiologic state of pregnancy that is marked by hemolysis, elevated liver enzymes & low platelet counts.
- Treatment for HELLP is maternal stabilization & correction of coagulopathy if needed.
- In the case of co-existing pre-eclampsia, treatment consists of fetal delivery as soon as safely possible.
- Anesthetic mgt should pay particular attention to coagulation status & platelet count.
- Sometimes epidurals are placed early, in anticipation of a continued precipitous drop in platelets.

CHECKLIST

- See "*Severe Pre-eclampsia*" chapter.
- Consider early epidural or general anesthesia.
- Wait for normalization of platelet count before removal of epidural catheter.

HEMOGLOBINOPATHIES

JEANNA VIOLA, MD
JANE BALLANTYNE, MD

FUNDAMENTAL KNOWLEDGE

- Sickle cell disease is caused by a mutation in the beta-globin gene that causes the synthesis of abnormal hemoglobin (Hgb S).
- Hgb S is abnormal because it "sickles" when it comes in contact w/ $PaO2 <40$.
  > Desaturated Hgb S molecules form stacks & alter the red cell's conformation, leading to damage, vaso-occlusion & an increased rate of clearance (half-life of these red cells is 10–20 days).
  > The oxyhemoglobin dissociation curve shifts to the right, favoring release of oxygen bound to hemoglobin at the tissue level.
- Homozygotes for Hgb S have sickle cell disease (0.5–1% of American Black population).
- Heterozygotes have sickle cell trait (8–10% of American Black population).

- Systemic effects
  - Vaso-occlusion & thrombosis in the CNS
  - Development of left ventricular hypertrophy & cardiomegaly (increased cardiac output & diastolic flow murmurs)
  - Pulmonary infarctions & atelectasis (acute chest syndrome)
  - Most sickle cell pts become asplenic in childhood & therefore are prone to infection w/ encapsulated organisms.
- Effects on pregnancy are related to the vaso-occlusive nature of the disease:
  - IUGR
  - Placental abruption
  - Fetal demise

STUDIES
- Diagnosed by Hgb electrophoresis

MANAGEMENT/INTERVENTIONS
- During a vaso-occlusive crisis
  - Maintain adequate hydration.
  - Administer supplemental oxygen.
  - Establish pain control w/ IV opioids. A combination of epidural opioid + bupivacaine may also be effective.
- Pts have an increased risk of acute chest syndrome, pneumonia, pulmonary embolism & vaso-occlusive crisis in the post-op period.
  - Maintain normothermia.
  - Maintain adequate hydration.
  - Avoid hypoxia & hypercarbia.
- Central neuraxial anesthesia (vs. general anesthesia) offers several advantages:
  - Peripheral vasodilation
  - Maintenance of pulmonary function
  - Decreased incidence of thromboembolic events
  - Decreased blood loss

CAVEATS AND PEARLS
- Hgb S shifts the oxyhemoglobin dissociation curve to the right, favoring release of oxygen to the tissues.
- Pts are at increased risk for a crisis, pneumonia & acute chest syndrome in the post-op period; maintain vigilance in pts who are post C-section or post-partum.
- Adequate hydration, normothermia & supplemental oxygen are important.
- Spinal & epidural anesthesia have advantages over GETA.

CHECKLIST
- Evaluate hemodynamic status & oxygen saturation.
- Obtain IV access to facilitate hydration.
- Apply supplemental oxygen.
- Raise OR temperature to comfortably warm.
- Prepare for vigilant monitoring of pts in post-op period.

HEMOLYTIC ANEMIAS

JEANNA VIOLA, MD
JANE BALLANTYNE, MD

FUNADMENTAL KNOWLEDGE

- Hemolytic anemias are divided into two categories:
    - Autoimmune
    - Drug-induced
        - Alpha-methyldopa (will induce warm IgG Abs in 10% of pts)
        - Quinine
        - Quinidine
        - PABA
        - Sulfonamides
        - Phenacetin
    - In both cases, antibodies are produced against erythrocytes, resulting in hemolysis.
    - Antibodies that react at body temperature are defined as warm & are usually IgG:
        - Lymphoma
        - Collagen vascular diseases such as lupus
        - Viral infections
- Antibodies that react at cooler temperatures are "cold agglutinins" & are usually IgM.

STUDIES

- Positive direct Coombs test: agglutination of the pt's red cells when exposed to animal serum that contains antibodies to IgG & C3
- Positive indirect Coombs test: agglutination of normal red cells when exposed to the pt's serum

MANAGEMENT/INTERVENTIONS

- Autoimmune hemolytic anemia
    - Treat w/ glucocorticoids to prevent hemolysis.
    - If steroid therapy fails, splenectomy is indicated.

➣ If disease is refractory to steroids & splenectomy, add azathioprine or cyclophosphamide immunosuppressive therapy.
- Regional anesthesia, general anesthesia are both options.
- Maintain body temp in pts w/ cold agglutinin disease.
- Avoid hypoxemia, acidosis.
- Avoid drugs known to activate complement if possible:
  ➣ Acetazolamide
  ➣ Magnesium compounds
  ➣ Protamine
- Prophylactic red cell transfusion may be considered after weighing risks vs. benefits.

CAVEATS AND PEARLS
- First-line treatment is administration of IV glucocorticoids.
- Avoid drugs that activate complement.
- Pts w/ hemolytic anemia may also have a collagen vascular disease or a blood dyscrasia.
- Regional anesthesia is not contraindicated in this pt population unless a concomitant thrombocytopenia or coagulopathy exists.

CHECKLIST
- Obtain direct and indirect Coombs tests if hemolytic anemia is suspected.
- Attempt to determine a cause of the hemolytic anemia; if it is drug-induced, stop the offending agent.
- Discontinue complement-activating drugs.
- Consider administration of glucocorticoids.
- Obtain type & cross if prophylactic PRBC transfusion will be used.
- Warm OR temp if pt has cold agglutinins disease.

HEPATIC ENCEPHALOPATHY

LAWRENCE WEINSTEIN, MD
DOUG RAINES, MD

FUNDAMENTAL KNOWLEDGE
- Reversible neurologic syndrome w/ symptoms ranging from mild confusion to coma
  ➣ Symptoms include mental obtundation, asterixis, fetor hepaticus
- Caused by buildup of ammonia & other toxins produced by bacteria in the gut

> Normally, these toxic substances are metabolized by the liver via the portal circulation before reaching the systemic circulation & the brain. In the setting of cirrhosis, ammonia & other toxins can reach the brain via porto-systemic shunts & also may not be sufficiently cleared due to hepatocellular dysfunction.

- Labs show elevated blood ammonia levels. Although it is not ammonia alone that is responsible for neurologic symptoms, elevated levels often correlate w/ symptoms.
- Encephalopathy verified by slowed or flattened waves on EEG
- Untreated, hepatic encephalopathy can result in cerebral edema, coma & death.

STUDIES
- Pathologic findings: glial hypertrophy, brain edema
- EEG consistent w/ metabolic encephalopathy
- Visual evoked potentials
- CT scan of head
- Venous ammonia levels

MANAGEMENT/INTERVENTIONS
- Treatment should be supportive & focus on decreasing amounts of ammonia & toxic metabolites entering the circulation.
  > Decrease dietary protein intake.
  > Oral lactulose decreases ammonia levels by lowering the intestinal pH & thus converting ammonia to ammonium, an ionized product that does not pass freely from the gut to the circulation.
  > Oral neomycin can kill enteric ammonia-producing bacteria, thereby decreasing the ammonia load in the gut.
- Upper GI bleeding from varices exacerbates encephalopathy by increasing protein (eg, Hgb) & thus protein load. Controlling such associated problems of cirrhosis can be helpful in reversing encephalopathy (see section on "*Portal Hypertension*").
- Take into account the pt's mental status & the effects of impaired cognition on an anesthetic plan.
- Restoration of mental status prior to anesthesia & surgery is preferred. In the case of a parturient, this may not be possible, as delivery is often something that cannot be delayed.
- For operative or vaginal delivery, regional anesthesia via spinal/ epidural is NOT absolutely contraindicated. However, mental deficit may make placement difficult if the pt is uncooperative.

➤ Prior to any regional technique in a liver failure pt, check coagulation labs & platelets & correct derangements prior to proceeding.

■ Encephalopathic pts often have a diminished gag reflex & are at higher risk for aspiration during induction & emergence from general anesthesia.

➤ Any induction should be rapid sequence w/ cricoid pressure. However, succinylcholine may be contraindicated in the presence of other derangements associated w/ cirrhosis & liver failure (renal failure, elevated potassium, chronic ICU status). Thus, a fast-acting non-depolarizing agent such as rocuronium should be used for relaxation. In general, use non-depolarizing agents cautiously

■ Severe hepatic encephalopathy is associated w/ cerebral edema & increased ICP.

➤ ICP monitoring w/ an intracranial bolt may be useful in general anesthesia. Strategies to minimize ICP:
  • Use of NS rather than LR helps prevent increasing edema due to its higher oncotic pressure.
  • Mannitol, an osmotic diuretic, can decrease ICP by shifting cerebral fluid intravascularly.
  • Although hyperventilation & consequent alkalosis can shift more ammonia across the blood-brain barrier, in the setting of acutely elevated ICP, it is a fast way to lower ICP.

➤ If ICP rises to the point where there is inadequate cerebral perfusion pressure, vasopressors may be necessary to raise systemic BP high enough to ensure adequate brain perfusion.

CAVEATS/PEARLS

■ Hepatic encephalopathy is reversible w/ appropriate treatment.
■ Supportive therapy is focused on lowering blood ammonia levels & toxic metabolites.
■ Altered mental status may make GETA & regional anesthesia more difficult.

CHECKLIST

■ Optimize blood ammonia levels preoperatively when possible.
■ Check coagulation status prior to regional anesthetic.
■ Beware of increased ICP.

HEPATITIS A

LAWRENCE WEINSTEIN, MD
DOUG RAINES, MD

FUNDAMENTAL KNOWLEDGE

- 1/1,000 incidence in pregnancy
- Transmitted via fecal-oral route. It is very contagious & people at greatest risk are those who traveled in developing nations.
- Hep A viremia is transient, so blood-borne transmission is extremely rare.
- Vertical transmission to the fetus is extremely rare.
- Incubation period 15–50 days
- Symptoms are usually mild, & the course tends to be self-limited.
- Does NOT progress to chronic hepatitis
- Can very rarely cause a fulminant hepatitis, w/ mortality rate for Hep A about 0.1%.
  - ➤ This incidence is higher when pts have pre-existing Hep C.

STUDIES

Serology of Diagnosis

- HAV IgM antibody is serologic marker. It is elevated early & persists for 6 months.
- HAV IgG rises early & persists for life, indicating immunity.

MANAGEMENT/INTERVENTIONS

- Treatment is generally supportive
- A Hep A vaccine is available.
- If symptoms are severe, Hep A immunoglobulin can be administered.

MANAGEMENT/INTERVENTION

- As w/ all liver disease pts, anesthetic decisions should be guided by the symptoms & manifestations of the liver process. Various manifestations will have differing effects on physiology & choice of anesthetic technique for labor or delivery.
  - ➤ If pt is coagulopathic, see the section on "*General Concepts.*"
  - ➤ If pt is cirrhotic, see sections on "*General Concepts,*" "*Cirrhosis,*" "*Portal Hypertension,*" "*Ascites,*" "*Hepatic Encephalopathy.*"
  - ➤ For general discussion of regional & general anesthesia considerations, see the section on "*General Concepts.*"

CAVEATS/PEARLS

- Viral hepatitis has a number of subtypes. Clinical course can range from mild, asymptomatic disease w/ full recovery to fulminant hepatitis w/ liver failure & death.
- Hep C is notable for its increased risk of progression to chronic hepatitis & cirrhosis.
- Diagnosis of viral hepatitis is based on serologic studies for viral antigens & antibodies.
- Prevention is based on either vaccination (for Hep A, B & D) or avoidance of exposure.
- Mgt is usually supportive.
- Anesthetic mgt is guided by physiologic manifestations of illness in each individual case.

CHECKLIST

- Understand acute or chronic nature of infection & impact on newborn.
- Studies & mgt depend on severity of compromise.

HEPATITIS B

LAWRENCE WEINSTEIN, MD
DOUG RAINES, MD

FUNDAMENTAL KNOWLEDGE

- 1–2/1,000 incidence in pregnancy
- Virus is blood-borne & transmitted commonly through sexual contact or direct exposure to infected blood (ie, needle stick, transfusion).
- Vertical transmission to infants is possible.
  - Timing of infection is important: women who are HBsAg & HBeAg positive at delivery have a 95% chance of vertical transmission.
  - In contrast, acute 1st-trimester infection w/o progression to chronic hepatitis has only a 10% risk of neonatal transmission.
  - Presence of anti-HBe antibodies reduces transmission risk to 25%.
- Nearly 2/3 of pts have subclinical disease & go on to clinical & serologic recovery.
- 20–25% develop clinical acute hepatitis; 99% of these recover & 1% go on to develop fulminant hepatitis & death.

■ Roughly 4% will have persistent infection.

➤ 10–33% of this group will develop chronic hepatitis. Of those, 25–50% progress to cirrhosis.

STUDIES

■ In acute hepatitis, serology will be positive for HBsAg, HBeAg & HBV-DNA.

■ Also in acute phase, IgM-anti-HBc & Anti HBe are detectable.

■ With resolution of acute illness & an absence of chronic disease, HBsAg levels decline to undetectable in 3–6 months.

■ After decline of HBsAg & resolution of acute symptoms, IgG-anti-HBs antibodies become detectable in the blood. This indicates serologic immunity.

■ If pt progresses to a chronic Hep B state, then HBsAg & HBV-DNA remain detectable in the blood.

MANAGEMENT/INTERVENTIONS

■ Supportive treatment for symptoms

■ HBV screening for all pregnant women

■ HBV vaccination for all newborns, regardless of maternal serology

■ If mother is HBsAg +, newborn should be vaccinated within 12 hours of delivery & receive HBV immune globulin as well.

■ Cesarean delivery does not alter the risk of vertical transmission, so delivery mode should be based on obstetrical criteria.

■ Universal Precautions are essential to avoid blood exposure & transmission to health care providers.

■ As w/ all liver disease pts, anesthetic decisions should be guided by the symptoms & manifestations of the liver process. Various manifestations will have differing effects on physiology & choice of anesthetic technique for labor or delivery.

➤ If pt is coagulopathic, see the section on *"General Concepts."*

➤ If pt is cirrhotic, see sections on *"General Concepts,"* *"Cirrhosis,"* *"Portal Hypertension,"* *"Ascites,"* *"Hepatic Encephalopathy."*

➤ For general discussion of regional & general anesthesia considerations, see the section on *"General Concepts."*

CAVEATS/PEARLS

■ Viral hepatitis has a number of subtypes. Clinical course can range from mild, asymptomatic disease w/ full recovery to fulminant hepatitis w/ liver failure & death.

■ Hepatitis C is notable for its increased risk of progression to chronic hepatitis & cirrhosis.

- Diagnosis of viral hepatitis is based on serologic studies for viral antigens & antibodies.
- Prevention is based on either vaccination (for Hep A, B & D) or avoidance of exposure.
- Mgt is usually supportive.
- Anesthetic mgt is guided by physiologic manifestations of illness in each individual case.

CHECKLIST
- Understand acute or chronic nature of infection & impact on newborn.
- Studies & mgt depend on severity of compromise.

HEPATITIS C

LAWRENCE WEINSTEIN, MD
DOUG RAINES, MD

FUNDAMENTAL KNOWLEDGE
- Incidence in pregnancy unknown
- Transmission is via blood contact (IV drug use, transfusion) or sexual contact.
- Vertical transmission is poorly studied; appears less common than w/ Hep B, though it is possible.
- Acute Hep C hepatitis tends to be mild; many cases go undiagnosed.
- Roughly 15% of cases resolve, but about 85% will progress to chronic hepatitis.
  - About 20% of those w/ chronic Hep C disease will progress to cirrhosis. However, the chance of a pt with cirrhotic chronic hepatitis maintaining a pregnancy is very slim.

STUDIES

Serology of diagnosis
- In acute infection, HCV-RNA is detectable, along w/ elevated serum transaminases.
- IgG & IgM-anti-HCV antibodies are present as HCV-RNA levels start to fall, as the acute phase begins to abate.
- With chronic Hep C infection, pts will have intermittent periods w/ detectable HCV-RNA, along w/ episodic elevations in serum transaminases.

MANAGEMENT/INTERVENTIONS

- Currently there is no vaccine for Hep C.
- Neonatal effects of Hep C are minimal, except for an increased risk of prematurity when contracted in the 3rd trimester.
- No formal newborn prophylactic recommendations, though some advise administration of Hep C immunoglobulin to neonates born to women w/ acute Hep C infection
- Alpha-interferon-2B can reduce HCV RNA titers & improve outcome in pts w/ chronic HCV infection, but it is not considered safe during pregnancy.
- Mode of delivery based on obstetric criteria
- Universal Precautions are essential to avoid blood exposure & transmission to health care providers.

As w/ all liver disease pts, anesthetic decisions should be guided by the symptoms & manifestations of the liver process. Various manifestations will have differing effects on physiology & choice of anesthetic technique for labor or delivery.

- If pt is coagulopathic, see the section on "*General Concepts.*"
- If pt is cirrhotic, see sections on "*General Concepts,*" "*Cirrhosis,*" "*Portal Hypertension,*" "*Ascites,*" "*Hepatic Encephalopathy.*"
- For general discussion of regional & general anesthesia considerations, see the section on "*General Concepts.*"

CAVEATS/PEARLS

- Viral hepatitis has a number of subtypes. Clinical course can range from mild, asymptomatic disease w/ full recovery to fulminant hepatitis w/ liver failure & death.
- Hep C is notable for its increased risk of progression to chronic hepatitis & cirrhosis.
- Diagnosis of viral hepatitis is based on serologic studies for viral antigens & antibodies.
- Prevention is based on either vaccination (for Hep A, B & D) or avoidance of exposure.
- Mgt is usually supportive.
- Anesthetic mgt is guided by physiologic manifestations of illness in each individual case.

CHECKLIST

- Understand acute or chronic nature of infection & impact on newborn.
- Studies & mgt depend on severity of compromise.

HEPATITIS D

LAWRENCE WEINSTEIN, MD
DOUG RAINES, MD

FUNDAMENTAL KNOWLEDGE

- Hep D causes clinical disease only when a pt also has Hep B virus.
- Transmission is via blood or sexual contact.
- Vertical transmission is possible.
- Co-infection w/ Hep B in a healthy individual usually results in a mild acute hepatitis w/ recovery. However, Hep D viral superinfection in a chronic Hep B virus carrier has a higher rate of fulminant hepatitis (7–10%) & chronic hepatitis & cirrhosis than does Hep B alone.
- Prevention should be based on effective Hep B vaccination, for Hep D does not cause clinical disease without concurrent Hep B infection.

STUDIES

N/A

MANAGEMENT/INTERVENTIONS

- As w/ all liver disease pts, anesthetic decisions should be guided by the symptoms & manifestations of the liver process. Various manifestations will have differing effects on physiology & choice of anesthetic technique for labor or delivery.
  - ➤ If pt is coagulopathic, see the section on *"General Concepts."*
  - ➤ If pt is cirrhotic, see sections on *"General Concepts," "Cirrhosis," "Portal Hypertension," "Ascites," "Hepatic Encephalopathy."*
  - ➤ For general discussion of regional & general anesthesia considerations, see the section on *"General Concepts."*

CAVEATS/PEARLS

- Viral hepatitis has a number of subtypes. Clinical course can range from mild, asymptomatic disease w/ full recovery to fulminant hepatitis w/ liver failure & death.
- Diagnosis of viral hepatitis is based on serologic studies for viral antigens & antibodies.
- Prevention is based on either vaccination (for Hep A, B & D) or avoidance of exposure.
- Mgt is usually supportive.
- Anesthetic mgt is guided by physiologic manifestations of illness in each individual case.

CHECKLIST

■ Understand acute or chronic nature of infection & impact on newborn.

■ Studies & mgt depend on severity of compromise.

HEPATITIS E

LAWRENCE WEINSTEIN, MD
DOUG RAINES, MD

FUNDAMENTAL KNOWLEDGE

■ Transmitted via fecal-oral route & not endemic in U.S.

■ Vertical transmission is possible.

■ In non-pregnant women, Hep E has a mild clinical course similar to Hep A.

■ In pregnancy, Hep E has significant maternal & neonatal morbidity & mortality, w/ maternal mortality on the order of 15–20%.

STUDIES

N/A

MANAGEMENT/INTERVENTIONS

■ As w/ all liver disease pts, anesthetic decisions should be guided by the symptoms & manifestations of the liver process. Various manifestations will have differing effects on physiology & choice of anesthetic technique for labor or delivery.

➤ If pt is coagulopathic, see the section on "*General Concepts.*"

➤ If pt is cirrhotic, see sections on "*General Concepts,*" "*Cirrhosis,*" "*Portal Hypertension,*" "*Ascites,*" "*Hepatic Encephalopathy.*"

  • For general discussion of regional & general anesthesia considerations, see the section on "*General Concepts.*"

CAVEATS/PEARLS

■ Viral hepatitis has a number of subtypes. Clinical course can range from mild, asymptomatic disease w/ full recovery to fulminant hepatitis w/ liver failure & death.

■ Diagnosis of viral hepatitis is based on serologic studies for viral antigens & antibodies.

■ Prevention is based on either vaccination (for Hep A, B & D) or avoidance of exposure.

■ Mgt is usually supportive.

■ Anesthetic mgt is guided by physiologic manifestations of illness in each individual case.

HEREDITARY MOTOR & SENSORY NEUROPATHY

MEREDITH ALBRECHT, MD; LISA LEFFERT, MD; AND MICHELE SZABO, MD

FUNDAMENTAL KNOWLEDGE

Definition
■ Heterogeneous group of inherited peripheral nerve diseases
■ Most common: Charcot-Marie-Tooth
■ Distal muscular atrophy & sensory neuropathy affecting lower, then upper extremities
■ Slow progressive degeneration of peripheral nerves & roots

Epidemiology
■ Generally inherited autosomal dominant
■ Estimated 1 in 2,500 incidence

Pathophysiology
■ Progressive neuropathic (peroneal) muscular atrophy

Clinical Manifestations
■ Two variants
■ Type I
  ➤ Early onset (10–20 years)
  ➤ Foot drop
  ➤ Lower extremity muscle wasting (peroneal & anterior tibialis)
  ➤ Decreased tendon reflexes & conduction velocities
  ➤ Sensory deficits "stocking & glove" distribution
  ➤ Demyelinating neuropathy
■ Type II
  ➤ Manifests in a similar manner
  ➤ Later onset w/ slower course
  ➤ Axonal degeneration
  ➤ Can present w/ only foot deformities

Effect of Pregnancy on Hereditary Neuropathy
■ Increases severity of symptoms in about 50% of pts w/ type I
■ No effect on type II
■ If symptom severity increases, usually resolves after delivery
■ Subsequent pregnancies can increase the magnitude of the exacerbation of symptoms w/ pregnancy.

- If it involves the intercostal muscles, the mechanical effects of the gravid uterus can worsen the degree of respiratory compromise.

Effect of Hereditary Neuropathy on Pregnancy & the Fetus
- No effect on pregnancy or fetus

STUDIES

History & Physical
- Weakness of feet & legs, later progressing to hands & forearms
- History of abnormal high-stepped gait w/ frequent tripping & falling
- Frequent foot deformity (pes cavus or high-arched feet)
- Careful motor & sensory neuronal exam focusing on lower extremities

Laboratory
- Genetic testing

Imaging
- None

Other
- Nerve conduction velocity studies
- EMG
- EKG to assess if cardiac conduction abnormalities present
- Pulmonary function tests to assess degree of respiratory compromise

MANAGEMENT/INTERVENTIONS

Medical Treatment
- Benefit from physical therapy
- Ankle-foot orthoses to alleviate foot drop
- If pt has intractable pain or difficulty walking, consider surgery.

Anesthesia
- Initial assessment
  - Careful neurologic exam documenting extent of disease
  - Assess respiratory function for signs of compromise.
- General anesthesia
  - Recommended if severe respiratory involvement
  - May need post-op ventilation if severe respiratory involvement
  - Most likely succinylcholine is safe
  - No increased incidence of malignant hyperthermia
- Regional anesthesia
  - Suitable in mildly involved cases
  - Scoliosis can increase the difficulty of the technique.

CAVEATS & PEARLS

- Heterogeneous collection of inherited peripheral neuropathies
- Complete neurologic exam is warranted to document preexisting dysfunction.
- General anesthesia recommended if significant pulmonary involvement
- Regional acceptable in most cases
- Succinylcholine generally safe
- No increased risk of malignant hyperthermia
- Normal response to non-depolarizing neuromuscular relaxants

CHECKLIST

- Conduct a thorough neurologic exam & document current deficits.
- Assess respiratory status (general anesthesia is recommended in cases of significant pulmonary involvement).
- Regional acceptable in most cases

HERPES SIMPLEX VIRUS

SISSELA PARK, MD
LAURA RILEY, MD

FUNDAMENTAL KNOWLEDGE

Introduction

- Herpes simplex virus (HSV)
  - ➤ Encapsulated double-stranded DNA virus
  - ➤ Infects susceptible mucosal surfaces
- Two types of HSV
  - ➤ HSV-1: predominantly oral
  - ➤ HSV-2: predominantly genital
  - ➤ Both can cause serious illness in the neonate.

Pathophysiology

- Incubation period of 2–10 days
- Primary infection
  - ➤ Focal vesicle formation
  - ➤ Pronounced cellular immune response
  - ➤ May also see:
    - Inguinal lymphadenopathy
    - Systemic flu-like symptoms: fever, myalgias, malaise, headache, nausea

- Usually lasts about 2 weeks
- Viral shedding period: 1–2 weeks
- Latent phase
  - Follows primary infection
  - Virus ascends peripheral sensory nerves.
  - Rests in nerve root ganglia
- Intermittent recurrent exacerbations
  - Stimulation unclear
  - Prodrome may precede the onset of lesions.
    - Tingling
    - Itching
    - Sacral dermatomal neuralgia
  - Frequency variable
  - 5- to 10-day course
  - Viral shedding period: 3–6 days
- Infection can be primary, recurrent or asymptomatic.
- Difficult to differentiate primary from recurrent infection
- Viral shedding occurs for a longer time w/ primary infection than w/ recurrent infection.
- Antibodies
  - Appear about 7 days after the start of the primary infection
  - Peak in 2–3 weeks
  - Usually detectable for life

Congenital HSV infection

- Extremely rare
- Usually appears within 72 hours of delivery
- Characteristic triad of signs
  - Skin vesicles/scarring
  - Eye involvement
    - Chorioretinitis
    - Microphthalmia
  - CNS abnormalities
    - Microcephaly
    - Hydranencephaly

Neonatal infection

- Can be vertically transmitted
- Morbidity & mortality decreased w/ prompt institution of IV acyclovir
- Greatest risk to fetus occurs w/ overt HSV infection at the time of labor

➤ Mechanism of infection is direct contact w/ infected vesicles.
■ Frequency depends on whether maternal infection is primary or recurrent.
  ➤ Viral inoculum in the genital tract is higher w/ primary infection.
  ➤ Maternal antibody is absent w/ primary infection.
  ➤ About 40% of infants delivered to women w/ primary infection will be infected.
■ Clinical manifestations
  ➤ Skin, eye & mouth disease
  ➤ Encephalitis
  ➤ Disseminated HSV

STUDIES
■ PCR assays are extremely sensitive in detecting low concentrations of viral DNA.
■ Culture of vesicular fluid
  ➤ Was the gold standard for HSV diagnosis before PCR
  ➤ Sensitivity 70–90%
■ Measurement of HSV1 & HSV2 specific antibodies to differentiate primary from recurrent disease
■ Primary infection: multiple painful lesions on an inflamed surface
  ➤ Lesions progress to ulcers.
  ➤ May be accompanied by adenopathy & fevers
■ Recurrent infection: more difficult to make a clinical diagnosis
  ➤ Genital lesions are more often unilateral, smaller & fewer.

MANAGEMENT/INTERVENTIONS
Obstetric
■ Ask pt about prior history of HSV at initial prenatal appointment.
■ If positive history of HSV, screen for other STDs.
■ Antiviral therapy during pregnancy
  ➤ Immunocompromised pts w/ disseminated infection: IV acyclovir
  ➤ Immunocompetent pts w/ primary HSV infection: oral acyclovir
    • Alternative regimens
      • Oral valacyclovir
      • Oral famciclovir
■ Consider suppressive treatment for women w/ frequent recurrent infection (from 36 weeks to delivery):
  ➤ Oral valacyclovir
  ➤ Oral acyclovir

- When pt is admitted for delivery
  - ➤ Ask about prodromal symptoms.
  - ➤ Examine pt for genital lesions.
  - ➤ Plan on vaginal delivery if no symptoms or lesions.
  - ➤ Perform cesarean if pt has prodromal symptoms or lesions.

Anesthetic mgt

Primary infection

- Concern of possible introduction of virus into CNS w/ possibility of disseminated disease
- Theoretically more likely in the setting of primary infection because there is transient viremia
- Safety of regional anesthesia in primary HSV has not been determined.
- Weigh risks of general anesthesia against risk of introducing virus into CNS w/ neuraxial blocks.

Recurrent infection

- Viremia is rare.
- Safety of neuraxial blocks has been documented in studies.
- Regional anesthesia contraindicated by the presence of an active lesion at the planned site for needle insertion

Reactivation of HSV-1

- Epidural dosing of opioids, particularly morphine, may reactivate thoracic & perioral HSV-1 lesions.
- Similar risk may exist w/ intrathecal opioids.
- Pathophysiology is unclear.
- No reported association btwn neuraxial opioids & recurrence of HSV-2

CAVEATS & PEARLS

- HSV is one of the most common STDs.
- Congenital HSV infection is very rare.
- High (60%) mortality rate w/ neonatal infection
- Ask pt about HSV history at initial prenatal appointment.
- Perform C-section if pt has prodromal symptoms or lesions when she is admitted for delivery.
- Introduction of virus into CNS w/ disseminated disease may be possible w/ regional anesthesia during a primary infection.
- Regional anesthesia is safe during recurrent infection so long as there is no active lesion at the planned needle insertion site.

■ Epidural dosing of narcotics (particularly morphine) may reactivate thoracic & perioral HSV lesions.

CHECKLIST
■ Determine pt's HSV history.
■ In setting of primary HSV infection, weigh risk of general anesthesia against risk of CNS introduction of virus.

HIV AND AIDS

SARAH WITT, MD
LAURA RILEY, MD

FUNDAMENTAL KNOWLEDGE

Epidemiology

HIV/AIDS has become a global pandemic since its first description in a case report of 4 homosexual men w/ *Pneumocystis carinii* pneumonia in 1981.

■ In the U.S., women of reproductive age are the fastest-growing population infected w/ HIV.
■ In 1995, HIV infection was the leading cause of death in the U.S. for people 25–44 years of age; in 1996 it was the third leading cause of death for U.S. women aged 25–44.

Most anesthesiologists will encounter HIV/AIDS pts at some point in their practice, including those caring for parturients in labor & delivery.

■ It is estimated that 25% of pts w/ HIV will need surgery, either obstetric or non-obstetric.
■ Anesthesiologists should be familiar w/ clinical presentations of HIV/AIDS, the effects of anti-retroviral & anti-opportunistic infection therapies & anesthetic & obstetric mgt of parturients.
■ HIV/AIDS & polysubstance abuse may be closely associated; the anesthesiologist must be aware of implications due to possible cocaine &/or heroin use.
■ HIV infection is also closely associated w/ lack of prenatal care, cigarette smoking & STDs.

Pathophysiology

HIV is a member of the family of human retroviruses of the genus Lentiviridae.

■ Strains include HIV-1 (most common in U.S.) & HIV-2.
■ HIV affects multiple organ systems.

- It is a neurotrophic virus; it infects the CNS early & can be isolated from CSF early in asymptomatic individuals.
- Characterized by cytopathic action, long latency period, persistent viremia
- Virus found in CSF, plasma, seminal & vaginal fluids, tears, saliva, urine, breast milk as well as synovial, pericardial & pleural fluid

CD+4 T lymphocytes & monocytes are the primary targets of HIV, but it also infects glial cells, gut endothelium, bone marrow progenitors & macrophages.

- T cells play a major role in cell-mediated immunity & B cells in humoral-mediated immunity.
- HIV causes impaired cell-mediated & humoral-mediated immunity (T cells are important for activation of B cells).
- Dysfunctions in cell- & humoral-mediated immunities make pts susceptible to bacterial, viral, fungal, parasitic & mycobacterial infection as well as some tumors.
- 98% of CD4+ T cells are located in lymph nodes, which are the major site of viral replication & T-cell destruction.
- Monocytes may serve as a long-term reservoir of HIV & may spread the virus to the brain & other organs.
- Although a pt may appear well (clinical latency), the virus is active & replicating throughout the entire course of infection.
- The latent period of infection can persist for up to 12 years.

AIDS

AIDS is defined when an HIV+ pt develops any one of the following AIDS indicator conditions:

- CD4+ T-cell count <200/microliter
- Opportunistic infections
    - Disseminated or extrapulmonary coccidioidomycosis
    - Disseminated or extrapulmonary histoplasmosis
    - Extrapulmonary cryptococcosis
    - *M. tuberculosis* at any site
    - Disseminated or extrapulmonary *Mycobacterium avium complex* or *Mycobacterium kansasii*
    - Cytomegalovirus (CMV) retinitis
    - Candidiasis of the esophagus or pulmonary system
    - Herpes simplex virus (HSV) bronchitis, pneumonitis or esophagitis
    - HSV mucocutaneous ulcer that persists >1 month
    - Cryptosporidiosis > 1 month

- Isosporiasis w/ diarrhea > 1 month
- *Pneumocystis carinii* pneumonia
- Recurrent *Salmonella*septicemia
- Cerebral toxoplasmosis
- Herpes simplex chronic ulcers (>1 month), bronchitis, pneumonitis, esophagitis
■ Neurologic disease
  - Progressive multifocal leukoencephalopathy
  - HIV encephalopathy
  - AIDS dementia
  - HIV wasting syndrome
■ Tumors
  - Kaposi's sarcoma
  - Primary CNS lymphoma
  - Invasive cervical cancer

Clinical Presentations of HIV: Systemic Abnormalities & Coexisting Diseases in HIV

Initial HIV infection
■ Most common signs & symptoms: fever, adenopathy, pharyngitis, rash, myalgias or arthralgias
■ An aseptic meningitis picture can occur w/ headaches & photophobia.
■ These are usually self-limited & resolve spontaneously in 1–3 weeks.
■ Chronic HIV infection: affects multiple organ systems

Neurologic abnormalities
■ Widely accepted that the CNS is infected early in the course of HIV infection, even in asymptomatic pts
■ Neurologic dysfunction is very common & caused by a primary effect of HIV itself or from opportunistic infections & tumors.

Neuropathies
■ Peripheral neuropathy is the most common neurologic complication in HIV pts.
  - Often occurs early, can be very debilitating & unresponsive to antiretroviral drug therapy (ART)
■ Several distinct neuropathy syndromes exist:
  - Most common is a "stocking-and-glove" pattern w/ numbness, painful dysesthesias & paresthesias
  - ART can cause a similar neuropathy that subsides when the drug is stopped.

➤ A chronic inflammatory, demyelinating polyneuropathy exists that is often responsive to corticosteroids, IVIG or plasmapheresis.

➤ Mononeuropathy multiplex can cause asymmetric weakness & sensory loss.

➤ Lumbosacral polyradiculopathy is less common & involves rapid progression of lower extremity weakness & loss of sphincter control.

➤ Autonomic neuropathy can cause syncope, postural hypotension or significant cardiovascular instability.

Spinal cord involvement in HIV

■ Vacuolar myelopathy is progressive, diffuse & painless degeneration causing sensory & gait disturbances w/ spasticity & hyperreflexia.

■ Acute cord myelopathies can be caused by tuberculous abscesses or viral infection (CMV or HSV).

Focal cerebral space-occupying lesions

Not uncommon but usually occur late in HIV/AIDS

■ Caused by cerebral toxoplasmosis & primary CNS lymphoma

■ May increase ICP & preclude neuraxial anesthesia

Meningitis

Can be from tuberculosis, *Cryptococcus neoformans*, metastatic lymphoma, direct infection of the meninges by HIV

Diffuse encephalitis

Usually occurs later in course of AIDS

■ Causes include CMV, HSV or *Toxoplasmosis* w/ impairment in both cognition & alertness. Progressive multifocal leukoencephalopathy (PML) is a viral disorder in AIDS that causes selective destruction of white matter tract.

AIDS dementia complex causes progressive impairment of cognition, motor function, behavioral changes, depression & can culminate in a vegetative state.

Cardiac abnormalities

■ Common & often clinically silent

■ Neoplastic or infectious involvement can lead to myocarditis, pericarditis or pericardial effusion.

■ IV drug abusers w/ HIV are at higher risk for infective endocarditis.

■ Pts w/ HIV can have accelerated arteriolosclerosis.

Pulmonary abnormalities

- Most abnormalities are caused by opportunistic infections or lymphoma causing pneumonitis, cavitary lung disease or abscesses.
- Endobronchial Kaposi's sarcoma can lead to significant hemoptysis.
- HIV can directly destroy the lung parenchyma & cause a syndrome similar to emphysema.
- Reactivation of latent *Mycobacterium tuberculosis* is common.
- Increased susceptibility to bacterial pneumonia from encapsulated organisms
- *Pneumocystis carinii* is a fungal organism that can cause pneumonia (PCP) & resemble adult respiratory distress syndrome (ARDS) w/ hypoxemia.
  - ➤ Chest x-ray & exam are often normal but usually show diffuse interstitial infiltrates.
  - ➤ Can predispose to pneumatocele formation & subsequent pneumothorax
  - ➤ Early steroid use may decrease progression to respiratory failure.
  - ➤ High-dose sulfamethoxazole-trimethoprim is treatment of choice.

Renal abnormalities

- A specific HIV nephropathy exists that produces focal segmental glomerular sclerosis (FSGS).
- May present early & can progress rapidly to end-stage renal disease (ESRD)
- Characterized by heavy proteinuria but rarely associated w/ hypertension or edema, allowing differentiation from pre-eclampsia
- Antiretroviral agents can lead to nephropathy & nephrolithiasis.
- Renal dysfunction can be exacerbated by volume depletion or recreational drug use (heroin).

Coagulation & hematologic abnormalities:

- Very common w/ all cell lines affected
- HIV-associated thrombocytopenia is similar to ITP, but bleeding complications are less common.
- Thrombocytopenia can occur early in HIV infection & usually responds to ART or IVIG.
- Presence of a lupus anticoagulant may prolong activated partial thromboplastin time (APTT), but this is thought to have little clinical significance.
- Liver dysfunction, commonly from hepatitis B & C, can impair coagulation.

■ Low-grade DIC has occurred in severely immunocompromised HIV pts.

■ Depletion of CD4+ lymphocytes & neutropenia predispose to opportunistic infections.

■ HIV-related anemia exacerbates the dilutional anemia of pregnancy.

GI abnormalities

■ Opportunistic infections of the pharynx or esophagus can cause tissue friability, make intubation difficult & increase the risk of aspiration.

■ Hepatobiliary disease is common & can lead to metabolic & coagulation derangements.

■ HIV enteropathy or bowel superinfections can cause severe, chronic diarrhea w/ volume depletion & electrolyte abnormalities.

Endocrine abnormalities

■ Opportunistic infections, the virion itself, neoplasms or antiretroviral/antimicrobial therapies can damage endocrine glands.

■ Diabetes mellitus is not uncommon due to pancreatic involvement.

■ Syndrome of inappropriate anti-diuretic hormone (SIADH) can occur due to opportunistic pulmonary infections or CNS pathology.

■ Protease inhibitor therapy can cause a hyperinsulinemic hypoglycemia.

■ Thyroid function abnormalities are common but clinical hypothyroidism is rare.

■ HIV pts often have a decreased adrenal stress response, w/ overt adrenal failure rare but serious.

Musculoskeletal abnormalities

■ The virion directly affects myofibers & can lead to myositis & a profound wasting syndrome.

■ Often associated w/ constitutional symptoms

Pain syndromes

■ Chronic pain syndromes similar to disseminated cancer pain are common, can affect almost any organ system & usually require a multidisciplinary approach for treatment.

■ Pain due to opportunistic infection or malignancy must be excluded.

■ Peripheral neuropathy is the most common.

Antiretroviral Therapy & the Parturient

Highly active antiretroviral therapy (HAART) has become very successful in treating HIV by decreasing the viral load.

- Overall, there is little significant evidence to suggest that HAART increases the rate of pregnancy complications.
- Pregnancy can affect timing, choice of therapy & dosing but is not considered a reason to postpone treatment.
- Although retrovirals are pregnancy category C, guidelines suggest pregnant women should receive the same therapy as if they were not pregnant.

There are 3 classes of antiretroviral agents; most have significant side effects & can interact w/ anesthetic agents.

- **Nucleoside analogue reverse transcriptase inhibitors (NRTI):** interfere w/ viral replication within host cells
  - Common side effects of this class include headache, GI disturbances, pancreatitis, elevated liver enzymes, insomnia, bone marrow suppression & peripheral neuropathy.
  - Can cause a clinical picture similar to severe gram-negative sepsis
  - Long-term therapy may cause myalgia, malaise, myopathy. Cessation of the agent usually reverses peripheral neuropathy.
    - Zidovudine (AZT, ZDV): first agent approved; can cause significant bone marrow depression w/ anemia & thrombocytopenia
    - Stavudine (D4T): can cause severe lactic acidosis
    - Zalcitabine (ddC)
    - Didanosine (ddi)
    - Lamivudine (3TC)
    - Adefovir: may cause acute tubular necrosis (ATN)
    - Abacavir
    - Tenofavir
- **Non-nucleotide reverse transcriptase inhibitors (NNRTI):** The major side effect is skin rash; can be as severe as Stevens-Johnson syndrome.
  - Nevirapine: causes cytochrome P450 induction & can increase the metabolism of many anesthetic, sedative & analgesic agents, thereby decreasing effective serum levels.
  - Efavirenz: potent teratogen; should not be used in pregnancy
  - Delavirdine
- **Protease inhibitors (PI)**
  - Side effects generally include GI disturbances, increased liver enzymes, altered glucose metabolism, peripheral neuropathy, lipodystrophy.
  - Usually inhibits the cytochrome P450 system & can cause elevated levels of many sedative medications (especially fentanyl, ketamine & midazolam) as well as many cardiac medications (amiodarone & quinidine) by decreasing their metabolism.

> Careful titration of meds is needed to prevent inadvertent overdose.
  - Saquinavir
  - Ritonavir
  - Indinavir (may cause nephrolithiasis)
  - Nelfinavir
  - Lopinavir/ritonavir

HIV/AIDS & Pregnancy

Effect of HIV on pregnancy outcomes

- Overall, there is little significant evidence to suggest that HIV or HAART increases the rate of pregnancy complications.
- No increased risk of fetal malformations in infants of HIV+ women
- Some studies have indicated that HIV+ women may be more likely to have an adverse pregnancy outcome than those uninfected, but confounding factors including substance abuse, poor nutrition & other STDs could account for the increased risk.
- Many studies in the U.S. & industrialized countries have noted no difference in incidence of low birthweight, preterm delivery, IUGR, SGA infants or 5-minute Apgar scores compared to those uninfected.
- In developing countries, some studies noted an association w/ HIV positivity & increased risk of preterm delivery & low birthweight.
- Pregnant women w/ advanced HIV infection can have serious infectious complications that could independently & adversely affect pregnancy outcomes.
- Data from a European collaborative study have shown that only 14% of HIV-infected pregnant women are severely immune compromised.

Effect of pregnancy on HIV progression

- There is no evidence that pregnancy alters or accelerates HIV progression, maternal mortality or viral load, especially when access to appropriate medical care is available.

Vertical transmission (mother to baby)

- Most common route for infection of children
- In the U.S., when transmission occurs, it occurs during labor & delivery in nearly 70% of cases, in utero 30%, & after delivery (breastfeeding) in the remainder.
- Elective cesarean delivery & AZT prophylaxis appear to have an additive effect in preventing vertical transmission.
- Maternal transmission rate is 0–2% w/ HAART.

- Elective cesarean delivery independent of ART decreases the risk of vertical transmission.
- Breast-feeding may double the rate of transmission & should be discouraged when bottle-feeding is safe.
- Risk factors for vertical transmission
  - Prolonged PROM (>4 hour)
  - Chorioamninitis
  - Presence of other STDs & hepatitis C
  - High maternal viral load, decreased CD4+ count (<400/microliter), advanced stage of disease
  - Obstetrical invasive procedures such as fetal scalp electrode or fetal scalp gas
  - Preterm delivery

STUDIES

HIV detection

ELISA confirmed by a Western blot against antibodies to viral P24 core antigen, as well as amplifying RNA/proviral DNA using PCR, can detect HIV seropositivity.

- Intervals up to 3 months after initial infection can occur before detectable levels of antibody are present.
  - Pts in this window period will have a negative test result but will be infectious (high viral load).
  - Pts may be infected w/ HIV but look clinically well.
- Viral load
  - Quantifies virus present & monitors response to ART
  - Levels usually correlate inversely w/ CD4+ T lymphocyte count.
  - Best predictor of disease progression & perinatal transmission
- Rapid HIV test
  - May be used for a parturient with no prenatal care in labor
  - If positive, antiretroviral agent(s) given in labor
  - Must be confirmed by Western blot after delivery

MANAGEMENT/INTERVENTIONS

Anesthetic effect on HIV

HIV infection ranges from asymptomatic to advanced disease w/ debilitation & multiorgan dysfunction. Limited information exists regarding the overall risk of anesthesia & surgery on pts w/ HIV/AIDS, but it is generally thought that HIV infection itself does not increase the risk for postprocedural complications, nor does anesthesia influence the natural progress of the disease.

- Necessary surgeries should not be limited in HIV/AIDS pts due to concern for subsequent complications.
- The ASA status, severity of opportunistic infections & degree of immunosuppression w/ the inherent surgical risk probably provide best measure of global risk.
- Some evidence does exist suggesting delayed wound healing irrespective of CD4+ count as well as an increased frequency of perioperative tachycardia & post-op fevers in pts w/ HIV, although the clinical significance is unknown.
- AMA declared that doctors have an ethical duty to treat HIV pts, & federal laws prohibit discrimination based on HIV status.

Preoperative evaluation

End-organ dysfunction, opportunistic infections, tumors, polysubstance abuse, STDs & ART may complicate the perioperative mgt of the HIV+ parturient. Assessment of coexisting disease using a thorough history, physical, lab studies & imaging prior to anesthesia is paramount.

- Detection of cardiac dysfunction is critical & EKG findings are often abnormal in pts w/ HIV. Transthoracic echocardiography or even coronary catheterization is indicated in those w/ symptoms. Invasive monitoring depends on the severity of cardiac dysfunction.
- Routine chest x-ray & EKG recommended
- Evaluate extent of neutropenia & thrombocytopenia.
- Chemistries for glucose, liver & renal function help assess extent of end-organ dysfunction.
- CD4+ count & viral load can reveal severity of HIV/AIDS as well as response to therapy.
- In pts w/ signs & symptoms of pulmonary dysfunction, consider ABGs & pulmonary function tests.
- Perform radiologic studies of brain or spinal cord to rule out compressive mass lesions in pts w/ neurologic symptoms.
- Thromboelastography (TEG) to evaluate platelet function & coagulation status may be useful prior to regional anesthesia.

Anesthetic technique

There are few studies evaluating anesthetic technique in HIV pts. Anesthetic or analgesic choice should be based on clinical obstetric indications, urgency & presence of coexisting disease, including coagulopathy & CNS mass lesions, but not HIV status alone.

- No reported perioperative complications or changes in immune function or viral load

- The stress response may be more profound after general anesthesia.
- General anesthesia & opiates may transiently decrease immune system function, but this is not thought to be significant in either healthy pts or those w/ HIV.
- In immunosuppressed & debilitated pts, weigh the risks & benefits btwn potential infections of the nervous system using regional against general anesthesia & possible prolonged mechanical ventilation. Also, many pts w/ pulmonary involvement or respiratory failure may not tolerate intercostal muscle blockade from regional anesthesia.
- Neurologic manifestations in HIV/AIDS can change rapidly, so carefully evaluate & document neurologic defects before anesthesia.

Comorbid conditions & multisystem disease can affect perioperative care

- Vomiting & diarrhea may cause volume depletion requiring replacement prior to induction of anesthesia.
- Decreased muscle mass & low albumin levels can have important pharmacokinetic implications requiring reduced dosages of medications.
- Consider pain consult for multidisciplinary approach to pt w/ chronic pain.
- Could need higher than normal doses of narcotics due to opioid tolerance or increased opiate metabolism due to antiretroviral therapy
- Immunosuppression requires careful aseptic technique.
- Consider potential difficult endotracheal intubation due to pharyngeal abnormalities.
- Increased incidence of extrapyramidal side effects w/ neuroleptic agents
- Shunting may be increased due to pulmonary pathology & increased FiO_2 may be required.
- Esophageal pathology could increase risk of aspiration.
- Respiratory tract is often hyperreactive in setting of pulmonary infection, & endotracheal intubation may exacerbate airway irritability.
- Increased sensitivity to CNS depressants in those w/ HIV-related mental status changes
- Opportunistic pulmonary infections may necessitate prolonged mechanical ventilation.
- Higher incidence of catheter sepsis exists in HIV population.

Regional anesthesia

- As HIV infects the CNS early in course of the disease, there is a minimal risk of introducing the virus to subarachnoid/epidural space, as it most likely is already present.
- Regional anesthesia is often technique of choice, but take into consideration the presence of neuropathies, local or CNS infection, mass lesions/ventricular dilations that increase ICP or coagulation abnormalities that could contraindicate neuraxial anesthesia.
- There is no evidence of increased infectious complications in parturients who receive regional anesthesia, & elective C-section w/ spinal anesthesia was not associated w/ perioperative complications.
- Short-term epidural catheter use in obstetrical anesthesia & analgesia is thought to have a much lower risk than long-term catheters placed for pain syndromes.
- Combined spinal-epidural technique (CSE) is thought to carry no increased risk.
- As in pts w/ chorioamnionitis or other maternal infections, pre-procedural anti-infection treatment is thought to allow for safe administration of regional anesthesia.
- In pts w/ cardiac dysfunction, cautiously conducted regional is often the technique of choice.

General anesthesia

General anesthesia is thought to be safe, but consider drug interactions w/ ART as well as dose adjustments for potential end-organ dysfunction, muscle wasting, mental status changes or concomitant drug abuse.

- Consider use of drugs such as etomidate, cis-atracurium, remifentanil & desflurane, as they are not dependent on CYP-450 system for metabolism.
- No reports of hyperkalemia or hyperpyrexia from succinylcholine use in HIV pts, even very debilitated ones

Miscellaneous

Contamination of equipment

- There is no evidence for airborne transmission of HIV & a very low likelihood of HIV transmission via an anesthesia machine.
- Consider circuit filters to prevent contamination from opportunistic pulmonary infections.
- Careful infection control is important.

Post Dural Puncture Headache

For treatment of PDPH, epidural blood patch w/ autologous blood has been used safely w/o increases in neurologic abnormalities, but only small numbers were studied. Because of this, some practitioners justify conservative mgt as first option, while others feel treatment of all anesthetic complications including PDPH should follow standards applied to non-HIV+ pts.

- IV hydration, oral & IV caffeine & 5-HT receptor agonist therapies are often used first.
- Postural nature should allay fears of bacterial meningitis.

CAVEATS/PEARLS

- Anesthesiologists will be faced w/ an increasing number of HIV-infected parturients who may present w/ various aspects & in various stages of this multisystem disease. Be familiar w/ clinical presentations of HIV/AIDS, the effects of anti-retroviral & anti-infection therapies & obstetric mgt of HIV+ parturients, as these have crucial implications to the safe administration of anesthesia.
- A multidisciplinary approach to care is critical. Infectious disease/AIDS specialists are now a common part of the obstetrical mgt group in many urban centers.
- Assessment of dysfunctions, opportunistic infections, tumors, polysubstance abuse, STDs & antiretroviral therapy w/ a thorough history, physical, lab studies & imaging prior to anesthesia is paramount.
- It is generally thought that HIV infection itself does not increase the risk for postprocedural complications, nor does anesthesia influence the natural progress of the disease.
- As HIV infects the CNS early in course of the disease, there is a minimal risk of introducing the virus to the subarachnoid/epidural space, as it most likely is already present.
- General anesthesia is thought to be safe, but consider drug interactions w/ potential antiretroviral therapy as well as dose adjustments for potential end-organ dysfunction, muscle wasting, mental status changes or concomitant drug abuse.
- Regional anesthesia is often the technique of choice, but consider the presence of neuropathies, local or CNS infection, mass lesions/ventricular dilation causing increased ICP or coagulation abnormalities that could contraindicate neuraxial anesthesia. Documentation of any neurologic deficits before performing anesthesia is paramount, as neurologic manifestations of HIV/AIDS can change rapidly.

- Vertical transmission (mother to baby) is the most common route for infection of children (transmission occurs during labor & delivery in nearly 70%, in utero 30% & after delivery [breast-feeding] in the remainder).
- Elective cesarean delivery & AZT prophylaxis appear to have an additive effect in preventing vertical transmission (maternal transmission rate is 0–2% w/ HAART).
- The preferred treatment of HIV-infected women is HAART to decrease viral load to <1,000 prior to delivery. If the viral load is <1000, vaginal delivery may be offered. If the viral load is undetectable, the maternal transmission rate is <2%.

CHECKLIST
- Detection of cardiac dysfunction is critical, & EKG findings are often abnormal in pts w/ HIV. Transthoracic echocardiography or even coronary catheterization is indicated in those w/ significant symptoms. Invasive monitoring depends on the severity of cardiac dysfunction.
- Routine chest x-ray & EKG recommended
- Evaluate extent of neutropenia & thrombocytopenia.
- Chemistries for glucose, liver & renal function help assess extent of end-organ dysfunction.
- CD4+ count & viral load can reveal severity of HIV/AIDS as well as response to therapy.
- In pts w/ signs & symptoms of pulmonary dysfunction, consider ABGs & pulmonary function tests.
- Perform radiologic studies of brain or spinal cord to rule out compressive mass lesions in pts w/ neurologic symptoms.
- Thromboelastography (TEG) to evaluate platelet function & coagulation status may be useful prior to regional anesthesia.

HYPERCOAGUABLE STATES & PATIENTS ON ANTICOAGULATION THERAPY

JEANNA VIOLA, MD
JANE BALLANTYNE, MD

FUNDAMENTAL KNOWLEDGE
- Parturient's risk of thrombosis increases due to the hypercoaguable state of pregnancy; pts w/ a hereditary predisposition to thrombosis are at even greater risk.

- Common hypercoaguable states: protein C, protein S & antithrombin III deficiencies, factor V Leiden disease & antiphospholipid antibody syndrome.
- Parturients w/ hypercoagulable syndromes are predisposed to placental compromise, risk of IUGR, placental abruption, severe premature pre-eclampsia, intrauterine fetal demise, placental infarction & recurrent miscarriages.
- Antiphospholipid syndromes
  - ➤ Lupus anticoagulant & anticardiolipin syndrome: antibodies are produced against proteins bound to anionic phospholipids in the plasma
  - ➤ Often accompanied by thrombocytopenia, but a hypercoaguable state predominates
  - ➤ Associated w/ a post-partum hemolytic uremic syndrome
- Factor V Leiden
  - ➤ Most common inheritable thrombophilia; accounts for 40–50% of cases
  - ➤ Factor V exists as an inactive cofactor, which is activated by thrombin to factor Va to convert prothrombin to thrombin.
  - ➤ Mutation in the Factor V gene (Leiden) causes resistance to factor Va breakdown by activated protein C; more thrombin is generated, causing a hypercoaguable state.
  - ➤ Heterozygotes for the Factor V Leiden gene mutation are 7× more likely to experience a thromboembolic event than controls (pts w/ normal factor V).
  - ➤ Homozygotes are 80× more likely to develop a thrombosis.
  - ➤ These pts are 16× more likely to develop a DVT during pregnancy or in the post-partum period than when they are not pregnant.
- Protein C deficiency
  - ➤ Protein C: vitamin K-dependent protein, synthesized in the liver
  - ➤ Gene is located on chromosome 2, closely related to the gene for factor IX.
  - ➤ Protein C is activated by thrombin bound to endothelial thrombomodulin. Activated protein C (APC) inactivates factors Va & VIIIa, which generate thrombin & activate factor X.
  - ➤ Protein C deficiency is an autosomal dominant mutation that occurs in two subtypes:
    - • Type 1: amount of protein C is 50% normal & is due to a missense or nonsense mutation

- Type 2: normal level of protein C in the plasma but decreased functional activity; caused by a point mutation that affects protein function
- ➤ Three syndromes associated w/ protein C deficiency are DVTs, neonatal purpura, warfarin-induced skin necrosis.
- ➤ Risks of placental compromise & risk of neonatal purpura in first day of life, ecchymoses, extensive arterial & venous thromboses & DIC
- ➤ Risk of thrombosis increased 7x compared to controls
- ■ Protein S deficiency
  - ➤ Protein S: vitamin K-dependent protein, synthesized by the liver & megakaryocytes. A cofactor for protein C.
  - ➤ Circulates in two forms, free (40–50%) & complement-bound
    - Only the free form acts as a cofactor for APC & inactivates Va & VIIIa, reducing thrombin activity.
    - Fibrinolysis is also enhanced & prothrombin activity inhibited via interactions w/ Va & Xa. Protein S deficiency pts have increased thrombin activity & are hypercoagulable.
  - ➤ Three subtypes of protein S deficiency
    - Type 1: levels of both total & free protein S are reduced to 50% normal
    - Type 2: total levels are normal but functional activity is decreased
    - Type 3 (also known as type 2a): normal levels of total protein S but reduced amount of free protein S; functional activity is reduced to approx. 40% of normal
- ■ Antithrombin III deficiency
  - ➤ Antithrombin III is also known as antithrombin (AT) or heparin cofactor 1.
  - ➤ A glycoprotein synthesized in the liver, like proteins C & S; a major inhibitor of thrombin & factors Xa & IXa
  - ➤ Two forms of antithrombin exist in the plasma: a latent, inactive form & an active monomer. One molecule of latent AT will bind to active monomer to form an inactive dimer.
  - ➤ AT activity is greatly augmented by heparin; thrombin is inactivated at a much greater rate.
  - ➤ AT III deficiency: autosomal dominant disease that occurs in two subtypes:
    - Type 1: decreased synthesis of AT III due to a deletion on the AT III gene. Associated w/ a 50% decrease in both amount & functional activity.

- Type 2: caused by a molecular defect in the protein, AT III levels are normal but functional activity is decreased.
- ➤ Risk of a thrombotic event in these pts is $8.1\times$ normal.
- Rarer causes of inherited thrombophilia
  - ➤ G20210A prothrombin gene mutation: risk of thrombosis during pregnancy is 4.6x normal
  - ➤ 4G/4G plasminogen activator inhibitor-1 mutation: modest increase in risk of thromboembolism
  - ➤ MHTFR T/T mutation: causes hyper-homocystinemia & is exacerbated by folate deficiency

STUDIES
- Antiphospholipid syndrome
  - ➤ Diagnosis is both clinical & laboratory.
  - ➤ Occurrence of one or more thrombotic events (venous or arterial) PLUS
  - ➤ Elevated PTT level, IgG or IgM anticardiolipin antibody, a false-positive syphilis test or the presence of anti-beta2 glycoprotein antibodies
- Factor V Leiden
  - ➤ Genetic testing
  - ➤ PTTs performed in presence & absence of a standard amount of APC (substance that inactivates normal factor Va). A ratio of the two values is obtained & this is compared to a standard, normalized value.
  - ➤ OR: dilution of pt's plasma (containing factor V Leiden) into factor V-deficient plasma & performing a PTT.
- Protein C deficiency
  - ➤ Electroimmunoassay, ELISA or radioimmunoassay to quantify amount of protein C in the plasma. Normal = 4 mcg/mL.
  - ➤ Southern copperhead snake venom activates protein C; it is mixed w/ the pt's serum & a PTT is measured.
  - ➤ Functional assays to detect type II also exist.
- Protein S deficiency
  - ➤ Test assesses both free & complement-bound levels of protein; however, values must be adjusted for pregnancy (40% less free protein S).
  - ➤ Free protein S is measured using monoclonal antibody-based assays & ligand sorbent assays.
  - ➤ The most reliable tests are radioimmunoassay & ELISA.

- Antithrombin III deficiency
  - ➤ Measure AT 3- heparin cofactor activity & quantity by immunoassay.
- G20210A prothrombin gene mutation: diagnosed using PCR
- 4G/4G plasminogen activator inhibitor-1 mutation: diagnosis is made by genotyping for this mutation
- MHTFR T/T mutation: diagnosis is made by quantification of the fasting homocysteine level & checking folate levels

MANAGEMENT/INTERVENTIONS

- Most pts are started on prophylaxis of 80 mg aspirin & low-dose heparin.
- If the pt has a thromboembolic event prior to pregnancy or a recurrence on the prophylaxis, she is anticoagulated w/ heparin (to therapeutic PTT level) & aspirin.
- Indications for when/if regional anesthesia can be safely performed depend on the specific anticoagulation regimen:
  - ➤ **Aspirin:** no monitoring of anticoagulation level available; no significant risk for placement or removal of catheter or dosing after catheter removal
  - ➤ **NSAIDs & COX-2 inhibitors** (Celebrex, Motrin, Naprosyn, Vioxx): no monitoring of anticoagulation level available; no significant risk for placement or removal of catheter or dosing after catheter removal
  - ➤ **Heparin SQ:** no monitoring of anticoagulation level available; no significant risk for placement or removal of catheter or dosing after catheter removal
  - ➤ **Heparin IV:** monitor anticoagulation level w/ PTT
    - Wait 2–4 hours after last dose to administer regional anesthesia.
    - Remove catheter 2–4 hours after postop dose was administered.
    - Restart medication 1 hour after catheter removal.
  - ➤ **Low-dose low-molecular-weight heparin** (dalteparin [Fragmin], enoxaparin [Lovenox], tinzaparin [Imnohep]): Factor Xa level monitoring available
    - Low dose is defined as <5,000 U QD Fragmin or <60 mg QD Lovenox.
    - Wait 12 hours after last dose to administer regional anesthesia.

- Remove catheter 12 hours after postop dose.
- Restart medication 2 hours after catheter removal.
- Single daily dosing should be started 6–8 hours postop.

➤ **High-dose low-molecular-weight heparin:** Factor Xa level monitoring available
  - High dose is defined as BID dosing of this medication.
  - Epidural catheters should be removed prior to initiation of BID dosing schedule.
  - Wait >24 hours after last dose to administer regional anesthesia.
  - Remove catheter prior to first dose; otherwise wait 24 hours.
  - Restart medication 2 hours after catheter removal.
  - BID dosing should be started >24 hours postop.

➤ **Warfarin** (Coumadin): monitor anticoagulation level by INR (<1.5, OK to proceed w/ regional)
  - Wait 3–5 days after last dose to administer regional; verify reversal of anticoagulation by checking INR.
  - Remove catheter when INR < 2.0.
  - Can restart medication on same day that catheter is removed.
  - Contraindicated in pregnancy due to transplacental transfer.

➤ **Tirofiban** (Aggrastat): no monitoring of anticoagulation level available
  - Wait 8 hours after last dose to administer regional anesthesia.
  - Remove catheter 8 hours after postop dose.
  - Restart medication 4 hours after catheter removal.

➤ **Abciximab** (Reopro): no monitoring of anticoagulation level available
  - Wait 48 hours after last dose to administer regional anesthesia.
  - Remove catheter 48 hours after postop dose.
  - Restart medication 12 hours after catheter removal.

➤ **Clopidogrel** (Plavix): no monitoring of anticoagulation level available
  - Wait 7 days after last dose to perform regional anesthesia.
  - Remove catheter within 24 hours of administration of last dose.
  - Restart medication 24 hours after catheter removal.
  - Clopidogrel has a 24- to 48-hour window to remove the catheter once the medication is given; if it has been >48 hours since dosing, you must wait 7 days to remove the catheter.

➤ **Eptifibatide** (Integrilin): no monitoring of anticoagulation level available
  - Wait 8 hours after last dose to administer regional anesthesia.

- Remove catheter 8 hours after postop dose.
- Restart medication 4 hours after catheter removal.
- **Thrombolytics** (streptokinase, alteplase): no monitoring of anticoagulation level available
  - Wait 10 days after last dose to administer regional anesthesia.
  - Remove catheter 10 days after postop dose.
  - Restart medication 10 days after catheter removal.
- **Ticlopidine** (Ticlid): no monitoring of anticoagulation level available
  - Wait 14 days after last dose to administer regional anesthesia.
  - Remove catheter 14 days after postop dose.
  - Restart medication 24 hours after catheter removal.
- **Fondaparinux** (Arixtra): no monitoring of anticoagulation level available
  - Wait >24 hours after last dose to perform regional anesthesia.
  - Remove catheter >24 hours after postop dose.
  - Restart medication 2 hours after catheter removal.
  - The above guidelines are suggested if Fondaparinux has been administered; however, this drug should not be given if regional anesthesia is anticipated.
- **Direct thrombin inhibitors** (desirudin, lepirudin, bivalirudin), **synthetic thrombin inhibitor** (Argatroban) & **fondaparinux** (Arixtra)
  - Spontaneous intracranial bleeding has been reported.
  - Due to the lack of information available, no assessment of risk can be made.
  - Avoid neuraxial anesthesia.
- If the pt is not on any anticoagulation, there is no contraindication to regional anesthesia.
- If a contraindication to regional anesthesia exists, IV opioid analgesia is provided during labor & general anesthesia is used for C-section.

CAVEATS AND PEARLS
- Many pts w/ a hypercoagulable syndrome are on anticoagulation therapy.
- Vigilance is required when initiating an epidural or spinal anesthetic as well as removing an epidural catheter.

- No restrictions are placed on administration of regional anesthesia to pts on NSAIDs, SQ heparin & ASA.
- Pts on anticoagulation therapy may still be candidates for regional anesthesia if the appropriate time interval has passed.
- Pts are prone to thromboembolic events such as DVT & PE; these diagnoses should remain high in the differential despite anticoagulant therapy.
- Pts w/ hypercoagulable syndromes are prone to placental compromise & pre-eclampsia; they may present for emergent C-section.

CHECKLIST
- Determine what anticoagulant regimen (drug name, amount, dosing schedule) pt is on.
- Determine when last dose of anticoagulant was given.
- Check coagulation indices of pts on anticoagulation regimens in preparation for labor or C-section.
- Check coagulation indices prior to epidural catheter removal.
- Careful airway assessment in preparation for GETA if regional anesthesia is contraindicated.
- Risk for thromboembolic events is high: monitor oxygen saturation & prepare to administer supplemental oxygen & support hemodynamics as necessary.

HYPERCORTISOLISM (CUSHING'S SYNDROME)

GRACE C. CHANG, MD, MBA; ROBERT A. PETERFREUND, MD, PHD; AND STEPHANIE L. LEE, MD, PHD

FUNDAMENTAL KNOWLEDGE

Adrenal Physiology
- Adrenal cortex secretes steroid hormones, including glucocorticoids; main hormones are cortisol and aldosterone.
- Adrenocorticotropic hormone (ACTH), secreted from the anterior pituitary, stimulates release of cortisol in response to stress & in a diurnal pattern.
- Function of cortisol
  - Affects carbohydrate, protein & fatty acid metabolism
  - Decreases cellular uptake of glucose
  - Promotes gluconeogenesis & hepatic glycogen synthesis

> Participates in conversion of norepinephrine to epinephrine
> Required for production of angiotensin II
> Acts as an anti-inflammatory agent
> Required for normal vascular tone
- Cushing's *disease* is overproduction of cortisol from adrenal cortical hyperfunction, driven by excess ACTH secretion from a pituitary tumor.
- Cushing's *syndrome* is hyperadrenalism from all other causes, most commonly iatrogenic, as a result of glucocorticoid administration.

Changes in Adrenal Physiology Associated w/ Pregnancy
- In normal pregnancy, high estrogen levels raise concentration of cortisol-binding globulin (CBG).
- Levels of maternal plasma cortisol & other corticosteroids increase from 12 weeks gestation to term & can reach 3–5× nonpregnant levels.
- Very high cortisol levels are observed, especially during 3rd trimester.
- Placenta also produces increasingly higher amounts of corticotropin-releasing hormone (CRHp), which is important during labor because of its vasodilator action.
- CRH-binding protein (CRH-BP) produced by the liver buffers the effects of CRHp levels to avoid pituitary/adrenal hyperstimulation.
- During last weeks of pregnancy, CRH-BP levels progressively drop, enabling more free CRHp to stimulate the pituitary-adrenal axis in preparation for labor.
- Serum & urinary cortisol levels will rise & these high levels of cortisol may lead to a misdiagnosis of Cushing's syndrome.
- Diurnal secretion of cortisol is preserved in normal pregnancy.

Epidemiology
- Pregnancy rarely occurs in pts w/ active Cushing's syndrome because high serum cortisol levels will block pituitary gonadotropin secretion, leading to anovulation & abnormal menstrual periods.
- Few cases of pregnancy complicated by Cushing's syndrome reported in the literature

Signs/Symptoms
- Truncal obesity w/ moon facies, supraclavicular fullness
- Hypertension
- Hyperglycemia

- Hypokalemia
- Excess intravascular volume
- Purple striae & acne
- Poor wound healing
- Diabetes mellitus
- Hypercoagulability w/ thromboembolism
- Mental status changes
- Benign intracranial hypertension
- Pancreatitis
- Peptic ulceration
- Glaucoma
- Infection
- Osteoporosis w/ propensity for fractures

Etiology
- Pituitary tumor
- Adrenal adenoma
- Bilateral adrenal micronodular hyperplasia
- Steroid therapy
- Carcinoids or tumors w/ ectopic production of ACTH

Maternal Complications
- Untreated, Cushing's syndrome is associated w/ high mortality rates (50% in 5 years).
- In pregnancy, 2/3 of women develop hypertension, which can lead to pre-eclampsia.
- 25% develop diabetes mellitus.
- Maternal mortality is 4%.

Fetal/Neonatal Complications
- 50% of newborns are premature.
- Mortality 25–40%

STUDIES
- Distinguish pts who develop Cushing's syndrome during pregnancy from pregnant pts w/ pre-existing Cushing's syndrome.
- Abnormal cortisol dexamethasone suppression test results may lead to misdiagnosis since serum & urine cortisol levels are high in pregnancy.
- Urinary free cortisol measurement is critical because it reflects cortisol secretion rate, despite a high rate of false-positive results.
- Absence of diurnal cortisol secretion is probably best test, since this is preserved in normal pregnancy.

MANAGEMENT/INTERVENTIONS

■ Surgical mgt rapidly reduces hypercortisolism.
  ➤ Adrenal tumors & pituitary adenomas have been surgically removed during pregnancy w/ excellent results.
  ➤ Surgery is ideally performed btwn weeks 12 & 29 of gestation.
■ Medical mgt
  ➤ Used in cases of surgical failure or if surgery is contraindicated
  ➤ Metyrapone is most widely used drug.
    • Crosses placenta but no neonatal congenital abnormalities reported
    • Can be started at 14 weeks gestation up to delivery
  ➤ Ketoconazole
    • No congenital malformations reported but can cause intrauterine growth restriction
    • Adrenal block is variable & replacement glucocorticoids should be given.

Anesthetic Management

■ Careful preanesthetic evaluation
■ Concentrate on mgt of diabetes mellitus, hypertension, fluid retention.
■ Preanesthetic check of electrolytes & glucose level
■ Careful positioning of pt since bone density is significantly decreased
■ Regional or general anesthesia can safely be administered.
■ Regional anesthesia has benefit of blunting stress response w/ labor.
■ Judicious use of nondepolarizing neuromuscular blocking agents
■ Monitor neuromuscular blockade w/ peripheral nerve stimulator.

CAVEATS/PEARLS

■ Pt may have associated muscle weakness & requirement for nondepolarizing muscle relaxants may be reduced.
■ Bone metabolism abnormal; pt may have premature osteoporosis, vertebral body collapse, pathologic fractures

CHECKLIST

■ Careful preanesthetic evaluation of associated diabetes mellitus, fluid retention & hypertension, as well as electrolytes & glucose
■ Document any pre-op fractures.
■ Carefully position pt to prevent fractures.
■ Judicious use of non-depolarizing muscle relaxants; monitor w/ peripheral nerve stimulator

HYPERPARATHYROIDISM

GRACE C. CHANG, MD, MBA; ROBERT A. PETERFREUND, MD, PHD; AND STEPHANIE L. LEE, MD, PHD

FUNDAMENTAL KNOWLEDGE

Parathyroid Physiology

- Parathyroid glands secrete parathyroid hormone (PTH), which maintains normal extracellular fluid concentration of calcium; calcium exists in ionized form (60%) or bound to albumin or organic acids (40%); the ionized form is biologically active.
- Role of calcium
  - Muscle contraction
  - Neurotransmission
  - Coagulation
  - Hormone secretion & action
- Role of PTH
  - Stimulates osteoclastic activity
  - Increases distal renal tubular reabsorption of calcium
  - Inhibits proximal renal tubular reabsorption of phosphate
- Role of calcitonin
  - Inactivates osteoclasts and causes mild natriuresis and calciuresis
  - Receptor structurally similar to PTH's
  - Involved in feedback loop w/ calcium to maintain homeostasis
- Role of vitamin D
  - Activated 1,25-dihydroxyvitamin D is necessary for active calcium transport from the gut.
  - Vitamin D precursor is made upon sun exposure of skin; sunblock preparations inhibit the synthesis of precursors.
  - Vitamin D precursor is first activated in the liver to the storage form, 25-hydroxyvitamin D, & finally fully activated in the kidney to 1,25-dihydroxyvitamin D.

Changes in Calcium Homeostasis Associated w/ Pregnancy

- PTH concentration increases from 1st to 2nd trimester, declines in 3rd trimester to the levels of 1st trimester, then significantly increases postpartum.
- Maternal concentrations of 1,25-vitamin D rise early in 1st trimester, remain high, then further increase during 3rd trimester; levels fall back to normal on the 3rd day postpartum.

- During pregnancy, there is high fetal uptake of ionized calcium across the placenta.
- During pregnancy, 25–30 g calcium is actively transported (across a placental-fetal calcium gradient of 1.0:1.4) to assist in fetal development & bone formation.
- Parathyroid hormone-related peptide (PTHrP) is the fetal equivalent of PTH & fetus derives supply from placenta & fetal parathyroid gland.
- Fetus uses PTHrP to maintain placental-fetal calcium gradient.
- After birth, placental supply of calcium abruptly stops, stimulating secretion of PTH & production of 1,25-vitamin D in neonate.

Definition
- Primary hyperparathyroidism occurs when the parathyroid gland is autonomously overactive.
- Secondary hyperparathyroidism is physiologic parathyroid response to low serum calcium level to maintain homeostasis, usually from vitamin D deficiency.

Epidemiology
- Prevalence of primary hyperparathyroidism 0.15% to as high as 1–1.4% when asymptomatic cases are included
- Incidence in pregnancy is low
- About 145 cases of primary hyperparathyroidism associated w/ pregnancy have been reported.
- True incidence is not known.

Signs/Symptoms
- Fatigue
- Anorexia
- Nausea/vomiting
- Polyuria
- Constipation
- Depression
- Blurred vision
- When serum calcium level is >13 mg/dL, risk of end-organ calcification increases & there may be nephrocalcinosis & renal calculi.
- Acutely ill pts may have cardiac dysrhythmias, osteopenia, pseudogout, muscle atrophy, conjunctival calcifications.
- At levels >14–15 mg/dL: hypercalcemic crisis (medical emergency) involving uremia, coma, cardiac arrest, death

DDx for Hypercalcemia Besides Hyperparathyroidism
- Malignancy (bone destruction or abnormal activation of bioactive 1,25-dihydroxyvitamin D)
- Immobilization
- Vitamin D intoxication
- Vitamin A intoxication
- Aluminum intoxication
- Idiopathic hypercalcemia
- Sarcoid/granulomatous diseases
- Hyperthyroidism
- Hypocalciuria
- Addison's disease
- Milk alkali syndrome
- Paget's disease
- Thiazide diuretics
- Dehydration

Maternal Complications
- Hyperparathyroidism during pregnancy is associated w/ a maternal complication rate as high as 67%.
- 24–36% incidence of nephrolithiasis w/ primary hyperparathyroidism during pregnancy
- Prevalence of pancreatitis 7–13%
- Hyperemesis gravidarum incidence is significantly increased.
- UTIs & pyelonephritis increased
- As many as 80% of pts may be asymptomatic, but still can progress to hypercalcemic crisis.
- Even if pt is well controlled, she can develop postpartum hypercalcemia when the fetal & placental drain of calcium has been removed.

Fetal Complications
- Incidence of fetal complications is as high as 80% in untreated mothers, as high as 53% in medically managed mothers.
- 27–31% neonatal death
- IUGR
- Low birthweight
- Preterm delivery
- Intrauterine fetal demise
- Postpartum neonatal hypocalcemic tetany is reported to occur in 50% of infants born to untreated mothers.
- Neonates do well if calcium supplementation is started promptly.

STUDIES

- Confirm elevated calcium level (>10.5 mg/dL after correction for albumin level) on at least 2 blood samples.
  - ➤ Biologically available calcium levels can be estimated if albumin levels are considered using the equation:
  - ➤ calcium = measured calcium + 0.8 * (4 − measured albumin)
  - ➤ Ionized calcium should be measured to eliminate variable of protein binding involved in total serum calcium levels.
- If hypercalcemia is confirmed, then iPTH assay should be performed.
- If iPTH level is elevated or in normal range, primary hyperparathyroidism has been confirmed because under normal conditions a high calcium level should lead to a very low iPTH level.
- Serum electrolytes, magnesium, phosphorus, renal function & urinary calcium should be measured to exclude renal dysfunction & benign familial hypocalciuric hypercalcemia.
- If indicated, rule out pancreatitis, nephrolithiasis, bone disease or peptic ulcer disease.
- Consider multiple endocrine neoplasia (MEN) 1 & 2a, as these syndromes are associated w/ hyperparathyroidism.
- A nuclear parathyroid scan is normally used for localization, but this is contraindicated in pregnancy.
- Ultrasound or MRI can be used to locate & identify adenomas prior to surgery to minimize the risk of unanticipated ectopic adenomas. CT scan localization should not be used during pregnancy.

MANAGEMENT/INTERVENTIONS

- Consider gestational age, success of medical mgt, presence of solitary adenoma & pt preference when deciding btwn medical & surgical mgt.
- Medical mgt
  - ➤ If pt is asymptomatic or calcium level is <12 mg/dL: increase oral fluids, decrease oral calcium intake, add loop diuretic to enhance calcium excretion.
  - ➤ Obtain surgical, pediatric & perinatal consults.
  - ➤ If pt is symptomatic & calcium level is >12 mg/dL, give IV hydration, follow & replete electrolytes, consider cardiac monitor, consider calcitonin/bisphosphonates.
- Calcitonin
  - ➤ Pregnancy category B medication that helps lower calcium levels through direct inhibition of osteoclastic function
  - ➤ Ideal for acutely lowering calcium levels

> Has greatest effect after single IV or IM injection
> Does not cross the placenta
> Used safely in pregnancy.

■ Oral phosphate
  > Category C medication
  > Therapeutic & safe if calcium times phosphate product is <60
  > Ectopic calcification if calcium times phosphate product is >60 & oral phosphate used long term
  > When given orally does not carry risk of IV calcium phosphate precipitation associated w/ IV phosphate administration
  > Standard dose 1.5–3.0 g daily; doses up to 7.5–9.0 g/day have been used successfully

■ Pamidronate (bisphosphonate)
  > Category C medication
  > Favored only in acutely ill pts
  > Teratogenic effects documented
  > Shown to cross the placenta
  > Unknown effects on fetal bone
  > May need to consider urgent parathyroidectomy if pt remains acutely ill

■ Surgical mgt
  > If diagnosis in 1st trimester & calcium levels are controlled medically, medical mgt is preferable.
  > Once pt is in the 2nd trimester, surgical intervention should be considered.
  > If pt prefers medical mgt, perinatal surveillance should include ultrasound, serial growth scans & antenatal testing.
  > If symptoms or hypercalcemia cannot be controlled at any time throughout the remainder of the pregnancy, surgical intervention should be strongly recommended.

Anesthetic Management
■ No evidence to suggest greater benefit w/ either regional or general anesthesia
■ Critical to maintain hydration & urine output; use loop diuretics if necessary
■ Monitor EKG for adverse cardiac effects (prolonged P-R interval, wide QRS complex, short Q-T interval).
■ If pt already has mental status changes, may require less anesthesia & sedation since at higher risk of aspiration

- Muscle relaxation: hypercalcemia may antagonize effects of non-depolarizing muscle relaxants
  - ➤ Reports describe increased sensitivity to succinylcholine & resistance to atracurium.
  - ➤ Because of unpredictability of effect, decrease initial relaxant dose & monitor w/ peripheral nerve stimulator.
- Carefully position pts during surgery as they are more prone to osteoporosis & at risk for pathologic fractures.

CAVEATS/PEARLS
- After parathyroidectomy, pt may develop hypocalcemia, leading to inspiratory stridor & airway compromise, as well as tetany; monitor pt carefully for signs & symptoms of hypocalcemia.
- Following parathyroidectomy, hypomagnesemia reduces parathyroid hormone secretion & may aggravate hypocalcemia.

CHECKLIST
- Thorough pre-op evaluation for signs & symptoms of hypercalcemia
- Monitor for hypercalcemic crisis.
- Use muscle relaxants carefully; monitor w/ peripheral nerve stimulator.
- Aggressive hydration, especially if calcium levels are very high, & follow urine output
- Monitor for EKG changes & hypertension.
- Prudent use of anesthesia & sedation
- After parathyroidectomy, monitor for airway compromise & signs of acute hypocalcemia.

HYPERTHYROIDISM

GRACE C. CHANG, MD, MBA; ROBERT A. PETERFREUND, MD, PHD; AND STEPHANIE L. LEE, MD, PHD

FUNDAMENTAL KNOWLEDGE
See "*Hypothyroidism*" for information about thyroid physiology during pregnancy.

Definition
- Abnormal increase in serum concentration of unbound or free thyroid hormones

Epidemiology
- Prevalence in general population is 0.2% to 1.9%, w/ female:male ratio 10:1.
- Prevalence is 0.05% to 0.2% in pregnancy.

Signs & Symptoms
- Hyperthyroid symptom scale is often used to follow clinical course of pts.
- Nervousness
- Tachycardia
- Sweating
- Heat intolerance
- Hyperactivity
- Tremor
- Weakness
- Hyperdynamic precordium
- Frequent stools
- Increased appetite
- Uncommon signs of Graves' disease include exophthalmos or infiltrative ophthalmopathy, pretibial myxedema or dermopathy
- Goiter
  - Thyroid gland 2–4× normal size
  - Usually symmetrical, but sometimes one lobe larger than the other
  - Thrill may be palpated & continuous bruit may be heard.
  - Pregnancy exerts mild subclinical increase in growth, even when iodine intake is sufficient.

Etiology
- Graves' disease (85–95% of hyperthyroid cases in pregnancy)
- Subacute thyroiditis
- Gestational trophoblastic neoplasia
- TSH-secreting pituitary tumor
- Toxic adenoma
- Toxic multinodular goiter
- Ectopic thyroid tissue
- Iatrogenic excessive thyroid hormone therapy

Pathophysiology
- Graves' disease is an autoimmune condition in which autoantibodies are developed against TSH receptors in the thyroid gland, resulting in augmentation or inhibition of TSH receptor function.

■ Natural course of Graves' in pregnancy: activation of disease in 1st half of pregnancy, remission in 2nd half, recurrence 1–6 months postpartum

■ Gestational trophoblastic neoplasms can be associated w/ high hCG concentrations, leading to TSH receptor activation & hyperthyroidism.

Complications

■ Increased rates of:
  ➤ Spontaneous abortion (8–14%)
  ➤ Preterm delivery (9–22%)
  ➤ Congenital goiter (3–7%)
  ➤ Pre-eclampsia
  ➤ IUGR
  ➤ Abnormal fetal thyroid function

STUDIES

■ Diagnosis depends on documentation of increase in serum concentration of unbound or free T4.

■ More common forms (Graves' disease, toxic adenoma, toxic multinodular goiter) can be differentiated from less common forms by a radioiodine uptake study (but this test is contraindicated during pregnancy).

■ Identification of TSH-receptor autoantibodies, antithyroid antibodies & thyroid peroxidase (TPO) antibody, w/ structural characterization of the gland using ultrasound, can help distinguish Graves' disease from toxic adenoma or multinodular goiter.

MANAGEMENT/INTERVENTIONS

■ Radioactive iodine: I-131 is contraindicated during pregnancy (all forms of iodine will cross the placenta & be taken up by the fetus) & lactation
  ➤ I-131 is taken up by thyroid gland & its therapeutic effect on Graves' disease is through local emission of beta-particle radiation w/ thyroid destruction.
  ➤ Hypothyroidism usually develops over a period of several months, requiring thyroid hormone replacement.
  ➤ Pregnancy should be delayed for 4–6 months after radioactive iodine therapy.
  ➤ Fetal thyroid gland begins to take up iodine at 10 weeks gestation; prior to this time the risk to the fetus is less well defined.

- Antithyroid meds: propylthiouracil (PTU) & methimazole (MMI)
  - Interfere w/ incorporation of iodine into thyroglobulin
  - PTU also inhibits iodothyronine deiodinase, which converts T4 to T3, in peripheral tissues
    - Some pts experience remission after administration of these drugs for 12–18 months.
    - Common complication is urticaria (5%).
    - Major complications of administration: agranulocytosis (0.1–0.5%) and hepatotoxicity
    - Maternal administration can lead to fetal hypothyroidism & goiter.
  - MMI is less protein-bound than PTU. PTU may cross the placenta less efficiently, making it the preferred drug during pregnancy.
    - MMI has rarely been associated w/ fetal scalp defect (cutis aplasia).
    - If fetal hypothyroidism develops, intra-amniotic injections of thyroxine have been described in individual case reports.
- Surgical therapy is controversial; reserved for pts who cannot, or are unwilling to, receive radioactive iodine or antithyroid meds, or for those who have failed medical mgt.
  - Preferred surgical procedure is subtotal thyroidectomy.
  - To reduce risk of precipitating thyroid storm, pts should receive pre-op glucocorticoids, beta blockers & iodine (short-term pre-op treatment should be safe for fetus).
  - Risk of surgery to fetus is unclear, but thyroidectomy should be delayed until the end of the 1st trimester & completion of organogenesis. If possible, plan surgery before the 3rd trimester to prevent inducing premature labor.
- Adjunctive therapies
  - Iodine (short term <2 weeks)
  - Radiocontrast agents (iopanoic acid)
  - Lithium
  - Glucocorticoids
  - Beta blockers to decrease cardiovascular responses to hyperthyroidism
- Thyroid storm
  - Life-threatening decompensation or exacerbation of severe hyperthyroidism; occurs in 2–4% of pregnant pts w/ untreated hyperthyroidism

➤ Signs/symptoms: fever out of proportion for infection, mental/emotional disturbances, tachycardia, tachypnea, diaphoresis, dehydration (from fever, vomiting, diaphoresis, diarrhea), hypotension resistant to pharmacotherapy; can be mistaken for malignant hyperthermia (although thyroid storm is not associated w/ rhabdomyolysis), neuroleptic malignant syndrome, sepsis, hemorrhage, drug or transfusion reactions

➤ W/o treatment, can progress to coma, multiorgan system failure, death; mortality rate was nearly 100% in early studies but has now decreased to <20–50% w/ recognition & improved therapy

➤ Mechanism unknown; could be caused by increased thyroid hormone & catecholamine secretion or precipitating event could augment thyroid hormone action by increasing circulating free fraction of thyroid hormones

➤ Thyroid storm associated w/ precipitating event in most cases; in pregnancy events could include infection, normal labor, hemorrhage, C-section & eclampsia

➤ Treatment of thyroid storm
  • General supportive measures
    • Cooling blanket & ice
    • Chlorpromazine or meperidine to decrease shivering
    • IV hydration
    • Glucose & electrolyte replacement
    • Oxygen
    • Glucocorticoids (dexamethasone 2 mg q6h IV or hydrocortisone 50–100 mg IV q8h), since pts w/ hyperthyroidism have a relative deficiency of endogenous glucocorticoid production
    • B-complex multivitamins
    • Antibiotic if infection is found
  • Reduction of synthesis & secretion of thyroid hormones
    • Antithyroid meds
      • PTU 300–400 mg PO q4h (preferred because it decreases thyroid hormone production & inhibits peripheral conversion of T4 to T3; PTU should be given at least 1 hr before iodine to prevent initial increase in iodine-induced synthesis
      • Methimazole orally 60–100 mg daily (decreases only thyroid hormone production)

- Iodine (sodium iodide 1 g IV or Lugol's solution 30 drops orally in 3 divided doses or supersaturated potassium iodide solution [SSKI] 5 drops PO q6h)
- High-dose glucocorticoids (inhibit both thyroid hormone production & conversion of T4 to T3)
- Reduction of peripheral conversion of T4 to T3
  - PTU
  - High-dose glucocorticoids
  - Radiographic contrast agents iopanoic acid or sodium ipodate 0.5 g PO bid
- Decrease in metabolic effects of thyroid hormones
  - Beta blockers
    - Propranolol 40–80 mg PO q6h or 2 mg IV q2–4h. Propranolol is the only beta blocker confirmed to inhibit peripheral conversion of T4 to T3; this is not related to its beta-blocking activity.
    - Esmolol: short-acting; better in pts who have cardiomyopathy from hyperthyroidism; can be used in pts who require more selective beta blockade, such as those w/ asthma; use results in fetal bradycardia & acidosis
    - In pregnant pts, use of beta blockers is associated w/ IUGR & preterm labor; if needed, propranolol is commonly prescribed in pregnancy.
    - Use esmolol when propanolol is contraindicated or when a short-acting beta blocker is necessary.
  - Calcium channel blockers: for pts intolerant of beta blockers
  - Plasma exchange
  - Diagnosis & treatment of precipitating illness

Anesthetic Management
- Either general or regional anesthesia can be safely administered.
- Consider glucocorticoid supplementation.
- Avoid meds resulting in tachycardia (eg, ketamine, atropine).
- Pts w/ exophthalmos need meticulous eye care to prevent corneal abrasions during general anesthesia.
- Deep pre-op sedation is controversial as it can increase maternal aspiration & neonatal depression.
- Pts may have respiratory muscle weakness; prudent use of muscle relaxants & reversal of muscle relaxants is important.

- Epinephrine & phenylephrine are safe to use in local anesthetics to decrease their uptake & toxicity.
- Phenylephrine may be a better choice as vasopressor instead of epinephrine for hypotension w/ regional anesthesia.

CAVEATS & PEARLS
- Goal is to make pt minimally hyperthyroid prior to delivery to ensure fetal euthyroidism. Treatment goal is free T4 in upper half of reference range w/ suppressed TSH.
- Thyroid storm is a medical emergency & may be precipitated by events associated w/ pregnancy: infection, normal labor, hemorrhage, C-section, eclampsia.

CHECKLIST
- Thorough airway evaluation, especially in pts w/ goiter
- Thorough cardiovascular pre-op evaluation, keeping in mind pt may have a hyperdynamic cardiovascular system & cardiomyopathy
- Assess volume status; pt may be volume deplete.
- Correct electrolyte abnormalities.
- Monitor for development of thyroid storm.
- In thyroid storm, give oral PTU, IV glucocorticoid, sodium iodide & propanolol & use general supportive measures.
- Pts having subtotal thyroidectomy should receive pre-op glucocorticoids, beta blockers & iodine to decrease risk of thyroid storm prior to normalizing thyroid hormone levels.

HYPOPARATHYROIDISM

GRACE C. CHANG, MD, MBA; ROBERT A. PETERFREUND, MD, PHD; AND STEPHANIE L. LEE, MD, PHD

FUNDAMENTAL KNOWLEDGE
See "*Hyperparathyroidism.*"

Definition
- Secretion of PTH is absent or deficient, or there is resistance in peripheral tissues to the effects of the hormone. Slow progression to hypocalcemia may have few, if any, neuroirritation symptoms. Acute development of hypocalcemia is usually associated w/ severe life-threatening symptoms.

Signs/Symptoms
- Acute hypocalcemia
  - Perioral paresthesias
  - Restlessness
  - Neuromuscular irritability (positive Chvostek sign or Trousseau sign)
  - Stridor, laryngeal spasm
  - Prolonged QT interval on EKG
  - Seizure
- Chronic hypocalcemia
  - Mental retardation
  - Calcification of basal ganglia
  - Obesity, short stature, short 4th & 5th metacarpals & metatarsals associated w/ McCune-Albright syndrome of pseudohypoparathyroidism
  - Prolonged QT interval on EKG
  - Osteoporosis

Etiology
- Decreased or absent PTH
  - Iatrogenic (parathyroid gland loss during thyroidectomy)
  - Parathyroidectomy to treat hyperplasia
  - Autoimmune (polyglandular autoimmune syndromes)
  - Idiopathic (DiGeorge syndrome)
- Resistance of peripheral tissues to effects of PTH
  - Pseudohypoparathyroidism
  - Hypomagnesemia
  - Chronic renal failure
  - Malabsorption
  - Anticonvulsant therapy (phenytoin)
  - Osteoblastic metastases
  - Acute pancreatitis

Maternal Complications
- Uterine irritability reduces resting potential & spike frequency of muscle fibers, possibly leading to preterm labor or abortion.

Fetal/Neonatal Complications
- Intrauterine fractures
- Fetal reactive hyperparathyroidism, predisposing to intracranial bleeding

- Neonatal rickets

STUDIES
- Serum calcium concentration & ionized calcium are best indicators.

MANAGEMENT/INTERVENTIONS
- Calcium supplementation is used in combination w/ calcitriol (1,25-dihydroxyvitamin D).
- Calcitriol
  - Absence of PTH impairs metabolism of endogenous 25-hydroxyvitamin D to 1,25-dihyroxyvitamin D; thus bioactive vitamin D, calcitriol, is used as a substitute.
  - Immediate & predictable bioavailability
  - Sufficiently short-acting so that if there is overtreatment, hypercalcemia will resolve quickly
- 25-hydroxyvitamin D (ergocalciferol)
  - Reports of teratogenicity in humans after overdosage
  - Risk of teratogenicity small as long as serum calcium & 1,25-dihydroxyvitamin D levels remain in normal range
  - Reduced activation of bioactive vitamin D w/ hypo- or hyperparathyroidism or chronic renal failure

Anesthetic Management
- Neither regional nor general anesthesia is contraindicated.
- Regional anesthesia may be preferable since it prevents hyper- or hypoventilation resulting in shifts of electrolytes.
- Avoid respiratory or metabolic alkalosis, since ionized calcium levels decline.
- Monitor serum electrolyte levels (especially calcium, magnesium, phosphate) & replete if necessary.
- In emergency (neuroirritative symptoms, laryngospasm, corrected calcium < 7 mg/dL), give 1 amp 10% calcium gluconate slowly IV over 10 minutes followed by 10 mg/kg (usually 10 amps in 500 cc D5W) over 6–10 hours by continuous infusion.
  - Rapid administration may lead to cardiac dysfunction or arrest.
  - Calcium gluconate is preferable to calcium chloride because it causes less tissue necrosis if extravasated.
- Closely monitor ionized calcium levels if giving rapid transfusion of blood or if metabolism or elimination of citrate is impaired by renal dysfunction, liver cirrhosis or hypothermia.

■ Monitor EKG closely for prolonged QT interval, which may precede cardiac dysrhythmias.

■ Non-depolarizing muscle relaxants are preferable since hypocalcemia is associated w/ decreased acetylcholine release.

■ Check coagulation studies since extreme hypocalcemia can affect clotting.

CAVEATS/PEARLS

■ Severe hypotension, myocardial dysfunction, congestive heart failure & elevated left ventricular pressures can be triggered by decreased ionized calcium.

■ Chronic hypocalcemia can produce muscle weakness due to decreased acetylcholine release.

■ Monitor for laryngospasm since acute hypocalcemia can lead to muscle spasms.

■ Hypomagnesemia may aggravate hypocalcemia.

■ Correct for albumin level when interpreting total calcium level.

■ Do not give calcium in same IV line as blood transfusion.

■ Do not give calcium w/ sodium bicarbonate.

■ Do not draw calcium level from same extremity as calcium infusion.

CHECKLIST

■ Carefully follow calcium levels, even during IV infusion.

■ Avoid respiratory or metabolic alkalosis.

■ Closely monitor EKG & BP.

■ Non-depolarizing muscle relaxants are preferable.

■ Monitor for inspiratory stridor & laryngospasm.

HYPOTHYROIDISM

GRACE C. CHANG, MD, MBA; ROBERT A. PETERFREUND, MD, PHD; AND STEPHANIE L. LEE, MD, PHD

FUNDAMENTAL KNOWLEDGE

Thyroid Physiology

■ Thyroid hormone regulates metabolic & developmental processes in every tissue, including the liver (calorigenesis & metabolism), kidneys, brain (somatic & nervous system development), pituitary, cardiac & skeletal muscle (increase in performance) & placenta.

- Thyrotropin-releasing hormone (TRH) is produced & released by hypothalamic neurons & stimulates secretion of thyroid-stimulating hormone (TSH) from anterior pituitary cells.
- TSH controls thyroid hormone synthesis & release, iodine uptake by the thyroid gland & iodine incorporation into tyrosine residues of thyroglobulin, a precursor protein of thyroid hormones.
- Thyroid hormones thyroxine, (T4) & 3,5,3'-triiodothyronine (T3), are formed in the thyroid gland under control of TSH.
- A high level of T3 & T4 will negatively feed back & inhibit secretion of TRH & TSH, reducing secretion of thyroid hormone.
- A low systemic level of thyroid hormone allows an increase in release of TRH & TSH, stimulating production & secretion of T3 & T4.
- In euthyroid pts, the ratio of secretion of T4:T3 is 10:1.
- 80% of circulating T3 is derived by deiodination of T4 in peripheral tissues such as kidneys or liver; systemic illness prevents this deiodination, causing the circulating T4:T3 ratio to be changed.
- Both hormones are usually bound (>99%) to plasma proteins (70–80% to thyroxine-binding globulin [TBG], 10–20% to thyroxine-binding prealbumin, 10–15% to albumin); only the unbound hormone fraction has biological activity.

Changes in Thyroid Physiology Associated w/ Pregnancy
- Serum concentration of TBG increases steadily until plateauing at 20 weeks gestation, when its level is 50% greater than in the nonpregnant state.
- The increase in TBG results in the pregnant euthyroid pt having a total T4 that is 150% of the reference range; the pregnant pt is euthyroid because serum concentrations of free T3 & T4 remain in normal range for non-pregnant pts.
- Human chorionic gonadotropin (hCG) has structural features similar to TSH; hCG levels rise after implantation, peak at 10–12 weeks gestation, then slightly decrease to a steady-state plateau; serum concentrations of TSH & hCG have an inverse relationship during pregnancy.
- Weak stimulation of TSH receptor by hCG results in approx. 12% of women w/ suppressed TSH but high-normal free T4 at the end of the 1st trimester.
- Maternal iodine availability decreases during pregnancy because of increased fetal uptake of iodine & increased maternal renal clearance; pts who live in geographic areas w/ iodine shortage may be predisposed to iodine deficiency, goiter & hypothyroidism.

Definition
- Abnormal decrease in serum concentration of unbound or free thyroid hormones

Epidemiology
- Prevalence in general population is 1.8–7.5%. More common in elderly.
- Prevalence in pregnancy is 2–3%

Signs & Symptoms
- Fatigue
- Hoarseness
- Paresthesias
- Cold intolerance
- Delayed relaxation of deep tendon reflexes
- Slow movements
- Coarse skin & hair
- Periorbital puffiness
- Bradycardia
- Diastolic hypertension
- Constipation

Etiology
- Primary hypothyroidism
  - Autoimmune (most common, Hashimoto's thyroiditis)
  - Iatrogenic (radioiodine therapy for hyperthyroidism, subtotal thyroidectomy or external neck radiation)
  - Drugs (iodine deficiency or excess, lithium, amiodarone, antithyroid drugs)
  - Congenital (dyshormonogenesis or thyroid gland agenesis)
- Secondary hypothyroidism
  - Pituitary dysfunction (irradiation, surgery, neoplasm, Sheehan's syndrome, idiopathic)
  - Hypothalamic dysfunction (irradiation, granulomatous disease, neoplasm)

Pathophysiology
- Primary hypothyroidism (more common than secondary) occurs w/ lack of thyroid hormone action at target organs & tissues.

Effect on Pregnancy
- Prevalence of hypothyroidism in pregnancy is lower than in the general population since hypothyroid women have a lower fertility rate

than euthyroid women, due to neuroendocrine & ovarian dysfunction.

■ Early diagnosis is important since treatment is associated w/ improved maternal & fetal outcomes.

■ Neonatal thyroid function is usually normal, unless mother & fetus have hypothyroidism due to iodine deficiency, & these neonates are readily identified through universal newborn screening for hypothyroidism.

■ Between 6 & 20 weeks gestation, approx. 50% of women are hypothyroid from autoimmune thyroiditis, & approx. 75–85% of women hypothyroid by surgical or radioactive iodine ablation require increase in T4 therapy by 25–75 mcg/day.

Complications
■ Increased incidence of:
  ➢ Spontaneous abortions (>2× rate in normal women)
  ➢ Perinatal mortality (>20%, includes stillbirths & neonatal deaths)
  ➢ Pre-eclampsia
  ➢ IUGR
  ➢ Placental abruption
  ➢ Postpartum hemorrhage
  ➢ Fetal distress during labor
  ➢ Poor somatic & intellectual development in offspring
■ Cognitive development is normal in those hypothyroid infants who receive thyroid hormone replacement within 6 weeks of birth.

STUDIES
■ Best screening test is measurement of serum TSH because in pts w/ hypothyroidism & intact feedback loop, there should be increased serum TSH in pts w/ primary hypothyroidism.

■ Diagnosis is confirmed w/ decreased serum concentration of free T4 or a free thyroxine index <150% of the normal reference range.

MANAGEMENT/INTERVENTIONS
■ Replacement therapy w/ oral thyroid hormone, levothyroxine (L-thyroxine)

■ Requires serial measurements of serum TSH after 4 weeks of a dose adjustment to allow for titration to appropriate dose

■ Pts on T4 therapy should have a TSH checked immediately after pregnancy is confirmed.

■ Myxedema coma

➤ Seen in winter when thermoregulatory stress on body is at its peak

➤ Symptoms include hypothermia & altered mental status.

➤ Associated w/ hyporesponsiveness to CO_2, congestive heart failure & exaggerated signs & symptoms of severe hypothyroidism

➤ Can be precipitated by surgery, drugs, trauma, infection

➤ Treatment: IV L-thyroxine (50–75% daily oral dose), but this is associated w/ a significant risk of myocardial ischemia

Anesthetic Management

■ Elective surgery rarely needs to be delayed to treat hypothyroidism.

■ Hypothyroidism is associated w/ myocardial dysfunction & coronary artery disease.

■ Hypothyroidism is associated w/ a reversible defect in hypoxic & hypercapnic ventilatory drives & sleep apnea.

■ Hyponatremia & anemia are often present, requiring careful fluid mgt, especially w/ free water.

■ General vs. regional anesthesia: no studies have compared safety & efficacy, but both are generally well tolerated in hypothyroidism

➤ General anesthesia

- Pt may have abnormal response to peripheral nerve stimulation during neuromuscular blockade; also can have paresthesias & increased peripheral nociceptive thresholds.
- Prolonged somatosensory evoked potential central conduction time is seen.
- Airway issues: potential problems include enlarged tongue, relaxed oropharyngeal tissues, poor gastric emptying
- Use sedatives & narcotics judiciously for general anesthesia & post-op analgesia because of increased sensitivity.

➤ Regional anesthesia

- Hypothyroidism is associated w/ qualitative platelet dysfunction; rare cause of acquired von Willebrand disease
- Epidural abscess is theoretical risk; no published case reports of this complication in pregnant pts

■ Give glucocorticoid supplementation for emergency procedures for theoretical risk of concomitant autoimmune adrenal insufficiency

CAVEATS/PEARLS

■ Anticipate airway issues as well as problems w/ hypoxic/hypercapnic ventilatory drives & obstructive sleep apnea post-op or after sedation is given.

- Goiter associated w/ hypothyroidism may compromise airway and reduce access to internal jugular veins.
- Be aware of signs & symptoms of myxedema coma.
- Anticipate sensitivity to narcotics & sedatives.
- Do a careful review of history, physical exam & lab results prior to choosing regional anesthesia, given risk of associated coagulopathy.

CHECKLIST
- Thorough preanesthetic evaluation, especially of cardiovascular, pulmonary & neurologic systems
- Review lab results; check for coagulopathy prior to selecting regional anesthesia; correct sodium & electrolyte abnormalities
- Thorough airway evaluation
- Document preexisting paresthesias prior to regional or general anesthesia.
- Judicious use of sedation & narcotics
- Consider stress-dose steroids for emergency procedures.

ICU CARE

KRISTOPHER DAVIGNON, MD
HARISH LECAMWASAM, MD

FUNDAMENTAL KNOWLEDGE
- While most parturients have uncomplicated pregnancies & deliveries, pregnancy, labor & delivery can be associated w/ significant morbidity & mortality.
- Even in a normal pregnancy, labor & delivery are associated w/ numerous alterations in maternal physiology.
- Clinicians managing the critically ill parturient must be aware of these changes & their clinical impact & implications.
- In general, 2 major types of parturients need ICU care:
  - ➤ Those w/ pre-existing conditions that require ICU monitoring to manage their physiology during labor & delivery
  - ➤ Those who acquire a condition during pregnancy that makes them unstable
- The ICU differs from a regular labor floor by the availability of specially trained nurses, respiratory therapists & physicians & by the availability of invasive monitors, vasopressor/inotropic support, mechanical ventilators & renal replacement therapy.

■ See individual chapters for management of specific disease states.
Studies, Management/Intervention, Caveats & Pearls, Checklist N/A

IDIOPATHIC POSTPARTUM RENAL FAILURE

JOSHUA WEBER, MD
PETER DUNN, MD

FUNDAMENTAL KNOWLEDGE
■ First described in 1968; about 200 cases reported
■ Appears 2 days to 10 weeks after normal delivery
■ Typically proceeded by URI or GI viral syndrome
■ Has been associated w/ ethinyl estradiol contraceptive use

Hallmarks
■ Acute renal failure
■ Microangiopathic hemolytic anemia
■ Thrombocytopenia

Complications
■ CHF
■ Bleeding
■ Seizures
■ Hypertension
■ High morbidity & mortality

STUDIES
■ Creatinine
■ BUN
■ Electrolytes
■ Creatinine clearance
■ CBC
■ Urinalysis

MANAGEMENT/INTERVENTIONS
Anesthetic mgt of idiopathic postpartum renal failure

Pre-op
■ Evaluate degree of renal dysfunction & hypertension.
■ Evaluate for anemia & electrolyte abnormalities.

Intraoperative mgt
■ Monitors: standard monitoring +/− arterial line +/− CVP

- Limit fluids in pts w/ marginal renal function to prevent volume overload.
- Use strict aseptic technique, as uremic pts are more prone to infection.

Regional anesthesia
- Uremia-induced platelet dysfunction leads to increased bleeding time.
- Pts may have thrombocytopenia from peripheral destruction of platelets.
- Increased toxicity from local anesthetics has been reported in pts w/ renal disease, but conflicting literature exists.
- Contraindications to regional technique: pt refusal, bacteremia, hypovolemia, hemorrhage, coagulopathy, neuropathy

General anesthesia
- Uremic pts may have hypersensitivity to CNS drugs due to increased permeability of blood-brain barrier.
- Uremia causes delayed gastric emptying & increased acidity, leading to increased risk of aspiration pneumonitis (consider sodium citrate, H2-receptor blocker, metoclopramide).
- Succinylcholine is relatively contraindicated, as it causes approx. 1 mEq/L increase in serum potassium, which may precipitate cardiac dysrhythmias.
- Use caution w/ drugs dependent on renal excretion (gallamine, vecuronium, pancuronium) & clearance (mivacurium, rocuronium).

CAVEATS/PEARLS
- Succinylcholine is relatively contraindicated, as it causes approx. 1 mEq/L increase in serum potassium, which may precipitate cardiac dysrhythmias.
- Use caution w/ drugs dependent on renal excretion (gallamine, vecuronium, pancuronium) & clearance (mivacurium, rocuronium).
- Cisatracurium is a good muscle relaxant for pts w/ renal dysfunction, as its clearance is independent of renal function (Hoffman degradation).
- Standard doses of anticholinesterases are used for reversal of neuromuscular blockade.
- Consider whether pt is likely to have platelet dysfunction (secondary to uremia) or significant peripheral neuropathy before doing regional anesthetic.

CHECKLIST

- Know OB history & postpartum plan.
- Document degree of renal dysfunction.
- Be prepared to treat hypertension.
- Consider effects of uremia, hypoalbuminemia, impaired renal metabolism & excretion when choosing meds.

IDIOPATHIC THROMBOCYTOPENIC PURPURA

JEANNA VIOLA, MD
JANE BALLANTYNE, MD

FUNDAMENTAL KNOWLEDGE

- Common in healthy young women; 0.01–0.02% incidence in parturients
- Anti-platelet antibodies (usually IgG) responsible for premature platelet destruction & impaired thrombopoiesis
- Isolated thrombocytopenia occurs in first trimester or precedes pregnancy.
- Platelet function may be improved, normal or impaired.
- Petechiae found at pressure points
- Risk of intracranial bleed
- Transplacental passage of antibodies leads to neonatal bleeding:
  - ➤ <5% have significant thrombocytopenia at birth (<50,000 plts)
  - ➤ 30–40% develop significant thrombocytopenia in first 2 days.
- Associated w/ family history of autoimmune disease

STUDIES

- CBC: thrombocytopenia but normal #s of RBCs & WBCs
- Blood smear: large, well-granulated platelets
- Bleeding time: normal platelet function despite decreased number
- Coagulation indices (PT, PTT): normal
- No specific lab test exists; identifying anti-platelet antibodies is helpful.

MANAGEMENT/INTERVENTIONS

- Early consultation w/ a hematologist is helpful.
- If mother is asymptomatic & platelets are >60–75,000 prior to delivery, no treatment is needed; regional anesthesia is considered safe.

■ With impaired hemostasis, a higher platelet count is desired prior to delivery. Consider:
  ➤ Prednisone 1 mg/kg preop & postop (steroids require 24–48 hours to affect platelet count)
  ➤ Intravenous immunoglobulin (IVIG) 2 g/kg over 2–5 days
  ➤ If pt fails to respond, consider splenectomy (2nd trimester preferred).
  ➤ Danazol & vincristine sometimes used in refractory cases
■ Sometimes IVIG (immunoglobulin) or a short course of steroids is given at 37–38 weeks to ensure adequate platelet count at delivery.
■ Obtain fetal scalp vein or percutaneous umbilical cord blood sample to check fetal platelet count.
  ➤ If fetal plts <50,000, consider C-section.
  ➤ Monitor neonates × 72h for evidence of bleeding.
■ NSAIDs are contraindicated in ITP pts.

CAVEATS AND PEARLS
■ Lack of bleeding problems in the history at a given platelet count is reassuring.
■ Differential diagnosis includes SLE, HIV, antiphospholipid antibodies.
■ When fetal plt count is <50,000, C-section is sometimes performed to decrease risk of neonatal intracranial trauma.
■ Spinal anesthesia is sometimes preferred to GETA (if plt count > 40,000) when there is fetal distress in a pt w/ a difficult airway.

CHECKLIST
■ Check platelet count on admission and shortly prior to C-section.
■ If plt count is in the "gray zone" (60–75,000), weigh risks & benefits of regional anesthesia vs. alternatives.
■ Consider PCA for labor analgesia.
■ Check airway & prepare for possible GETA.
■ Prepare for transfusions if indicated.

IMPLANTABLE CARDIOVERTER DEFIBRILLATORS

JASMIN FIELD, MD
DWIGHT GEHA, MD

FUNDAMENTAL KNOWLEDGE
■ ICDs were first used in humans in 1980.

- ➤ Currently >30,000 placed each year
- ➤ Prevalence in women of childbearing age will likely increase w/:
  - Increasing evidence that devices are well tolerated by mother & fetus
  - Increased survival of pts w/ life-threatening arrhythmias
- ■ Indicated for prevention of sudden cardiac death due to VF or VT
  - ➤ VT often precedes VF & can be stable or unstable.
  - ➤ Unless spontaneously resolved, the only way to correct VF is w/ electricity.
  - ➤ Most common causes of VT/VF are structural heart disease & conductive abnormalities.
  - ➤ Pts w/ history of previous episodes of VT/VF due to non-reversible issues should get an ICD placed promptly.
  - ➤ Pts w/ conditions w/ high risk for VT/VF also may benefit:
    - Severe LV dysfunction
    - CHF
    - Hypertrophic cardiomyopathy
    - Long QT syndrome
    - Complex ventricular ectopy
- ■ ICDs are made up of 3 components
  - ➤ Sensing electrodes
    - Placed in RV
    - Detect length of cardiac cycle
  - ➤ Defibrillating electrodes
    - 2 electrodes create a circuit (anode & cathode).
    - One electrode is usually an RV or SVC coil but can be subcutaneous.
    - One electrode is within the generator case.
  - ➤ Pulse generator
    - Contains electronic circuitry, 3-volt battery & a high-voltage capacitor that can deliver a 750-joule shock.
- ■ ICDs have many functions:
  - ➤ Defibrillating (high-energy shock)
    - Can give up to 6 shocks
    - Increases pt's sympathetic tone
  - ➤ Cardioversion (low-energy shock)
  - ➤ Most ICDs also have pacing capabilities.
    - Dual-chamber device
    - Atrial sense/pace lead placed in right atrial appendage
    - Anti-tachycardia & anti-bradycardia pacing (DDDR)

➤ Monitoring/memory for interrogation & mgt
  • Heart rate is continuously monitored.
  • Therapies are delivered whenever programmed rate is exceeded.
■ In the OR, the defibrillating capabilities can be turned off using a magnet, but pacing capabilities will be preserved.
  ➤ During most non-cardiothoracic surgeries, magnet inhibition of ICD therapy is recommended.
  ➤ Pts should be monitored continuously, w/ external defibrillation immediately available while magnet is in place.
  ➤ Application of the magnet inhibits tachycardia therapy/detection only.
  ➤ Most ICDs are designed to reactivate (detect rates & deliver treatments) immediately on removal of the magnet.
  ➤ The magnet should be placed directly over the ICD device for inhibition.
    • Various manufacturers make ICDs that emit various sounds when inhibited.
    • Some ICDs make no noise at all.
  ➤ The magnet should be taped in place to prevent it from moving inadvertently, as most ICDs are fully active as soon as the magnet is removed.
  ➤ Application of the magnet cannot change the mode of pacing function.
■ All ICD pts should have an ID card that identifies the device manufacturer & the physician following the pt for ICD-related issues. Knowing the manufacturer is essential to knowing how the device will respond to the magnet.

STUDIES

History & physical exam
■ Device type, lead type, location of ICD leads & generator
■ Chest x-ray can confirm location of leads & device as needed.
■ Any recent shocks or syncopal episodes
■ Date of last interrogation

Noninvasive programmed stimulation (NIPS)
■ Performed the day after ICD placement & then once a year or surrounding any discharges or misfiring of ICDs
  ➤ Light general anesthesia w/ propofol, spontaneous ventilation & standard monitors is safe in most pts, but standard airway

concerns for anesthesia in advanced pregnancy & the gravid uterus apply.

➤ NIPS have been done safely in pregnant pts, although data are limited.

■ Replacement generators are necessary every 6 years, or more frequently if pts experience frequent shocks or require higher defibrillation thresholds.

MANAGEMENT/INTERVENTIONS

Anesthesia for initial placement of ICD

■ Standard monitors

■ Sedation is sufficient for initial part of procedure, depending on stage of pregnancy.

➤ Leads are advanced through subclavian or cephalic veins under fluoroscopy.
  • Mother & fetus should be shielded w/ lead.
  • Duration of fluoroscopy should be minimized if possible.

➤ Local anesthetic is given for making a subcutaneous pocket in subpectoral or abdominal tissue.

■ During placement, the device must be tested for:

➤ Pacing threshold

➤ Pacing lead impedance

➤ Defibrillatory threshold

➤ Shocking electrode impedance

➤ Cardioversion threshold & impedance

■ VF is induced during testing phase of ICD placement.

➤ External defibrillator pads are placed in case the ICD fails.

➤ Light general anesthesia is induced.
  • Spontaneous ventilation w/ oxygen via face mask is usually sufficient for non-pregnant pts, w/ bag valve mask used as needed.
  • Though most pts do not need an LMA or ETT, the pt in later stages of pregnancy must be treated as a full stomach & should be intubated w/ cuffed endotracheal tube.
  • A viable fetus should be monitored continuously.

➤ Programmed VF is induced via a wand placed over the device externally. Time to VF sensing & defibrillation threshold is then evaluated.

➤ Hypotension is treated w/ phenylephrine & ephedrine.

ICD alternatives for treating pts at risk for SCD
- Ablation (see "Arrhythmias")
- Anti-arrhythmic drugs (see "Arrhythmias")
- Cardiac transplant

Management of pregnant pt w/ ICD in place
- Labor & vaginal delivery do not require disabling of ICD.
- For C-section & any surgical procedure, electromagnetic interference (EMI) can adversely effect ICD via:
  - ➤ Inappropriate shocks
  - ➤ Device reprogramming
  - ➤ Pacing & shock inhibition
  - ➤ Myocardial injury at electrode sites
- Prior to any surgery, the following precautions should be taken:
  - ➤ External defibrillating pads must be applied prior to placing magnet & should be placed away from existing leads & generator.
  - ➤ Electrocautery should be limited to short bursts in bipolar mode.
  - ➤ Electrocautery grounding pads should be placed far away from ICD leads & generator.
  - ➤ Defibrillating capacity should be disabled via application of a magnet.
    - For most modern ICDs, backup pacing capabilities should still be intact w/ magnet on.
    - If the pt has any unstable rhythms during the procedure, remove magnet to allow shock. External defibrillating pads are used for backup defibrillation.
  - ➤ Most ICDs resume defibrillation capacity when magnet is removed, but some older models require removal followed by reapplication for reactivation, or followed by reprogramming.
  - ➤ EP services should be consulted preop & postop (also before delivery & postpartum) for interrogation & to determine if reprogramming is required.

CAVEATS & PEARLS
- Fast heart rate can be misinterpreted by ICD as an episode of VF, causing shocks to be delivered inappropriately.
- ICDs cannot currently distinguish well between VT & SVT.
- Until recently, pts w/ existing ICDs were cautioned against getting pregnant because of insufficient data on risks to fetus.

- Discharge of the ICD has been associated w/ (though not always proven to be causative):
  - Preterm labor/low birthweight
  - Abruption
  - Fetal loss
- In a 1997 retrospective analysis of 44 women w/ ICDs in place who became pregnant, Natale et al showed the relative safety & efficacy of ICDs in pregnant women:
  - Pregnancy, labor & delivery did not increase the rate of ICD-related complications, ICD device fractures or discharges/shocks.
  - ICD therapy did not significantly increase maternal or fetal complications:
    - 82% had no complications.
    - 18% had complications that were not always clearly causative & did not occur at a rate significantly higher than normal pregnant women.
    - >85% of babies were born healthy, no different than general population.
    - No erosions or migrations occurred, even though 96% of the pts had abdominally implanted generators.
- Leads are placed under fluoroscopy.
  - Fetus can be protected from radiation exposure w/ lead shielding.
  - Adverse outcomes due to radiation have not been documented.

CHECKLIST
- Document device type, manufacturer, physician following, lead type & location of ICD (pt should have an ID card that gives information on all of the above).
- Ask pt about any recent shocks or episodes of syncope.
- Ask when device was last interrogated.
- Full stomach of pregnancy means general anesthesia w/ proper control of airway during placement & interrogation of ICD.
- Viable fetus must be continuously monitored during placement & interrogation of ICD.
- ICDs do not need to be turned off for labor or vaginal deliveries.
- ICDs should be turned off w/ application of a magnet during any surgical procedure where electrocautery will be used.
- External defibrillator pads should be placed prior to application of magnets; note & avoid location of ICD & leads.

■ Surgeons should be encouraged to use bipolar cautery only & to avoid prolonged periods of EMI.

EP services should be consulted for preop/postop (antepartum/postpartum) interrogation of ICD, w/ evaluation of potential need for reprogramming.

INFLUENZA

SISSELA PARK, MD
LAURA RILEY, MD

FUNDAMENTAL KNOWLEDGE

■ Influenza caused by RNA virus from Orthomyxoviridae family
  ➤ Influenza A
  ➤ Influenza B
  ➤ Influenza C
■ Most serious type is A.
  ➤ Acute onset after 1- to 4-day incubation period
  ➤ Symptoms include:
    • Fever
    • Coryza
    • Malaise
    • Cough
    • Headache
  ➤ Usually self-limited
  ➤ If illness lasts >5 days during pregnancy, suspect complications such as pneumonia.
■ Influenza pneumonia
  ➤ Result of either viral infection of lungs or secondary bacterial infection
  ➤ Can be fatal
  ➤ Quick progression from unilateral to diffuse bilateral disease
  ➤ Pt may develop respiratory failure requiring intubation & mechanical ventilation.

STUDIES

■ Influenza A & influenza B are identified by nucleoprotein antigenic reactions.
■ Can be further classified by hemagglutinin & neuraminidase antigens
■ Chest x-ray if pneumonia is suspected

MANAGEMENT/INTERVENTIONS

Prevention
- Vaccination
- Is safe in pregnancy
- Recommended for all pregnant women during flu season
- Flumist is not safe since it uses a live virus.

Influenza pneumonia
- Supportive care to decrease fever
- Antibiotics to treat secondary infections
- Antiviral agents

CAVEATS & PEARLS
- If pt is sick w/ influenza for 5 or more days, suspect pneumonia.
- Influenza pneumonia
  - ➤ Can be fatal
  - ➤ Quick progression from unilateral to bilateral disease
- Vaccination is safe & recommended for all pregnant pts during the flu season.

CHECKLIST
- Pregnant pts w/ influenza pneumonia can develop respiratory failure & need intubation.
- Encourage pregnant pts to get vaccinated.

INFORMED CONSENT

LATA POTTURI, MD
ADELE VIGUERA, MD

FUNDAMENTAL KNOWLEDGE
- Informed consent is a process by which a fully informed pt can make decisions about her health care. The following elements are usually discussed: procedure or treatment options, risks & benefits of the procedure or treatment options, alternatives to the procedure, risks & benefits of all alternatives, assessment of pt understanding & acceptance or refusal of the procedure or treatment options. A pt must be deemed competent & consent must be voluntary. All discussions should be carried on in layperson's terms.
- Studies have examined the ability of a pt in labor to give informed consent. Although many laboring pts were later unable to remember

the actual informed consent process, these pts were deemed competent to make informed decisions & give voluntary consent.

■ Rarely in obstetrics, pts will have received premedication or pain medication prior to giving informed consent. Premedication affects the informed consent process only if the pt is unable to verbalize understanding of the treatment or procedures being discussed & is unable to make informed decisions. Often, premedication or pain medication can alleviate duress & actually enhance a pt's ability to make decisions. Sedation or pain medication should not be withheld from a suffering pt in order to obtain consent. Pregnant minors are allowed to participate in the informed consent process, make informed decisions & sign forms on their own behalf.

STUDIES
■ Assess the pt's ability to understand the situation, understand the risks associated w/ the decision at hand & communicate a decision based on that understanding. When this is unclear, a psychiatric consultation can be helpful.

MANAGEMENT & INTERVENTIONS
■ When a pt is determined to be incapacitated or incompetent to make health care decisions, a surrogate decision maker must be appointed. A hierarchy of appropriate decision makers is defined by law. If no appropriate surrogate is available, the physicians are expected to act in the best interest of the pt until a surrogate is found or appointed.
■ Pt consent can be "presumed" in emergency situations when the pt is unconscious or incompetent & no surrogate decision maker is available.
■ A pt always has the right to refuse information & treatment as long as she is competent & verbalizes understanding of her decisions.

CAVEATS & PEARLS
Determine who can appoint & serve as surrogate decision makers beforehand.

CHECKLIST
■ Determine if the pt can provide informed consent.
■ Discuss treatment, risks & benefits of every procedure as part of obtaining informed consent. Ask the pt if she has any specific concerns. Answer all questions truthfully & in layperson's terms.
■ If there is any question regarding the pt's competency, consult a psychiatrist.

■ If the pt is incapacitated, seek advice from a psychiatrist & seek a surrogate decision maker. If no surrogate decision maker is found, make every effort to act in the pt's best interest until a surrogate decision maker is found.

INTRA-AMNIOTIC INFECTION

SISSELA PARK, MD
LAURA RILEY, MD

FUNDAMENTAL KNOWLEDGE

Definition
■ Also known as chorioamnionitis, amnionitis, amniotic fluid infection
■ Infection that involves the amniotic fluid, placenta, amnionic membranes &/or uterus
■ One of the most common infections in pregnancy
■ Incidence of intra-amniotic infection is higher in preterm deliveries.

Pathogenesis
■ Most cases are due to ascending infection, in which bacteria gain access to amniotic cavity & fetus through the cervix after rupture of the membranes.
■ Instances of intra-amniotic infection w/ intact membranes due to hematogenous spread of organism
■ Contamination from invasive procedure such as:
  ➤ Amniocentesis
  ➤ Cerclage
  ➤ Chorionic villus sampling

Risk factors
■ Nulliparity
■ Preterm labor
■ Internal fetal or uterine monitoring
■ Meconium-stained amniotic fluid
■ Cervical colonization (gonorrhea or group B streptococcus)
■ Bacterial vaginosis
■ PROM
■ Prolonged duration of membrane rupture
■ Prolonged duration of labor

- Larger number of vaginal exams after membrane rupture
- Young age of mother

Maternal complications
- Common complications
  - Bacteremia
  - Dysfunctional labor patterns
  - Higher incidence of cesarean delivery
  - Hemorrhage
- More serious complications
  - Coagulopathy
  - Septic shock
  - Adult respiratory distress syndrome
  - These are low risk in the setting of broad-spectrum antibiotics & modern medical facilities.
- Increased risk of surgical complications from cesarean delivery, such as:
  - Hemorrhage
  - Wound infection
- Hemorrhage as a result of impaired myometrial contraction/atony
- Bacteremia in about 5%–10% of pts w/ intra-amniotic infection
  - Slightly higher rate when intra-amniotic infection is due to:
    - Group B streptococcus (18%)
    - *E. coli* (15%)
- Dystocia
  - Pathophysiology for abnormal labor in the setting of intra-amniotic infection is poorly understood.
  - Two possible reasons dystocia is associated w/ intra-amniotic infection:
    - Abnormal labor patterns/prolonged labor predisposes to infection (ie, intra-amniotic infection).
    - Intra-amniotic infection leads to abnormal labor.

Fetal complications
- Neonatal morbidity
  - Reduced but not eliminated by antibiotics
- Fetal infection
  - Risk is 10–20% when mother has intra-amniotic infection.
  - Preterm & low-birthweight infants are more commonly affected than full-term or normal-birthweight infants.
- Sepsis

- Pneumonia
- Respiratory distress syndrome
- Perinatal asphyxia
- Intraventricular hemorrhage
- Cerebral palsy
- Neurodevelopmental delay

STUDIES
- Diagnosis of intra-amniotic infection requires a high index of suspicion.
- Clinical diagnosis
  - Usually based on the presence of maternal fever & at least 2 of the following:
    - Maternal leukocytosis (>15,000 cells/cubic mm)
    - Maternal tachycardia (>100 bpm)
    - Fetal tachycardia (>160 bpm)
    - Uterine tenderness
    - Foul odor of amniotic fluid
  - Clinical criteria for intra-amniotic infection are neither specific nor sensitive.
- Amniotic fluid culture
  - Gold standard for documenting intra-amniotic infection
  - Results available after 48–72 hours, so helpful only in the postpartum mgt of women suspected of having intra-amniotic infection
  - Multiple organisms are seen on culture from pregnancies complicated by intra-amniotic infection, including:
    - Group B streptococci
    - *E. coli*
    - Enterococci
    - *Gardnerella vaginalis*
    - *Peptostreptococcus* species
    - *Bacteroides* species
    - *Clostridium* species
    - *Fusobacterium* species
    - Gram-negative anaerobes
    - *Mycoplasma hominis*
- Gram stain: when positive for bacteria & leukocytes, it is suspicious for intra-amniotic infection
- Glucose level: abnormal result is a good predictor of positive amniotic fluid culture in women w/ suspected intra-amniotic infection

- Leukocyte esterase levels: when detected, it provides a sensitivity & specificity >90% according to some studies
- Cytokine immunoassays
  - Can detect the cytokines interleukin-6, interleukin-1, interleukin- 8 & tumor necrosis factor-alpha
  - Elevation of these cytokines is associated w/ intra-amniotic infection.
  - Can help predict positive amniotic fluid cultures
  - Limited clinical usefulness due to:
    - Invasive nature of specimen collection
    - Complexity of assays
    - Lack of standards across different labs
    - Relatively high false-positive rate
  - Used mostly in research settings

MANAGEMENT/INTERVENTIONS

Antibiotics

- In recent studies, use of intrapartum antibiotics was associated w/ decreased maternal & neonatal morbidity.
- Usual treatment is broad-spectrum antibiotics that cover beta-lactamase-producing anaerobes.
- Most common
  - Ampicillin 2 g q6h w/ gentamicin 1.5 mg/kg q8h in mothers w/ normal kidney function
  - Found to be safe & effective
- Alternative single-agent regimens
  - Ampicillin-sulbactam 3g q6h
  - Ticarcillin-clavulanate 3.1 g q4h
  - Cefoxitin 2g q6h
- Anaerobe coverage decreases failure rates in post-cesarean endometritis.
  - Some clinicians add clindamycin (900 mg q8h) to the primary regimen after cord clamping in women undergoing C-section.
- Continue antibiotics until pt is clinically better & afebrile for 24–48 hours.

Delivery

- Minimal evidence that cesarean delivery offers an improved outcome over vaginal delivery
- Use standard obstetric indications in determining the delivery method.

- Cesarean delivery is more common in women w/ intra-amniotic infection. Likely explanations include:
  - ➤ Intra-amniotic infection is often seen in women w/ dystocia.
  - ➤ Uterus affected by intra-amniotic infection is less sensitive to oxytocin.

CAVEATS & PEARLS
- Intra-amniotic infection is an infection that involves the amniotic fluid, placenta, chorioamnionic membranes &/or uterus.
- Diagnosis of intra-amniotic infection is usually based on the presence of maternal fever & at least 2 of the following:
  - ➤ Maternal leukocytosis (>15,000 cells/cubic mm)
  - ➤ Maternal tachycardia (>100 bpm)
  - ➤ Fetal tachycardia (>160 bpm)
  - ➤ Uterine tenderness
  - ➤ Foul odor of amniotic fluid
- Use of intrapartum antibiotics is associated w/ decreased maternal & neonatal morbidity.
- Dystocia is common in women w/ intra-amniotic infection.

CHECKLIST
- Consider the presence of intra-amniotic infection in febrile pregnant women.
- Be prepared for fetal resuscitation in the setting of intra-amniotic infection.

INTRACRANIAL ANEURYSM

MEREDITH ALBRECHT, MD
MICHELE SZABO, MD

FUNDAMENTAL KNOWLEDGE

Definition
- An abnormal bulging outward of one of the arteries in the brain. Often discovered when aneurysm ruptures, typically into the subarachnoid space, causing a subarachnoid hemorrhage (SAH).

Epidemiology
- Prevalence of spontaneous SAH during pregnancy: 1–5 in 10,000
- Prevalence of rupture in age-matched non-pregnant population: 0.02–1 in 10,000
- Third leading cause of maternal death, according to some reports

Pathophysiology
- Aneurysms typically occur at bifurcation of large arteries at the base of the brain.
- Unclear why aneurysms develop
- Likely combination of intrinsic & extrinsic factors; the disease is associated w/:
  - Hypertension
  - Smoking
  - Family history of aneurysms
  - Polycystic kidney disease
- Aneurysmal rupture w/ SAH is a devastating disease.
- Maternal mortality rate: 30–50%, reported as high as 83%
- Causes of mortality
  - Aneurysmal re-rupture: maternal mortality rate of 70%
  - Vasospasm
    - Occurs 4–14 days following hemorrhage
    - Prolonged focal, reversible arterial narrowing
    - Causes cerebral ischemia +/− infarction
  - Pulmonary embolism

Clinical Manifestations
- Symptoms & signs vary; severity depends on extent of bleeding.
- Neurologic
- At the time of rupture:
  - Headache: "worst of my life"
  - Nausea, vomiting
  - Meningismus or neck stiffness
  - Loss of consciousness: occurs in 50% of pts
    - 15% will die before reaching the hospital.
- At the time of admission to hospital
  - Pt may be alert w/ headache, or comatose.
  - Neurologic condition related to severity of initial injury
  - Condition can worsen w/ rebleeding or w/ development of hydrocephalus.
- 4–14 days following admission, vasospasm may develop.
  - Worsening level of consciousness
  - Focal neurologic deficit
- Seizures often occur.
- Pulmonary
  - Aspiration pneumonia, usually at time of SAH-induced unconsciousness
  - "Neurogenic" pulmonary edema

- Cardiac
  - Massive sympathetic "surge" at time of aneurysmal rupture
  - Can cause cardiac dysfunction (eg, global hypokinesis & cardiogenic shock). More likely to occur in pts w/ worse neurologic injury.
- DVT

Effect of pregnancy on intracerebral aneurysm
- Pregnancy confers increased risk of rupture 5x that of non-pregnant women of same age.
- Incidence of rupture increases w/ advancing maternal age & as gestation progresses.
- Following SAH, maternal mortality rate is similar to general population.

Effect of SAH on pregnancy & fetus
- Fetal mortality rate: 17% overall
- Fetal mortality rate following maternal antepartum surgery for aneurysm clipping: 5%
- Fetal mortality in pts not undergoing surgery: 27%

STUDIES
History & physical
- Determine presence of preexisting risk factors: hypertension, smoking, polycystic kidney disease.
- Neurologic: determine prior course of the neurologic disease
  - Neurologic status upon admission
  - Evidence for rebleeding
  - Evidence of or treatment for hydrocephalus
  - Presence of seizures
- Pulmonary: determine oxygen saturation (current & during event, if known) & look for evidence of possible aspiration or "neurogenic" pulmonary edema.
- Cardiac: examine for evidence of cardiac dysfunction
  - History of pulmonary edema
  - Abnormal ECG
  - Hypotension
- Determine ideal blood pressure parameters.

Imaging
- CT scan
  - Initial diagnostic procedure of choice for pregnant pt

- ➤ Amount of blood is related to severity of bleed & subsequent risk of neurologic complications.
- ➤ Shielded fetus, safe radiation exposure
- ■ CT angiography
  - ➤ Ideal method to identify suspected vascular lesions
  - ➤ Avoids increased complications of invasive angiography
  - ➤ Contrast dye does not cross placenta, physiologically inert; considered safe for fetus.
  - ➤ Contrast dye is a diuretic, so hydrate pt well.
  - ➤ Shield fetus from radiation exposure.
- ■ Cerebral angiography
  - ➤ Shielded fetus, safe radiation exposure
  - ➤ Contrast agents pose little risk for fetus.
  - ➤ Hydrate well to prevent maternal & fetal dehydration; contrast dye is a diuretic.
- ■ MRI
  - ➤ No long-term data on fetal outcome
  - ➤ Generally avoided during 1st trimester
  - ➤ Gadolinium crosses the placenta.
  - ➤ No reported adverse effects of fetal exposure to gadolinium
  - ➤ Most advise against gadolinium use during pregnancy; not FDA approved for this purpose
- ■ Chest radiograph: if suspicious of associated pulmonary disease process

Other
- ■ EKG: look for evidence of cardiac involvement w/ SAH
- ■ BUN/Cr: following IV contrast studies & if suspect polycystic kidney disease
- ■ Check electrolytes; may be abnormal due to diuretic effects of dye, SIADH or cerebral salt-wasting syndrome associated w/ SAH
- ■ Type & crossmatch blood; check for antibodies to prevent any surgical delay.
- ■ Serum anticonvulsant levels

MANAGEMENT/INTERVENTIONS

Surgical
- ■ Unruptured: incidentally discovered aneurysm
  - ➤ Pregnancy confers increased risk of rupture.
  - ➤ Risk increases w/ increased gestation.
  - ➤ Substantial risk of SAH to mother & fetus

> Many recommend elective surgical/endovascular treatment as soon as feasible following fetal organogenesis
- Following SAH
  > Maternal mortality rate following surgical treatment, 11%
  > Maternal mortality rate for those not undergoing surgery, 63%
  > Neurosurgical/endovascular treatment is done ASAP following medical stabilization.
  > Data for endovascular Rx not yet available
- External ventricular drainage: may be placed in pts who develop hydrocephalus (SAH can block reabsorption of CSF)

Medical
- Stabilization of blood pressure is critical.
  > Hypertension increases risk of aneurysmal re-bleed.
  > Treat nausea & vomiting; these increase BP.
  > Treat headache to prevent hypertension.
    • Avoid oversedation, which obscures neurologic exam.
- Avoid hypotension.
  > Treat headaches, nausea & vomiting before employing antihypertensive.
  > Use antihypertensives cautiously.
  > Hypotension can lead to cerebral ischemia.
  > Worsens neurologic injury
  > Decreases uterine-placental blood flow
- Sodium nitroprusside: used successfully in pregnant pts w/ SAH
- Hydralazine: data support use as first-line therapy for pregnant pts w/ severe hypertension
- Labetalol: reasonable data support that it is safe for the fetus & effective for mother
- Nimodipine
  > Calcium channel blocker
  > Improves outcome following SAH, decreases risk of cerebral ischemia caused by vasospasm
  > Can cause mild decrease in BP
  > Animal studies: associated w/ congenital malformations & IUGR
  > Human studies lacking
- Anticonvulsants
  > All are established teratogens; greatest risk during 1st trimester
  > Risk of maternal & fetal hypoxia & acidosis associated w/ seizure justifies their use in SAH pt at risk for seizure.
  > Drug pharmacokinetics are altered during pregnancy, so check serum anticonvulsant levels.

> Interfere w/ folic acid & vitamin K metabolism; give supplementation

Anesthesia

1) For non-urgent craniotomy & clipping of an unruptured aneurysm
- Administer prophylactic antibiotics.
- Monitor BP w/ an arterial line.
- Consider placement of CVP for monitoring as well as for medication infusion.
- Prevent hypertension.
  > Increase depth of anesthesia
  > Treat w/ antihypertensive such as labetalol or sodium nitroprusside.
- Reports of safe induction accomplished w/ pentothal, propofol, succinylcholine & narcotic titrated to prevent a hypertensive response to intubation
- Potential for large blood loss should aneurysm rupture
  > Establish sufficient large-bore IV access.
  > Have blood products readily available.
- Provide "brain relaxation" to facilitate surgical exposure.
  > Lumbar spinal drain
    • Decreases ventricular size
    • First choice for brain relaxation
  > Most avoid furosemide & mannitol in the elective case as these meds have the potential to cause transient fetal dehydration.
- Induced mild hypothermia
  > Used for possible "brain protection"
  > Used for brain relaxation
  > Reported safe for fetus
- Emergence: plan anesthetic around prompt emergence, facilitating an early neurologic exam
- OB consult to determine appropriate fetal monitoring
2) For the urgent craniotomy for aneurysm clipping following SAH w/o concurrent C-section
- Administer prophylactic antibiotics.
- Urgent OB consult if feasible (do not delay surgery)
- Direct measurement of arterial pressure w/ A-line
  > Hypertension increases risk of re-bleed, which is associated w/ 70% mortality rate.
  > Hypotension worsens neurologic injury & decreases uterine-placental blood flow.
- CVP recommended as time permits

➤ Helps facilitate adequate hydration; reduces likelihood of hypotension, particularly w/ induction
➤ More reliable & safe route of administration of potent vasodilators/pressors

■ Prevention of hypertension until aneurysm is secure is of paramount importance!
➤ Deepen the anesthetic w/ additional narcotic or increased concentration of inhalational agent.
➤ Nitroprusside & labetalol should be readily available.

■ Induction
➤ Goals: avoid hypertension, hypotension, inadequate muscle relaxation; prevent aspiration
➤ "Modified" rapid sequence induction
➤ Goal is to minimize cough, response to pain that would increase ICP.
  • Maintain cricoid pressure.
  • Induction w/ pentothal or propofol
  • Muscle relaxation w/ rocuronium (assuming normal airway anatomy); monitor TOF to ensure adequate relaxation for intubation
  • Ventilate as needed to maintain oxygenation & "normocarbia"
  • Add narcotic as necessary to help blunt hypertensive response to intubation.

■ Maintenance
➤ Goals: prevent hypertension until the aneurysm is secure, avoid hypotension at all times
➤ There is no evidence that one anesthetic is superior to others.
➤ Normovolemia facilitates the prevention of hypotension.

■ Emergence: plan for prompt emergence that permits early neurologic exam
➤ Extubation is dependent on usual extubation criteria & pt's neurologic status.
➤ Evaluate, but do not always extubate these pts.

■ Prepare for potential large blood loss.
➤ Establish adequate large-bore IV access.
➤ Have blood readily available for transfusion. Do not transfuse Rh+ blood to Rh- mother.
➤ Should there be an aneurysmal rupture, goal is always to maintain BP >100 mmHg systolic. Aggressively resuscitate w/ blood & vasopressors.

■ Provide adequate "brain" relaxation.

➤ Lumbar CSF drainage catheter can be placed to decrease CSF volume.
  • First-line choice for brain relaxation in pregnant pt; avoids use of mannitol
  • Neurosurgical procedure
  • Indicated if there is no risk for brain herniation
  • Do not drain until dura is open to avoid brain shift & rupture of aneurysm.
➤ Mannitol
  • Osmotic diuretic
  • Effective in treating intracranial hypertension & providing brain relaxation
  • Can increase fetal plasma osmolality & cause transient fetal dehydration
  • Fetal outcome data are limited.
  • Limited use for life-threatening elevated ICP or when CSF drainage is ineffective
➤ Furosemide
  • Not at effective as mannitol
  • Causes less fetal dehydration than mannitol
➤ Hyperventilation
  • Reliably reduces ICP
  • Marked hyperventilation causes uteroplacental vasoconstriction, resulting in fetal hypoxia & acidosis.
  • Thought that reduction in cardiac output caused by positive-pressure ventilation is the likely cause of observed decreased uterine blood flow & not alkalosis per se
  • Used when there is evidence of increased ICP; adverse effects on fetus minimized w/ normovolemia & low airway pressure
■ Provide "brain" protection.
➤ Risk of cerebral ischemia when parent vessel is clipped
➤ Induced hypothermia is used by some centers; track record of safety for mother & fetus
➤ Induced hypertension to improve collateral flow when temporary clip is on & as directed by the neurosurgeon
■ Fetal heart rate monitoring as per obstetric consult
■ If labor begins during craniotomy & delivery is imminent
➤ Suspend intracranial procedure.
➤ C-section if indicated.
➤ After delivery of the infant, anesthesia may be modified as required for the neurosurgical procedure.

3) For urgent craniotomy for aneurysm clipping w/ concurrent C-section
- Same guidelines as above except:
  - ➤ C-section should precede the craniotomy except if maternal transtentorial herniation.
  - ➤ Narcotic-induced neonatal depression can be readily reversed w/ naloxone.
  - ➤ Fetal dehydration secondary to mannitol can be treated w/ fluids.
  - ➤ Following delivery, measures such as mannitol & hyperventilation can be used to reduce ICP or provide improved brain relaxation.
  - ➤ Oxytocin
    - Effect in pts w/ intracranial vascular lesions is unclear; likely to cause cerebral vasoconstriction.
    - Can cause maternal hypotension; vigilant attention to BP needed
    - Has been used clinically in these circumstances w/o adverse effect
  - ➤ Check for uterine bleeding at regular intervals throughout the craniotomy.
4) Anesthesia for a C-section in pt w/ unsecured unruptured aneurysm
- Rarely, a pt has an inoperable intravascular lesion.
- Arterial line
- Epidural preferred; avoids potential for Valsalva during intubation
- Establish block slowly.
- Allows continuous neurologic monitoring
5) For pt w/ a clipped & secure aneurysm
- No special anesthetic considerations for either labor & vaginal delivery or C-section

CAVEATS & PEARLS
- SAH is a catastrophic disease w/ significant maternal & fetal mortality.
- Arrange obstetric consult.
- Maternal & fetal anesthetic requirements have the potential to conflict & should be balanced via ongoing discussions w/ the neurosurgeon & obstetrician.
- Maternal hypertension & hypotension significantly contribute to maternal morbidity & mortality.
- Check neurologic status frequently; pt can deteriorate quickly.
- Inform neurosurgeon of anesthetic plan & establish means of emergency contact.

CHECKLIST

- Have resuscitation equipment readily available; pts can deteriorate quickly!
- Have antihypertensive drugs drawn up & readily available.
- Have pressors readily available.
- Be prepared for large blood loss should pt come to the OR. If transfusion needed & mother Rh negative, do not transfuse Rh-positive blood.
- Be prepared to treat a seizure.
- Administer prophylactic antibiotics for craniotomy.
- Arrange obstetric consult.

INTRACRANIAL ARTERIOVENOUS MALFORMATIONS

MEREDITH ALBRECHT, MD
MICHELE SZABO, MD

FUNDAMENTAL KNOWLEDGE

Definition
- Intracerebral vascular lesion w/ abnormal direct connection of small arteries to veins w/o intervening capillary bed

Epidemiology
- Incidence of symptomatic AVMs: 1 per 100,000 population
- Incidence of AVMs in pregnant pts is equal to their respective frequencies in age-matched non-pregnant counterparts.
- Most commonly present btwn 20–45 years of age

Pathogenesis
- Thought to be a congenital lesion caused by disrupted vasculogenesis
- The abnormal vascular plexus progressively dilates over time, making it more prone to rupture.
- Once an AVM becomes symptomatic, its annual rate of rupture is 2–3%.

Clinical manifestations
- Intracerebral hemorrhage, 38–86% of pts
- Seizure, 4–46% of pts
- Focal neurologic deficit, 4–23% of pts
- Specific neurologic symptoms depend on the location of the AVM & the severity of bleed.

> Small AVM & hemorrhage may present w/ headache or new-onset seizure.

> Large hemorrhage may have potential for herniation & coma.

Effect of pregnancy on AVMs

- Risk of first hemorrhage during pregnancy same as non-gravid population

- Condition of pregnant pt following hemorrhage is worse: 57% stuporous or comatose

- Incidence of re-hemorrhage from AVM is higher in pregnant pts.
  > 25% of pregnant pts re-hemorrhage during pregnancy.
  > 3–6% of general population re-hemorrhage in year following first rupture.

- Overall maternal mortality rate: 28% vs. 10% in non-pregnant population

Effect of AVM on pregnancy & fetus

- Fetal mortality rate 14%

- Possible teratogenic & carcinogenic effects of radiation during diagnostic testing

- Possible teratogenic effects of drug therapy

STUDIES

History & physical

- These are typically young, previously healthy individuals.

- Neurologic
  > Obtain history of presentation, intervening therapy & complications.
  > Mental status exam
  > Examine for & document neurologic deficits.
  > Document if associated seizures & anticonvulsant therapy.

Imaging

- Do not avoid appropriate diagnostic testing because of perceived risk to fetus, as AVM hemorrhage can be life-threatening.

- CT scan
  > Usually initial diagnostic procedure of choice for pregnant pt
  > Appropriately shielded fetus, safe radiation exposure

- CT angiography
  > Ideal method to identify suspected vascular lesions
  > Avoids complications of invasive angiography
  > Contrast dye does not cross placenta, physiologically inert; considered safe for fetus.

➤ Contrast dye is a diuretic, so hydrate pt well.
➤ Shield fetus from radiation exposure.
■ Cerebral angiography
➤ Gold standard for diagnosis & defining anatomy of AVM for resection or endovascular treatment
➤ Shielded fetus, safe radiation exposure
➤ Contrast agents pose little risk for fetus.
➤ Hydrate well to prevent maternal & fetal dehydration; contrast dye is a diuretic.
■ MRI
➤ No long-term data on fetal outcome
➤ MRI generally avoided during 1st trimester
➤ MRI contrast agent, gadolinium, crosses the placenta.
➤ No reported adverse effects of fetal exposure to gadolinium
➤ Nevertheless, most advise against contrast use during pregnancy unless clinically necessary (not FDA approved for this use).

Other
■ Check plasma level of anticonvulsant.
■ Type & crossmatch blood if presenting for a neurosurgical procedure.

MANAGEMENT/INTERVENTIONS
■ Acute medical mgt of intracranial hemorrhage in pregnant pt w/ AVM: similar to non-pregnant pt
➤ Hemodynamic stabilization
➤ Strict control of seizures
➤ Prevention of complications
■ Neurosurgical mgt
➤ Benefit of surgical treatment during pregnancy is less clear.
➤ Surgery prevents re-hemorrhage yet has no proven benefit to maternal or fetal mortality rate.
➤ AVMs are complex, heterogeneous lesions w/ varying degrees of surgical risk.
• Decision to operate is individualized & based on neurosurgical considerations, such as:
• Emergency surgery to evacuate a hematoma that is causing neurologic compromise
• Elective resection during pregnancy in neurologically stable pt w/ easily accessible, low-risk lesion
• Delay resection of large, complex lesion that might require multiple modalities of treatment until the post-partum period.

- Alternate treatment modalities
  - Endovascular therapy & radiosurgery
  - Neither confers immediate protection against re-hemorrhage.
- Anticonvulsants are given to all pts as risk of seizure is high.
  - All are established teratogens, w/ greatest risk during 1st trimester.
  - Risk of maternal & fetal hypoxia & acidosis associated w/ seizure justifies their use in pt at risk for seizure.
  - Drug pharmacokinetics are altered during pregnancy, so check serum anticonvulsant levels.
  - Interfere w/ folic acid & vitamin K metabolism, so give supplementation.

Anesthesia

1) For the pt who is neurologically stable w/ either an unruptured or untreated AVM
- Mode of delivery: vaginal vs. cesarean section has little influence on outcome & remains controversial
- Many advocate regional anesthesia.
  - Prevents or attenuates increases in venous pressure associated w/ Valsalva maneuvers
  - Permits continuous neurologic monitoring
  - Anecdotal case reports suggest that it is "safe."
  - Administer local anesthetic solution slowly into the epidural space; rapid administration can produce an increase in ICP.
2) For the pt undergoing emergency craniotomy for evacuation of life-threatening intracerebral hematoma
- General anesthesia
- Pt is assumed to have markedly increased ICP.
- Major determinant of maternal outcome: time to evacuation of hematoma
- Rapid sequence induction
  - Pentothal or propofol, succinylcholine (unless pt has paresis > 48 hrs), narcotic or IV lidocaine to blunt BP response to intubation
  - Effects of succinylcholine on ICP are short-lived & attenuated w/ prior administration of pentothal (advantage of rapid onset outweighs its potential transient adverse effect on ICP).
- Hypotension &/or hypoxia will dramatically worsen neurologic injury; treat aggressively.
- Hyperventilation is indicated in life-threatening intracranial emergency; cease once hematoma is resected if brain is not swollen.

➤ Reliably reduces ICP
➤ Marked hyperventilation causes uteroplacental vasoconstriction, resulting in fetal hypoxia & acidosis.
➤ Thought that reduction in cardiac output caused by positive-pressure ventilation is likely the cause of decreased uterine blood flow & not alkalosis per se
➤ Used when there is evidence of increased ICP. Adverse effects on fetus minimized w/ normovolemia & low airway pressures.
■ Mannitol is indicated to treat life-threatening emergency.
➤ Potential to cause temporary fetal dehydration
➤ Fetal outcome data are limited.
➤ Anecdotal case reports suggest it is safe for these circumstances.
■ Choice of maintenance anesthetic agent should include need for rapid emergence.
■ Very large-bore IV access; these cases have the potential for large amount of blood loss, particularly if resection of the AVM is attempted
■ Have blood readily available for transfusion.
■ Arterial line as time permits
■ If a concurrent C-section is planned
➤ Life-saving craniotomy should be performed first.
➤ Follow same recommendations as above & be prepared to treat the mannitol-induced fetal dehydration & narcotic-induced respiratory depression
➤ Fetal monitoring as per OB recommendation
➤ If labor begins during craniotomy & delivery is imminent
  • Suspend intracranial procedure.
  • Delivery plan as per obstetrician
➤ Oxytocin
  • Effect in pts w/ intracranial vascular lesions is unclear; likely to cause cerebral vasoconstriction
  • Can cause maternal hypotension; vigilant attention to BP needed
  • Has been used clinically in these circumstances w/o adverse effect
➤ After delivery of the infant, anesthesia may be modified as required for the neurosurgical procedure.
3) For the pregnant pt undergoing craniotomy for non-emergent resection of AVM
■ General anesthesia
■ ICP is not elevated

- Direct arterial BP measurement w/ A-line
- Consider CVP.
- Controlled, "modified" rapid sequence induction
  - Cricoid pressure
  - Graded doses of pentothal or propofol
  - Titrated doses of narcotic to prevent hypertensive response to intubation
  - Rocuronium: monitor w/ TOF to ensure twitch suppression to prevent Valsalva response to intubation
- Potential for large blood loss
  - Gauge amount w/ neurosurgeon.
  - Large-bore IV access
  - Blood readily available for transfusion (if transfusion needed & pt is Rh negative, do not transfuse w/ Rh-positive blood)
- Brain "relaxation"
  - Lumbar CSF drainage recommended; usually provides sufficient relaxation & avoids use of mannitol or furosemide
  - Mannitol only if swelling or perfusion pressure breakthrough occurs
- Choice of maintenance anesthetic agent should include need for rapid emergence.
- Should perfusion pressure breakthrough occur:
  - Keep systolic blood pressure <100 mm Hg.
  - Labetalol, hydralazine & nitroprusside are safe by anecdotal report.
  - Give short-acting barbiturate to induce a barbiturate coma if brain swelling is severe.
- For pts on anticonvulsants
  - Shorter duration of neuromuscular blockade
  - Decreased sensitivity to narcotics
- If a concurrent C-section is planned
  - The C-section should precede the craniotomy.
  - Prevention of hypertension is less important in the neurologically stable pt w/ presumed normal ICP; consider using less or little narcotic for induction.
  - Oxytocin
    - Effect in pts w/ intracranial vascular lesions is unclear; likely to cause cerebral vasoconstriction.
    - Can cause maternal hypotension; vigilant attention to BP needed
    - Has been used clinically in these circumstances w/o adverse effect

➤ Check for uterine bleeding at regular intervals throughout the craniotomy.

CAVEATS & PEARLS
■ Anesthetic mgt is largely determined by the acuity of the neurologic disease process.
■ AVMs are complex, heterogeneous & potentially high-risk lesions & their mgt is individualized & largely determined by neurologic considerations.
■ Identify & inform the pt's neurosurgeon of your anesthetic plans. Determine most efficient means of emergency contact.
■ AVM resection has the potential to be associated w/ large blood loss, so plan appropriately.
■ Check serum anticonvulsant levels.

CHECKLIST
■ Prophylactic antibiotics before craniotomy
■ Sufficient IV access for resuscitation
■ Blood products available (if transfusion needed & pt is Rh negative, do not transfuse w/ Rh-positive blood)
■ Have equipment & medications available to treat seizure.

INTRAHEPATIC CHOLESTASIS OF PREGNANCY

LAWRENCE WEINSTEIN, MD
DOUG RAINES, MD

FUNDAMENTAL KNOWLEDGE
Intrahepatic cholestasis of pregnancy is a disorder of the 2nd & 3rd trimesters, characterized by pruritus & elevated serum bile acid concentrations.

Epidemiology & pathogenesis
■ Incidence 0.2–4%, w/ some geographic variability. For example, it is increased in Bolivia & among the Araucanos Indians in Chile.
■ The cause of intrahepatic cholestasis of pregnancy is not known, though likely a combination of genetic & hormonal factors is involved.
➤ Evidence for a genetic role come from cases of recurrent familial intrahepatic cholestasis of pregnancy. Heterozygous mutations in the MDR3 gene (which codes for a canalicular phospholipids translocator involved in biliary secretion of phospholipids) have

been found in a large family in which six women all had at least one episode of intrahepatic cholestasis of pregnancy.

➤ Estrogens cause cholestasis & likely play a role in intrahepatic cholestasis of pregnancy. Estrogen levels are at their peak during the 3rd trimester, the time at which intrahepatic cholestasis of pregnancy is most often seen. Intrahepatic cholestasis of pregnancy is also more common w/ twin pregnancies, characterized by higher levels of circulating estrogens.

➤ Progesterone administration may be a risk factor for intrahepatic cholestasis of pregnancy. Accumulation of progesterone metabolites can result in saturation of the hepatic transport systems used for those compounds' biliary excretion.

Clinical manifestations

■ Intrahepatic cholestasis of pregnancy is marked by pruritus. Itching is usually generalized but can predominate on the palms & soles, w/ worst symptoms at night.

■ Other symptoms, such as abdominal pain, encephalopathy & other hallmarks of liver failure, are uncommon & should prompt a workup for a different pathology.

■ Physical exam is unremarkable, though 10–20% of pts may develop jaundice, typically after the onset of pruritus.

➤ Jaundice w/o itching is rare in intrahepatic cholestasis of pregnancy; if itching is absent, evaluate for other causes of jaundice.

Diagnosis

■ Diagnosis is after 30 weeks gestation & based on pruritus & the presence of elevated serum bile acids &/or aminotransferases.

■ Rule out other hepatic/biliary pathology.

■ The presence of pruritus is essential, as it helps distinguish intrahepatic cholestasis of pregnancy from other conditions w/ elevated liver enzymes (eg, HELLP syndrome).

■ Ultrasound shows a LACK of biliary ductile dilation, as would be expected w/ an obstructive process.

Though not necessary for diagnosis, liver biopsy shows cholestasis without inflammation. Bile plugs in hepatocytes & canaliculi are prominent in zone 3, w/ portal tracts unaffected.

STUDIES

Lab data

■ Serum total bile acid concentrations are increased. This may be the only lab abnormality seen.

> Cholic acid increases more than chenodeoxycholic acid. This causes an increase in the cholic/chenodeoxycholic acid ratio when compared w/ pregnant women without intrahepatic cholestasis of pregnancy.

■ Other lab values consistent w/ cholestasis may be present.
> Alkaline phosphatase may increase up to 4–5× normal.
> Total & direct bilirubin concentrations may be high, though total bilirubin rarely exceeds 6 mg/dL in intrahepatic cholestasis of pregnancy.
> Significantly, gamma glutamyl transpeptidase (GGTP) levels are normal or only very slightly elevated.
> Serum aminotransferases can be elevated, w/ values of up to 1,000 U/L.
> PT is normal; an elevated value reflects a vitamin K deficiency secondary to cholestasis.

MANAGEMENT/INTERVENTIONS

■ Treatment is aimed at reducing symptoms & preventing maternal or fetal complications.
■ Ursodeoxycholic acid is a synthetic bile acid that increases bile flow & is used to relieve pruritus & improve liver biochemical tests in cholestatic liver diseases. It has been shown to improve symptoms & decrease serum bilirubin & AST levels without deleteriously affecting maternal or fetal outcomes.
■ Cholestyramine (8–16 g/day) decreases absorption of bile salts in the ileum. Doses should be started low & increased slowly. The effect on pruritus is limited, & it may cause steatorrhea & exacerbate vitamin K deficiency.
■ If cholestasis is severe, pts may have fat-soluble vitamin deficiency.
> If vitamin K deficiency is severe, PT may be elevated & can be an issue for peripartum hemorrhage.
> Vitamin K should be repleted prior to delivery if possible. If a parturient needs urgent delivery in the setting of an elevated PT, then FFP might become necessary to prevent excessive blood loss.

Maternal outcome

■ Maternal prognosis is good.
■ Pruritus disappears within a few days of delivery, & serum bile acid concentrations normalize.
■ Women generally have no lasting hepatic sequelae.
■ Increased risk for intrahepatic cholestasis of pregnancy in subsequent pregnancies (60–70%)

■ Rarely, oral contraceptive use by women w/ a history of intrahepatic cholestasis of pregnancy causes cholestasis & pruritus.

■ Delivery should occur by 38 weeks in most pts w/ intrahepatic cholestasis of pregnancy but should be considered at 36 weeks or even sooner if cholestasis is severe.

Fetal outcome

■ Significant risks for fetus
  ➤ Prematurity: incidence varies widely among studies (6–60%). Increased incidence may partially be due to the greater percentage of multiple pregnancies having intrahepatic cholestasis of pregnancy.
  ➤ Meconium-stained amniotic fluid
  ➤ Fetal demise: causes of fetal demise in intrahepatic cholestasis of pregnancy are unknown. It is rare before the 9th month & there is currently no good test to reliably predict risk of fetal demise.
  ➤ Best approach to avoiding infant morbidity & mortality is early delivery.
  ➤ Timing guided by maternal symptoms (pruritus) & gestational maturity

■ Anesthetic mgt for ICP, & indeed for all liver disease of pregnancy, should be guided by the symptoms & manifestations of the liver process. Various manifestations will have differing effects on physiology & choice of anesthetic technique for labor or delivery. Frequently, intrahepatic cholestasis of pregnancy results in minimal liver pathology that is of significance to the anesthesiologist.

■ For general discussion of regional & general anesthesia considerations, see the section on "*General Concepts.*"

CAVEATS/PEARLS

■ Intrahepatic cholestasis of pregnancy is a disorder of late pregnancy, characterized by pruritus & elevated serum bile acid concentrations.

■ Treatment is based on alleviating maternal symptoms & can involve ursodeoxycholic acid or cholestyramine.

■ Liver failure is not typical, though coagulopathy may be present due to vitamin K malabsorption.

■ Anesthetic mgt can usually proceed as usual for the parturient, though attention should be given to coagulation status prior to any regional techniques.

CHECKLIST
- Usual pre-anesthetic labs as dictated by clinical history
- Rule out clinical history of coagulopathy.

INTRAPARTUM ASSESSMENT

ANJALI KAIMAL, MD
LORI BERKOWITZ, MD

FUNDAMENTAL KNOWLEDGE
- Continuous fetal monitoring and intermittent auscultation are the methods for monitoring a fetus during labor.
- There is no difference in intrapartum fetal death rate, Apgar scores, rates of long-term neurologic impairment or cerebral palsy btwn the two methods.
- In one trial, continuous monitoring led to better prediction of fetal acidemia at birth.
- The disadvantage of continuous monitoring is that it leads to a higher rate of operative vaginal delivery & cesarean section without an improvement in neonatal outcome.
- Fetal heart rate (FHR) can be monitored using an external ultrasonographic monitor or by using an internal lead.
- The external monitor detects the frequency of heart valve movement; the heart rate is calculated by a computer that averages several consecutive beat-to-beat frequencies. There is more baseline variability inherent in this method as opposed to a fetal ECG detected by an internal electrode.
- The electrode is placed on the fetal scalp, w/ a second electrode on the mother's body to eliminate interference. The fetal heart rate is calculated based on R-R intervals, providing accurate measurement of beat-to-beat variability.

STUDIES

FHR Assessment
FHR assessment consists of identifying patterns indicative of fetal well-being & patterns that may be associated w/ adverse neonatal outcomes.
- Reassuring patterns:
  - Baseline FHR 120–160 bpm
  - Absence of fetal heart rate decelerations: Mild, transient episodes of hypoxia lead to bradycardia, either as variable or late

decelerations depending on the etiology (cord compression or fetoplacental insufficiency)

➤ Age-appropriate fetal heart accelerations: Advancing gestational age is associated w/ increased frequency & amplitude of FHR increases. Before 30 weeks' gestation, accelerations are typically 10 bpm for 10 seconds as opposed to 15 bpm for 15 seconds. Hypoxemia leads to a loss of the normal sympathetic response to movement & accelerations are absent.

➤ Normal FHR variability: FHR variability results from sympathetic & parasympathetic nervous system input. Parasympathetic influence increases w/ gestational age; therefore, the absence of variability is abnormal after 28 weeks.

■ Nonreassuring patterns:

➤ Late decelerations: In this case, the nadir of the deceleration occurs after the peak of the contraction. Late decelerations w/ absent variability are particularly concerning.

➤ Variable decelerations: Intermittent mild or moderate variable decelerations w/ a quick return to baseline likely result from cord compression & are not worrisome. In contrast, deep, repetitive, severe variables can be associated w/ a fall in pH.

➤ Absent variability: Loss of variability is thought to result from cerebral hypoxia & acidosis & signifies that the compensatory mechanisms to maintain adequate oxygenation to the brain have failed.

■ Distress patterns:

➤ Severe bradycardia: FHR <100 bpm for a prolonged time in the absence of drugs, heart block or hypothermia

➤ Tachycardia w/ diminished variability, esp. when associated w/ other nonreassuring patterns & in the absence of maternal fever

Fetal scalp stimulation

Absence of acidosis (pH > 7.20) is confirmed if an acceleration can be elicited by stimulating the fetal vertex w/ a finger or an Allis clamp during a vaginal exam.

Fetal scalp blood sampling

■ Fetal scalp blood sampling may provide useful information when a tracing is difficult to interpret, esp. when delivery is imminent.

■ The pH of scalp blood is the same as the pH of capillary blood, which is lower than the umbilical vein pH.

■ A sample is obtained by cleaning the scalp, making a small nick in the skin & using a capillary tube to obtain a sample.

Meconium-stained amniotic fluid

■ Meconium-stained amniotic fluid has been associated w/ nonreassuring fetal status, but it is also common in fetuses w/o compromise.

■ Meconium is first evident in the fetal intestine at 70–85 days' gestation. It is composed of water w/ primary bile acids.

■ Meconium is seldom passed before 34 weeks. As the fetus matures, the innervation of the bowel increases; some have suggested that the passage of meconium is a normal result of this maturation process.

■ Studies have also suggested that lower oxygen saturation is correlated w/ meconium passage, as well as variable decelerations. The pathophysiology of these connections is not well understood.

■ The incidence of meconium at delivery at term is 7–22%; it approaches 40% in post-term pregnancies.

■ The presence & consistency of meconium has not been correlated w/ fetal compromise.

■ The presence of meconium alone does not imply fetal distress unless it is correlated w/ other worrisome findings.

■ Meconium aspiration syndrome develops in 2–8% of infants delivered through amniotic-stained fluid. Effects can range from mild neonatal tachypnea to severe respiratory distress. The pathophysiology involves mechanical obstruction & chemical pneumonitis. Pulmonary vasculospasm can lead to pulmonary hypertension; respiratory distress may be worsened by inhibition of surfactant's surface tension-reducing properties by meconium.

■ In many cases, extracorporeal membrane oxygenation (ECMO) is required to maintain oxygenation & prevent barotrauma.

MANAGEMENT/INTERVENTIONS

See "*Non-reassuring Fetal Heart Rate Tracing*" chapter.

FHR Assessment

Abnormalities of the fetal heart tracing must be interpreted in light of the clinical scenario.

The incidence of abnormal or variant heart rate patterns is much higher than the incidence of severe acidosis, seizures or cerebral palsy.

■ Late decelerations must be repetitive to be considered ominous. Interventions to correct maternal hypovolemia or increase blood flow to the uterus such as fluid resuscitation, blood pressure support or correction of hyperstimulation may lead to resolution of late decelerations. The majority of term fetuses will tolerate 30 minutes of late decelerations w/o decompensation. The presence of late decelerations w/ absent variability suggests decompensation & necessitates immediate delivery.

■ Mild to moderate variable decelerations may be relieved by maternal position change. It is unlikely that the fetus will decompensate in the setting of mild to moderate decelerations; the danger is that the decelerations will become severe. Severe repetitive variables may be treated w/ amnioinfusion. If the severe variable decelerations persist, decompensation may occur after 30 minutes. In the presence of severe variables, the tracing must be monitored for the development of decreased beat-to-beat variability or late decelerations, indicating decompensation.

■ A bradycardia in the 100–110 range w/ good variability can be tolerated by the fetus for some time. The lower the bradycardia, the greater the likelihood of fetal compromise. A heart rate <60 is highly predictive of asphyxial compromise.

Fetal scalp stimulation
FHR acceleration in response to scalp stimulation is most useful in helping to rule out fetal acidemia. However, failure to elicit an acceleration should be interpreted w/ caution; continued monitoring is suggested, w/ operative delivery or fetal scalp blood sampling if the worrisome pattern persists.

Fetal scalp blood sampling
Pathologic acidemia is defined as <7.20. Values 7.20–7.25 are considered borderline & warrant resampling in 30 minutes. Values <7.20 are considered non-reassuring & expedient delivery is recommended.

Meconium-stained amniotic fluid
In cases of thick meconium, amnioinfusion has been proposed to decrease the incidence of meconium aspiration syndrome. While this was initially thought to be due to a dilutional effect, it may be that by reducing cord compression & deep variables, normal oxygenation is restored, decreasing in utero fetal gasping.

DeLee suctioning after the delivery of the head but before the delivery of the thorax has been shown to reduce the incidence & severity of meconium aspiration syndrome. However, this does not remove meconium aspirated in utero. Laryngoscopic visualization of the vocal cords w/ endotracheal suctioning if necessary is performed after delivery in neonates who are depressed or born through particulate meconium.

CAVEATS/PEARLS

- Continuous fetal monitoring & intermittent auscultation are the methods for monitoring a fetus during labor. There is no difference in intrapartum fetal death rate, Apgar scores, long-term neurologic impairment or cerebral palsy between the two methods.
- FHR assessment consists of identifying patterns of fetal well-being & patterns that may be associated w/ adverse neonatal outcomes.
- A baseline of 120–160, the absence of decelerations, the presence of accelerations & normal heart rate variability are reassuring.
- Late decelerations, variable decelerations & absent variability are nonreassuring patterns.
- Severe bradycardia and tachycardia w/ absent variability are distress patterns.
- The presence of accelerations in response to scalp stimulation indicates a non-acidotic fetus.
- A fetal scalp pH of <7.20 indicates pathologic acidemia & warrants expedient delivery. A pH of >7.25 is reassuring.
- The presence of meconium alone does not indicate fetal distress unless it is correlated w/ other worrisome findings.
- Amnioinfusion decreases the incidence of meconium aspiration syndrome.
- DeLee suctioning after delivery of the head & before the delivery of the thorax reduces the incidence & severity of meconium aspiration.

CHECKLIST

- Assess the fetal heart tracing for reassuring & nonreassuring patterns.
- Obtain additional information by performing scalp stimulation or getting a fetal scalp pH.
- Repeat testing or proceed w/ delivery based on results.
- Consider amnioinfusion for thick meconium, esp. in the setting of deep variable decelerations.

Plan for DeLee suction on the perineum if meconium is present. Be prepared to intubate if the baby is depressed at birth.

ISCHEMIA & MI IN PREGNANCY

JASMIN FIELD, MD
DWIGHT GEHA, MD

FUNDAMENTAL KNOWLEDGE

As many Western cultures continue to gravitate toward childbearing later in life & technologies supporting this trend improve, we will likely see an increasing incidence of comorbidities in parturients, for whom significant cardiovascular disease may be unmasked by the demands of pregnancy.

- Overall incidence of MI during pregnancy in the U.S. is estimated at 1 in 10,000–30,000 deliveries.
  - Most often in first or second pregnancies
  - Most often in third trimester or puerperium
  - Most often in left anterior descending artery distribution w/ injury to anterior wall
  - Average age of parturient 32 years
  - >50% of pts w/ MI have no coronary artery disease on cardiac catheterization.
- Risk factors for coronary artery disease & MI
  - Cigarette smoking
  - Diabetes
  - Hypertension
  - High cholesterol
  - Obesity
  - Family history of premature CV disease
  - Toxemia of pregnancy
  - Use of oral contraceptives
  - Use of cocaine
- Maternal mortality from MI estimated at 20–30%
  - Data on outcome for survivors not readily available in the literature
  - Many cases of ischemia during pregnancy w/ transient EKG changes & SMALL troponin I leaks report no sequelae at 6 weeks follow-up & beyond.
  - Some sources have suggested mortality for MI within 2 weeks of labor is as high as 45%.
- Though ischemic heart disease is very rare in women of childbearing age, pregnancy raises the relative risk.

➤ Incidence of MI in the U.S. not associated w/ pregnancy is exceedingly rare in women <35 years of age & extremely rare <45 years.

➤ According to Ros et al, in a population-based Swedish cohort of >1 million births from 1987 to 1995, the relative risk of peripartum MI essentially doubled in the third trimester & then increased *exponentially* in the 1–2 days before & after delivery.

■ Several small studies have shown that 25–81% of women experience some kind of EKG changes suggestive of ischemia during uncomplicated C-section.

➤ EKG changes generally thought to be artifactual or normal variants associated w/ the changes of pregnancy, labor & delivery

➤ Difficult to determine clinical significance prior to use of troponin I as marker of cell injury (CK & CKMB levels are abnormal during pregnancy), so data are quite limited.

➤ Moran et al reported that in 26 pts undergoing elective C-section (using IV bolus of oxytocin 10 IU immediately after delivery):

• 42% of pts had perioperative chest pain requiring opioid analgesia.

• 82% of pts w/ chest pain had ST segment changes.

• 8% (n = 2) of pts w/ ST changes & chest pain had mildly positive levels of troponin I.

• Study results have been criticized in light of potentially confounding factors of relatively large IV bolus of oxytocin.

Antepartum ischemia

■ Increased myocardial oxygen demand

➤ Increased intravascular volume & heart rate

➤ Anemia of pregnancy, etc.

■ Atherosclerotic disease most commonly found in parturients w/ antepartum MI (58%).

➤ Stresses may make atherosclerotic plaques more likely to rupture.

➤ More common in pts w/ risk factors such as advanced age, smoking, family history of premature CV disease, hypercoagulable disorders, diabetes, familial hypercholesterolemia, substance abuse.

■ Thromboembolism

■ Malignant arrhythmias

➤ Hormonal changes contribute.

➤ Electrolytes can be disturbed by long labor, eclampsia/pre-eclampsia & its treatment.
■ Substance abuse
  ➤ Cocaine causes:
    • Premature atherosclerosis
    • Coronary artery vasospasm
    • EKG changes in intervals & voltage
    • Severe hypertension w/ general anesthesia
    • Severe hypotension w/ neuraxial blockade
    • Systolic dysfunction from myocardial ischemia
    • Diastolic dysfunction from chronically increased sympathetic tone
  ➤ Pregnant women are more sensitive to toxic effects of cocaine.

Peripartum ischemia
■ Normal coronary arteries were found in 75% of pts w/ acute peripartum MI.
■ Vasospasm is frequently considered to be contributory.
  ➤ Hypothesized risk factors for severe coronary vasospasm in parturients:
    • Age >30
    • Smoking
    • Alcohol abuse
    • History of migraines
    • Asian population has higher incidence than Caucasian.
  ➤ Transient spasm leads to clot or plaque rupture more easily in hypercoagulable state.
  ➤ Can be caused by meds or stress & usually resolves spontaneously
  ➤ Responds to intracoronary artery injection of nitroglycerin
■ Increased myocardial oxygen demand coupled w/ decreased supply also potentially contributes to peripartum MI.
  ➤ Each uterine contraction adds 300–500 cc of uterine blood back into maternal circulation.
  ➤ Heart rate, BP & cardiac output increase.
  ➤ Pain causes release of catecholamines & other hormones.
  ➤ Anemia of pregnancy, etc.
■ Emboli
  ➤ Thromboemboli due to hypercoagulability
  ➤ Amniotic fluid emboli
  ➤ Venous air emboli can occur during externalization of uterus in C-section deliveries

Meds commonly given peripartum that may contribute to peripartum ischemia

- Oxytocin
  - ➤ Rapid IV bolus of doses as small as 5 IU synthetic oxytocin during uncomplicated, elective C-section have been reported to cause chest pain, nausea/vomiting & shortness of breath associated w/ significant EKG changes & elevated levels of troponin.
  - ➤ Most pts w/ cardiac injury from Pitocin are found to have normal coronaries on cardiac catheterization.
  - ➤ Proposed mechanisms include coronary arterial spasm & vasodilatation of vascular smooth muscle causing diastolic hypotension & decreased coronary perfusion in the face of increased demand & anemia of pregnancy.
- Ergometrine or methylergonovine
  - ➤ Potent vasoconstrictor used in promoting coronary vasospasm for diagnostic purposes
    - Decreases luminal diameter by 20%
    - Vasospasm may last for hours.
    - With IV injection, onset of spasm is rapid, but can be delayed approximately 20 minutes w/ IM injection.
  - ➤ Used for constriction of uterine musculature & vessels after delivery of placenta
    - After second dose of Pitocin inadequately controls hemorrhage/improves uterine tone, IM 0.2 mg is standard dose.
    - Most often given by anesthesiologist at surgeon's request
    - Sutaria et al reported acute MI after 0.5 mg IM methylergonovine for vaginal delivery in pt w/ previously asymptomatic & undiagnosed three-vessel coronary artery atherosclerosis (found on subsequent cardiac catheterization).
    - There are multiple reports of normal coronaries & presumed vasospasm causing MI in the parturient.
  - ➤ Coronary vasospasm can be treated w/ intra-coronary nitroglycerin & supportive care
- Calcium channel blockers
  - ➤ Used for tocolysis & hypertension
  - ➤ Hypotension & reflex tachycardia associated w/ recommended doses of ritodrine & nifedipine for tocolysis of preterm labor have caused non-Q wave MI w/ chest pain, EKG changes & positive enzymes in otherwise healthy young women.
  - ➤ Long-term sequelae were not documented.

➤ Proposed mechanisms include physiologic changes of pregnancy causing stronger reactions to meds well tolerated by the non-pregnant pt.

■ Spinal anesthesia
➤ Several papers report cardiac arrest after spinal anesthesia (for elective C-section) in association w/ hypovolemia & hypotension.
➤ Preload or "co-load" of volume around the time of intrathecal injection is recommended.
➤ Appropriate peripartum use of ephedrine & phenylephrine has not been shown to contribute to ischemia via vasoconstriction & should be used liberally to maintain normal BP.

■ Epidural anesthesia
➤ Associated vasodilation & hypotension disturb balance of oxygen supply & demand, though symptoms are generally less severe & abrupt than w/ spinal anesthesia.
➤ Vasovagal episodes during difficult epidural placements are not uncommon.
  • Staying in the upright seated position for epidural placement during true vasovagal episodes w/ associated bradycardia & hypotension can result in asystolic arrest.
  • Pt should be immediately placed in left uterine displacement position w/ elevation of lower extremities & oxygen via face mask, fluid bolus & treatment w/ ephedrine as indicated.

Postpartum ischemia
■ Approx. 100 cases of postpartum MI are reported in medical literature.
■ The most commonly reported cause of postpartum MI is spontaneous coronary artery dissection (33%).
➤ Hormonal effects on connective tissue make dissection much more common than in non-pregnant pts.
➤ Urgent/emergent cardiac angiography, catheterization & CABG w/ cardiopulmonary bypass are often necessary for repair.

■ Hemorrhage w/ both vaginal & cesarean delivery may contribute to increased myocardial demand & has been associated w/ postpartum MI.
➤ See "*Postpartum Hemorrhage.*"
➤ Severe postpartum hemorrhage is one of the leading causes of obstetrically related maternal morbidity & mortality in the U.S. & throughout much of the world.

- Occurs in 2–3% of all deliveries
- Accounts for >100,000 obstetric deaths (25% of total) annually in the world
- A leading cause of maternal death despite ICU care
➤ In a Jan. 2004 study in *Anesthesiology*, Karpati et al. looked at 55 pts w/ severe postpartum hemorrhagic shock receiving intensive care:
  - 28 pts (51%) had EKG changes suggesting ischemia, elevated levels of troponin I & decreased myocardial contractility.
  - Severity of symptoms & presence of enzyme leak correlated w/ severity of hemorrhage, low hemoglobin counts & use of inotropic support.
  - Independent risk factors for myocardial ischemia included low blood pressure, increased heart rate & exogenous catecholamines.
  - Uterotonic agents (oxytocin, sulprostone & ergometrine given specifically by slow IV infusion w/o rapid IV bolus) hypothesized to contribute to coronary vasoconstriction & potential cardiac arrest or ischemia did not correlate significantly w/ myocardial damage in these pts.

Heart failure
- ▪ In the parturient, heart failure is usually caused by valvular disease or cardiomyopathy but can be due to decompensation of significant acute coronary syndromes.
- ▪ Treatment goals include:
  ➤ Optimization of hemodynamics
  ➤ Afterload reduction & control of hypertension
  ➤ Aggressive correction of pulmonary congestion
  ➤ Rx: digoxin, diuretics, vasodilators, sodium restriction

STUDIES
- ▪ History & physical exam
  ➤ Identify risk factors & family history.
  ➤ Evidence of hemodynamic compromise?
  ➤ Activity level, exercise tolerance
  ➤ Frequency, duration, severity, associated events
  ➤ Previous medical evaluation/treatment
- ▪ Family history
  ➤ Syncope
  ➤ Sudden cardiac death

- ➤ Premature cardiac disease
- ➤ Familial hypercholesterolemia
- ■ EKG
  - ➤ Suggestive of ischemia
  - ➤ Arrhythmia perhaps contributing to ischemia
- ■ Lab values
  - ➤ Chemistry, CBC, electrolytes, cholesterol panel, endocrine panel, pre-eclampsia labs
  - ➤ Cardiac enzymes
    - • Troponin I is the only myocardial marker that is reliably negative during pregnancy w/o cardiac injury.
    - • CK & CKMB fractions are abnormal at some point in all pregnancies, independent of myocardial cell death.
    - • Check troponin w/ onset of symptoms & follow for peak & resolution.
- ■ Chest x-ray
  - ➤ Heart size
  - ➤ Pulmonary edema, pleural effusion, etc.
- ■ Echo
  - ➤ Uses deflections of ultrasound waves to give a 2-dimensional picture of the heart. Provides information on:
    - • Valvular disease
    - • Chamber size, wall motion abnormalities, wall thickness
    - • Systolic, diastolic function & estimated ejection fraction
    - • Pericardium & great vessels
  - ➤ Doppler uses ultrasound deflected off RBCs to gather information about volume & flow.
- ■ Exercise tolerance test/stress echo
  - ➤ EKG & echo performed during exercise or pharmacologically induced cardiac stress
    - • Provides information on flow through coronary arteries & valves & on how the heart responds to potential ischemia
    - • Many pregnant women are not capable of nor encouraged to perform strenuous exercise, so pharmacologic induction is preferred.
    - • Dobutamine 5–10 mcg/kg/min given to increase systolic myocardial contraction
- ■ Nuclear scans
  - ➤ Radioactive isotopes that emit gamma rays during decay are injected into the bloodstream. Special cameras can then

image myocardium & vessels & size, function & perfusion of the heart.

- Commonly used isotopes: technetium 99m (or ^{99m}Tc sestamibi) & thallium 201
- Multiple images are collected, under resting & stressed conditions, often over a 2-day protocol, allowing areas at risk for ischemia to be identified; demonstrates reversible ischemia.
- Sestamibi 99m scans tend to give better images but are more expensive.
- Fetal radiation exposure is <0.01 Gy.

■ Cardiac catheterization & CTA of coronary vessels
➤ Indicated for pregnant pts w/ signs & symptoms suggestive of unstable or progressive ischemia, usually in addition to potential risk factors such as advanced age, family history, smoking, obesity, diabetes, etc.
➤ Risks of clinical picture must outweigh risk of an invasive procedure w/ potential for serious complications & known radiation exposure.
- Fetal radiation exposure usually <0.01 Gy.
- Difficult or prolonged procedures can deliver 0.05–0.10 Gy.
- Considering termination of pregnancy is recommended at doses >0.05 Gy.
➤ Other risks include maternal bleeding, infection & arrhythmia.

MANAGEMENT/INTERVENTIONS
Pharmacologic management of ischemic disease in pregnancy Most drugs are FDA pregnancy risk category C, but medications most commonly used for listed indications w/ demonstrated safety & lack of adverse outcomes are listed in bold.

■ Beta blockers: rate control, anti-hypertensive
➤ **Propranolol**
➤ **Metoprolol**
➤ Atenolol
➤ Bisoprolol
➤ Bucindolol
➤ Labetalol
➤ Nadolol
■ Low-dose aspirin
■ Calcium channel blockers
➤ Verapamil

- **Lidocaine** (see "*Arrhythmias*")
- Inotropy
  - **Norepinephrine** & epinephrine are used for critical pts as indicated.
  - Dopamine & dobutamine have limited utility during pregnancy.
  - **Digoxin**
    - Can improve ventricular contractility & rate control
    - Can be used in pregnancy, class C
    - Does cross placenta, is secreted in breast milk
- Diuretics
  - Decrease edema, paroxysmal nocturnal dyspnea, dyspnea on exertion
  - Use only if sodium restriction has failed
  - Class C
- Vasodilators can reduce afterload & improve cardiac output.
  - Hydralazine
  - IV nitroglycerin
  - IV nitroprusside
    - Last-resort medication for cardiogenic shock that does not respond to inotropic treatment
    - Can cause toxicity to fetus; thus, dose & duration of therapy should be minimized
- Anticoagulation for chronic atrial fib
- Cardiovascular meds to **avoid** in pregnancy
  - ACE inhibitors & ARB
    - Contraindicated due to fetal effects
  - Amiodarone
    - Evidence of fetal malformations

Interventions for ischemic disease in pregnancy
- Thrombolysis
  - Options include tissue plasminogen activator (tPA) & streptokinase.
  - Several case studies suggest satisfactory perinatal outcome in thrombolytic therapy for acute MI in the second & third trimesters.
  - Third-trimester administration of thrombolytics should be accompanied by continuous fetal monitoring & is controversial because:
    - No operative procedure may be done for 10 days after tPA; thus, women close to term may not be candidates for urgent/

emergent C-section after tPA & would be strongly discouraged from this treatment.
  - Thrombolytics cannot be used for MI intrapartum or immediately postpartum.
- ➤ Benefits of tPA
  - May work more rapidly than cardiac cath can be completed
  - No radiation exposure to fetus
  - Short half-life
  - Large molecular weight (unlikely to cross placenta)
- ➤ Complications
  - Maternal hemorrhage
  - Abruption
  - Preterm labor
  - Fetal loss
- ■ Cardiac catheterization
  - ➤ Diagnostic & potentially therapeutic
  - ➤ Reperfusion strategies
    - Percutaneous transluminal coronary angioplasty (PTCA)
    - Stenting
    - Intra-coronary nitroglycerin for vasospasm
  - ➤ Has been used for intrapartum & immediately postpartum MI w/o reported complication to mother or fetus
  - ➤ Fetal shielding during fluoroscopy reduces risks associated w/ radiation exposure.
- ■ Intra-aortic balloon pump
  - ➤ Increases coronary perfusion
  - ➤ Temporary intervention prior to permanent intervention (cath vs. surgery)
  - ➤ Complications
    - Infection
    - Injury to vessels causing ischemia to the leg in as many as 20% of pts w/ intra-aortic balloon pump
    - Hemorrhage
    - Arrhythmia
    - Hypotension
    - Nerve injury
- ■ Surgical revascularization via coronary artery bypass grafting (CABG)
  - ➤ Cardiopulmonary bypass machine requires large doses of heparin; thus, a minimum 12-hour interval is recommended after emergent cesarean for ongoing maternal ischemia prior to CABG w/ CPB to reduce the risk of bleeding.

➤ CPB during gestation
  • Not generally associated w/ increased maternal risk
  • Risk of fetal loss reported 17–33%
➤ Off-pump CABG allows for much smaller doses of heparin & lowers potential risks associated w/ CPB.

Anesthetic management of parturient w/ known ischemic cardiovascular disease

■ For all scenarios, minimizing imbalance between myocardial oxygen supply & demand is key.
  ➤ Avoid derangements in BP, heart rate, oxygenation.
    • In a recent randomized, double-blinded, controlled trial, Warwick et al. reported that phenylephrine infusion at 100 mcg/min for 3 min immediately after spinal anesthesia for C-section significantly decreased frequency, magnitude & incidence of hypotension over treating SAP <80% of baseline (checked every minute) w/ a 100-mcg bolus (P < 0.0001).
  ➤ Left uterine displacement to avoid aortocaval compression in supine position after 24 weeks' gestation
  ➤ Minimize pain & anxiety.
  ➤ Minimize exertion & Valsalva, work of contractions & the reflex urge to bear down w/ contractions.
■ Plan invasive, continuous hemodynamic monitoring, esp. for the pt w/ high likelihood of ongoing ischemia or unstable angina.
■ Avoid oxytocin for labor induction/augmentation.
■ Avoid methylergonovine in the postpartum period.
■ Determine vaginal vs. C-section for delivery on an individual basis.
  ➤ Selection must optimize health of the mother, then baby.
  ➤ There is a tendency toward vaginally assisted births.
  ➤ Assisted vaginal deliveries eliminate risks of surgery & surgical anesthesia.
    • Epidural anesthetic derangements in hemodynamics tend to be more subtle than w/ spinal anesthesia.
    • Supplemental oxygen required
    • Left lateral position for vaginal delivery
    • Pain, anxiety & hemodynamic changes must be minimized.
  ➤ Most pts w/ CAD can tolerate assisted vaginal deliveries.
■ Elective C-section reduces the stress of prolonged labor & allows controlled timing of delivery w/o medication or intervention for induction of labor.

➤ If possible, surgical procedures should be avoided for 2–3 weeks post-MI to allow for healing of myocardial injury.

➤ C-section is indicated in pts w/ ongoing unstable ischemia or hemodynamic compromise.

■ Plan for postop ICU care & for the possibility of postop intubation.

CAVEATS & PEARLS

■ Common to many reported cases of ischemia, MI & arrest in the parturient are multifactorial issues/dynamics related to the normal physiologic cardiovascular changes of pregnancy plus the additional imbalance of myocardial oxygen supply & demand.

➤ Hypotension from meds or hemorrhage

➤ Anemia

➤ Coronary artery disease or spasm

➤ Thromboembolism, etc.

■ Many complications may be easily preventable w/ a high index of suspicion & low threshold for monitoring, diagnostics & intervention.

■ Good outcomes are facilitated by early identification of significant cardiovascular events, risk factors for cardiovascular compromise & a multidisciplinary approach to care.

➤ Both cardiac & obstetric surgical teams should be available in the OR for any obstetric or cardiac surgical procedures on a mother w/ a viable fetus.

➤ Consult cardiology early!

■ Chest pain, nausea/vomiting, anxiety & shortness of breath are common during uncomplicated C-sections & are predominantly thought to be benign. Though the majority of symptoms have been proven clinically insignificant & not associated w/ myocardial injury, recent studies have documented true myocardial damage in as many as half of the parturients w/ chest pain associated w/ EKG changes during C-section.

➤ Young age, lack of comorbidities & lack of known coronary artery disease were **not** cardioprotective factors in the face of severe hemorrhage, coronary vasospasm & coronary dissection

➤ Recommendations for myocardial protection include early & aggressive use of uterotonics via slow IV infusion for control of hemorrhage.

■ Any imbalance in myocardial oxygen supply & demand can cause myocardial ischemia during pregnancy, even in pts w/ normal coronaries & normal coagulation status when not pregnant.

CHECKLIST

- Uterotonic agents should be given by slow IV infusion as opposed to rapid IV bolus, but should be given early.
- Aggressive, early volume resuscitation is crucial in severe hemorrhage, w/ specific attention to:
  - ➤ Restoration of hemoglobin levels
  - ➤ Restoration of normal BP
  - ➤ Minimizing tachycardia
  - ➤ Restoring imbalance in myocardial oxygen supply & demand
- Be aware of cardiovascular disease risk factors that may contribute to potential for myocardial ischemia in an otherwise young, healthy parturient.
- Recognize potential for unmasking of unknown disease via normal physiologic changes of pregnancy in previously healthy pts.
- Take chest pain & EKG changes suggestive of ischemia seriously, even in the healthy parturient, while recognizing that more than half of symptoms will not be associated w/ myocardial injury.
- In pregnant pts, troponin I must be used exclusively as the marker for myocardial injury; do not use CK or CKMB. Follow levels for 24–48 hours to watch peak & duration of elevation.
- Immediate interventions for parturients w/ acute MI potentially include medical mgt, thrombolysis, cardiac catheterization & surgical correction of lesions.
- In pts w/ unstable angina and/or acute MI w/ significant coronary artery disease & ongoing injury or hemodynamic compromise, consider therapeutic abortion or immediate early delivery of the fetus >24 weeks' gestational age.
  - ➤ Therapeutic abortion & C-section must be performed w/ cardioprotective anesthesia relevant to pt's clinical status.
    - Minimize hemodynamic derangements.
    - Appropriate resuscitation/volume replacement
    - Invasive/continuous monitoring as indicated
    - Vasopressors as indicated
    - Have pacing & defibrillating capabilities easily accessible.
- While many reports suggest that most parturients w/ cardiac events do well long term, w/ recovery of functional status, data are lacking on outcomes in pts w/ MI or cardiac arrest during pregnancy.

Subsequent pregnancies will produce similar or progressive symptoms w/o specific intervention & active mgt of cardiac disease.

LANDRY-GUILLAIN-BARRÉ SYNDROME (GB) OR ACUTE INFAMMATORY DEMYELINATING POLYRADICULOPATHY

MEREDITH ALBRECHT, MD; LISA LEFFERT, MD; AND MICHELE SZABO, MD

FUNDAMENTAL KNOWLEDGE

Definition
- Inflammatory demyelinating illness

Epidemiology
- 2.3/100,000 women; 1.2/100,000 males
- Increased incidence in older (>60) versus younger (<18)
- Incidence in pregnant females- similar to general population

Pathophysiology
- Etiology unknown
- Preceded by a viral infection or vaccination (generally antirabies & influenza) in 2/3 of pts
- Acute inflammatory polyradiculoneuropathy affecting peripheral nerves & roots w/ patchy demyelination

Clinical manifestations
- Presents w/ weakness first of the limbs, then the trunk, neck & facial muscles
- Loss of reflexes, motor paralysis & respiratory failure can occur.
- Symptoms peak at 2 to 3 weeks.
- Majority of pts recover completely by 6 months.
- 10% residual disability
- 3% mortality due to increased risk of aspiration pneumonitis & respiratory failure, autonomic involvement w/ cardiac arrhythmia

Effect of pregnancy on GB
- GB not exacerbated during pregnancy
- Increased incidence of respiratory complications most likely due to the gravid uterus
- Mechanical ventilation due to GB: 33% in pregnant vs. 16% of non-pregnant pts
- Mortality due to GB doubled if GB contracted during 3rd trimester
- Remote history of GB can be associated w/ a 5% risk of relapse.

Effect of GB on pregnancy & the fetus
- Pregnancy & delivery unaffected by GB
- No increase in spontaneous abortion

- In severe cases during the 3rd trimester there is an increased incidence of premature births.
- Uterine contractions are unaffected, but assisted delivery is frequently needed due to skeletal muscle weakness.

STUDIES

History & physical
- Flaccid ascending quadriparesis
- Sensory symptoms of pain, numbness & paresthesia
- Areflexia

Laboratory
- CSF protein concentration increased
- Cell count normal or mildly elevated

Other
- Abnormal nerve conduction studies showing slowing
- Respiratory status assessed by pulmonary function tests, specifically forced vital capacity & forced expiratory volume

MANAGEMENT/INTERVENTIONS

Medical treatment
- Treatment is supportive, maintaining respiratory & nutritional status.
- If respiratory compromise, then mechanical ventilation may be necessary:
  - ➤ Use left uterine displacement to limit aortocaval compression.
  - ➤ Avoid hyperventilation.
- Plasmapheresis early in the course of GB (1st week) can decrease severity & length of the illness & is safe in pregnancy.
- IV gamma globulin can be useful.
- Steroids have not been proven useful.
- Improvement can be seen in 3 to 4 weeks but complete recovery may take months.
- DVT prophylaxis

Anesthesia
- Initial assessment
  - ➤ Differentiate severe from mild GB.
  - ➤ Assess pt's degree of respiratory compromise.
  - ➤ Remote history of GB can be associated w/ persistent diminished respiratory status & 5% risk of relapse.

- Regional anesthesia
  - ➤ Well tolerated in cases of mild GB
- General anesthesia
  - ➤ Necessary for ventilatory support in cases of severe GB
  - ➤ Autonomic dysfunction present in cases of severe GB, resulting in vascular instability & arrhythmias during induction & intubation
  - ➤ Pts sensitive to neuromuscular blocking agents & neuromuscular function should be monitored.
  - ➤ Avoid succinylcholine due to the increased risk of hyperkalemia.

CAVEATS & PEARLS

- GB is not exacerbated by pregnancy.
- Fetus is unaffected by GB.
- Increased risk of mortality of GB during pregnancy is due to respiratory compromise.
- Remote history of GB is associated w/ a 5% risk of relapse during pregnancy.
- Increased incidence of instrument-assisted delivery
- Epidural acceptable in cases of mild GB
- General anesthesia necessary in cases of severe GB w/ respiratory compromise
- Vascular instability & arrhythmias may be present in severe cases of GB w/ induction & intubation.

CHECKLIST

- Conduct a thorough neurologic exam & document current deficits.
- Assess respiratory status.
- Epidural anesthesia acceptable for mild cases of GB
- Severe cases of GB w/ respiratory compromise require general anesthesia.
- GB pts sensitive to neuromuscular blockers
- Avoid succinylcholine.
- DVT prophylaxis

LOCAL ANESTHETIC PHARMACOLOGY

ADRIAN HAMBURGER, MD; LISA LEFFERT, MD; AND WEI CHAO, MD

FUNDAMENTAL KNOWLEDGE

Mechanism of action

Local anesthetics are compounds that reversibly prevent the conduction of action potentials along nerves, primarily by directly inhibiting voltage-gated sodium channels. Some local anesthetics also inhibit potassium channels, but at high concentrations. Inhibition of resting potassium current may enhance nerve impulse-blocking activity of local anesthetic & increase its potency.

■ Structure/properties: Local anesthetics structurally have a hydrophobic group (typically a benzene ring) attached to a hydrophilic group (typically a tertiary amine) via either an ester $(-O-C=O)$ or an amide $(-NH-C=O)$ bond (mnemonic: amides contain two "i"s, esters contain only one "i").

1. Esters: tetracaine, procaine, chloroprocaine, cocaine, benzocaine

2. Amides: lidocaine, mepivacaine, prilocaine, bupivacaine, etidocaine, dibucaine

3. Storage properties: Local anesthetics are mostly weak bases & tend to be only weakly soluble. To provide an adequate storage & delivery medium they are combined w/ hydrochloric acid to form water-soluble salts (acidic solutions w/ pH 4.5–5.5, depending on the manufacturer). This acidic environment promotes prolonged stability of both the local anesthetic & any accompanying vasoconstrictor such as epinephrine.

4. Racemic vs. pure: Mepivacaine, bupivacaine & ropivacaine have levo-isomers & dextro-isomers. Typically these are available as racemic mixtures, except for ropivacaine, which is marketed only as a levo-isomer. Bupivacaine can also be obtained as a pure levo-isomer. The difference is clinically significant. For example, the levo-isomer of bupivacaine has a lethal dose far higher than its dextro-isomer & hence is less cardiotoxic.

5. Protein-binding changes during pregnancy: During pregnancy there is a decrease in serum protein concentration, especially albumin due to dilution and/or consumption. The decrease in serum protein results in a higher free fraction of the drug.

6. Potency: Potency is determined by lipid solubility of the compound. The more lipophilic molecules are more concentrated in the bilayer of the nerve membrane & have easier access to the sodium channel receptor

7. pKa/pH/speed of onset: The pKa of a local anesthetic is the pH at which half of the drug is present in its ionized form & the other half in its non-ionized form. Local anesthetics w/ a pKa closer to physiologic pH have a higher concentration of non-ionized molecules, can permeate the cell membrane more readily, and thus have faster onset. Since most local anesthetics have

a pKa > 7.0[TU1], the onset of action is slower in an acidic environment (due to the acidic storage medium or the acidic tissues in the setting of infection) wherein a larger amount of the compound is ionized. Alkalinizing the solution of local anesthetic by adding sodium bicarbonate (maintaining a 1:20 to 1:10 ratio) increases the speed of onset by increasing the amount of non-ionized molecule. In a study of brachial plexus blocks, alkalinization was shown to prolong the block as well. Adding sodium bicarbonate to the lidocaine solution used for local skin infiltration can decrease the pain of the injection. Adding sodium bicarbonate to bupivacaine can cause the solution to precipitate.

■ Response of different nerve fibers: Smaller, unmyelinated nerve (sympathetic & dorsal root C fibers, A-delta fibers, preganglionic sympathetic B fibers) fibers are more easily penetrated by local anesthetics than are larger, myelinated nerves (A-alpha, A-beta, A-gamma motor fibers). This partially explains the loss of pain & temperature response before the loss of pressure, motor & proprioception sensation in the anesthetized nerve.

Kinetics
■ Absorption
1. Systemic: Systemic absorption is dependent on blood flow to the site of injection: areas w/ high perfusion will have a higher uptake of the local anesthetic. Intravenous > tracheal > intercostals > caudal > paracervical > epidural > brachial plexus > sciatic & femoral > subcutaneous
2. Placental transfer: Non-ionized local anesthetics cross the placenta & enter the fetal circulation. Chloroprocaine is the exception due to the rapidity of maternal metabolism by plasma cholinesterases. Several factors increase the transfer of local anesthetic to the fetus:
   • Large dose
   • Low maternal protein levels (as local anesthetics, especially amides, are highly protein bound)
   • High lipid solubility
   • Acidemia in the fetus (as may occur in the setting of compromised uteroplacental blood flow)
3. Vasoconstriction: The addition of a vasoconstrictor allows a local anesthetic to remain in contact w/ the nerve for a longer time. The constriction of surrounding blood vessels slows systemic

absorption of local anesthetic. The most common additive is epinephrine at a concentration between 1:200,000 & 1:100,000 or 5–10 mcg/mL. Epinephrine can have a dual action on blood vessels: whereas skin & cutaneous vessels become constricted, muscle vessels may become constricted or dilated.

4. Onset of action: Onset of local anesthesia is affected by the pKa of drugs (drugs with lower pKa values have a shorter onset time for block), the proximity of the injectate to the target nerve & the concentration, volume & degree of ionization of the local anesthetic.
   - Rapid onset: lidocaine, mepivacaine, chloroprocaine, etidocaine
   - Medium onset: prilocaine
   - Slow onset: bupivacaine, procaine, tetracaine

5. Baricity: The baricity determines direction of migration of the local anesthetic within the intrathecal space. The clinical effect of baricity is affected by the pt's position. Hyperbaric local anesthetic solutions tend to follow gravity; hypobaric local anesthetics tend to go in the opposite direction.

■ Dosage: Excessive risk of systemic toxicity occurs at the following doses (in parentheses indicates w/ epinephrine):
   ➤ Lidocaine: 4 mg/kg (7 mg/kg)*
   ➤ Mepivacaine: 5 mg/kg (7 mg/kg)*
   ➤ Chloroprocaine: 10 mg/kg (15 mg/kg)*
   ➤ Etidocaine: 2.5 mg/kg (4 mg/kg)*
   ➤ Prilocaine: 5 mg/kg (7.5 mg/kg)*
   ➤ Bupivacaine: 2.5 mg/kg (3 mg/kg)*
   ➤ Procaine: 8 mg/kg (10 mg/kg)*
   ➤ Tetracaine: 1.5 mg/kg (2.5 mg/kg)*
   *Disclaimer: These are not the recommended doses for regional anesthesia applications.

■ Dosage in pregnancy: Pregnant patients require a 20–30% lower dose of local anesthetic to achieve the same anesthesia as a nonparturient. Proposed explanations for this observation include:
   ➤ Increased progesterone levels
   ➤ Pregnancy-related changes in diffusion barriers
   ➤ Pregnancy related changes in the endogenous analgesic system

■ Distribution: Distribution is dependent on blood flow/reservoir of organs. Initially the most highly perfused organs (brain, lung, liver, heart, kidney) receive the highest concentration of the local anesthetic, w/ a slower distribution to organs w/ lower blood flow (muscle, fat).

■ Metabolism

1. Ester: Ester local anesthetics undergo breakdown of the ester bond connecting the benzene ring & the side chain via plasma esterases, by plasma cholinesterases (i.e., pseudocholinesterase).

2. Amide: Amide local anesthetics are bound to hepatic endoplasmic reticulum, where they undergo dealkylation followed by hydrolysis. The amide local anesthetics are also extensively protein bound; thus, changes in plasma proteins will affect presentation of amide local anesthetics to the liver for metabolism. Hepatic failure is a relative contraindication to the use of amide local anesthetics. The lungs are capable of metabolizing & eliminating local anesthetics (primarily amides), as they can extract local anesthetics from circulation.

3. Pseudocholinesterase deficiency: Some pts have abnormal genetic variants of pseudocholinesterase. Atypical plasma pseudocholinesterase lacks the ability to hydrolyze the ester bond in local anesthetics such as chloroprocaine & tetracaine. This dysfunction can be assessed in vitro with the administration of dibucaine. In normal patients, dibucaine inhibits 80% of pseudocholinesterase function, while it inhibits only 20% of atypical pseudocholinesterase function. This provides a "Dibucaine" number, which can be used to predict if increased length of time will be required for recovery from drugs requiring pseudocholinesterase for metabolism. A pt w/ a pseudocholinesterase deficiency will have a delayed recovery from ester-type local anesthetics.

■ Duration of action

➤ Short (20–45 minutes): procaine, chloroprocaine

➤ Intermediate (60–180 minutes): lidocaine, mepivacaine

➤ Long (360–600 minutes): bupivacaine, etidocaine, ropivacaine, tetracaine

■ The data suggest that the addition of epinephrine lowers absorption rates of the long-acting agents somewhat less effectively than of the short-acting agents.

■ Elimination: Most local anesthetics undergo complete metabolism & only a very small fraction is excreted unchanged in the urine.

Local anesthetic effects/toxicities

■ Neurologic

➤ CNS: With systemic absorption, the CNS is exposed to progressively increasing levels of local anesthetics. As local anesthetics cross the blood-brain barrier, they depress neuronal activity. Initially a mild excitatory phase characterized by dysphoria, tremors & restlessness is created w/ depression of inhibitory neurons. Common early signs of systemic toxicity include perioral numbness, tinnitus, drowsiness, lightheadedness & a metallic taste. As the CNS concentration increases, tonic-clonic convulsions followed by loss of airway & respiratory reflexes occur. Mgt of CNS toxicity is primarily supportive, w/ discontinuation of the local anesthetic, increasing the seizure threshold w/ the administration of benzodiazepines or barbiturates & airway mgt (including initial hyperventilation).

➤ Peripheral nervous system

• Neuromuscular junction/ganglionic synapse: Infiltration of the local anesthetic into the neuromuscular junction or the ganglionic synapse can lead to the blockade of skeletal muscle response or ganglionic blockade via inhibition of the ion channel of the acetylcholine receptor.

• Cauda equina syndrome: The syndrome consists of sensory anesthesia, rectal & urethral sphincter dysfunction as well as marked lower extremity weakness. Cauda equina syndrome has been reported after continuous spinal anesthetics via micro-catheters. It has been postulated that neuronal damage in these cases is secondary to the pooling of high concentrations of drug at the cauda equina.

• Transient neurologic symptoms/transient radicular irritation (TNS/TRI): Transient neurologic symptoms are described as a constellation of symptoms characterized as burning radicular pain experienced in the lower extremities, lower back & buttocks that typically appears within 24 hours following recovery from spinal anesthesia, w/ full recovery from symptoms within 7 days. It is attributed to radicular irritation by intrathecal lidocaine > mepivacaine > bupivacaine. Obesity, prolonged lithotomy position & outpatient surgery are considered to be risk factors.

• Anterior spinal artery syndrome: The anterior spinal artery is a long anastomotic channel that supplies blood to the anterior two thirds of the spinal cord. Occlusion can be seen in the event of vasospasm or trauma from spinal anesthesia or from hypoperfusion secondary to hypotension. This is a very rare phenomenon. Acutely it manifests as flaccid muscle tone & areflexia & progresses to loss of pain & temperature sensation w/ preservation of proprioception & vibration sense. The clinical diagnosis can be supported w/ MRI evidence of anterior spinal cord ischemia or infarct.

- Cardiac: Systemic absorption of local anesthetics can have toxic effects on the myocardium, including direct depression of myocardial contractility & impaired cardiac automaticity & conduction of cardiac impulses. Local anesthetics dilate the vasculature via direct smooth muscle relaxation. It is relatively rare to see ventricular tachycardia or fibrillation w/ most local anesthetic toxicities, bupivacaine being the exception. Inadvertent intravascular injection of bupivacaine can lead to severe cardiac compromise including hypotension, atrioventricular blockade & ventricular dysrhythmias, worsened by the lowered threshold seen in pregnancy, hypoxia & acidosis. Since it was found that the majority of cardiac toxicity is due to the dextro-isomer of bupivacaine, many centers are choosing to use the levo-isomer of bupivacaine. The most common adverse cardiac reactions, however, are usually those associated with epinephrine when there is systemic absorption or direct intravascular injection of the epinephrine-containing solution.

- Allergic: Rarely a pt has a hypersensitivity reaction to local anesthetics. This is most commonly seen w/ ester local anesthetics that are broken down to metabolites that are related to para-aminobenzoic acid (PABA), a well-known allergen. The subsequent reaction can range from a mild allergic dermatitis to a full-blown allergic reaction, including bronchospasm & hemodynamic collapse. A far more common cause of hypersensitivity reaction is the added preservatives (i.e., methylparaben) & associated compounds. For pts who are thought to have a hypersensitivity, either to ester local anesthetics or their preservatives, the recommendation is to use a preservative-free, amide-based local anesthetic. There is no known cross-sensitivity btwn the different classes of local anesthetics. Consider using preservative-free meperidine (Demerol) for subarachnoid block (e.g., 1 mg/kg) in patients who exhibit hypersensitivity reactions to local anesthetics. Demerol is chemically unrelated to local anesthetics but has weak local anesthetic properties.

■ Immunologic: It is felt that local anesthetics interfere w/ proper neutrophil/phagocyte function & therefore may have an effect on wound healing.

■ Hematologic/coagulopathic: High doses of prilocaine or benzocaine can lead to the accumulation of a metabolite (ortho-toluidine) that is capable of converting hemoglobin to methemoglobin. Methemoglobinemia is characterized by cyanosis & discoloration of blood. This can be managed w/ the administration of methylene blue. Pts w/ G6PD deficiency may actually have a worsening of their symptoms upon administration of methylene blue due to hemolysis & worsening methemoglobinemia.

Preservatives

■ Antimicrobial: Multiple-dose vials typically contain up to 0.1% methylparaben as an antimicrobial that is effective against gram-positive bacteria as well as fungi.

Stabilizers: Stabilizing agents such as preservatives & antioxidants are frequently added to prolong shelf life. Commonly used stabilizers include sodium metabisulfite (in low concentrations), citric acid, ascorbic acid, EDTA & monothioglycerol. Studies & case reports have shown sodium metabisulfite to be an allergen as well as a neurotoxin.

STUDIES

■ Consider allergy testing (when no longer pregnant) in pts who report a history of allergy to local anesthetics.

■ The Dibucaine number can be used to predict if an increased length of time will be required for recovery from drugs requiring pseudo-cholinesterase for metabolism.

MANAGEMENT/INTERVENTIONS

See the "Regional Anesthesia" chapter and the Obstetric Anesthesia Formulary.

CAVEATS/PEARLS

■ Potency: The more potent local anesthetics tend to be more lipid soluble. The lipophilic local anesthetics will more readily traverse cell membranes & will bind to intracellular sites.

■ Onset of action: The closer the pKa value to physiologic pH, the greater the percentage of the uncharged form of the local anesthetic & thus the more rapid onset of action. With some local anesthetics, the addition of sodium bicarbonate to alkalinize the solution will speed the onset of action due to the larger percentage of non-ionized drug available to penetrate nerve cells.

■ Ultimately it is the charged or ionized form of the drug that actively binds at intracellular receptors.

■ Duration of action: Greater protein binding leads to a longer duration of action. It has been also found that the more potent/more lipid-soluble local anesthetics have greater protein binding.

■ Systemic absorption: Intravenous > tracheal > intercostal > caudal > paracervical > epidural > brachial plexus > sciatic/femoral > subcutaneous

■ Ion trapping: In the setting of an acidotic fetus, a greater percentage of ionized drug is retained in fetal circulation & cannot return to maternal circulation. This phenomenon, most commonly seen w/ amide local anesthetics, can theoretically result in toxic concentrations of local anesthetic in the fetus.

■ Methemoglobinemia: Ortho-toluidine, one of the metabolites of prilocaine & benzocaine, leads to the conversion of hemoglobin to methemoglobin.

■ Local anesthetics w/ added epinephrine: Many preparations contain metabisulfite as a preservative & therefore should be avoided in pts w/ sulfite allergies. Epinephrine is a useful adjunct in increasing the duration of block.

■ Consider using preservative-free meperidine (Demerol) for subarachnoid block (e.g., 1 mg/kg) in pts who exhibit hypersensitivity reactions to local anesthetics.

■ Adding sodium bicarbonate to the lidocaine for skin wheal can decrease the burning or stinging sensation experienced by the pt.

CHECKLIST

■ Monitor total doses of local anesthetic used to minimize the changes of systemic toxicity.

■ Check pt's history for reports of hypersensitivity/allergic reactions to local anesthetics or associated preservatives.

■ Check pt's history for evidence of pseudocholinesterase deficiency, which can result in prolonged blockade.

MASSIVE BLOOD TRANSFUSION

JEANNA VIOLA, MD
JANE BALLANTYNE, MD

FUNDAMENTAL KNOWLEDGE
- Factors V and VIII are depleted in stored blood.
- Diffuse microvascular bleeding
- Inadequate # of functioning plts

STUDIES
- Increased PT, PTT
- Abnormal TEG (thromboelastogram)
- Assay factors V & VIII: <20% normal
- Fibrinogen <50 mg/dL

MANAGEMENT/INTERVENTIONS
- Replenish as needed: factor, FFP, plts

CAVEATS AND PEARLS
- Massive transfusion of stored products can also cause acid-base imbalances & affect potassium & calcium levels.
- Normalize pt's temp.

CHECKLIST
- Check compatibility of transfused blood.
- Verify oxygen-carrying capacity has been achieved through transfusion.
- Replenish deficient components.
- Watch for signs/symptoms of acute transfusion reaction.

MATERNAL HYDROCEPHALUS

MEREDITH ALBRECHT, MD
MICHELE SZABO, MD

FUNDAMENTAL KNOWLEDGE
Definition
- Condition characterized by increased CSF volume & dilation of the cerebral ventricles

Pathophysiology
- Variety of etiologies

- Obstruction of CSF outflow (non-communicating hydrocephalus): congenital malformations or obstructing mass lesion
- Altered CSF dynamics (communicating hydrocephalus): overproduction or defective reabsorption of CSF

Epidemiology
- 1 per 1,000 births
- 85% survive to reproductive age.
- 60–70% near normal intelligence

Clinical Manifestations
- Headache
- Nausea & vomiting
- Blurred or double vision
- Problems w/ balance, coordination, gait or urination
- Memory loss
- Irritability
- Drowsiness or altered mental status
- If ICP rise is rapid & severe
    - Ischemic brain damage can occur when cerebral perfusion pressure (MAP-ICP) < 60 mm Hg
    - Herniation can occur.

Effect of pregnancy on hydrocephalus
- Approx. 75% pts w/ indwelling shunts reported to experience neurologic complications
- Physiologic changes of pregnancy alone can cause neurologic symptoms:
    - Pregnancy causes increase in brain water content.
    - Pregnancy causes intracranial venous distention.
    - The increase in intracranial volume may not be well tolerated in the hydrocephalic pt w/ preexisting decreased intracranial compliance.
- Intra-abdominal pressure increases & may alter shunt function.
- Causes of neurologic complications
    - Partial malfunctioning shunt/deterioration w/ physiologic changes of pregnancy
    - Shunt malfunction
    - Brain tumor expansion during pregnancy

Effect of hydrocephalus on fetus
- None per se

- If maternal hydrocephalus is associated w/ neural tube defect, higher incidence of defect in fetus
- If on anticonvulsants: teratogenic potential

STUDIES

History & Physical
- Obtain neurologic history & course during pregnancy.
  - ➤ Determine underlying cause for hydrocephalus.
  - ➤ Presence of symptoms of increased ICP
  - ➤ Associated seizure disorder
- Perform a thorough neurologic exam; highlight the mental status evaluation.

Imaging
- Preconception MRI or CT scan
  - ➤ Useful for comparing ventricular size
  - ➤ May predict pt's compliance: larger ventricles will have less compliance
- MRI or CT scan w/ onset of symptoms
  - ➤ Evidence of dilated ventricles &/or mass lesion
- Shuntogram to determine shunt patency

Other
- Indwelling shunt can be tapped to determine ICP & status of shunt function
- Symptoms may mimic eclampsia; perform tests to rule out eclampsia.

MANAGEMENT/INTERVENTIONS

Medical Treatment
- Indicated when ventricular size is unchanged w/ functioning shunt
- Symptoms: presumed due to physiologic changes of pregnancy
  - ➤ Bed rest
  - ➤ Fluid restriction
  - ➤ Steroids in severe cases
  - ➤ Diuretics in severe cases

Surgical Treatment
- Indicated in presence of enlarging ventricles or shunt obstruction
- VP shunt placement or revision is definitive therapy.
- VP shunt for 1st & 2nd trimester, VA (atrial) shunt 3rd trimester (avoid abdominal surgery)

■ Acute hydrocephalus w/ altered mental status is a neurosurgical emergency.
  ➤ Immediate VP shunt revision or external ventricular drainage
  ➤ Avoid C-section if possible; subsequent adhesions may obstruct shunt.

Anesthesia

■ Choice is based on neurologic status as well as obstetrical considerations.
■ Anesthetic goal is to prevent or minimize increases in ICP & to avoid hypoxemia or hypotension, which could exacerbate neurologic injury.

General

■ Technique of choice if:
  ➤ Pt is neurologically deteriorating
  ➤ Pt is stable but has risk of herniation w/ inadvertent dural puncture (non-communicating hydrocephalus)
■ For the nonurgent C-section
  ➤ "Modified" rapid sequence induction w/ cricoid pressure, rocuronium
  ➤ Positive-pressure ventilation during induction to maintain oxygenation & normocarbia
  ➤ Adequate depth of anesthesia during induction to prevent Valsalva response to noxious stimuli such as coughing w/ intubation
  ➤ Choice of maintenance anesthetic agent should reflect the need for rapid emergence: low-dose isoflurane & nitrous oxide is reasonable.
■ In setting of acute hydrocephalus w/ impending herniation or altered sensorium:
  ➤ ICP is presumed to be significantly elevated.
  ➤ Goal is to aggressively treat intracranial hypertension, anesthetize & prepare the pt as rapidly as possible.
  ➤ Rapid sequence induction
    • Thiopental or propofol
    • Succinylcholine: used for its rapid & reliable onset of action; its ICP effects are transient & self-limited & attenuated by prior administration of pentothal
  ➤ Hyperventilation
    • Remains most reliable therapy to reduce ICP acutely

- Has the potential to decrease uterine placental blood flow via mechanism of positive-pressure ventilation-induced decrease in cardiac output
- Benefits of hyperventilation outweigh risks during a neurosurgical emergency.
  ➤ Administer mannitol.
    - Effective in reducing ICP
    - Can cause fetal dehydration (thought to be a temporary effect)
    - Anecdotal case reports suggest its use is safe for these emergency situations.
- ■ Treat hypotension aggressively.
  ➤ Insult is cerebral ischemia. Keep cerebral perfusion pressure (CPP) > 60 mm Hg.
- ■ If possible, have pt awake for neurologic exam at conclusion of procedure.

Regional
- ■ Epidural anesthesia preferred in neurologically stable pts
  ➤ Safe in pts w/ communicating hydrocephalus
  ➤ May result in herniation in pts w/ non-communicating hydrocephalus
  ➤ Facilitates vaginal delivery w/ minimal Valsalva if forceps/vacuum is used
    - For second stage of labor, dose epidural to produce dense block.

CAVEATS & PEARLS
- ■ Mgt primarily determined by course of the neurologic disease
- ■ Consult pt's neurosurgeon when composing anesthetic plan; determine means of emergency contact should pt deteriorate neurologically.
- ■ With help of neurosurgeon, determine cause of hydrocephalus & whether pt is at risk for herniation w/ intentional or unintentional dural puncture.
- ■ Avoid regional (spinal or epidural) in pts at risk for herniation w/ dural puncture.

CHECKLIST
- ■ Administer prophylactic antibiotics for labor & delivery if shunt in situ.

■ With help of neurosurgeon, assess risk of herniation & determine course of action if neurologic deterioration occurs.

MATERNAL HYDROPS

JEANNA VIOLA, MD
JANE BALLANTYNE, MD

FUNDAMENTAL KNOWLEDGE
■ Fetal hydrops may be transmitted to the mother.
■ Etiology of maternal hydrops is unknown.
■ Fetal hydrops may occur due to isoimmunization, viral infection, alpha thalassemia or other causes.
■ Pts present w/ features of pre-eclampsia such as hypertension, proteinuria, pulmonary edema, anemia, uremia.

STUDIES
■ Largely a clinical diagnosis made in conjunction w/ knowledge of the presence of fetal hydrops

MANAGEMENT/INTERVENTIONS
■ Delivery of the hydropic fetus & placenta
■ Pts may become hemodynamically unstable, requiring resuscitation measures & insertion of arterial & central catheters.
■ Use of epidural catheters in these pts should be accompanied by slow, incremental injection of local anesthetic & cautious fluid-loading to prevent hemodynamic compromise.

CAVEATS AND PEARLS
■ Syndrome may mimic pre-eclampsia.
■ Treatment is delivery of the hydropic fetus & placenta.
■ Pts can become hemodynamically unstable; prepare for invasive monitoring.

CHECKLIST
■ Obtain blood sample for type & cross in case transfusion of blood products is necessary.
■ Careful evaluation of airway, as GETA likely needed for C-section
■ Obtain & set up invasive hemodynamic monitors such as arterial catheter & central catheter transducers.

MATERNAL RESUSCITATION

SHYAM PAREKH, MD; LEE WESNER, MD; AND RICHARD PINO, MD

FUNDAMENTAL KNOWLEDGE

Emergency cardiac care for the pregnant woman

- Incidence of cardiac arrest in pregnancy estimated to be 1:30,000
- Successful resuscitation requires thorough understanding of the physiologic changes seen in pregnancy.
  - ➤ The gravid uterus of late pregnancy makes successful resuscitation difficult because of increased intrathoracic pressure, reduced venous return & obstruction of the aortic flow in the abdominal aorta; all 3 are exacerbated in the supine position.
- Cardiovascular changes w/ pregnancy
  - ➤ Increased cardiac output (CO)
    - After 10th week of gestation, CO is increased by 1.0–1.5 L/min.
    - Pt position may greatly affect CO.
    - Supine positioning may decrease CO 30–40% due to aortocaval compression.
  - ➤ Increased heart rate, peaking at 20 bpm above pre-pregnant baseline
  - ➤ Decreased systolic BP, typically 10–15 mm Hg below prepregnant levels
  - ➤ Physiologic anemia of pregnancy: by 34 weeks plasma volume increases 40%, but RBC volume increases to a lesser extent
  - ➤ All of these changes make recognition of hypovolemia & bleeding difficult when based upon hypotension, tachycardia & Hct.
  - ➤ Physiologic "shunting": gravid uterus accounts for 10% of the cardiac output. This may lead to difficulty w/ effective resuscitation, especially w/ Cardiopulmonary Resuscitation-Emergency Cardiac Care (CPR-ECC).
  - ➤ External cardiac massage may generate only about 30% of the pregnant pt's normal CO.
- Respiratory changes w/ pregnancy
  - ➤ Rapid desaturation during apnea
    - Increased oxygen consumption
    - Decreased FRC
  - ➤ Increased minute ventilation, mainly due to increased tidal volume
  - ➤ Increased risk of aspiration & difficult airway mgt

- Pregnancy-specific considerations for CPR & Advanced Cardiac Life Support (ACLS)
  - For brevity, this chapter will not include treatment of myocardial infarction as an etiology for a cardiac arrest since it is rare in pregnancy.
  - The goal of resuscitation is the safety & well-being of the mother, although the well-being of the fetus is obviously desirable.
  - The well-being of the mother & that of the fetus are best served by following ACLS protocols w/ the modifications listed.
  - **Consideration of C-section within 5 minutes of arrest is of primary importance. Prompt operative delivery may improve mother & fetal outcomes!**
  - Key interventions to prevent arrest in a near-arrest situation
    - Reduce aortocaval compression.
      - Place pregnant female in left lateral decubitus position, or right lateral decubitus if no improvement on left side (this helps displace the gravid uterus off the great vessels).
      - Also consider placing the rescuer's (or assistant's) knees or a wedge under the pt's right flank/back to produce a tilt to the left.
      - Manually displacing the gravid uterus may also be useful.
    - Give 100% oxygen.
    - Administer fluid bolus.
    - Reevaluate drugs being given (eg, possibility of epidural infusion of local anesthetic actually being intravascular, magnesium sulfate infusion, etc.)
  - BLS modifications during arrest
    - Aortocaval compression will make CPR ineffective.
    - Reduce aortocaval compression.
  - ACLS modifications during arrest
    - Consider possible causes of arrest that are more pregnancy-specific:
      - Amniotic fluid embolism
      - Air embolism
      - Venous thromboembolic disease/pulmonary embolism
      - Drug toxicity
        - Magnesium sulfate
        - Intravascular administration of local anesthetics given through epidural catheter
        - Narcotics (including epidural)
        - Recreational drugs

- Antibiotics (rapid infusion of vancomycin, allergies, etc.)
- Congestive cardiomyopathy
- Eclampsia
- Aortic dissection
- Trauma
- Hemorrhage
- Prompt operative delivery

STUDIES
- ECG
  - ➤ Rapid interpretation is essential to provide appropriate mgt of arresting pt using ACLS protocol.
    - "Quick look" via the defibrillator paddles or pads
    - 3-, 5- or 12-lead ECG
- FHR monitoring
  - ➤ May be instituted if feasible & not obstructive of resuscitative efforts
  - ➤ Maternal resuscitation personnel & resources must not be distracted or diverted by FHR monitoring efforts.

MANAGEMENT/INTERVENTIONS
This section provides basic information for resuscitation of adults w/ emphasis on the obstetrical pt.
- Protocols described below follow the evidence-based "Guidelines 2000 for Cardiopulmonary Resuscitation & Emergency Cardiovascular Care," w/ modifications for the obstetric service.
- Anesthesiologist role in cardiac emergency
  - ➤ Anesthesiologist responsibilities include knowing ACLS algorithms & managing people & resources effectively.
    - The anesthesiologist should strive to maintain global awareness in an event, delegate tasks to appropriate personnel & instill a sense of calm & order.
- **Cardiac Arrest**
  - ➤ Diagnosis
    - ECG might reveal ventricular tachycardia (VT), ventricular fibrillation (VF), pulseless electrical activity (PEA) or asystole.
      - PEA: organized ECG is present w/o pulse or BP
    - The absence of a palpable pulse in a major artery (eg, carotid, femoral) in an unconscious, unmonitored pt is diagnostic of a cardiac arrest.

- Usually made swiftly in the obstetrical unit because of the high nurse-to-patient ratio
- Pathophysiology
  - Cardiac arrest leads to cessation of effective blood flow (notably placental)
    - Tissue hypoxia
    - Anaerobic metabolism: leads to acidosis
    - Accumulation of cellular wastes
  - Organ function is compromised; permanent damage to the fetus or death ensues unless the condition is reversed within minutes.
  - Systemic vasodilatation from acidosis & a decrease in responsiveness to the actions of endogenous & exogenous catecholamines.
  - Acidosis may cause pulmonary vasoconstriction.
  - Reperfusion injury: following resuscitation, organ dysfunction may be exacerbated.
- Basic Life Support
  - Includes basic techniques taught to the general public but applies equally to in-hospital situations
  - Cardiac arrest is suspected in any person unexpectedly found unconscious.
  - If the subject is unarousable, the ABCDs (Airway, Breathing, Circulation, Defibrillation) of resuscitation should be followed after first calling for assistance or activating the hospital's medical emergency "code" system.
  - EMS should be activated before attempts at resuscitation in cases of submersion or near-drowning, arrest secondary to trauma & drug overdose.
  - Airway & breathing
    - Spontaneous ventilation is evaluated by observation, auscultation & tactile sensation.
      - Aided by repositioning: head-tilt chin-lift or jaw-thrust maneuvers
      - Aided by insertion of an oropharyngeal or nasopharyngeal airway
    - In the absence of effective spontaneous ventilation
      - Rescue breathing or ventilation by bag-valve mask w/ 100% O_2
      - Two slow breaths at low airway pressures are used initially to limit gastric distention, followed by 10–12 breaths/min.

- If a foreign-body obstruction is considered as the reason for failed ventilation in the parturient, chest compressions are given.
- The Heimlich maneuver is relatively contraindicated in pregnancy.

➤ **Circulation**
- The circulation is assessed by palpation of the carotid, radial or femoral artery pulse for 5–10 seconds.
  - The presence of a pulse does not necessarily mean adequate perfusion is present.
- Maintenance of FHR is an indication of adequate maternal BP.
- In the absence of a palpable pulse, artificial circulation should be instituted w/ external chest compressions by the rescuer.
  - The pt should be on a firm surface (eg, backboard) w/ the head on the same level as the thorax.
  - Left tilt of the thorax
    - Folded blankets placed under the backboard
    - Rescuer's thighs under the pt's back, when in kneeling position
    - Cardiff wedge: a device used to facilitate CPR in a pt w/ a gravid uterus
  - Place the heel of one hand on the pt's sternum two finger-breadths above the xiphoid process & the other hand either on top of the first w/ interlocked fingers, or grasping the wrist of the first hand.
  - Shoulders positioned directly over the pt, elbows locked
  - Sternal depression
    - Depth of 3.5–5 cm (normal-sized adult)
    - 1:1 compression-relaxation ratio
    - Rate of 100 compressions/min
  - Chest compression-ventilation ratio is 15:2 for resuscitation w/ 1 or >1 rescuer.

➤ **Defibrillation**
- The major determinant of a successful resuscitation is VF.
- VF is the most likely etiology of a cardiac arrest in adults, though in the pregnant female, pregnancy-specific factors, such as amniotic fluid embolus, may play a larger role.
- Public access defibrillation programs (PAD) have now enabled "Level I" responders (eg, fire personnel, police, security guards, airline attendants) to employ readily accessible automated external defibrillators (AEDs).

➤ **Reassessment**
- If no spontaneous circulation after 3 shocks, or w/ a "no shock indicated" on AED, continue CPR for 1 minute followed by another ECG analysis.
- Cardiopulmonary activity should be checked via carotid, femoral or radial pulse after the first 4 cycles & every several minutes thereafter if an AED is not used or if defibrillation is not indicated.

■ **ACLS:** definitive treatment of cardiac arrest w/ endotracheal intubation, electrical defibrillation & pharmacologic intervention

➤ Successful resuscitation may be possible only w/ immediate operative delivery of the fetus.
- Decreases the fraction of cardiac output supplying the uterus
- Decreases the amount of aortocaval compression
- May improve the outcome for the fetus

➤ **Intubation**
- Swift control of the airway
- Performed by the most experienced person present, provided this does not delay defibrillation
- Optimize oxygenation & removal of carbon dioxide during resuscitation.
- Nonphysical examination technique to confirm endotracheal (ET) tube placement
  - Qualitative end-tidal CO_2 indicator
  - Esophageal detector device
  - Capnograph
  - Capnometer
- ET tube must be secured after confirmation of placement.
- ET intubation should not interrupt ventilation for >30 seconds.
- ET tube may be used to deliver epinephrine, lidocaine & atropine if IV access has not been established, but NOT $NaCO_3$.
  - Peak drug concentrations are lower w/ the ET vs. IV.
  - Use higher doses (2–3×) diluted in 10 mL sterile saline.

➤ **Defibrillation**
- VT & VF are the most common arrhythmias associated w/ a cardiac arrest.
- Electrical defibrillation is the priority & must be administered as soon as a conventional defibrillator can be brought to the pt.

- Early defibrillation (<5 min after arrest) is a well-established high-priority goal.
- Only for a witnessed cardiac arrest, & if a defibrillator is not quickly available, is an immediate solitary precordial thump recommended.
- 3 shocks can be delivered in rapid succession.
  - Decrease in transthoracic impedance w/ each shock
- The energy levels used for defibrillation depend on the type of defibrillator used.
- **Monophasic waveform defibrillators:** unidirectional current
  - Energy level for the initial series of unsynchronized monophasic damped sinusoidal (MDS) shocks is 200 joules (J) followed by 300 J & 360 J, if needed.
  - Subsequent shocks at 360 J are repeated after every pharmacologic intervention.
    - For recurrent VF following a successful defibrillation, the lowest energy level that was previously useful should be tried first.
    - The person operating the defibrillator is responsible for ensuring that members of the resuscitation team are not in contact w/ the pt during defibrillation.
- **Biphasic waveform defibrillators:** current flows in a positive direction, followed by reversal of current flow in the negative direction
  - Optimal biphasic energy to terminate VF has not been determined.
    - Repeated shocks at 200 J or less appear to be at least as effective as monophasic 200 J, 300 J & 360 J.
    - Each defibrillator manufacturer uses a proprietary biphasic waveform; the manufacturer's recommendations may be followed in selecting an energy level for each shock.
- **Cardioversion**
  - Synchronized MDS shocks of 50–100 J are used for supraventricular arrhythmias such as paroxysmal supraventricular tachycardia (PSVT) & atrial flutter.
  - Hemodynamically stable VT & atrial fibrillation (AF) can be cardioverted using 100-J MDS as the starting point.
  - Optimal energy levels for biphasic defibrillators have not been clearly determined; at least one clinical trial has shown that a 120-J biphasic waveform was superior to a 200-J MDS conventional waveform in synchronized cardioversion of AF.

- **Pacing**
  - High-grade heart block w/ profound bradycardia is an etiology of cardiac arrest.
  - Temporary pacing should be used when the heart rate does not increase w/ pharmacologic therapy.
    - Transcutaneous pacing is the easiest method to increase the ventricular rate, though sedation of the pt may be necessary.
    - Esophageal pacing is efficacious for sinus bradycardia w/ maintained atrioventricular (A-V) conduction.
    - Useful intraoperatively for bradycardia-related hypotension in otherwise stable pts
    - Transvenous pacing via a temporary wire into the right heart
      - Used to increase heart rate
      - Technically more difficult
      - More secure & reliable for longer periods
      - Special pacing pulmonary artery catheters are capable of A-V pacing.
- **IV access**
  - Imperative for a successful resuscitation
  - Central circulation is the most desirable route of access: internal or external jugular, subclavian or femoral veins
    - Provide more rapid delivery of drugs to the site of action in the body
    - Very few OB pts already have central venous catheters placed.
  - Peripheral catheters
    - May take a prolonged period of time to circulate to the site of action, especially in physiologic states of low or no CO.
    - Antecubital veins are adequate when an appropriate volume is used to flush the meds toward the central circulation.
  - Fluid replacement is indicated for pts w/ known or suspected intravascular volume depletion.
  - Choice of crystalloid, colloid or blood products can be made based on the clinical context & laboratory data available at the time of resuscitation.
- **Drugs**
  - Pt may already be taking meds that affect cardiopulmonary status.

- Meds must be identified & continued or stopped based on clinical situation.
  - For instance, bolus doses of magnesium may lead to hypotension & cardiac arrest.
  - Pt w/ stable SVT on a dopamine infusion may require reduction in the rate of infusion to bring the heart rate to a normal level.
- The drugs described below are used in ACLS protocols for the treatment of hemodynamic instability & arrhythmias.
- The safety of many of these drugs in pregnancy has not been established.
- The paramount goal of successful maternal resuscitation precludes changing the pharmacologic recommendations in the ACLS protocols.
  - **Adenosine**
    - Slows A-V nodal conduction & interrupts A-V node reentry pathways to convert narrow-complex tachycardias & wide-complex tachycardias w/ *confirmed* supraventricular origin to a sinus rhythm
    - 6 mg rapid IV bolus. 5-second half-life.
    - Untoward effects may include vasodilation, angina, bronchospasm & arrhythmias.
  - **Amiodarone**
    - Most versatile drug in the ACLS algorithms; properties of all four classes of antiarrhythmics
    - Dose for the treatment of unstable VT & VF is 300 mg administered rapidly.
    - Untoward effects may include bradycardia & hypotension
  - **Atropine**
    - May be useful in treatment of hemodynamically significant bradycardia or A-V block occurring at the nodal level
    - 0.5 mg repeated q3–5min to a total dose of 0.04 mg/kg
    - Atropine should not be used when Mobitz type II block is suspected.
  - **Beta-adrenergic blocking drugs** (atenolol, metoprolol, propranolol)
    - May be useful in pts w/ unstable angina & myocardial infarction, acute treatment of PSVT, AF, atrial flutter & ectopic atrial tachycardia
    - Dosing varies based on specific drug.

- Contraindications include 2nd- or 3rd-degree heart block, hypotension, severe congestive heart failure.
- Use caution in pts w/ reactive airway disease or sinus bradycardia.
- **Calcium chloride**
  - Indicated during cardiac arrest only when hyperkalemia, hypermagnesemia, hypocalcemia or toxicity from calcium channel blockers is suspected
  - Calcium chloride, 2–4 mg/kg IV
  - May cause extravasation necrosis
- **Calcium channel blockers** (verapamil & diltiazem)
  - Used to treat hemodynamically stable narrow-complex PSVTs unresponsive to vagal maneuvers or adenosine
  - Dosing varies based on specific drug.
  - Can cause hypotension, exacerbation of congestive heart failure, bradycardia & enhancement of accessory conduction in pts w/ Wolff-Parkinson-White syndrome
- **Dopamine**
  - Indicated for bradycardia in which atropine is ineffective
  - Active at various receptors: dopaminergic (generally at doses <2 mcg/kg/min), beta (2–5 mcg/kg/min) & alpha (5–10 mcg/kg/min)
  - May induce tachyarrhythmias
- **Epinephrine**
  - Produces compensatory shunting of blood toward brain & heart by alpha-adrenergic activity
  - 1.0 mg IV repeated q3–5min for cardiac arrest. ET tube dosing also effective.
  - May cause extravasation necrosis
- **Isoproterenol**
  - Second-line drug w/ beta-1 & beta-2 agonist activity
  - IV infusion at 2–10 mcg/min titrated to heart rate
  - May cause hypotension
- **Lidocaine**
  - Used for ventricular arrhythmias, but a second choice compared w/ amiodarone, procainamide & sotalol
  - Initial dose during a cardiac arrest: 1.0–1.5 mg/kg IV
  - Decrease dosing for reduced cardiac output, hepatic dysfunction, prolonged lidocaine infusion or advanced age

- **Magnesium**
  - Used to treat drug-induced torsades de pointes even in absence of magnesium deficiency
  - Dose for emergent administration: 1–2 g
  - May precipitate refractory VF as well as exacerbate hypokalemia, hypotension & bradycardia
- **Oxygen**
  - Administered to all cardiac arrest victims
  - 100% by bag-valve mask or ET ventilation; to hemodynamically stable pts by face mask
- **Procainamide**
  - Can convert AF & atrial flutter to sinus rhythm, control the ventricular response to SVT, secondary to accessory pathways, & convert wide complex tachycardias of unknown origin
  - Loading dose: continuous infusion of 20–30 mg/min
  - Contraindicated for overdose of TCAs or antiarrhythmics. May lead to hypotension & QRS complex widening by 50%.
- **Sodium bicarbonate**
  - Used when ACLS has failed in presence of severe preexisting metabolic acidosis & for the treatment of hyperkalemia or TCA or phenobarbital overdose
  - Administration is detrimental in most cardiac arrests because it creates a paradoxical intracellular acidosis.
  - 1 mEq/kg IV
- **Vasopressin**
  - Alternative to epinephrine during the treatment of VF
  - Single dose of 40 units
  - May lead to anaphylaxis or bronchospasm
- ➤ **Specific ACLS protocols**

Algorithm 1: Protocol for ventricular fibrillation (VF)
1. Cardiac arrest
2. BLS algorithm
3. Assess rhythm
4. VF/pulseless VT
5. Defibrillate, 200, 300, 360 joules monophasic (equivalent biphasic)
6. CPR if VF, pulseless VT
7. Secure airway
8. Consider DDx
9. Establish IV access

10. Epinephrine 1:10,000, 1 mg IV, q3–5min (defibrillate after each epinephrine administration), OR vasopressin 40 U IV once
11. Defibrillate (use the lowest voltage that was successful w/ initial defibrillation)
12. Amiodarone 300 mg IV push (amiodarone is diluted in 20–30 mL saline or D5W). If successful, an infusion of 1 mg/min for 6 hr followed by 0.5 mg/hr is given. An additional dose of 150 mg IV push can be administered if VF or pulseless VT recurs. Max dose: 2.2 g over 24 hr.
13. Magnesium sulfate, 1–2 g IV (especially for hypomagnesemia; polymorphic VT [torsades de pointes])
14. Defibrillate
15. Procainamide, 20–30 mg/min IV for refractory VF (max dose: 17 mg/kg or termination w/ arrhythmia suppression, hypotension, or QRS width prolongation of >50%. If successful, infuse at 2 mg/kg/hr)

Algorithm 2: Protocol for Asystole
1. Cardiac arrest
2. BLS algorithm
3. Assess rhythm
4. If rhythm is unclear & possible VF, defibrillate as for VF
5. Asystole
6. Secure airway
7. Establish IV access
8. Transcutaneous pacing
9. Epinephrine 1:10,000, 1 mg IV q3–5min
10. Intubate when possible
11. Atropine, 1 mg IV q3–5min (total dose 0.04 mg/kg)

Algorithm 3: Protocol for Pulseless Electrical Activity (PEA)
1. Organized ECG activity w/o pulse
2. CPR, IV access, intubation
3. Consider underlying cause:
   a. Amniotic fluid embolus (give oxygen & volume, otherwise supportive care)
   b. Hypovolemia (give volume)
   c. Tension pneumothorax (relieve pressure)
   d. Hypoxemia (give oxygen)
   e. Cardiac tamponade (perform pericardiocentesis)
   f. Hypokalemia (give potassium)
   g. Pre-existing bicarbonate-responsive metabolic acidosis (give bicarbonate)

    h. Drug overdose (give treatment appropriate to substance)
    i. Massive myocardial infarction (appropriate therapy including heparin, thrombolysis, intra-aortic balloon pump, etc)
4. Epinephrine 1:10,000, IV q3–5min
5. Atropine 1 mg IV (if slow PEA rate; for a total dose of 0.04 mg/kg)

Algorithm 4: Protocol for Unstable Tachycardia
1. Tachycardia
    a. Ventricular tachycardia
    b. Wide-complex, of unknown type
    c. Paroxysmal supraventricular tachycardia
    d. Atrial fibrillation
    e. Atrial flutter
2. If accompanied by:
    a. Chest pain
    b. Dyspnea
    c. Hypotension
    d. Decreased level of consciousness
    e. Pulmonary edema
    f. Congestive heart failure
    g. Acute myocardial infarction
    h. Hypoxemia
    i. Ventricular rate >150 bpm
3. Administer appropriate sedation & have resuscitation equipment present
4. Synchronous cardioversion (50, 100, 200, 300, 360 joules monophasic [equivalent biphasic])

Algorithm 5: Protocol for Stable Tachycardia
1. Stable tachycardia: depending on type, go to 2, 3, or 4
2. Narrow-complex tachycardia
    a. Vagal maneuvers
    b. Adenosine for conversion to sinus rhythm or for diagnosis of rhythm w/o conversion
    c. If rhythm is atrial fibrillation or atrial flutter
        i. Rate control w/ diltiazem or beta-blocker or digoxin
        ii. Rate control & conversion w/ amiodarone or procainamide
        iii. Conversion w/ DC cardioversion or ibutilide
    d. If rhythm is supraventricular tachycardia with EF $\geq$40%
        i. And arrhythmia is junctional: administer amiodarone, beta-blocker or diltiazem/verapamil

    ii. And arrhythmia is paroxysmal: administer diltiazem/verapamil, or beta-blocker or digoxin; DC cardioversion; consider procainamide, amiodarone or sotalol

    iii. And arrhythmia is ectopic or multifocal atrial: administer diltiazem/verapamil, beta-blocker or amiodarone

  e. If rhythm is supraventricular tachycardia with EF <40%

    i. And arrhythmia is junctional: administer amiodarone

    ii. And arrhythmia is paroxysmal: administer amiodarone, digoxin or diltiazem

    iii. And arrhythmia is ectopic or multifocal atrial: administer amiodarone or diltiazem

3. Wide-complex tachycardia of unknown type

  a. Place esophageal lead for clarification (go to 2 or 4)

  b. Consider clinical information (go to 2 or 4; if unknown go to 4)

4. Ventricular tachycardia (VT)

  a. Monophasic VT : consider cardioversion

    i. If EF $\geq$40%: preferred meds are procainamide & sotalol; acceptable meds are amiodarone & lidocaine

    ii. If EF <40%: amiodarone (150 mg) or lidocaine (0.5–0.75 mg/kg) or synchronized cardioversion

  b. Polymorphic VT: consider cardioversion

    i. If EF $\geq$40% & normal baseline Q-T interval: treat ischemia, correct electrolytes, consider one of the following: beta-blocker, lidocaine, amiodarone, procainamide, sotalol

    ii. With prolonged baseline Q-T interval: consider torsades, correct electrolytes, consider the following: magnesium, overdrive pacing, isoproterenol, phenytoin, lidocaine

Algorithm 6: Protocol for Bradycardia

1. Slow heart rate (60 bpm)
2. Consider the mechanism:
  a. Sinus or junctional
  b. Second-degree A-V block, type I
  c. Second-degree A-V block, type II
  d. Third-degree A-V block
3. Are there serious signs or symptoms? (chest pain, dyspnea, reduced level of consciousness, hypotension, CHF, pulmonary congestion, shock)
  a. No
    i. Observe

    ii. Have a transcutaneous pacer available in case symptoms develop

    iii. Prepare for transvenous pacer placement

  b. Yes

    i. Administer atropine 0.5–1.0 mg IV

    ii. Transcutaneous pacing

    iii. Dopamine (titration to effect; begin at 150 mcg/min)

    iv. Epinephrine 2–10 mcg/min

    v. Prepare for transvenous pacer placement

➤ **Open-chest direct cardiac compression**

- Used at institutions w/ appropriate resources to manage penetrating chest trauma, abdominal trauma w/ cardiac arrest, pericardial tamponade, hypothermia & pulmonary embolism
- Indicated for individuals w/ anatomic deformities of the chest that prevent adequate closed-chest compression
- Use would be accompanied by immediate operative delivery of the fetus.

➤ **Termination of CPR**

- No absolute guidelines to determine when to stop an unsuccessful resuscitation
- Exceedingly low probability of survival after 30 minutes
- The anesthesiologist or other physician in charge determines when the pt has died due to the failure of the cardiovascular system to respond to adequately applied BLS & ACLS.
- Meticulous documentation of the resuscitation, including the reasons for terminating the effort.

CAVEATS & PEARLS

- Prompt operative delivery may improve maternal & fetal outcomes.
- Ensure everyone is clear prior to defibrillation or cardioversion.
- The team leader during CPR-ECC must have a solid grasp of ACLS algorithms, integrate all available information, execute plan & maintain order.
- Administration of $NaCO_3$ may cause intracellular acidosis by diffusion of CO_2 intracellularly once $NaCO_3$ forms carbonic acid & dissociates into CO_2 & H_2O.
- IV access is important but should not take priority over initial airway mgt, chest compressions or defibrillation.
- Peripheral infusions of drugs should be flushed w/ 20 cc of fluid since peripheral blood flow is decreased during cardiac arrest.
- Management of CPR-ECC is a team effort; coordination is imperative.

CHECKLIST
- Recognize cardiac arrest.
  - ➤ Person collapses/possible cardiac arrest
  - ➤ Assess responsiveness.
- Primary ABCD survey
  - ➤ Activate emergency response or hospital "code" system.
  - ➤ Call for defibrillator.
  - ➤ Assess breathing (look, listen, feel).
  - ➤ If not breathing, give 2 slow breaths.
  - ➤ Circulation: assess pulse; if no pulse, position pt & start chest compressions
  - ➤ Defibrillation: attach defibrillator or monitor if available, continue chest compressions
    - If VF/VT, attempt defibrillation.
    - If not VF/VT, continue CPR & begin secondary ABC survey.
- Memorize BCLS & ACLS algorithms. People's lives may be saved if you memorize & effectively implement them!

MECHANICAL VENTILATION

KRISTOPHER DAVIGNON, MD
HARISH LECAMWASAM, MD

FUNDAMENTAL KNOWLEDGE
- Mechanical ventilation provides support for gas exchange.
- Hypoventilation or hypoxemia is the most common reason for institution of mechanical ventilation.
- Basic goals of mechanical ventilation
  - ➤ Provide adequate alveolar ventilation
  - ➤ Provide adequate oxygenation
  - ➤ Avoid traumatic lung injury (ventilator-associated lung injury [VILI]) by not overdistending the lung (using high inspiratory pressures or tidal volumes) & using positive-end expiratory pressure (PEEP) to maintain alveolar recruitment
  - ➤ Optimize pt-ventilator synchrony
- **Phase variables**
  - ➤ Trigger variable: starts inspiration. This may be a flow or pressure variable. Its sensitivity is set to allow the pt to trigger the ventilator easily but not to allow triggering in the absence of effort by the pt.

➤ Control or limit variable: remains constant throughout inspiration regardless of impedance. This variable is either a pressure or volume.

➤ Cycle variable: terminates inspiration. Most commonly is volume, time or flow.

■ **Basic modes of ventilation**

➤ SIMV (synchronized intermittent mandatory ventilation)

- Patient receives a mandatory minute ventilation as determined by a set rate as well as a set volume (and flow) or set pressure (and inspiratory time).
- Breaths are synchronized w/ pt's inspiratory effort.
- Between mandatory breaths the pt is allowed to breathe spontaneously. These spontaneous breaths are not supported unless an additional mode of ventilation (pressure support) is added.

➤ A/C (Assist/Control)

- Pt receives a mandatory minute ventilation as determined by a set rate as well as a set volume (Volume Control) or set inspiratory pressure (Pressure Control).
- Breaths are synchronized w/ pt's inspiratory effort. If pt triggers a breath between mandatory breaths, the ventilator delivers a breath identical to the mandatory breaths (either a volume- or a pressure-controlled breath).
- If a pt is not breathing at a rate greater than the minimum rate set, A/C & SIMV are identical.

➤ CPAP (continuous positive airway pressure)

- No mandatory minute ventilation is set. Spontaneous respirations are assisted by a set pressure.
- If the pressure during inspiration is set higher than the pressure during expiration, this is termed pressure support ventilation (PSV).
- With PSV or CPAP the tidal volume, inspiratory time & flow can all vary from breath to breath. The tidal volume is determined by the amount of pressure support, the inspiratory effort of the pt & the compliance/resistive characteristics of the lung.

➤ Positive end-expiratory pressure (PEEP)

- Not a mode of ventilation
- Defined as the pressure in the airway at end-expiration
- PEEP is used to prevent alveolar collapse & maintain functional residual capacity, or to optimize the compliance of the lung & chest wall.

- PEEP may be used in an effort to optimize oxygenation, lower the delivered inspiratory concentration of oxygen (FiO2) & help protect the lung from VILI.
- PEEP can decrease cardiac output & result in cardiovascular compromise. PEEP can also worsen oxygenation in the setting of intracardiac shunts or w/ inhomogeneous lung disease by overdistending healthy lung, increasing pulmonary vascular resistance & increasing intrapulmonary shunt.

➤ Peak inspiratory pressure (PIP)
- The maximum pressure measured during the inspiratory phase
- The PIP typically represents the pressure imparted onto the conducting airways (trachea, bronchi).
- High peak inspiratory pressures in the setting of normal plateau pressures indicate increased airway resistance. Common causes include secretions, bronchospasm or a narrow endotracheal tube.

➤ Plateau pressure (Pplat)
- The pressure measured during an end-inspiratory pause
- When flow is 0 (during a pause), pressure equilibrates btwn the ventilator & the alveolus. Thus, this pressure typically represents the pressure conducted to the alveolus. It is always equal to or lower than the PIP.
- Risk of alveolar injury is thought to be significant if this pressure is >30 cm H2O. (Note that this pressure can only be measured in the pt not making inspiratory efforts.)

STUDIES

■ PaO2 & PaCO2 from ABGs can be used to assess adequacy of oxygenation & ventilation. Arterial pH can help in determining whether changes in PaCO2 are acute or chronic. A mild respiratory acidosis is usually well tolerated by pts & "permissive hypercapnia" has become one strategy used to avoid excessive tidal volumes & the associated VILI.

■ Chest radiography is useful to determine appropriate endotracheal tube placement (usually approx. 3 cm proximal to the carina). The CXR may also help identify the etiology of the respiratory failure (pneumothorax, pulmonary edema, pneumonia, pleural effusion or atelectasis).

■ Pulse oximetry provides a noninvasive measurement of arterial oxygen saturation.

MANAGEMENT & INTERVENTIONS

- Mode of ventilation
  - ➤ Several modes of mechanical ventilation exist. The goals of mechanical ventilation have been previously discussed.
  - ➤ Choice of mode is primarily dependent on institutional bias. In fact, w/ appropriate manipulation, the ventilator-delivered breath can be made to look identical in either volume- or pressure-limited modes.
  - ➤ Current literature does not support any one mode of ventilation over another. Pts not spontaneously breathing or breathing inadequately to achieve an appropriate alveolar ventilation will need a mode of ventilation that allows a set respiratory rate (A/C or SIMV). Others may tolerate PSV.
  - ➤ No matter what mode of ventilation is chosen, it is prudent to limit alveolar pressure to less than 30 cm H2O & tidal volumes to 6–8 mL/kg. In addition, PEEP should be used. These interventions limit traumatic injury to the lung.
- Oxygenation
  - ➤ Poor oxygenation has many etiologies. The etiology should be investigated so that treatment can be instituted.
  - ➤ In general, 3 parameters set on the ventilator can be manipulated to improve hypoxemia due to interstitial lung disease. However, these maneuvers may worsen some causes of hypoxemia (ie, pneumothorax or VSD w/ right-to-left shunt).
    - Increase in FiO2
    - Increase in PEEP
    - Increase in inspiratory time
  - ➤ Alternate maneuvers used to improve oxygenation
    - Recruitment maneuver
      - May help eliminate atelectatic lung & increase functional residual capacity
      - Performed w/ a sustained inspiration of 30–40 cm H2O for 30 seconds
      - Consider the hemodynamic effects of a recruitment maneuver in pts w/ compliant lungs or low intravascular volume prior to instituting one.
      - Current evidence shows recruitment maneuvers produce only short-term improvement in oxygenation, w/o improvement in morbidity or mortality.
    - Prone positioning
      - Has been shown to improve PaO2 in pts w/ adult respiratory distress syndrome (ARDS) w/o mortality benefit

- Given the difficulty that would be associated w/ placing a parturient in the prone position, sandbags can be placed on the chest while supine.
- Inhaled nitric oxide (INO)
  - Concentrations of up to 20 PPM can be used.
  - Current evidence supports the use of INO as a temporary bridge to support oxygenation until lung injury recovers.
  - Outcome data do not show consistent improvement in morbidity or mortality w/ INO.

■ Ventilation
  ➤ Hypoventilation leading to hypercapnia & respiratory acidosis can result from many diseases of the respiratory system. Treatment of the primary pathology, if available, should be initiated.
  ➤ In general, modest hypercapnia (pCO2 <60) & respiratory acidosis (pH >7.20) is tolerated to permit lung-protective ventilation strategies.

■ **Weaning**
  ➤ As the disease process that initiated the need for mechanical ventilation improves, evaluate the pt's need for continued support.
  ➤ Several strategies of weaning ventilator support & extubation have been extensively studied. There is no gold standard for weaning or universally accepted extubation criteria.
  ➤ Most clinicians, based on their level of familiarity & comfort, use either a pressure support wean or spontaneous breathing trials to wean pts from ventilatory support.
  ➤ Consider confounding problems (eg, hemodynamic stability, need for transport for diagnostic studies, continued volume resuscitation or delirium) prior to extubation.

CAVEATS & PEARLS
■ **Auto-PEEP:** In certain clinical scenarios the pressure in the alveolus at the end of expiration may not be equivalent to the pressure measured by the ventilator at the same point in time. The ventilator measures pressure in the expiratory limb. If there is an obstruction to flow btwn the alveolus & the expiratory limb & flow does not stop prior to the next breath, the pressure measured will not reflect that at the alveolus. High levels of unrecognized auto-PEEP can result in impaired triggering of a ventilator, increased work of breathing during assisted ventilation & cardiovascular collapse from decreased venous return.

CHECKLIST

- Confirm appropriate position of endotracheal tube.
- Confirm Pplat < 30 H2O & tidal volume 6–8 mL/kg w/ minimum 5 cm H2O of PEEP.
- Obtain pulse oximetry &/or arterial pO2 to determine adequacy of oxygenation & adjust PEEP & FiO2 as needed.
- Obtain arterial pH & pCO2 to assess adequacy of ventilation & adjust minute ventilation as appropriate.
- Consider use of aerosolized bronchodilators.

MECONIUM

RICHARD ARCHULETA, MD
SANDRA WEINREB, MD

FUNDAMENTAL KNOWLEDGE

Meconium is the first intestinal discharge of the newborn.

- Usually present in fetal GI tract at around 31 weeks of gestation
- Meconium is thick, viscous & greenish & consists of desquamated epithelial cells, bile & mucus.
- Meconium occurs in amniotic fluid in approximately 10–15% of deliveries.
- Meconium is usually passed within the first few hours after birth, always within 48 hours in normal infants.

Meconium-stained amniotic fluid is a risk factor for meconium aspiration & perinatal asphyxia.

STUDIES

- Be aware of signs of intrauterine fetal distress (poor heart rate variability, extremes of heart rate, scalp pH <7.2), which may increase the likelihood of meconium expression into the amniotic fluid.
- At birth, observe amniotic fluid for meconium.
- Observe respiratory efforts after initial airway suctioning.

MANAGEMENT/INTERVENTIONS

- Neonates w/ meconium-stained amniotic fluid should receive airway suctioning (nose, mouth, oropharynx; see "*Routine Newborn Care*") after delivery of the head but before delivery of the shoulders.
- After initial airway suctioning, immediately evaluate neonatal respiratory effort, muscle tone & heart rate.

➤ If neonate is vigorous (strong respiratory efforts, good muscle tone, heart rate >100), continue w/ routine care (see "*Routine Newborn Care*").
➤ If neonate is depressed w/ poor or absent respiratory effort, poor muscle tone or poor color:
  • Delay drying & stimulation to prevent spontaneous aspiration of meconium into lungs.
  • Place neonate in warm environment (ie, radiant warmer).
  • Perform laryngoscopy (Miller 0 for premature neonate, Miller 1 for term infant), examine hypopharynx & suction residual meconium in hypopharynx.
  • Intubate & apply suction to the endotracheal tube (2.5–3.0 mm for premature neonate, 3.5 mm for term infant) w/ meconium aspirator as it is withdrawn from the trachea.
    • Use negative pressure <100 mm Hg.
    • Repeat intubation & suction until little meconium remains or neonatal heart rate/oxygen saturation drops, necessitating further resuscitation.
  • Perform resuscitation as needed (see "Resuscitation of the Neonate").
    • When the neonate has good oxygenation & heart rate >100, gently pass orogastric tube to empty the stomach of meconium & reduce the potential for future meconium aspiration.

CAVEATS & PEARLS
■ Meconium passage is usually delayed in low-weight infants (especially in those <1,500 g).
■ 20–30% of neonates w/ meconium-stained amniotic fluid will have meconium in their trachea despite initial suctioning & the absence of spontaneous respirations.
■ Positive-pressure ventilation may be necessary before the trachea is cleared of all meconium.
  ➤ Neonate may begin to become hypoxic before all meconium can be suctioned & require PPV.
  ➤ Neonate may become bradycardic in response to deep suctioning & require PPV.

CHECKLIST
Observe delivery of neonate for meconium-stained amniotic fluid & vigorousness of neonate.

- If neonate is vigorous (strong respiratory efforts, good muscle tone, heart rate >100), continue w/ routine care.
- If neonate is depressed:
  - ➤ Delay drying & stimulation of neonate.
  - ➤ Perform laryngoscopy & suction hypopharynx of meconium.
  - ➤ Intubate trachea & withdraw w/ suction repeatedly until either little meconium remains or neonatal heart rate/oxygenation necessitates further resuscitation.
  - ➤ Perform resuscitation as needed (see *"Resuscitation of the Neonate"*).

MERALGIA PARESTHETICA

MEREDITH ALBRECHT, MD; LISA LEFFERT, MD; AND MICHELE SZABO, MD

FUNDAMENTAL KNOWLEDGE

Definition
- Compression of the lateral femoral cutaneous nerve

Epidemiology
- 4.3 per 10,000 person-years
- Associated w/ carpal tunnel & pregnancy

Pathophysiology
- Entrapment of the lateral femoral cutaneous nerve as it passes around the anterior superior iliac spine or through the inguinal ligament
- Obesity & exaggerated lordosis of pregnancy may increase the stretch on the nerve, predisposing it to compression/entrapment.

Clinical Manifestations
- Pain & numbness in the lateral aspect of the thigh
- No motor weakness
- Symptoms typically present after the 1st trimester.
- Symptoms remit spontaneously after the pregnancy is completed (within 3 months).
- May occur as a post-partum neurapraxia

Effect of Pregnancy on Meralgia Paresthetica
- Associated w/ an increased incidence

Effect of Meralgia Paresthetica on Pregnancy & the Fetus
- No effect on pregnancy or fetus

STUDIES

History & Physical
- Careful neurologic exam
- Pain & numbness in distribution of the lateral femoral cutaneous nerve
- No motor weakness

Laboratory
- None

Imaging
- None

MANAGEMENT/INTERVENTIONS

Medical Treatment
- Conservative therapy
  - ➤ Minimize periods of standing.
  - ➤ Eliminate tight clothing.
  - ➤ Oral analgesics
- In severe cases surgery may be necessary.

Anesthesia
- Regional anesthesia does not alter disease course.

CAVEATS & PEARLS
- Compression of the lateral femoral cutaneous nerve
- Pain & numbness in distribution of the lateral femoral cutaneous nerve
- No motor weakness
- May occur as a post-partum neurapraxia

CHECKLIST
- Careful physical exam to document neurologic deficits

MITRAL REGURGITATION

MATTHEW CIRIGLIANO, MD
DWIGHT GEHA, MD

FUNDAMENTAL KNOWLEDGE
The major causes of mitral regurgitation (MR) are mitral valve prolapse, rheumatic heart disease, infective endocarditis, collagen vascular disease, cardiomyopathy & ischemic heart disease.

■ In surgical series, mitral valve prolapse is the most common cause of MR. In the parturient, the most common cause of MR is mitral valve prolapse. In general, MR is well tolerated in pregnancy.

The mitral valve apparatus consists of the mitral annulus, anterior leaflet, posterior leaflet, chordae tendineae, the papillary muscles & the supporting L ventricle, L atrium & aortic walls; MR may result when any of these structures are altered structurally or functionally.

■ With MR, the L atrium dilates to compensate for increased regurgitant volume from the L ventricle. Depending on the time course, the L atrium may dilate sufficiently to accommodate the extra volume without an increase in L atrial pressure. With acute MR or in the presence of chronic MR a dramatic increase in intravascular volume or systemic vascular resistance (SVR), the L atrium does not dilate sufficiently & increased L atrial pressures & possibly pulmonary edema may result.

■ In the pregnant woman w/ MR, the L atrium may overdistend as blood is introduced into this chamber from both the pulmonary veins & the L ventricle during the cardiac cycle. The problem of L atrial volume overload is made worse during pregnancy, as the blood volume increases. Blood volume increases by 30–50% due to increases in plasma volume in response to progesterone & due to increased red cell mass production. Immediately after delivery, the maternal blood volume increases acutely. The uterus contracts & returns uterine blood to the systemic circulation. The vena cava decompresses, facilitating venous return.

■ The problem of L atrial volume overload in some ways is compensated during pregnancy. The heart rate increases during pregnancy. An increased heart rate decreases time spent in systole for each given contraction, thus decreasing the time for regurgitant blood flow from the left ventricle into the L atrium. During pregnancy, the resting heart rate increases by 10–20 bpm. The SVR decreases during pregnancy, facilitating forward flow of blood out of the L ventricle instead of back into the L atrium.

■ As the L atrium overdistends w/ blood, problems can manifest in the lung. An acute increase in blood volume into the L atrium will transmit pressure back into the lungs due to the poor compliance of this chamber. Increased postcapillary pressure in the lung will lead to extravasation of fluid, manifesting as pulmonary edema & dyspnea. As the L atrium overdistends w/ blood, problems will manifest in the pulmonary circulation & R ventricle. In the chronic setting, the L atrium may dilate, but L atrial & consequently pulmonary artery pressure will increase. Increased pulmonary artery pressure leads to compensatory R ventricular hypertrophy. Increased pulmonary artery pressure will limit the ability of the body to compensate for changes in cardiac output & SVR w/ a change in pulmonary vascular resistance. As the L atrium overdistends, problems will manifest w/ the L atrium.

■ Patients w/ L atrial dilation are prone to atrial fib. Pts w/ atrial fib have decreased ability to empty the L atrium due to loss of a coordinated atrial contraction at the end of diastole.

■ The L ventricle may or may not be affected, depending on the progression of the disease. Early in the disease, the L ventricular wall stress & pressure remain normal. Late in the disease, the L ventricle may dilate & hypertrophy.

■ In the setting of MR, there may be inadequate cardiac output. During systole, a portion of the stroke volume does not enter the systemic circulation; rather, it enters the L atrium. Decreased ventricular filling (venous return) yields a smaller cardiac output. A smaller cardiac output may be insufficient for the parturient or the fetus: cardiac output on average increases by 50% during pregnancy to satisfy increased metabolic demands.

STUDIES

Several sources of information or studies may be used to arrive at a diagnosis of MR.

■ A history of symptoms consistent w/ L atrial volume overload causing pulmonary edema suggests that a pt may have valvular disease. The pt may report dyspnea, hemoptysis, chest pain, weakness & fatigue secondary to a low cardiac output. Auscultation may reveal evidence of MR: MR produces a systolic murmur that radiates to the axilla. The murmur is holosystolic. A widely split S2 may occur.

■ EKG may reveal evidence of a volume-overloaded L atrium & L ventricle.

➤ Atrial enlargement, characterized by:
  • A wide P wave in lead II that lasts >0.12 seconds
  • Deeply inverted terminal component in lead V_1
  • Notched, slurred P waves in leads I, II

➤ Consistent w/ an enlarged L atrium, EKG may reveal atrial fib.

➤ Late in the disease the EKG may reveal evidence of L ventricular hypertrophy from dilatation & volume overload: L axis deviation, increased QRS voltage. Voltage criteria for L ventricular hypertrophy include R wave in AVL >12 mm; R wave in I >15 mm; sum of S wave in V_1 or V_2 plus R wave in V5 or V_6 equal to or greater than 35 mm.

➤ Consistent w/ elevated pulmonary artery pressures, EKG may show R ventricular hypertrophy late in disease, which is characterized by tall R waves in V_1 though V_3; deep S waves in leads I, L, V_5 & V_6; R axis deviation.

■ Chest x-ray may reveal pulmonary edema, enlarged L atrium, cardiomegaly.

■ Echocardiography is the best study for evaluating & characterizing mitral regurgitation. The lesion can be examined in real time. The severity of mitral regurgitation can be assessed. Valve leaflet morphology can be evaluated. Mechanisms of mitral regurgitation can be determined.

➤ Echocardiography is indicated when a diastolic murmur is auscultated, when a continuous murmur is auscultated, when a loud systolic murmur is auscultated, when the murmur is associated w/ symptoms & when the murmur is associated w/ an abnormal ECG.

■ A pulmonary artery catheter may reveal a prominent V wave w/ a wide pulse pressure in severe MR.

Echocardiographic & angiographic criteria for evaluating the severity of MR are varied but well defined. Nonetheless, it is difficult to offer prognostic information for the parturient w/ MR based on diagnostic studies; MR can have a long, slow progression w/ only symptoms of fatigue until symptoms of failure w/ CHF & low cardiac output develop. At that point, irreversible L ventricular dysfunction will have developed.

■ The American College of Cardiology & American Heart Association have classified maternal & fetal risk during pregnancy based on the type of valvular abnormality in conjunction w/ the New York Heart Association functional class

➤ NYNA functional classification for congestive heart failure:

• Class I: Pts have no limitation of activities, no symptoms from ordinary activities

• Class II: Pts have slight, mild limitation of activity; pts are comfortable w/ mild exertion.

• Class III: Pts have marked limitation of activity & are comfortable only at rest.

• Class IV: Pts should be at complete rest, confined to bed; any physical activity brings discomfort; symptoms occur at rest.

➤ Associated w/ a low maternal & fetal risk: MR in the setting of NYHA class I or II symptoms w/ normal L ventricular function

➤ Associated w/ a high maternal & fetal risk: MR in the setting of NYHA class III or IV symptoms; MR in the setting of severe pulmonary hypertension; MR in the setting of reduced L ventricular function (estimated ejection fraction <40%).

■ Angiographic & echocardiographic descriptors of the degree of backflow across the mitral valve provide the definition of severe MR.

➤ Pts w/ severe symptomatic MR have a poor outcome, w/ an average mortality rate of 5% per year.

➤ Poor outcome for severe MR in the long term (years), but the physiologic changes associated w/ pregnancy may allow the parturient to do well in the short term.

MANAGEMENT/INTERVENTIONS

Medical mgt

■ Time course for evaluation by a cardiologist:

➤ During pregnancy, women w/ valvular heart disease should be evaluated once each trimester for presence or worsening of symptoms & if there is a change in symptoms to assess for any deterioration in maternal cardiac status.

➤ The American College of Cardiology & American Heart Association recommend that women w/ high-risk cardiac lesions undergo full evaluation prior to & during pregnancy.

■ During the antepartum period, treatment goals for the pt w/ mild or moderate symptoms focus on:

• Treatment of volume overload to avoid or treat pulmonary edema: diuretic therapy w/ a loop or thiazide diuretic while avoiding hypovolemia & uteroplacental hypoperfusion; avoidance of excessive salt, which will increase intravascular volume

➤ Avoid bradycardia. An increase in diastolic time will increase L ventricular filling & thus the regurgitant volume per cardiac cycle.

• Atrial fib should be aggressively treated as the loss of the atrial contraction will decrease atrial emptying & may lead to pulmonary congestion.

• Atrial fib w/ hemodynamic instability and/or pulmonary edema requires cardioversion.

• Atrial fib w/o hemodynamic instability should be rate-controlled pharmacologically. Beta blockers are safe for use in pregnancy. Digoxin depresses atrioventricular conduction & thus an excessively high ventricular rate & is safe for use in pregnancy. Calcium channel blockers block activated & inactivated calcium channels in the sinoatrial & atrioventricular node. Peripheral vasodilation is a side effect. Calcium channel blockers are safe for use in pregnancy. Cardioversion often is performed when pharmacologic therapy fails to control the ventricular response to atrial fib.

- Medications that have a suppressive effect on atrial fib may be prescribed to the parturient in the antepartum period.

  Procainamide, a sodium channel blocking drug (class I), may cause direct myocardial depression & may cause reduced peripheral vascular resistance. It is safe for use in pregnancy.

  Quinidine, a sodium channel blocking drug (class I), depresses pacemaker rate, including ectopic pacemaker. It depresses conduction & excitability & has alpha receptor blocking properties & may cause vasodilatation & a reflex increase in sinoatrial node rate. It is safe for use in pregnancy.

  Amiodarone, a blocker of sodium, potassium & calcium channels, suppresses supraventricular & ventricular arrhythmias. It may cause peripheral vascular dilation through alpha-blocking effects & may cause bradycardia. It is *not* safe for use in pregnancy because it is associated w/ IUGR, prematurity, fetal hypothyroidism.

- Patients in atrial fib will need to be anticoagulated. When the onset of atrial fib cannot be determined, the pt should not be cardioverted until she has been anticoagulated for a sufficient period of time as determined by her cardiologist (unless she is hemodynamically unstable).

- All parturients are at increased risk of thromboembolic disease; the parturient w/ MR is at even greater risk. Pts may be taking anticoagulant medication during the antepartum period. Atrial fib increases the risk of thromboembolic disease still further.

During the antepartum period, pts may undergo surgical correction of their regurgitant mitral valve if they are symptomatic.

- ■ Valve repair is preferred to valve replacement for pts w/ MR:
  - ➤ Superior hemodynamics & ventricular function
  - ➤ Avoids need for long-term anticoagulation
  - ➤ Valve repair feasibility is highest in pts w/ mitral valve prolapse
  - ➤ Valve repair has significantly better long-term outcome.
- ■ In pts w/ symptomatic MR w/o severe L ventricular dysfunction, surgical intervention is indicated.
- ■ In asymptomatic pts w/ MR, surgical intervention should be performed before the onset of irreversible ventricular dysfunction. No randomized trials have assessed optimal timing for non-pregnant

pts. Onset of irreversible ventricular dysfunction is likely to be some time long after delivery for the parturient.

Obstetric concerns for the mgt of the pt w/ MR in the peripartum period are as follows:

- Vaginal delivery should proceed w/ invasive hemodynamic monitoring if the pt has had severe symptomatic MR during pregnancy

  During the second stage of labor, the obstetric goal is to avoid maneuvers that worsen MR symptoms. Valsalva maneuver may result in sudden increase in SVR & is thus avoided. The obstetrician usually discourages maternal expulsive efforts during the second stage of labor to avoid Valsalva. Uterine contractions will facilitate fetal descent. The parturient should avoid pushing. Low forceps and vacuum extraction are techniques used to facilitate delivery after fetal descent.

- C-section is performed only when there are obstetrical indications for such a mode of delivery.

- The American College of Cardiology/American Heart Association guidelines for the mgt of pts w/ valvular heart disease recommend that antibiotic prophylaxis be provided for pts w/ MR to prevent endocarditis. Recommendations are that antibiotic prophylaxis be provided for dental procedures & certain respiratory, GI & GU procedures (listed in the ACC/AHA guidelines). Antibiotic prophylaxis for endocarditis is not recommended for routine vaginal delivery or for C-section.

The goals of anesthetic mgt are the same as during the antepartum period: Avoid conditions that exacerbate MR & facilitate conditions that improve the symptoms of MR.

- Maintain a normal to increased heart rate to decrease diastolic time. This will decrease the time during systole for regurgitation into the L atrium. This will decrease the available stroke volume per cardiac cycle available for regurgitation into the L atrium.

- Administer agents that have a favorable side effect profile & avoid agents with an unfavorable side effect profile in relation to heart rate (ephedrine preferred to phenylephrine, meperidine may be the preferred opioid; although ketamine is not associated w/ bradycardia, it is associated w/ increased SVR & as such would not offer a favorable side effect profile).

- Aggressively treat atrial fib (maintain normal sinus rhythm). Cardioversion is always indicated if new-onset atrial fib causes hemodynamic instability. Treat a rapid ventricular rate: IV beta blockers, IV calcium channel blockers, IV digoxin.

■ Maintain cardiac output. Maintain a normal to increased heart rate to avoid L atrial volume overload. Maintain venous return. Avoid compression of the inferior vena cava w/ the uterus; maintain left uterine displacement. Avoid insufficient intravascular volume while avoiding volume overload. If a central venous catheter is in situ, optimize the central venous pressure to allow for sufficient systolic BP while avoiding pulmonary edema. If a pulmonary artery catheter is in situ, optimize pulmonary capillary wedge pressure to maximize cardiac output while avoiding pulmonary edema. Avoid an increase in pulmonary vascular resistance: avoid pain, hypoxia, hypercarbia, acidosis. Boluses of oxytocin, methylergonovine & 15 methyl prostaglandin F2-alpha may result in increased pulmonary vascular resistance.

➤ Maintain a decreased afterload. An increase in SVR may increase the regurgitant fraction. An increase in SVR may decrease cardiac output. The decreased SVR associated w/ pregnancy benefits patients w/ this lesion. Avoid uterine compression of the aorta, as this will increase SVR. Neuraxial analgesia/anesthesia will provide a decrease in SVR & is well tolerated by pts w/ this lesion. Neuraxial analgesia/anesthesia may prevent increases in SVR associated w/ pain. Neuraxial techniques promote forward flow of blood & thus may decrease pulmonary congestion

• General anesthesia w/ a volatile agent will provide a decrease in SVR & is well tolerated by the parturient w/ MR. Isoflurane & sevoflurane decrease SVR the most of the volatile agents.

• Halothane produces myocardial depression much more than a decrease in SVR & is a poor choice if other volatile agents are available.

• Pharmacologic agents may be necessary to decrease SVR: sodium nitroprusside; hydralazine (dilates arterioles & not veins; reflex increase in heart rate is a favorable side effect for the parturient w/ MR); nitroglycerin (use w/ caution as this agent may promote uterine relaxation).

• Avoid ACE inhibitors until after delivery as they cause renal damage in the fetus during all trimesters, esp. the second & the third.

■ Avoid pulmonary congestion. Maintain a normal to increased heart rate. Maintain cardiac output. Treat volume overload. Pt may be taking diuretics; missed doses may lead to volume overload. During labor, SVR may increase due to pain, which will impede forward blood flow. Treat the pain of labor: epidural analgesia will decrease pain as well as SVR; IV opioids; intrathecal opioids. Increase the venous capacitance when indicated. Immediately after delivery, intravascular volume increases dramatically as the uterus contracts; the heart may be unable to accommodate the large increase in blood volume. Immediately after delivery, compression on the inferior vena cava decreases, which facilitates venous return. Vasodilators will facilitate the accommodation of the mobilized blood volume: nitroprusside, epidurally administered local anesthetics, hydralazine, nitroglycerin (use w/ caution, causes myometrial relaxation). Blood loss during vaginal delivery & C-section may be efficacious for treating pulmonary congestion. Blood loss during vaginal delivery is typically 300–400 cc; blood loss during C-section is typically 800 to 1,000 cc.

CAVEATS/PEARLS

- MR is usually well tolerated by the parturient. The increased heart rate & the decreased SVR that accompany pregnancy are favorable to the patient w/ MR
- Early administration of epidural analgesia during labor prevents a pain-mediated increase in SVR, which may exacerbate MR.
- The obstetrician usually discourages maternal expulsive efforts during the second stage of labor to avoid Valsalva & its associated increase in SVR.
- Hydralazine is an excellent choice for afterload reduction, as it is associated w/ an increase in heart rate, which may benefit the pt w/ MR.
- Avoid ACE inhibitors for afterload reduction until after delivery, as they are associated w/ several adverse fetal effects.
- Nitroglycerin will provide afterload reduction but may cause deleterious uterine relaxation.

CHECKLIST

- Ascertain if the pt has had symptoms of pulmonary congestion or heart failure during pregnancy.
- Review meds that the pt may be taking for rate control, atrial fib suppressive therapy & symptoms of heart failure.
- Obtain echocardiographic data to characterize MR severity if there has been a significant change in the pt's symptoms.
- Pt is high risk if she has MR w/ New York Heart Association class III or IV symptoms; mitral valve disease resulting in pulmonary

hypertension; or mitral valve disease w/ L ventricular systolic dysfunction.

■ Women who are at high risk should have invasive monitoring during labor & delivery, as this is the period w/ the greatest magnitude in change w/ regard to hemodynamics.

■ If GU procedures are to be performed other than routine vaginal delivery or C-section, administer prophylactic antibiotics to prevent endocarditis from bacteremia.

■ C-section is performed only when there are obstetrical indications for such a mode of delivery.

■ During anesthetic mgt, maintain normal to increased heart rate to avoid L atrial volume overload. Maintain venous return. Maintain a decreased afterload. Consider epidural labor analgesia for vaginal delivery. Consider epidural anesthesia for cesarean delivery. Consider isoflurane, sevoflurane & desflurane rather than halothane for general anesthesia. Consider vasodilators as necessary, but avoid ACE inhibitors.

MITRAL STENOSIS

MATTHEW CIRIGLIANO, MD
DWIGHT GEHA, MD

FUNDAMENTAL KNOWLEDGE
Mitral stenosis (MS) is the most common valvular lesion of significance in pregnant women.

■ MS is most commonly due to rheumatic heart disease.

➤ For those w/ a history of rheumatic heart disease, MS is the most common lesion.

➤ Roughly 90% of pregnant women w/ a history of rheumatic heart disease have this lesion.

• In developed countries the incidence of rheumatic heart disease has decreased; as such, it is an uncommon problem in the U.S.

• Some believe the decreased incidence is due to the effect of improved socioeconomic conditions. Others point to the change in the prevalence of the hemolytic streptococcal pathogen.

• In Asia & Africa, MS due to rheumatic heart disease is still a common problem.

- Other causes of MS include congenital abnormalities & endocarditis.

A stenotic mitral valve due to anatomic distortion alters the normal physiology of the parturient.

■ The mitral valve diseased by rheumatic heart disease is anatomically distorted.
  ➣ The valve may be fused along the edges of the cusps, creating a "fish-mouth valve," or along the commissures.
  ➣ The chordae tendineae may be fused. Calcium may accumulate on the leaflets, cusps & annulus.

■ Multiple variations of valve morphology may exist, but the end result is the same: a decreased valve area. A normal valve area at the valve orifice is 4–6 cm^2. Symptoms often develop when the orifice area decreases to 2 cm^2 or less. When the orifice area approaches 1 cm^2, MS is characterized as severe.

■ A stenotic mitral valve may prevent the heart from providing an adequate cardiac output. A stenotic mitral valve may impede filling of the L ventricle by offering a smaller orifice for egress of blood from the L atrium into the L ventricle during diastole. Decreased ventricular filling yields a smaller stroke volume. Decreased ventricular filling (venous return) yields a lower cardiac output.

■ A reduced cardiac output may be insufficient for the parturient, as it has been well studied that in pregnant women w/ normal heart valves, cardiac output will increase by 40–50% to satisfy increased metabolic demands. In women w/ normal cardiac physiology, the cardiac output is often increased above the pre-labor flow during labor & delivery.

■ A stenotic valve prevents emptying of the L atrium by offering a smaller orifice for blood to egress from the L atrium into the L ventricle during diastole. The problem of inadequate L atrial emptying is made worse during pregnancy as the blood volume increases. Blood volume increases by 30–50% due to increases in plasma volume & increased red cell mass. The maternal blood volume increases acutely immediately after delivery. Immediately after delivery the uterus contracts & returns uterine blood to the systemic circulation. The vena cava decompresses, facilitating venous return.

■ The problem of inadequate L atrial emptying is made worse during pregnancy as the heart rate increases. During pregnancy, the resting heart rate increases by 10–20 bpm. As heart rate increases, time spent in diastole decreases, thus decreasing time for egress of blood into the ventricle.

■ As the L atrium overdistends w/ blood, the increased L atrial pressure will eventually be manifested in the lung. An increase in blood volume into the L atrium will transmit pressure back into the lungs due to the poor compliance of this heart chamber. Increased postcapillary pressure in the lung causes extravasation of fluid, which manifests as pulmonary edema, dyspnea & hemoptysis.

■ As the L atrium overdistends w/ blood, problems will manifest in the pulmonary circulation & the R ventricle. In the chronic setting, the L atrium dilates & L atrial & pulmonary artery pressures increase. Increased pulmonary artery pressures lead to compensatory R ventricular hypertrophy & enlargement. Increased pulmonary artery pressures will limit the ability of the body to compensate for changes in cardiac output & systemic vascular resistance by altering pulmonary vascular resistance.

■ As the L atrium overdistends, problems will manifest w/ the L atrium. Pts w/ L atrial dilation are prone to atrial fibrillation. Pts w/ atrial fib have decreased ability to empty the L atrium of its volume load due to loss of a coordinated atrial contraction at the end of diastole.

STUDIES

History, physical exam and laboratory studies are used to arrive at a diagnosis of MS.

■ A history of symptoms consistent w/ L atrial volume overload causing pulmonary edema suggests that a pt may have valvular disease.

➤ Pts may report dyspnea or orthopnea. Pts may report hemoptysis (occurs secondary to rupture of dilated bronchial veins), blood-tinged sputum secondary to pulmonary edema. Pts may report chest pain. In roughly 25% of parturients w/ MS, pregnancy will unmask the lesion by eliciting symptoms. A severely dilated L atrium may lead to hoarseness (Ortner's syndrome) as the L recurrent laryngeal nerve is compressed.

■ Auscultation may reveal evidence of MS.

➤ MS produces a diastolic murmur. One may hear a loud S_1 secondary to quick closure of valve leaflets at the end of diastole. One may auscultate an opening snap: The opening snap is characterized as high-pitched. The snap occurs immediately after S_2 due to abrupt mitral valve opening. One may note an audible S_4.

■ EKG reveals evidence of a volume-overloaded L atrium.

➤ Atrial enlargement may be noted.

• There may be a wide P wave in lead II that lasts >0.12 seconds.

- There may be a deeply inverted terminal component in lead V_1
➤ Atrial fibrillation
➤ R ventricular hypertrophy, which is characterized by:
  - Tall R waves in V_1 though V_3
  - Deep S waves in leads I, L, V_5 & V_6
  - Right axis deviation
■ Chest x-ray may reveal L atrial enlargement, pulmonary edema.
■ Echocardiography is the best tool for evaluating & characterizing MS.
  ➤ The lesion can be examined in real-time & valve morphology can be examined. The valve area can be calculated for prognostication. A transmitral valve gradient can be measured for prognostication.
  ➤ Echocardiography is indicated when a diastolic murmur is auscultated, a continuous murmur is auscultated, a loud systolic murmur is auscultated, the murmur is associated w/ symptoms or the murmur is associated w/ an abnormal EKG.

Several sources of information or studies may be used to offer a prognosis for how the pregnant pt w/ MS will fare.
■ The presence & severity of symptoms associated w/ MS offer information on how the parturient may fare during her pregnancy.
  ➤ Clark et al. reported a mortality rate <1% in parturients who had minimal symptoms associated w/ MS in their study of labor & delivery in the presence of MS.
  ➤ Pts who have had a previous episode of pulmonary congestion are believed to be at increased risk for cardiac complications during pregnancy.
    - The parturient will be at increased risk for pulmonary edema during pregnancy.
    - She runs a higher risk of mortality during or after pregnancy, w/ the greatest risk of maternal death during labor & the postpartum period.
  ➤ The American College of Cardiology & American Heart Association have classified maternal & fetal risk during pregnancy based on the type of valvular abnormality in conjunction w/ the New York Heart Association functional class.
    - NYHA functional classification for congestive heart failure
      - Class I: Pts have no limitation of activities & no symptoms from ordinary activities.
      - Class II: Pts are comfortable w/ mild exertion.

- Class III: Pts have marked limitation of activity; they are comfortable only at rest.
- Class IV: Any physical activity brings discomfort; symptoms occur at rest.
- Associated w/ a low maternal & fetal risk: mild to moderate MS (mitral valve area >1.5 cm^2 w/ a gradient <5 mmHg) w/ NYHA class I symptoms
- Associated w/ a high maternal & fetal risk: MS w/ NYHA class II, III or IV symptoms
- Most pts w/ moderate to severe MS exhibit a worsening of 1 or 2 classes in NYHA functional status during pregnancy.

➤ Silversides et al. found that symptom presence prior to pregnancy had little to do w/ risk of cardiac complications (defined as pulmonary edema, arrhythmia, chest pain) during pregnancy in a study of 80 parturients w/ MS secondary to rheumatic heart disease. Asymptomatic parturients had a complication rate of 35%. Symptomatic parturients had a complication rate of 33%. These findings suggest that the absence of symptoms in a pt w/ MS diagnosed prior to pregnancy does not necessarily categorize that patient as low risk, in contrast to the study by Clark et al.

■ The valve area associated w/ MS may provide prognostic information; as such, it should be determined via echocardiography.

➤ The American College of Cardiology & American Heart Association define the severity of MS according to valve area as determined by echocardiography:
- Mild: Valve area >1.5 cm^2
- Moderate: Valve area 1.0–1.5 cm^2
- Severe: Valve area <1.0 cm^2

➤ In a study of 80 parturients w/ MS secondary to rheumatic heart disease, Silversides et al. reported that moderate or severe MS, as determined at the time of the first antenatal echocardiogram, is an independent predictor of cardiac complications.
- Odds ratio of 3.4 (95% confidence interval 1.2–10.0)
- Cardiac complication defined as pulmonary edema, arrhythmia, chest pain

➤ In the same study by Silversides et al., the severity of stenosis as defined by American College of Cardiology/American Heart Association guidelines was directly proportional to the rate of cardiac complications. Mild MS had a cardiac complication rate of 26% (11/42 parturients). Moderate MS had a cardiac complication orate of 38% (11/29 parturients). Severe MS had a cardiac complication rate of 67% (6/9 parturients).

➤ Barbosa et al. noted that a mitral valve area of <1.5 cm^2 & an abnormal functional class prior to pregnancy was a predictor for adverse outcome.

MANAGEMENT/INTERVENTIONS

Medical mgt

■ Time course for evaluation by a cardiologist
  ➤ During pregnancy, women w/ valvular heart disease should be evaluated:
    • Once each trimester for presence or worsening of symptoms
    • If there is a change in symptoms to assess for any deterioration in maternal cardiac status
  ➤ American College of Cardiology & American Heart Association recommend that women w/ high-risk cardiac lesions undergo full evaluation prior to & during pregnancy (this includes MS).
■ During the antepartum period, treatment goals for the patient w/ mild or moderate symptoms focus on:
  ➤ Treatment of volume overload to avoid or treat pulmonary edema
    • Reduction of physical activity to limit increases in heart rate & systemic vascular resistance that accompany catecholamine release
    • Avoidance of excessive salt, which will increase intravascular volume
    • Careful use of diuretic therapy w/ a loop diuretic or thiazide diuretics Aggressive diuretic therapy can cause hypovolemia & reduced uteroplacental perfusion
  ➤ Achieving an increase in diastolic time to increase L atrial emptying
    • Beta blockers are prescribed to decrease heart rate, which increases the diastolic time interval for each cardiac cycle.
      • In a study in the *American Journal of Obstetrics & Gynecology*, Kasab et al. studied the effects of propranolol & atenolol in the parturient. This study showed a decreased incidence of maternal pulmonary edema w/ beta-blocker therapy. The study did not show adverse effects on the fetus or neonate.
    • Atrial fib w/ rapid ventricular rate should be aggressively treated, as an increased heart rate will limit diastolic time & L atrial emptying.

- Atrial fib w/ hemodynamic instability and/or pulmonary edema requires cardioversion.
- Atrial fib w/o hemodynamic instability should be rate-controlled pharmacologically.
  - Beta blockers have antiarrhythmic properties by their beta receptor-blocking action & direct membrane effects. Digoxin has a cardioselective vagomimetic effect that depresses atrioventricular conduction & thus an excessively high ventricular rate. Digoxin increases inotropy, which may improve symptoms of heart failure. Digoxin is safe for use during pregnancy. Calcium channel blockers block activated & inactivated calcium channels in the sinoatrial & atrioventricular node; peripheral vasodilation is a side effect. Calcium channel blockers are safe for use during pregnancy.
  - Cardioversion often is performed when pharmacologic therapy fails to control the ventricular response to atrial fib.
- Meds that have a suppressive effect on atrial fib may be prescribed to the parturient in the antepartum period.
  - Procainamide is a sodium channel blocking drug (class I) that may cause direct myocardial depression & may cause reduced peripheral vascular resistance. It is safe for use during pregnancy.
  - Quinidine is a sodium channel blocking drug (class I) that decreases the pacemaker rate & decreases conduction & excitability. It has alpha receptor-blocking properties & may cause vasodilatation & a reflex increase in sinoatrial node rate. It is safe for use during pregnancy.
  - Amiodarone is a blocker of sodium, potassium & calcium channels. It suppresses supraventricular & ventricular arrhythmias. It may cause peripheral vascular dilation through alpha-blocking effects & may cause bradycardia. It is *not* listed as safe for use in pregnancy due to risk of hypothyroidism in the fetus as well as IUGR & prematurity.
- Pts in atrial fib need to be anticoagulated.
- When the onset of atrial fib cannot be determined, the pt should not undergo cardioversion until she has been anticoagulated for a sufficient period of time as determined by her cardiologist (unless she is hemodynamically unstable);

TEE-guided cardioversion can be attempted if the onset of atrial fib is within 48 hrs.

- The parturient w/ MS is at increased risk of thromboembolic disease. Pts may be taking anticoagulant medication during the antepartum period.

■ During the antepartum period, pts may undergo surgical correction or palliation of their stenotic mitral valve.

➤ Surgery is recommended if significant MS is recognized before pregnancy (NYHA class II or greater, valve area < 1.5 cm^2).

- Parturients who undergo surgical correction of significant MS prior to pregnancy appear to tolerate pregnancy w/ fewer complications than similar women treated medically. The ideal time for surgery is during the second trimester. The mitral valve may be replaced or repaired or a commissurotomy performed.

➤ Mitral commissurotomy is preferred to valve replacement.

- The ideal time for this procedure is during the second trimester, though severe symptoms should prompt this procedure no matter the gestational age of the fetus. Commissurotomy will delay the progression of MS but will not cure the disease. Maternal outcomes parallel those of nonpregnant women who have mitral valve surgery, but fetal loss is significant. In a study by Bernal et al., fetal loss ranged from 10% to 30% during/after cardiac surgery w/ cardiopulmonary bypass. Becker et al. examined the outcomes of 101 closed mitral commissurotomies during pregnancy; no maternal deaths were noted but 3 fetal demises occurred.
- Closed mitral commissurotomy is associated w/ only minimal risk to the fetus.

➤ Mitral balloon valvuloplasty is an alternative procedure to valve repair, replacement, or closed commissurotomy.

- Mitral balloon valvuloplasty avoids open-chest surgery as well as the risks of anesthesia & surgery for both mother & fetus. This procedure is palliative: it serves as a bridge to eventual repair after delivery. It provides a delay in the progression of MS. It usually is performed during the second trimester, though it can be performed at any time if symptoms are severe. This procedure has been associated w/ normal subsequent deliveries w/ excellent fetal outcomes.
  - Exposure of fetus to radiation is a risk. To limit the exposure to radiation, this procedure has been performed under guidance of transesophageal echocardiography.

- Case reports have shown marked improvement in the mitral valve area. Onderoglu et al. reported two cases involving mitral balloon valvuloplasty for parturients w/ severe MS. One case showed an improvement in valve area from 0.9 cm^2 to 2.3 cm^2 w/ a decrease in gradient from 18 mm Hg to 3 mm Hg. In another case, the valve area increased from 1.1 cm^2 to 2.1 cm^2 w/ no complications.

■ Obstetric concerns for the mgt of the pt w/ mitral valve disease in the peripartum period are as follows:

➤ Vaginal delivery should proceed w/ invasive hemodynamic monitoring if the pt has had symptomatic MS during pregnancy.

➤ During the second stage of labor, the obstetric goal is to avoid maneuvers that worsen MS symptoms. The Valsalva maneuver may increase venous return & should be avoided. Maternal expulsive efforts during the second stage of labor are discouraged so as to avoid Valsalva. Uterine contractions will facilitate fetal descent. The parturient should avoid pushing. Low forceps and vacuum extraction are techniques used to facilitate delivery after fetal descent.

➤ C-section is performed only when there are obstetrical indications for such a mode of delivery.

➤ The American College of Cardiology/American Heart Association guidelines for the mgt of pts w/ valvular heart disease recommend that antibiotic prophylaxis be provided for MS pts to prevent endocarditis.

  - Recommendations are that antibiotic prophylaxis be provided for dental procedures & certain respiratory, GI & GU procedures; a list is given in the ACC/AHA guidelines.
  - Antibiotic prophylaxis for endocarditis is not recommended for routine vaginal delivery or C-section.

■ The goals of anesthetic mgt are the same as during the antepartum period: Avoid conditions that exacerbate MS symptoms & facilitate conditions that improve MS symptoms.

➤ Maintain a normal to slow heart rate to increase diastolic time. This will facilitate L atrial emptying & L ventricular filling.

➤ Administer agents to decrease heart rate when indicated (beta blockers, calcium channel blockers). With regard to heart rate, administer agents that have a favorable side effect profile & avoid agents with unfavorable side effects (phenylephrine instead of ephedrine; milrinone instead of dopamine or dobutamine; succinylcholine instead of pancuronium; opioids instead of ketamine; avoid atropine, glycopyrrolate, meperidine).

- Aggressively treat atrial fib (maintain normal sinus rhythm). Cardioversion is always indicated if new-onset atrial fib causes hemodynamic instability. Treat rapid ventricular rate: IV beta blockers, IV calcium channel blockers; IV digoxin.

➤ Maintain cardiac output. Maintain normal to slow heart rate to optimize ventricular filling (see above). Maintain venous return. Avoid aortocaval compression. Avoid insufficient intravascular volume while avoiding volume overload. If a central venous catheter is in situ, optimize central venous pressure to allow for sufficient systolic BP while avoiding pulmonary edema. If a pulmonary artery catheter is in situ, optimize pulmonary capillary wedge pressure to maximize cardiac output while avoiding pulmonary edema. Avoid an increase in pulmonary vascular resistance. Avoid pain, hypoxia, hypercarbia, acidosis. Boluses of oxytocin, methylergonovine or 15 methyl prostaglandin F2-alpha may result in increased pulmonary vascular resistance.

- Maintain adequate systemic vascular resistance for sufficient perfusion pressure. Insufficient perfusion pressure at the level of the coronary ostia will limit coronary flow. Insufficient perfusion pressure can lead to lactic acidosis, which in turn may decrease cardiac output. The pt w/ MS has limited ability to increase cardiac output to maintain perfusion pressure if systemic vascular resistance decreases. Avoid spinal anesthesia, as it is associated w/ a precipitous drop in systemic vascular resistance. Dose epidural catheters carefully, paying close attention to the development of hypotension and/or signs & symptoms consistent w/ an insufficient cardiac output. Consider weaker concentrations of local anesthetic for epidural analgesia. Consider the use of combined spinal-epidural technique. Prior intrathecal administration of an opioid may permit smaller doses of epidural local anesthetics. The presence of an epidural catheter facilitates the provision of perineal anesthesia during the second stage of labor. The presence of an epidural catheter facilitates the provision of perineal anesthesia for episiotomy repair.

➤ Avoid pulmonary congestion. Maintain normal to slow heart rate. Maintain cardiac output. Treat volume overload. The pt w/ a history of congestive heart failure during pregnancy may benefit from a pulmonary artery catheter to optimize volume status, as hypovolemia & hypervolemia are both deleterious. The pt may be taking diuretics: missed doses may lead to volume overload. During labor, systemic & pulmonary vascular resistance may increase due to pain, which will impede forward flow. Treat the pain of labor: epidural analgesia, IV opioids, intrathecal opioids. Increase the venous capacitance when indicated: immediately after delivery, intravascular volume increases dramatically as the uterus contracts; heart may be unable to accommodate to large increase in blood volume. Immediately after delivery, compression of the inferior vena cava decreases, which facilitates venous return. Vasodilators will facilitate the accommodation of the mobilized blood volume: nitroprusside; epidurally administered local anesthetics; hydralazine (reflex tachycardia may be deleterious for patient); nitroglycerin (use w/ caution, causes uterine relaxation). Blood loss during vaginal delivery & C-section may be efficacious for treating pulmonary congestion. Blood loss during vaginal delivery is typically 300–400 cc; blood loss during C-section is typically 800–1,000 cc.

CAVEATS / PEARLS
- MS is the most common valvular lesion of significance in pregnant women.
- Pts w/ MS will worsen 1 or 2 NYHA functional status classes during pregnancy.
- If the pt has had a previous episode of pulmonary congestion, she is at increased risk for cardiac complications during pregnancy.
- Some anesthesiologists choose not to include epinephrine in the test dose for epidural catheter position so as to avoid sudden-onset tachycardia if the catheter is intravenous.
- Atrial fib w/ rapid ventricular rate should be aggressively treated, as an increased heart rate will limit diastolic time & L atrial emptying.
- Use synchronized cardioversion for atrial fib if the pt is hemodynamically unstable.
- Vaginal delivery should proceed w/ invasive hemodynamic monitoring if the pt has had symptomatic MS during pregnancy.
- Maternal expulsive efforts during the second stage of labor are discouraged to avoid Valsalva.
- Avoid spinal anesthesia, as it is associated w/ a precipitous drop in systemic vascular resistance.

CHECKLIST
- Determine whether the patient has had symptoms of pulmonary congestion, atrial fib or heart failure during pregnancy.

- Obtain echocardiographic data to characterize the severity of MS if it has not been obtained during pregnancy.
- The pt is high risk if:
  - ➤ She has MS w/ NYHA class II, III or IV symptoms
  - ➤ She has aortic valve disease resulting in pulmonary hypertension
  - ➤ She has aortic valve disease w/ L ventricular systolic dysfunction
- Review meds that the patient may have been taking for rate control, atrial fib suppressive therapy, symptoms of heart failure & anticoagulation.
- Women w/ moderate to severe MS by echocardiography or w/ symptoms associated w/ MS should have invasive monitoring during labor & delivery, as this is the period w/ the greatest magnitude in change w/ regard to hemodynamics.
- If GU procedures are to be performed other than routine vaginal delivery or C-section, administer prophylactic antibiotics to prevent endocarditis from bacteremia.
- C-section is performed only when there are obstetrical indications for such a mode of delivery.
- During anesthetic mgt:
  - ➤ Maintain a normal to slow heart rate.
  - ➤ Treat the pain of labor.
  - ➤ Administer agents that have a favorable side effect profile & avoid agents with unfavorable side effects (phenylephrine instead of ephedrine; milrinone instead of dopamine or dobutamine; succinylcholine instead of pancuronium; opioids instead of ketamine; avoid atropine, glycopyrrolate, meperidine).
  - ➤ Aggressively treat atrial fib.
- Maintain adequate systemic vascular resistance. Avoid spinal anesthesia. Avoid abrupt decreases in systemic vascular resistance while dosing epidural catheters w/ local anesthetic.

MITRAL VALVE PROLAPSE SYNDROME

MATTHEW CIRIGLIANO, MD
DWIGHT GEHA, MD

FUNDAMENTAL KNOWLEDGE

- Mitral valve prolapse (MVP) syndrome occurs when there is systolic billowing of one or both mitral leaflets into the L atrium during systole. MVP may or may not be associated w/ mitral regurgitation, but it is the most common cause of significant mitral regurgitation in the U.S. (40–60% of all cases). MVP is the most common form of valvular heart disease, occurring in 2–3% of the population. MVP occurs twice as often in females than males. Serious mitral regurgitation occurs more frequently in elderly men than young women w/ MVP syndrome.

■ Primary MVP is due to myxomatous degeneration of the mitral valve. Weakening of the valve cusp leads to expansion of the cusp & valve redundancy. The chordae tendineae elongate, furthering prolapse, & are prone to rupture. This anatomic group represents 15–20% of pts w/ MVP. Pts w/ primary MVP often develop significant mitral regurgitation, ultimately requiring mitral valve surgery. MVP is the most common predisposing cardiac diagnosis in endocarditis.

■ Secondary causes of MVP include papillary muscle ischemia w/ acute coronary syndrome, endocarditis, postinflammatory changes from rheumatic fever, hypertrophic cardiomyopathy w/ a small L ventricular cavity & altered papillary muscle alignment.

■ Several medical conditions are associated w/ MVP: von Willebrand disease, Ehlers-Danlos syndrome, kyphoscoliosis, pectus excavatum, osteogenesis imperfecta, myotonic dystrophy, Marfan syndrome.

■ For a discussion of the fundamentals of the pathophysiology of mitral regurgitation, see the chapter "*Mitral Regurgitation.*"

STUDIES

Several sources of information or studies may be used to arrive at a diagnosis of MVP. Most pts w/ MVP are asymptomatic, but pts who have symptoms may report palpitations, chest pain, anxiety, fatigue & dyspnea, lightheadedness, visual changes, symptoms consistent w/ transient ischemic attack, symptoms associated w/ mitral regurgitation (see chapter "*Mitral Regurgitation*").

■ Auscultation may reveal evidence of MVP. One may hear the characteristic midsystolic click of MVP:

➤ High-pitched sound of short duration

➤ The clicks change in their timing during the cardiac cycle from beat to beat.

➤ The click occurs during systole when mitral valve leaflets enter the atrium & the mitral valve apparatus suddenly tenses.

➤ There may be a late systolic murmur as well: medium- to high-pitched, heard at the apex of the heart, of varying volumes.

- ➤ The intensity of a murmur associated w/ MVP may decrease during pregnancy. The maternal intravascular volume expands during pregnancy. Increased L ventricular volume increases the relative dimension of the L ventricle to the mitral valve annulus. The change in relative dimension decreases the degree of prolapse.
- ➤ Systemic vascular resistance (SVR) decreases during pregnancy. Decreased SVR promotes forward blood flow. Increased forward flow decreases MVP.
- ▪ EKG
  - ➤ EKG may reveal evidence of a volume-overloaded L atrium & L ventricle, which is consistent w/ mitral regurgitation (see the chapter "*Mitral Regurgitation*"). ECG is usually normal, however. Paroxysmal supraventricular tachycardia is the most common tachyarrhythmia associated w/ MVP. Ventricular arrhythmias have been implicated in rare cases of sudden death.
- ▪ Chest x-ray may reveal an enlarged L atrium, pulmonary edema, cardiomegaly.
- ▪ Echocardiography may be used to characterize MVP & any associated mitral valve regurgitation. Though at present there is no consensus on the 2-D echocardiographic criteria for MVP, it remains the most useful noninvasive test for characterizing MVP. The American College of Cardiology & American Heart Association list the following as class I indications for obtaining 2-D echocardiography for a pt w/ MVP:
  - • Diagnosis of MVP
  - • Assessment of hemodynamic severity of possible associated mitral regurgitation
  - • Assessment of ventricular compensation
  - ➤ Careful measurements are critical because mitral valve area calculation by Doppler may be inaccurate during pregnancy.
- ▪ A pulmonary artery catheter may reveal a prominent V wave w/ a wide pulse pressure w/ severe mitral regurgitation, if it is present w/ MVP.

The American College of Cardiology & the American Heart Association have classified maternal & fetal risk during pregnancy based on the type of valvular abnormality in conjunction w/ the New York Heart Association functional class.

- ▪ NYHA functional classification for congestive heart failure:
  - ➤ Class I: Pts have no limitation of activities, no symptoms from ordinary activities.

➣ Class II: Pts have slight, mild limitation of activity; pts are comfortable w/ mild exertion.

➣ Class III: Pts have marked limitation of activity; they are comfortable only at rest.

➣ Class IV: Pts should be at complete rest, confined to bed; any physical activity brings discomfort; symptoms occur at rest.

■ Associated w/ a low maternal & fetal risk: MVP w/ no mitral regurgitation; MVP w/ mild to moderate mitral regurgitation in the setting of normal L ventricular systolic function

■ Associated w/ a high maternal & fetal risk: MVP w/ mitral regurgitation in the setting of NYHA class III or IV symptoms; mitral valve disease resulting in severe pulmonary hypertension; mitral valve disease w/ a depressed L ventricular systolic dysfunction (estimated ejection fraction <40%)

MANAGEMENT/INTERVENTIONS

Medical mgt

■ Time course for evaluation by a cardiologist:

➣ During pregnancy, women w/ valvular heart disease should be evaluated once each trimester for presence or worsening of symptoms & if there is a change in symptoms to assess for any deterioration in maternal cardiac status.

➣ The American College of Cardiology & the American Heart Association recommend that women w/ high-risk cardiac lesions undergo full evaluation prior to & during pregnancy.

■ Reassurance is the mgt plan for most pts w/ MVP, as most are asymptomatic.

■ Some pts may require beta blockers to treat arrhythmias, chest pain & palpitations associated w/ MVP.

■ A subset of pts will have associated mitral valve regurgitation. See the chapter "*Mitral Regurgitation*" for details of medical mgt.

■ Antibiotic prophylaxis for prevention of endocarditis is recommended by the American College of Cardiology/American Heart Association for procedures associated w/ bacteremia. Recommendations are that antibiotic prophylaxis be provided for dental procedures & certain respiratory, GI & GU procedures, as listed in the ACC/AHA guidelines. Antibiotic prophylaxis for endocarditis is not recommended for routine vaginal delivery or C-section.

■ Daily aspirin therapy is recommended by the American College of Cardiology/American Heart Association for pts w/ documented focal neurologic events in the setting of MVP who are in sinus rhythm & do not have atrial thrombi.

Surgical considerations are the same as those for mitral valve regurgitation; see the chapter "*Mitral Regurgitation.*"

Obstetric mgt is routine for most pts w/ MVP. Most pts w/ MVP tolerate pregnancy very well. There is no increased risk of obstetric complications or fetal distress in the setting of MVP. For pts w/ moderate to severe mitral regurgitation associated w/ MVP, see the obstetric management section of the chapter "*Mitral Regurgitation.*"

See the chapter "*Mitral Regurgitation*" for the anesthetic management of pts w/ MVP who have mitral regurgitation.

CAVEATS/PEARLS

■ MVP is usually well tolerated by the parturient.

■ Sympathomimetic agonists should probably be avoided in the parturient w/ MVP due to the high incidence of arrhythmias in these pts. Ephedrine may precipitate or exacerbate tachyarrhythmias. Treat hypotension w/ small bolus doses of phenylephrine. Some may choose not to include epinephrine in the epidural catheter test dose.

■ Likewise, one should avoid agents that sensitize the myocardium to catecholamines, such as halothane.

CHECKLIST

■ Ascertain if the pt has symptoms of mitral regurgitation secondary to MVP.

■ Review meds that the pt may be taking for rate control, atrial fib suppressive therapy & symptoms of heart failure if mitral regurgitation is present.

■ Obtain echocardiographic data to ascertain presence & if applicable severity of mitral regurgitation if there has been a significant change in the pt's symptoms.

■ Pt is high risk if she has mitral regurgitation w/ NYHA class III or IV symptoms; mitral valve disease resulting in pulmonary hypertension; or mitral valve disease w/ L ventricular systolic dysfunction.

■ Women who are at high risk should have invasive monitoring during labor & delivery, as this is the period w/ the greatest magnitude in change w/ regard to hemodynamics.

■ If the pt has echo-documented MVP & GU procedures are to be performed other than routine vaginal delivery or C-section, administer prophylactic antibiotics to prevent endocarditis from bacteremia.

- C-section is performed only when there are obstetrical indications for such a mode of delivery.
- During anesthetic mgt, avoid sympathomimetic agents if possible. For pts w/ mitral regurgitation is present, see the chapter "*Mitral Regurgitation.*"

MULTIPLE GESTATIONS

THERESA CHANG, MD
YANDONG JIANG, MD, PhD

FUNDAMENTAL KNOWLEDGE

Definition

- Multiple gestations refers to a pregnancy in which 2 or more fetuses are present in the uterine cavity. There are generally 2 categories of twins: monozygotes & dizygotes. Monozygotic twins occur when a single fertilized ovum divides & develops into 2 distinct individuals after a number of divisions. Such twins are usually identical. Rarely, mutations occur that cause differences phenotypically. Dizygotic twins occur when 2 separate ova are fertilized & each individual twin is genetically distinct.

Epidemiology

- Multiple gestations occur in about 1.5% of all births. The number of multiple gestational births is increasing, which in turn means higher rates of both maternal & neonatal morbidity & mortality. The frequency of monozygotes does not relate to maternal characteristics (age or parity). Dizygotic twins, however, are associated w/ multiple episodes of ovulation. The frequency differs among races & within countries. Dizygotic birth rates also augmented w/ increased maternal age & increased parity. Another factor is the use of IVF & embryo transfer (see "*Assisted Reproductive Technology*").

Etiology (inc. ART technology, ovulation induction therapy)

- The cause of monozygotic twinning is unknown. Although there seems to be a correlation w/ ART & monozygotic twinning, the explanation for this occurrence has not yet been elucidated. Dizygotic twinning seems to result from an increased ovulation of multiple follicles. Serum follicle-stimulating hormone (FSH) levels control ovulation & appear to correlate w/ rates of dizygotic births. Medications used in ART, including clomiphene citrate & other gonadotropins used to induce ovulation, are also associated w/ an increased rate of twinning. IVF is linked to a higher order of multiple gestations, depending on the number of embryos transferred.

Placentation

■ Twins are categorized by the types of membranes they acquire. Normally in pregnancy, the sac of a singleton pregnancy contains an outer chorion & an inner amnion. In dizygotic twins, each twin develops within a similar sac because both blastocysts have their own placentas, especially if the implantation of the blastocysts is far enough apart from each other. They will thus have separate chorions & amnions. If they implant side by side, however, fusion of the placental disks may occur, but they will still have separate amnions & chorions. Unlike dizygotic twins, monozygotic twins typically have a single chorion surrounding 1 or 2 amnions, although they can have 2 amnions & 2 chorions. In most cases of monochorionic placentas, there is a communication btwn the blood vessels of the fetal circulations. Placentation in monozygotic pregnancy depends on the cleavage of the fertilized ovum. If twinning occurs in the first 2–3 days, then it comes before chorionic formation. Thus, 2 chorions & 2 amnions are formed. After the third day, however, a monochorionic placenta occurs. If the split occurs btwn day 3 and 8, there will be 2 amnions. Btwn day 8 and 13, there will only be 1 amnion. With higher orders of multiple gestations (e.g., triplets, quadruplets), monochorionic & dichorionic placentations may coexist.

Physiologic changes & maternal complications

■ Multiple gestations accelerate the physiologic changes that occur w/ pregnancy from a cardiovascular & pulmonary standpoint. In particular, increased uterine size secondary to multiple gestation leads to decreased TLC & FRC; thus O2 desaturation occurs at a faster rate after induction of anesthesia. After 30 weeks' gestation, women w/ multiple fetuses have an increased risk for difficult intubation & mask ventilation. The maternal heart rate increases by approximately 15% & the PVR decrease is greater in multigestational pregnancies. The total plasma volume increases (which is related to the fetal number) & because the maternal RBC volume increases only minimally, there is a relative dilutional anemia. Cardiac output is increased as a result of this increase in stroke volume & heart rate. The overall oxygen demand is increased. The physiologic changes in other systems such as the GI tract, CNS & GU tract closely resemble the changes in pregnant women w/ a single fetus.

Aside from the basic physiologic changes that occur w/ multiple gestational pregnancies, there has been an associated increase in the number of maternal comorbid illnesses as well, including gestational hypertension, preeclampsia, anemia, gestational diabetes & placental abruption. Such medical problems have also been linked to higher-order gestations but present more severely & in atypical manners.

Complications unique to multiple gestations

■ Multiple gestational pregnancies are considered high risk. Both perinatal morbidity & mortality have been greater in twins or higher-order multiples compared to singletons. This has been secondary to the high incidence of low-birthweight infants, IUGR, congenital anomalies, the increased number of preterm deliveries & IUGR, cord accidents & malpresentations. The risks to the mother are also higher, including a higher incidence of placenta previa, abruptio placentae & preeclampsia. Approx. 10% of perinatal deaths result from multiple gestations, which is 4× higher than that in singleton pregnancies. Most of the complications arise from preterm delivery, but other complications are common as well, including congenital anomalies, polyhydramnios, cord entanglement, umbilical cord prolapse, IUGR, twin-twin transfusion & malpresentation. Those complications that are specific to multiple gestations are listed here.

■ Twin-twin transfusion (TTT)

➤ TTT is a complex cardiovascular complication in monochorionic twin pregnancies in which one twin becomes the donor & the other twin becomes the recipient of blood that circulates btwn them. This occurs when deep arteriovenous vascular malformations in a monochorionic placenta allow the passage of blood btwn the pair. In such cases, the donor twin is smaller & is at higher risk for IUGR & anemia. On the other hand, the recipient is plethoric & is at risk for volume overload & CHF. If untreated, it is associated w/ a high perinatal mortality & morbidity. It is diagnosed by ultrasound in the mid-trimester after serial scanning every 2–4 weeks. An increased frequency of scanning should occur once minor amniotic fluid discordance is noticed. Treatment includes decompression amniocentesis, interruption of placental vessel communication, amniotic septostomy & selective feticide.

■ Vanishing twin syndrome

➤ Approx. 50% of twin pregnancies identified in the first trimester result in the birth of 2 babies. In some cases, a single fetal death in early pregnancy occurs w/ good outcome for the surviving fetus. It usually presents as vaginal bleeding, although many pts are asymptomatic.

■ Fetal death in utero

➤ Other multigestational pregnancies result in the death of a twin in the late second or third trimester. This is different from the vanishing twin syndrome because in most circumstances of fetal death in utero, there is considerable morbidity to the remaining twin. Most of the IUFDs are detected on routine ultrasound. Serial ultrasounds are then routinely performed for the evaluation of fetal growth & development. The cause of the loss of the deceased fetus is usually unknown. Contributing factors to demise include TTT in monochorionic pregnancies & cord entanglement in monoamniotic twins. The demise of one fetus may increase the risk of unfavorable events in the remaining fetus, such as neurologic injury & preterm delivery in mono- & dichorionic pregnancies. Mgt of the remainder of the pregnancy depends on maternal & fetal complications as well as gestational age & fetal lung maturity. Pts need close monitoring for evidence of preterm labor. Corticosteroid administration is advocated to enhance fetal lung maturity btwn 24 & 34 weeks. Consider elective delivery at 37–38 weeks or once fetal lung maturity is noted.

■ Discordant twin growth

➤ Growth discordance occurs when there is a difference in growth btwn twins or higher-order multiple gestations. In the past, it has been associated as an independent risk factor for neonatal hypoglycemia. In the long term there has been a question of the smaller twins having a lower IQ. Overall, however, there is no conclusive evidence that this affects long-term neurodevelopmental outcome.

➤ Fetal complications

• IUGR

➤ Studies have indicated that the rate of fetal growth slows in the third trimester (30–32 weeks) when compared to singletons. For triplets, growth slows at 27–28 weeks. Most of this slowing has been thought to be secondary to a competition for nutrients. Any comorbid condition that prevents the delivery of adequate nutritional support, including placentation, preeclampsia or diabetes, further affects growth. Consistently this has correlated w/ decreased abdominal circumferences of the mother, likely indicating uteroplacental insufficiency. Overall survival is at least in part determined by relative birthweight & gestational age.

- Prematurity

➤ Multiple gestational pregnancies result in a high rate of preterm birth. This corresponds to a high rate of low birthweight. Because of such circumstances, there are associated complications including respiratory distress syndrome, intraventricular hemorrhage & necrotizing enterocolitis. After taking into account the differences in gestational age, it appears that twins experience the same rates of these complications as singletons, implying that reducing the incidence of premature birth would decrease twin comorbidity & mortality.

- Congenital Anomalies

➤ When fetal abnormalities are detected in one of the fetuses in multiple gestations, couples have several options: complete termination of the pregnancy, selective termination of the affected fetus or expectant mgt.

STUDIES

Ultrasound

■ Ultrasound screening helps in the diagnosis of multiple gestations early in pregnancy & w/ a near 100% accuracy. It has the greatest level of sensitivity & specificity & should be performed once there is a question of multiple gestations. It is usually suspected when the uterus is larger than what is expected from a patient's size according to dates. Furthermore, ultrasound is useful in determining any structural abnormalities, in determining amnionicity & chorionicity, in recognizing fetuses that might need fetal or early neonatal therapy & in detecting fetal abnormalities that may affect decision-making in overall pregnancy mgt (including early pregnancy termination).

Serum marker screening

■ Maternal serum marker screening is not as helpful in twins & higher-order multiples as it is in singletons. Altered serum levels of certain markers from an affected fetus will be brought closer to the mean by the presence of unaffected fetuses. Levels of maternal serum markers are usually doubled in women w/ twins than in those w/ single fetuses. Singletons that arise as a result of ART, however, have elevated beta-hCG levels (increased by 21%). Second-trimester screening is also limited. Levels of serum markers such as alpha-fetoprotein, beta-hCG & unconjugated estriol were not exactly twice as high for twins as for singletons.

MANAGEMENT/INTERVENTIONS

Antepartum care

■ Corticosteroid administration

➤ Women experiencing preterm labor prior to 34 weeks' gestation or those w/ PPROM at less than 30–32 weeks' gestation should be given corticosteroids to induce fetal lung maturity & decrease perinatal complications. Twin outcome studies have shown that nonpresenting twins are more likely to develop hyaline membrane disease & respiratory problems & often require more oxygen therapy than the presenting infant.

■ Fetal surveillance

➤ Retrospective studies have shown that nonstress tests are equally efficacious in multiples as they are in singletons in recognizing those affected by IUGR, those at risk for hypoxia & those w/ a higher risk for perinatal mortality. Such monitoring is indicated in those at higher risk (e.g., those w/ IUGR, abnormal fluid volumes, growth discordance, PIH, fetal anomalies & other complications affecting at least 1 fetus). Although nonstress tests have not been shown to be beneficial in uncomplicated multiples, they are routinely performed in pts w/ inadequate ultrasound evaluations to rule out IUGR or fetal growth discordance.

■ Predicting preterm delivery

➤ Having the ability to predict those w/ the highest chance of preterm delivery allows resources to be used efficiently & avoids potential side effects associated w/ unnecessary treatments.

  • Endovaginal ultrasound cervical length
    • Reduced cervical length of <2.5 cm has been associated w/ an increased risk of preterm birth between weeks 24 & 28 in multiple gestations. Several measurements have been used in different studies; thus, no specific length is absolutely predictive. However, a measurement <2.0 cm in the early second trimester is highly associated w/ preterm birth.

  • Digital cervical assessment
    • Because digital cervical assessments are easy to perform, inexpensive & helpful when an experienced provider performs this assessment, such an exam is likely most useful. No increase in bleeding, PPROM, preterm birth or risk of chorioamnionitis associated w/ this assessment has been shown in women w/ twins or higher-order multiples. When cervical scoring is used, it has been valuable in determining

the risk for preterm delivery, but no data have shown that it improves perinatal outcome.
- Cervical/vaginal fetal fibronectin
  - This complex adhesion molecule is normally found in vaginal secretions before 20 weeks' gestation. After 20 weeks, it disappears because of the obliteration of the extra-amniotic space & approximation of the chorion & decidual surface. Disruption of the maternal-fetal interface after 20 weeks leads to an elevated level of these proteins in maternal cervical or vaginal secretions. The test has been shown to be more clinically useful in ruling out preterm delivery in pts who are symptomatic. Studies have shown that it has a >97% negative predictive value for preterm birth when taken from 1–3 weeks of the test, thus avoiding unnecessary interventions in both singleton & twin pregnancies.

Intrapartum care
- Monitoring
  - Continuous monitoring w/ FHR monitoring & ultrasound to estimate relative fetal weights, to evaluate the presentation of each fetus & to assess the remaining fetus btwn deliveries is crucial in the delivery of multiple gestations.
- Timing of delivery
  - To decide when delivery should occur, consider birthweight & gestational age. Some recommend delivery of uncomplicated pregnancies electively at 38 weeks & no later than 39 weeks. Prolonged pregnancy beyond this time increases the risk of fetal complications w/o any improvement in outcome. Pregnancies w/ presumed difficulties secondary to IUGR, growth discordance or maternal disorders require an earlier delivery date (usually around 36–37 weeks or earlier if the pt has severe preeclampsia or non-reassuring fetal stress testing). For pts w/ gestational diabetes, pregestational diabetes or poor dating, an amniocentesis for fetal lung maturity helps to determine fetal lung maturity prior to an elective delivery before 36 weeks. The data are unclear about the timing of delivery for triplets. One study has shown that the nadir of fetal mortality occurs when fetuses are delivered at a weight from 1,900 to 2,200 g & at gestational age 34–35 weeks. The mortality risk rises significantly after a gestational age of 37 weeks. Those w/ complications (e.g., IUGR, growth discordance, preeclampsia) are usually delivered earlier. An amniocentesis to assess fetal lung maturity should be taken no later than 34 weeks

in pregnancies affected by gestational diabetes, pregestational diabetes or poor dating.

■ Route of delivery (presentation/higher-order multiples)

➤ At any time during the pregnancy, regardless of the position of the fetus, emergent operative vaginal procedures may be necessary. Most reports show that the most common presentation in labor is vertex-vertex, but there has been significant variation depending on the decade of birth & the country of origin. Because size & position of the fetuses are crucial, several actions must take place during labor mgt. The presentation & fetal weights must be determined; then, after delivery of the first fetus, ultrasound evaluation is again necessary. Not only may the presentation of the remaining twin after delivery of the first twin change, but the FHR may be monitored & external version may be performed if the second twin is not in the desired position. A dual-channel monitor that records the FHR of both fetuses must be used. A decision for the type of delivery must be made according to the presentation of the fetuses & the presence of maternal/fetal complications.

• Vertex-vertex

• The most common presentation is the vertex-vertex position. Reports show that most of the cases are delivered vaginally. For those w/ the usual obstetric indications for C-section delivery, C-section was performed on both fetuses. In <10% of cases, unexpected events such as cord prolapse, fetal distress, abruption & malpresentation led to a cesarean delivery for only the second fetus after initial vaginal delivery of the first.

• Twin A vertex, twin B nonvertex

• Options for delivery of the fetuses in this circumstance include C-section, vaginal delivery of both after external version of twin B or breech extraction of twin B.

If version of twin B is attempted, there appears to be comparable success rates compared to singleton versions, but the number of complications is significantly higher. Possible causes for the adverse consequences include higher likelihood of prematurity, advanced cervical dilation or limited experience w/ intrapartum external version.

A possibly safer option for a nonvertex twin B is to perform breech extraction of the second fetus. To avoid unfavorable consequences, this should be executed only if the second fetus weighs at least 1,700–2,000 g.

The last option for vertex/nonvertex presentations is a C-section, but the risk of such a procedure still remains. The febrile morbidity associated w/ C-section is considerably higher than that w/ vaginal/breech delivery.

- Twin A nonvertex, twin B other
- This is the least common presentation for twins. Compared w/ other presentations, these fetuses are at risk for fetal entanglement & death w/ attempted vaginal delivery. Risk factors for entanglement include twin A breech & twin B vertex, IUGR, birth weight <2,000 g & IUFD of one fetus. Prevention of complications includes external version of twin A or more commonly C-section. Breech delivery of twin A is possible as some studies show, but only if the actual weight of the fetus is at least 1,500 g. Risk for entanglement is high if this criterion has not been met.

➤ Delivery of higher-order multiples
- C-section is the recommended mode of delivery in higher-order multiples, since a vaginal delivery might require physical manipulation of a potentially premature fetus to extract the fetus during delivery. If vaginal delivery is attempted, it is generally understood that the fetuses be at least 1,500 g, w/ the first 2 fetuses in the vertex position.

➤ Interval btwn vaginal deliveries
- If the first twin is delivered vaginally, the second twin usually delivers spontaneously within 15 minutes; most deliver within 30 minutes. IV oxytocin may be administered in mothers w/ inadequate uterine contractions 10 minutes after the first delivery. A prolonged delay btwn the deliveries of twins can lead to development of uterine inertia, a rapidly closing uterus, umbilical cord prolapse & placental abruption. With the wide availability of fetal monitoring & safe birthing mgt, there is no need to deliver the second twin 30 minutes after the first.

■ Anesthesia for multiple gestations
➤ Physiologic changes related to multiple gestations
- Cardiovascular system
  - Because there is such a large increase in cardiac output secondary to both the increased heart rate & stroke volume in parturients w/ multiple gestations, there is limited reserve for the heart to compensate for decreased systemic vascular resistance to maintain an adequate perfusion pressure.

Therefore, w/ neuraxial anesthesia, be prepared to manage potential hypotension w/ medications such as ephedrine. Furthermore, aortocaval compression is increased in multiple gestations because of the elevated pressure on the venous system of the abdomen & lower extremities. This may cause fetal compromise w/o maternal hypotension; thus, lateral uterine displacement & close monitoring of the fetuses are crucial.

- Respiratory system
  - Changes in the respiratory system are also likely amplified in those w/ multiple gestations. Because of the increased uterine size, there is a corresponding decrease in FRC that causes accelerated desaturation while the pt is supine & during induction of anesthesia. The minute ventilation & tidal volumes are increased secondary to the stimulation of the respiratory centers by progesterone, but again the reserve is very limited. Lastly, the changes that occur w/ a singleton pregnancy are still significant in those w/ multiple gestations. The airway is susceptible to becoming edematous & friable & the potential for difficulty w/ intubation remains a substantial problem.
- Other changes
  - Additional physiologic factors that the anesthesiologist should be aware of are the following:
  - Decreased lower esophageal sphincter tone secondary to increased progesterone levels places the pt at risk for aspiration during intubation.
  - Decreased intrathecal CSF volume in the lumbar area makes these parturients more susceptible to high spinals than those w/ singleton pregnancies.
- ➤ Preterm labor
  - Medications
    - Be knowledgeable about the medications used to prevent preterm labor. Ritodrine & terbutaline (β-sympathomimetics) can cause maternal hypotension, tachycardia, hyperglycemia, hypokalemia & pulmonary edema. Pulmonary edema in particular appears to occur more commonly when terbutaline is administered along w/ corticosteroids or normal saline. Anesthesiologists must be aware of these potential complications & the possible need for respiratory support.

- Anesthesia
  - Regional anesthesia has been shown to cause a decrease in perinatal mortality. This might be due to inhibition of expulsive efforts on delivery by the mother & thus avoidance of early delivery, as well as a relaxed pelvic floor.
- Preeclampsia
  - Multiple gestation is a known risk factor for pregnancy-induced hypertension & preeclampsia. Women w/ twin gestations are at least 2x more likely to develop a hypertensive disorder than those w/ a singleton, & this rate increases w/ the number of fetuses involved. Other factors that may increase the risk for PIH include parity & the use of ART in pregnancy. Symptoms of preeclampsia include headaches, epigastric pain, visual problems & HELLP. Be aware of the potential for prolonged effects of neuromuscular blockers & exaggerated hypotension during regional anesthesia secondary to diminished intravascular volume & increased responsiveness to sympathomimetics. Thrombocytopenia (<100,000) might affect one's decision for epidural/spinal placement, even though no well-established guidelines for platelet count & regional anesthesia have been established to balance the benefits of regional anesthesia & the risk of epidural hematoma formation. Such a risk for bleeding might lead the clinician to choose general anesthesia for delivery during a C-section, which in & of itself increases the probability of anesthesia-related maternal death.
- Maternal hemorrhage
  - The risk for maternal hemorrhage is elevated in multiple gestations. This is secondary to the increased number of placental abruptions & placenta previas in twins (as well as risk factors for abruption such as PROM, eclampsia & polyhydramnios). The average blood loss in a vaginal twin delivery resembles that of a repeat C-section & is about 2× that of a singleton delivery, likely because of uterine atony. Whatever the cause for excessive bleeding, be prepared to help in maintaining hemodynamic stability & repletion of blood products. Actively ensure that adequate access is achieved early on & that cross-matched blood is available. Agents to maintain persistent uterine tone such as oxytocin, methylergonovine, prostaglandin F2 or misoprostol must also be available.
- Anesthesia for vaginal delivery of multiple gestations

- Although triplet & higher-order multiple gestations are delivered by C-section, twin deliveries are still controversial. As noted earlier, considerations are usually based on the position of the twins. As always, the type of anesthetic is determined by the presence of maternal comorbidities. Generally if there are no contraindications, regional anesthesia is advantageous. Not only are maternal expulsive efforts suppressed, but the comfort of a regional anesthetic may also facilitate version of the second twin if twin B is not vertex. The convenience of an epidural in particular extends to its use either in the OR or during vaginal delivery.

➤ Anesthesia for C-section for multiple gestation

- Regional & general anesthetics are options for the cesarean delivery of multiple fetuses. The risk for maternal mortality is observed to be approx. $17\times$ higher when general is administered, but this is confounded by the fact that many of the general anesthetics are done under emergent, non-ideal circumstances. With regional anesthesia, watch for the increased spread of spinal medications, the greater potential for maternal hypotension when supine & the predisposition toward respiratory compromise. Consider large-bore IV access, the availability of cross-matched blood & a back-up plan should emergency airway mgt become necessary.

CAVEATS/PEARLS

- The number of multiple gestational births is increasing, possibly as a result of the increase in maternal age & difference in parity as well as technological advances related to ART.
- Complications unique to multiple gestational pregnancies include:

  Loss of one fetus either early in the pregnancy (vanishing twin syndrome) or during the second or third trimester (fetal death in utero); the latter may cause significant morbidity in the remaining fetuses

  TTT, in which deep AVMs in a monochorionic placenta allow the passage of blood from one twin to the other, causing adverse outcomes in both twins in different ways

  Monoamniotic twins: complications related to congenital anomalies, TTT, cord entanglements, IUGR, preterm delivery & IUFD become issues

  Discordant twin growth: a difference in growth between twins & higher-order multiples may lead to hypoglycemia & deficits in neurodevelopmental outcome.

- Other complications relating to multiple gestations include the potential for IUGR, prematurity & congenital anomalies.
- Diagnosis of multiple gestations is primarily via ultrasound screening. Serum screens may also give indications regarding potential fetal complications.
- Antepartum care for those w/ multifetal pregnancies is important. Regular fetal surveillance is essential in determining fetuses at higher risk for complications.
- The delivery of twins depends primarily on the presentation of the fetuses. Higher-order gestations are usually delivered by C-section. If there are no contraindications, regional anesthesia is preferred in most cases. Be aware of the predisposition in those w/ multiple gestations toward hypotension when regional anesthetics are performed, as well as the increased sensitivity to spinal anesthetics.
- If a general anesthetic is administered, be aware of the increased risk for maternal mortality, & the need for back-up airway mgt should an emergency occur.

CHECKLIST
- Know obstetric plan for delivery.
- Be familiar w/ pt's history/physical, as these pts are at higher risk for needing operative delivery.
- Reconfirm adequacy of labor epidural near time of anticipated delivery. Reinforce sensory blockade if necessary, appreciating the significant possibility of operative delivery.
- Beware of postop complications, including hemorrhage related to uterine atony.

MULTIPLE SCLEROSIS (MS)

MEREDITH ALBRECHT, MD
MICHELE SZABO, MD

FUNDAMENTAL KNOWLEDGE

Definition
- Chronic demyelinating disease characterized by plaques of inflammatory demyelination scattered throughout the CNS white matter in brain & spinal cord

Epidemiology
- 3–8 per 1,000 in U.S.

- Ratio of female:male, 3:2
- Incidence peaks in the 3rd decade of life.

Pathophysiology
- Etiology unknown. Potential causes include:
  - Immunologic response to viral infection triggering an autoimmune response
  - Environmental: specifics unknown
  - Genetic: familial clusters, but not thought to be hereditary.
  - Perhaps due to common histocompatibility antigen
  - Geographic: decreased incidence in equatorial regions
- Pathologic findings throughout CNS (brain & spinal cord)
  - Inflammatory plaques of perivascular lymphocytic infiltration, demyelination, gliosis, aberrant remyelination

Clinical Manifestations
- Diagnosis: multiple criteria:
  - Neurologic deficits attributable to white matter lesions
  - Lesions present in >1 area of the CNS
  - Neurologic deficits of variable onset & location
- Two general clinical patterns
  - Relapsing-remitting: attacks appear abruptly & resolve over several months
  - Chronic progressive
- Common symptoms (in order of frequency)
  - Motor weakness
  - Spasticity &/or hyperreflexia
  - Impaired vision, including diplopia
  - Sphincter dysfunction, especially bladder & bowel
  - Ataxia
  - Paresthesias
  - Dysarthria
  - Mental disturbance, including emotional liability
  - Pain
  - Vertigo
  - Dysphagia
  - Convulsions
  - Decreased hearing
  - Tinnitus
- Exacerbations provoked by
  - Stress
  - Rise in core body temp
  - Infection

Effect of Pregnancy on MS
- Pregnancy does not negatively affect long-term outcome of MS.
- Decreased relapses & exacerbations during pregnancy may be due to immunosuppression.
- Increased relapse rate during delivery & in first 3–6 months postpartum (up to 3× higher), likely due to factors such as stress, fatigue, fever.

Effect of MS on Pregnancy & Fetus
- Does not affect fertility
- Does not adversely affect pregnancy (no increase in preterm labor, difficult delivery, birth defects or stillbirth)
- Severe MS associated w/ paraplegia can cause autonomic dysreflexia during delivery (see "*Spinal Cord Injuries*").

STUDIES

History & Physical
- Signs (from most to least common)
  - ➤ Spasticity &/or hyperreflexia
  - ➤ Babinski sign
  - ➤ Absent abdominal reflex
  - ➤ Dysmetria
  - ➤ Nystagmus
  - ➤ Impairment of vibratory, position or pain sensation
  - ➤ Facial weakness
  - ➤ Impairment of touch or temperature sensation
  - ➤ Altered consciousness
- Lab/CSF
  - ➤ Elevated protein
  - ➤ Mild lymphocytic pleocytosis
  - ➤ Elevated immunoglobulin G
  - ➤ Increased gamma-globulin
  - ➤ Oligoclonal bands
  - ➤ Elevated myelin basic protein
- Evoked potentials have prolonged conduction time due to demyelination.

Imaging
- Classic finding on MRI is white matter plaques (T2 hyperintense white matter lesions w/ gadolinium enhancement of active plaques)

MANAGEMENT/INTERVENTIONS

Medical Treatment

- Immunosuppressive therapy
  - ➤ Glucocorticoids (eg, ACTH, prednisone or methylprednisolone) can be used to treat severe exacerbations.
  - ➤ Beta-interferon reduces the exacerbation rate & long-term progression of disease in relapsing-remitting MS. Avoid during pregnancy.
  - ➤ Cytotoxic agents (cyclosporine, azathioprine, cyclophosphamide, methotrexate) can be used to treat chronic progressive MS. Avoid during pregnancy since these medications are teratogens.
  - ➤ Immunosuppressive therapy is contraindicated in nursing mothers due to the risk of bone marrow or adrenal suppression in the infant.
- Symptomatic therapy
  - ➤ Muscle spasms: baclofen, diazepam (avoid during pregnancy), dantrolene
  - ➤ Urinary retention: anticholinergic such as imipramine. Increased incidence of UTI may necessitate antibiotic prophylaxis w/ ampicillin or nitrofurantoin.
  - ➤ Fatigue: amantadine

Anesthesia

- Pre-delivery assessment
  - ➤ Note pt's degree of compromise & document preexisting neurologic deficits.
  - ➤ Assess respiratory function, and reserve
- During labor and delivery:
  - ➤ Increased incidence of relapse at time of delivery regardless of type of anesthesia
  - ➤ Administer stress-dose steroids if chronic steroid therapy.
  - ➤ Maternal exhaustion during delivery may require operative or assisted vaginal delivery.
  - ➤ Avoid hyperpyrexia.
- General anesthesia
  - ➤ Does not increase the risk of a relapse compared w/ regional anesthesia
  - ➤ Avoid succinylcholine if severe musculoskeletal involvement due to risk of hyperkalemia
  - ➤ May be necessary if pt has respiratory compromise

- Regional anesthesia
  - ➤ There is a theoretical risk of local anesthetics at high concentrations (ie, bupivacaine >0.25%) causing inflammation & damaging nerves. However, there are many examples in the literature of epidural anesthesia & spinal anesthesia w/o complications.

CAVEATS & PEARLS
- The course of MS is not adversely affected by pregnancy.
- In most cases MS does not affect fertility.
- In most cases MS does not adversely affect the pregnancy.
- Labor & delivery does exacerbate MS.
- Avoid hyperpyrexia.
- Either general or regional anesthesia may be used safely.
- Use dilute concentrations of local anesthetics in epidural infusion (bupivacaine 0.25% or less).

CHECKLIST
- Conduct thorough neurological exam & document current deficits.
- Assess respiratory status.
- Inform pt of increased incidence of relapse during delivery & post-partum period.
- Use dilute concentrations of local anesthetic (0.25% or less for epidural anesthesia).
- Administer stress-dose steroids during labor & delivery if pt is chronically on steroid therapy.
- Actively avoid and aggressively treat hyperpyrexia.

MUSCULAR DYSTROPHY

MEREDITH ALBRECHT, MD; LISA LEFFERT, MD; AND MICHELE SZABO, MD

FUNDAMENTAL KNOWLEDGE

Definition
- Relatively normal muscle function early in life
- Progressive degenerations of skeletal muscle w/ intact innervation

Epidemiology
- For Duchenne's (most common type), 1/3,300 male births
- Sex-linked recessive trait
- Although most pts are boys, there are some well-documented cases in girls.
- For Becker's: 1/33,000 male births (X-linked)

- Emery-Dreifuss dystrophy (X-linked)
- Congenital muscular dystrophy: syndrome of muscular dystrophy at birth

Pathophysiology
- Variable muscle fiber size w/ increased amounts of fibrous connective tissue & muscle atrophy
- Most involve abnormal types of dystrophin (muscle fiber protein)

Clinical Manifestations
- Duchenne's
  - Gower's sign: pt uses hands to climb up legs to arise from the floor
  - Usually wheelchair-bound after 3–10 years, w/ death at 5–20 years
  - Cardiac anomalies: arrhythmias, MVP, fibrosis of myocardium
  - Present in high proportion (50–70%) but clinically significant in roughly 10% in the terminal phase of disease
  - Respiratory dysfunction, scoliosis, pulmonary infection
- Becker's
  - Distinguishable from Duchenne's by its later onset (mean age 12 years), more benign course
  - Average age of death 42 years; pneumonia most common cause of death
- Emery-Dreifuss
  - Involves biceps & triceps in upper extremities, distal muscles in lower extremities
  - Slow progression of disease
  - Sudden death common btwn ages 30–60
  - Cardiac manifestations include cardiomyopathy.
- Congenital: benign & disabling subtypes exist

Effect of Pregnancy on Muscular Dystrophy
- Can worsen effect of the illness on the pulmonary system

Effect of Muscular Dystrophy on Pregnancy & the Fetus
- Increased incidence of operative & instrumented delivery
- No increase in adverse outcomes

STUDIES

History & Physical
- Normal muscle function early in life
- Slowly progressive muscle weakness w/ intact innervation

Laboratory
- CPK, SGOT, LDH, SGPT (values increased)

Imaging
- None

Other
- Muscle biopsy
- EMG studies
- Pulmonary function tests to assess extent of restrictive disease
- EKG/ECHO to elucidate conduction abnormalities, cardiomyopathy

MANAGEMENT/INTERVENTIONS

Medical Treatment
- In Duchenne's, some evidence that verapamil helps the symptoms of the disease.
- Supportive care
- Physical therapy
- May require respiratory support

Anesthesia
- Predelivery assessment
  - Careful physical exam to document preexisting deficits
  - Carefully assess extent of pulmonary/cardiac involvement.
  - Severe disease can cause both airway & spinal abnormalities.
  - Careful airway exam, especially w/ nemaline myopathy.
- General anesthesia
  - Many reports of cardiac arrests in pts w/ Duchenne's during or immediately after anesthesia; thought to be secondary to a hypermetabolic syndrome similar to malignant hyperthermia (MH)
  - Prudent to avoid MH-triggering agents: succinylcholine or halogenated anesthetics
  - Normal response to non-depolarizing muscle relaxants
  - Careful neuromuscular monitoring recommended
  - Post-op ventilatory support may be necessary.
- Regional anesthesia
  - Recommended if possible
  - Level of block should be extended slowly, focusing on pulmonary function

CAVEATS & PEARLS
- Increased incidence of operative & instrumented delivery

- Pregnancy can worsen pulmonary dysfunction of the disease.
- Avoid use of MH-triggering agents (succinylcholine & inhalational anesthetics), as pts may be susceptible to a hypermetabolic syndrome.
- Depending on variant, there will be a differential degree of cardiac involvement (conduction defects, cardiomyopathy).
- Depending on variant, there will be a differential degree of muscle involvement.

CHECKLIST

- Careful physical exam focusing on pulmonary function & airway
- EKG to investigate cardiac conduction abnormalities; echocardiogram if cardiomyopathy is suspected
- Physical exam to document preexisting muscle deficits
- Consider regional anesthesia if possible, but pt may have kyphoscoliosis.
- Carefully monitor pulmonary function during anesthesia.
- General anesthesia should avoid MH-triggering agents, as pts are prone to hypermetabolic state.
- Careful neuromuscular monitoring

MYASTHENIA GRAVIS: MANAGEMENT OF THE PARTURIENT WITH AUTOIMMUNE DISEASE

AUGUST CHANG, MD
MIRIAM HARNETT, MD

FUNDAMENTAL KNOWLEDGE

Definition

- Chronic autoimmune disease affecting neuromuscular transmission

Epidemiology

- Prevalence: 1 in 10,000 to 50,000
- Male:female 1:2–3
- Peak onset: 3rd decade for women & 5th decade for men

Pathophysiology

- Underlying defect is an autoantibody-mediated reduction in the number of available nicotinic acetylcholine receptors at the post-synaptic neuromuscular junction of skeletal muscle
- However, 10–20% pts w/ clinical evidence of MG have no detectable antibody

- No definite correlation btwn antibody level & disease activity

Clinical manifestations
- Characterized by episodes of muscle weakness & rapid fatigability of striated muscle w/ repetitive activity
- Smooth & cardiac muscle unaffected
- Most common clinical manifestations
  - Thymic hyperplasia
  - Diplopia
  - Ptosis
  - Dysarthria
  - Generalized weakness
  - Dysphagia
  - Dyspnea
- Remissions & exacerbations are unpredictable
- Classification according to disease severity
  - I: Ocular myasthenia only
  - IIA: Mild, generalized myasthenia w/ slow progression, no respiratory crises, responsive to drug therapy
  - IIB: Moderate, generalized myasthenia w/ severe skeletal & bulbar involvement, no respiratory crises, inadequate response to drug therapy
  - III: Acute, rapid deterioration (<6 months), respiratory crises, poor response to drug therapy, high mortality
  - IV: Late, severe myasthenia, progressive over 2 years from class I to II, respiratory crises, high mortality
- Diagnosis: no single test adequate
  1. Acetylcholine receptor antibody assay
  2. Edrophonium test
  3. Electromyography

Effect on pregnancy & fetus
- Does not effect uterine activity or duration of labor because uterus is smooth muscle
- No evidence of increased rate of spontaneous abortions
- Preterm delivery rate btwn 13–41% reported
- Congenital malformations, unrelated to meds, attributed to prolonged fetal immobilization
  - Fetal akinesia deformation sequence due to congenital myopathies & neuropathies
  - Multiple ankyloses, craniofacial dysmorphism, pulmonary hypoplasia & growth retardation

- Transplacental passage of autoantibodies leads to neonatal MG in 10–20%
  - No correlation btwn incidence of neonatal MG & antibody titers
  - Weak cry, poor sucking, hypotonia, occasionally respiratory insufficiency occur btwn a few hours & a few days after birth & may persist for 3 weeks to 3 months
  - Both antibodies & maternal anticholinesterase drugs pass into breast milk

STUDIES

History & Physical
- Evaluate for signs & symptoms of ocular, bulbar & respiratory involvement
  - Ptosis & diplopia
  - Dysphagia
  - Dyspnea on exertion & at rest

Imaging
- Chest radiograph: evaluate for evidence of chronic aspiration
- Fetal ultrasound: evaluate for signs of decreased fetal movement

Other
- Pre-op measure of muscle strength for post-op comparison
  - Electromyogram
  - Train-of-four
- Pulmonary function testing & ABGs: consider if there is evidence of respiratory compromise
- ECG: case reports of focal myocardial necrosis
- Fetal kick-counts

MANAGEMENT/INTERVENTIONS

Medical treatment
- Anticholinesterase drugs: first line & safe during pregnancy
  - Neostigmine
    - Most commonly used anticholinesterase
    - Duration 2–3 hrs
    - Dosing: 0.5 mg IV, 1.5 mg SC, 0.7 mg IM, 15 mg PO
  - Pyridostigmine
    - Preferred over neostigmine because it has fewer muscarinic side effects
    - Duration 4–6 hrs
    - Dosing: 2 mg IV, 3 mg IM, 60 mg PO

- ➤ Dosage may need to be increased due to increased intravascular volume, increased renal clearance, hepatic stasis
- ➤ Parenteral administration avoids potential problem of variable gastric absorption
- ➤ Both neostigmine & pyridostigmine are quaternary amines & do not readily cross placenta
- ➤ Symptoms of overdose include nausea, vomiting, abdominal cramps, diarrhea, increased salivary/tear duct secretions
- ➤ Cholinergic crisis
  - Excess of muscarinic effects of anticholinergic medication resulting in muscle weakness, respiratory failure
  - Can be mistaken for myasthenic crisis
  - Differentiate by administration of short-acting edrophonium 1–2 mg IV; there is a dramatic improvement in myasthenic crisis but not cholinergic crisis
- ■ Corticosteroids
  - ➤ No evidence of teratogenicity
  - ➤ Inactivation by placental 11-beta-OH-dehydrogenase results in low fetal levels of active drug
  - ➤ May precipitate gestational diabetes mellitus & hypertension
  - ➤ Longer-term adverse effects
    - Osteoporosis
    - GI ulceration
    - Impaired immunity
    - Adrenal suppression
- ■ Azathioprine
  - ➤ No evidence of teratogenicity, but has been associated w/reversible neonatal lymphopenia, decreased serum immunoglobulin levels, decreased thymic size
- ■ Cyclosporin A
  - ➤ Higher incidence of spontaneous abortion or preterm delivery
- ■ Myasthenic crisis
  - ➤ High-dose IVIG & plasmapheresis are safe during pregnancy

Surgical
- ■ Thymectomy
  - ➤ Reason for improvement unclear but helps approx. 96% of pts w/ complete remission (46%) & asymptomatic or improved symptoms (50%)

Anesthesia
- ■ General anesthesia

➤ Involved muscles are very sensitive to non-depolarizing muscle relaxants, while uninvolved muscles are more resistant to their effects

➤ Avoid muscle relaxants if possible

➤ If required, use agents w/ short half-life, starting at about 10% of the usual dose

➤ Mivacurium is relatively contraindicated because it is metabolized by pseudocholinesterase

➤ Slowed metabolism of succinylcholine in pts on anticholinesterase therapy

➤ Duration of muscle relaxants is unpredictable in setting of anticholinesterase drugs

➤ Volatile halogenated anesthetics potentiate muscle relaxation

➤ Reverse neuromuscular blockade using incremental doses of neostigmine or pyridostigmine to avoid cholinergic crisis

➤ Using a nerve stimulator is essential

➤ Predictors for need of post-op ventilation
1. Duration of MG >6 yrs
2. History of chronic respiratory disease
3. Pyridostigmine dose >750 mg/day
4. Pre-op vital capacity <2.9 L

➤ Other factors identified
1. Female gender
2. $FEF_{25-75\%}$ <3.3 L/sec & <85% predicted
3. FVC <2.6 L/sec & <78% predicted
4. $MEF_{50\%}$ <3.9 L/sec & <80% predicted

➤ Regional anesthesia
• Amide-type local anesthetics are thought to be safer than ester-type agents because of decreased plasma cholinesterase activity in pts on anticholinesterase therapy resulting in unpredictable, prolonged half-life

➤ For cesarean delivery, a regional technique is usually preferred unless there is significant respiratory involvement that dictates securing the airway, because a high regional block may result in respiratory insufficiency

➤ Increased anticholinesterase medication may be required during labor due to increased physical & emotional stresses

➤ Use caution w/ opioid administration in pts w/ respiratory involvement

➤ Skin infiltration w/ local anesthetic can be used to help reduce post-op pain

➤ Stress-dose steroids during labor & delivery for pts currently on steroid therapy

CAVEATS & PEARLS

■ Differentiate between myasthenic & cholinergic crises w/ edrophonium test

➤ Improvement in symptoms in myasthenic crisis

■ Exacerbation of myasthenic symptoms w/ tocolytics: magnesium, terbutaline, ritodrine, aminoglycosides, tetracyclines, polymyxin, propanolol, quinidine

➤ Magnesium sulfate is contraindicated because hypermagnesemia potentiates neuromuscular block by inhibiting the release of acetylcholine

■ Amide-type local anesthetics are thought to be safer than ester-type agents because plasma cholinesterase activity may be decreased in MG pts, resulting in unpredictable, prolonged half-life

■ Involved muscles are very sensitive to non-depolarizing muscle relaxants, while uninvolved muscles are more resistant to their effects

■ Avoid muscle relaxants if possible because of unpredictable duration

■ Take particular care w/ opioids & other meds that may cause respiratory depression

CHECKLIST

■ Pre-op measure of muscle strength for post-op comparison

■ Discuss possibility of post-op intubation & ventilation

■ Nerve stimulator essential

■ Have anticholinesterase drugs, including edrophonium, readily available

■ Stress-dose steroids during labor & delivery for pts currently on steroid therapy

---

MYASTHENIA GRAVIS: MANAGEMENT OF THE PARTURIENT WITH NEUROLOGIC DISEASE

MEREDITH ALBRECHT, MD; LISA LEFFERT, MD; AND MICHELE SZABO, MD

FUNDAMENTAL KNOWLEDGE

Definition

■ Autoimmune disorder characterized by episodes of muscle weakness worsened by activity

Epidemiology

- 1 in 7,500
- In women, onset peaks btwn 20–30 years old.
- Women affected 3:1 vs. males in the age group 20–30 years old

Pathophysiology

- Antibodies against the nicotinic acetylcholine receptor on the neuromuscular endplate of skeletal muscle
- Antibodies cause acetylcholine receptor blockade & destruction.
- Reduction in the number of receptors results in weakness of muscle contraction.
- Smooth & cardiac muscles are unaffected.

Clinical Manifestations

- Weakness & fatigability of muscles
- Decreased amount of acetylcholine released during successive nerve impulses, causing increasing weakness w/ repetitive nerve stimulation ("myasthenic fatigue")
- Improves after sleep
- Increased muscle fatigue w/ repetitive activity
- Clinical course is variable, w/ exacerbations & remissions.
- Remissions rarely complete or permanent
- Associated w/ thymic hyperplasia and thymic tumors in 10% of pts
Associated w/ other autoimmune disorders (rheumatoid arthritis, polymyositis)
- Unrelated infections may precipitate crisis.
- 3–8% of pts w/ hyperthyroidism

Effect of Pregnancy on Myasthenia Gravis

- Variable: one third improve, one third see no change, one third worsen
- One third of pts relapse post-partum.
- Pregnancy can increase respiratory compromise due to the disease.
- Dose of anticholinergic agents may have to be altered during pregnancy.
- Myasthenia crises must be treated aggressively.
- During labor, an IV infusion of anticholinesterase may be necessary.
- Magnesium sulfate administration can worsen symptoms.

Effect of Myasthenia Gravis on Pregnancy & the Fetus

- Increased perinatal mortality
- Increased incidence of preterm labor

- Anticholinesterases can cause premature labor. Any dosage changes should be done in conjunction w/ monitoring of uterine activity.
- 1st stage of labor unaltered
- 2nd stage of labor prolonged
- Increased incidence of instrumented deliveries
- Neonatal myasthenia gravis
  - 16% of infants of mothers w/ myasthenia
  - Maternal antibodies to the acetylcholine receptor are transferred across the placenta.
  - Symptoms present in the first 4 days of life
  - Infants have feeding problems, hypotonia & respiratory difficulty.
  - Symptoms resolve over 2–4 weeks as antibodies are metabolized.
  - Anticholinesterase therapy may initially be required to control symptoms.

STUDIES

History & Physical
- Weakness increased w/ prolonged effort
- Cranial muscles involved early in course (lids & extraocular)
  - Diplopia
  - Ptosis
- Facial weakness: "snarling" expression when attempting to smile
- Speech: nasal timbre or "mushy" quality
- Difficulty in swallowing
- Limb weakness proximal may be asymmetric
- Deep tendon reflexes preserved
- Preserved sensation

Laboratory
- Presence of anti-acetylcholine receptor antibodies (in 85% of pts)

Imaging
- None

Other
- Edrophonium test: 10 (2, then 8) mg IV results in decreased muscle weakness in minutes
- EMG w/ repetitive nerve stimulation: decremental responses
- Pulmonary function tests: to assess extent of respiratory involvement

MANAGEMENT/INTERVENTIONS

Medical Treatment
- Thymectomy
  - Improves 96% of pts

➤ 46% of pts experience complete remission.
- Meds
  ➤ Anticholinesterase agents: neostigmine, pyridostigmine
  ➤ Immunosuppressive agents: corticosteroids, azathioprine, cyclosporine
- Plasmapheresis
- IV immunoglobulin
- For Eaton-Lambert:
  ➤ Plasmapheresis
  ➤ Immunosuppression
  ➤ Diaminopyridine: blocks potassium channels, prolonged depolarization
  ➤ Pyridostigmine: anticholinesterase
- Differentiation of crises (involve respiratory failure)
  ➤ Cholinergic: excess of muscarinic effects of anticholinesterase meds
  ➤ Myasthenic: worsening of the disease
- Distinguish btwn cholinergic & myasthenic crises w/ edrophonium, which improves only myasthenic crisis.
- Meds that typically worsen symptoms
  ➤ Neuromuscular blocking agents
  ➤ Quinidine
  ➤ Propranolol
  ➤ Aminoglycoside antibiotics
  ➤ Tocolytic agents (magnesium, terbutaline, ritodrine)

Anesthesia
- Predelivery assessment
  ➤ Physical exam focusing on respiratory & bulbar involvement
  ➤ Pulmonary function tests if respiratory involvement
  ➤ Respiratory involvement leads to a heightened opioid effect.
- General anesthesia
  ➤ Risk of aspiration increased
  ➤ Aspiration prophylaxis (H2 antagonists, sodium citrate, metoclopramide) recommended
  ➤ If significant degree of bulbar or respiratory compromise, general endotracheal anesthesia has advantage of securing the airway.
  ➤ Muscle relaxants have an unpredictable effect.
    • Pts are very sensitive to nondepolarizing agents.
    • Succinylcholine has a prolonged effect (slow metabolism).
    • Monitor neuromuscular blockade.
  ➤ If pt is taking anticholinesterases:

> May require post-op ventilation; risk factors:
  - Duration of myasthenia >6 years
  - History of chronic respiratory disease
  - Pyridostigmine dose >750 mg/day
  - Vital capacity <2.9 L
  - Forced vital capacity <2.6 L/sec
- Regional anesthesia
  > If pt is w/o respiratory compromise, preferred method
  > Anticholinesterases decrease plasma cholinesterase activity, leading to prolonged half-life of ester local anesthetics.
  > Amide local anesthetics preferred
  > Ester local anesthetics acceptable in spinal anesthesia (small amount)
- Post-partum, pt may require adjustment of anticholinesterase dosage.

CAVEATS & PEARLS
- Autoimmune illness w/ production of antibodies to acetylcholine receptors
- Muscle weakness worsened by activity
- Can be worsened or improved by pregnancy
- Pregnancy can worsen respiratory involvement.
- Associated w/ increased preterm labor & perinatal mortality
- Anticholinesterase dosage may have to be altered during pregnancy & post-partum.
- Magnesium sulfate may exacerbate symptoms.
- Tocolysis may cause a crisis.
- Cholinergic vs. myasthenic crisis can be differentiated by edrophonium challenge.
- Increased aspiration risk
- Regional anesthesia preferred if feasible; avoid large doses of ester local anesthetics
- Unpredictable response to neuromuscular blocking agents
- If respiratory involvement, pt may require post-op ventilation after general anesthesia.
- Neonatal myasthenia gravis may occur in infant due to maternal antibodies.

CHECKLIST
- Careful physical exam, assessing degree of weakness & pulmonary involvement

- Pulmonary function tests if there is pulmonary involvement
- Aspiration prophylaxis
- If significant respiratory involvement, general anesthesia recommended
- Carefully monitor neuromuscular blockade (succinylcholine has a prolonged effect; pts are also sensitive to non-depolarizing muscle relaxants).
- Recommend using only short-duration neuromuscular blocking agents.
- Post-op ventilation may be necessary after general anesthesia.
- Avoid use of ester local anesthetics due to prolonged half-life, except in spinals.
- If pt goes into crisis, the edrophonium test will differentiate cholinergic from myasthenic.
- Closely observe newborn's respiratory status for signs of neonatal myasthenia gravis.

MYOTONIA & MYOTONIC DYSTROPHY (STEINERT'S, BATTEN-CURSCHMANN'S & HOFFMAN'S DISEASE)

MEREDITH ALBRECHT, MD; LISA LEFFERT, MD; AND MICHELE SZABO, MD

FUNDAMENTAL KNOWLEDGE

Definition
- Myotonia: prolongation of muscle contraction caused by sustained muscle firing
- Progressive wasting of facial, neck & distal limb muscles

Epidemiology
- Autosomal dominant
- Onset in 2nd or 3rd decade
- 2–6 cases per 100,000 births

Pathophysiology
- Abnormal chloride conductance of the muscle fiber membrane
- Reduced ability of the sodium channels to inactivate
- Genetic defect: expanded CTG repeat in a protein kinase on chromosome 19
- Pathology
  - ➤ Myopathic features
    - Prominent type I fiber atrophy

- Increased central mucleation
- Chains of nuclei
- Ring fibers

Clinical Manifestations

- Myotonia
- Progressive wasting of facial, neck & distal limb muscles
- Pharyngeal, laryngeal muscles & diaphragm can be involved.
- Frontal balding
- Cataracts
- Diminished insulin sensitivity
- Cardiac disease, esp. of the conduction system (50% incidence)
- Mitral regurgitation & cardiomyopathy
- Abnormal insulin response
- GI paresis
- Esophageal incompetence

Effect of Pregnancy on Myotonic Dystrophy

- Symptoms can be unchanged or worsened by pregnancy.

Effect of Myotonic Dystrophy on Pregnancy & the Fetus

- Associated w/ hypogonadism
- Increased risk of premature labor & spontaneous abortion
- Increased incidence of fetal death
- Tocolysis can provoke the symptoms of myotonia.
- Prolonged 2nd stage of labor can occur as disease can involve uterine muscles.
- Increased incidence of instrumented deliveries
- Increased incidence of polyhydramnios/fetal hydrops
- Increased incidence of postpartum hemorrhage & retained placenta
- Congenital myotonic dystrophy can present in child presenting w/ respiratory distress, hypotonia &/or feeding difficulties.

STUDIES

History & Physical

- "Hatchet" face: ptosis, jaw slackness, temporal/masseter wasting often present
- Test myotonia by having pt tightly grip an object & then attempt to suddenly release it.
- Myotonia can be induced by:
  - Cold
  - Shivering
  - Surgical/mechanical stimulation
  - Anesthetic agents

Assess signs/symptoms of pulmonary & cardiac involvement (mitral regurgitation & cardiomyopathy).

Laboratory
- None

Imaging
- None

Other
- EMG: myotonic dive-bomber bursts
- Muscle biopsy
- EKG may reveal cardiac conduction defects.

MANAGEMENT/INTERVENTIONS

Medical Treatment
- Membrane-active meds to decrease myotonia
  - Phenytoin
  - Mexiletine
- For acute myotonic crisis
  - IV quinidine
  - IV steroids
  - IV dantrolene

Anesthesia
- Predelivery
  - Prophylaxis against aspiration (H2 antagonists, sodium citrate, metoclopramide)
  - Carefully maintain temp, as cold/shivering can trigger myotonic crisis.
  - Warm IV fluids
- General anesthesia
  - Succinylcholine can cause prolonged myotonia.
  - Variable response to non-depolarizing neuromuscular blocking agents
  - Nerve stimulators can trigger myotonic episodes.
  - Pain upon propofol injection can trigger a myotonic episode.
  - Heightened depressive response to opioids can occur.
  - Anticholinesterases can also precipitate myotonia.
- Regional anesthesia
  - Preferred if possible
  - Avoid shivering.

- Postdelivery
  - ➤ Increased incidence of uterine atony & postpartum hemorrhage if uterine involvement

CAVEATS & PEARLS

- Myotonia is a prolonged contraction of muscles after stimulation.
- Myotonia can be triggered by cold, shivering, surgical/mechanical stimulation, anesthesia.
- Can be associated w/ cardiac conduction abnormalities, mitral regurgitation & cardiomyopathy.
- Involvement of laryngeal muscles increases risk of aspiration.
- Uterine involvement can be present.
- Increased risk of spontaneous abortion & premature labor
- Tocolysis can trigger myotonia.
- Increased incidence of prolonged labor & instrumented deliveries
- Avoid succinylcholine.
- Anticholinesterases can also precipitate myotonia.
- Regional anesthesia preferred
- Carefully assess pulmonary status during labor/delivery.
- Variable response to non-depolarizing neuromuscular blocking agents
- Heightened response to opioids
- Increased incidence of uterine atony & postpartum hemorrhage
- May be able to treat myotonia w/ direct local anesthetic administration

CHECKLIST

- Careful physical exam focusing on:
  - ➤ Assessing myotonia by having pt grip tightly & then suddenly release
  - ➤ Pulmonary capacity, possibly pulmonary function tests
  - ➤ Signs/symptoms of mitral regurgitation
  - ➤ Document preexisting muscular deficits.
- EKG to investigate cardiac conduction abnormalities
- Aspiration prophylaxis
- Avoid cold/shivering.
- Warm IV fluids.
- Avoid succinylcholine.
- Avoid reversal agents.
- Avoid triggers of myotonic episodes.
  - ➤ Cold/shivering

➤ Fasciculation due to depolarizing neuromuscular blockers
➤ Pain due to propofol injection
➤ Pain due to surgery
➤ Pain due to neuromuscular twitch monitoring
■ Consider treating uterine atony w/ direct local anesthetic administration.
■ Carefully observe newborn for signs of congenital myotonic dystrophy.

NEONATAL AIRWAY MANAGEMENT

RICHARD ARCHULETA, MD
SANDRA WEINREB, MD

FUNDAMENTAL KNOWLEDGE
Effective oxygenation & ventilation is essential to the resuscitation of neonates.
■ Cardiovascular resuscitation is rarely needed because effective oxygenation & ventilation is successful in the large majority of cases.
■ Hypoxia & hypercapnia promote acidosis, decreased myocardial performance (bradycardia & decreased contractility) & eventual cardiovascular collapse.
If oxygen flow by & physical stimulation are insufficient (neonate continues to display poor respiratory effort, heart rate <100 &/or continued central cyanosis despite supplemental O2), PPV will be required.
PPV
■ Should initially be applied using a mask & bag unless an endotracheal tube (ETT) is initially indicated
  ➤ Intubation indications
    • Bag & mask ventilation is ineffective or prolonged
    • Neonate requires ongoing PPV
    • Meconium-stained amniotic fluid (see "*Meconium*")
    • Delivery of medications tracheally
    • Chest compressions
■ Neonatal masks
  ➤ Several neonatal masks should be available & selected so that:
    • The neonate's nose & mouth are covered
    • The mask does not impinge on the eyes or extend over the chin

- A tight seal should be obtained w/o having to apply excessive pressure to the mask

■ Neonatal bags
➤ Select a bag so you can judge the small tidal volumes required for neonates (6–8 cc/kg), but also one that can sustain inflation pressure for at least 1 second.
- Bag volume should be 500–750 cc.
- Use either a self-inflating bag w/ an intake valve & oxygen reservoir, or a flow-inflating bag w/ a pressure manometer.
- If there is a pressure release valve, set it btwn 30 & 35 cm H2O.

If tracheal intubation is required, the correct equipment should be selected:

■ Weight <1,000 g
➤ Age
- <28 wks
➤ Laryngoscope blade
- 0
➤ ETT
- 2.5 mm
➤ Depth from lips
- 6.5–7 cm

■ Weight 1,000–2,000 g
➤ Age
- 28–34 weeks
➤ Laryngoscope blade
- 0
➤ ETT
- 3.0 mm
➤ Depth from lips
- 7–8 cm

■ Weight 2,000–3,000 g
➤ Age
- 34–38 weeks
➤ Laryngoscope blade
- 0–1
➤ ETT
- 3.0–3.5 mm
➤ Depth from lips
- 8–9 cm

■ Weight >3,000 g
➤ Age
- >38 wks
➤ Laryngoscope blade
- 1
➤ ETT
- 3.5–4.0 mm
➤ Depth from lips
- 10–11 cm

■ The above table provides a rough correlation between weight & age. If there is a discrepancy (eg, IUGR), select equipment using neonatal weight.

LMAs are very useful if difficult mask ventilation or endotracheal intubation occurs.

■ Common size for term newborns is size 1.
■ Can be used for PPV in term newborns
■ Little data regarding use in preterm infants

STUDIES

Continue to evaluate neonate's respiration, heart rate & color at least every 30 seconds until neonate's respiratory status has stabilized.

MANAGEMENT/INTERVENTIONS

Apply appropriately sized face mask to neonate w/ either a self-inflating bag or a flow-inflating bag.

Applied airway pressure w/ bag & mask

1. For first breath, apply 30–40 cm $H2O$ w/ recruitment maneuver (held for several seconds)
2. Subsequent breaths
   a. Apply up to 20–30 cm $H2O$
   b. Deliver breaths w/ slight pauses to maintain recruitment

Applied breathing rate

- 40–60 breaths per minute w/o chest compressions
- 30 breaths per minute w/ chest compressions

Evaluation

1. If neonate clinically improves w/ 30 seconds of PPV w/ bag & mask (cyanosis improves, spontaneous respiratory effort improves, etc.), then continue bag & mask PPV as needed & insert 8F orogastric tube after prolonged (several minutes) bag & mask ventilation to relieve resultant elevated gastric pressures.
2. If neonate does not clinically improve w/ 30 seconds of bag & mask ventilation, consider endotracheal intubation.

Intubation indications

- Bag & mask ventilation is ineffective or prolonged
- Neonate requires ongoing PPV
- Meconium-stained amniotic fluid (see "*Meconium*")
- Delivery of medications tracheally
- Chest compressions

Intubation

1. Select appropriate equipment according to table above
   a. Ensure laryngoscope is working properly (should have been checked during preparation; see "*Preparation for Newborn Resuscitation*").
   b. Make sure ETTs 1 size larger & 1 size smaller are available if neonate does not match initial selection of ETT.

2. Only personnel skilled in laryngoscopy should attempt neonatal intubation. The neonatal larynx is anterior & intubation is often aided by gentle cricoid pressure.
3. Intubation technique
   a. Position left hand for laryngoscopy as follows:
      1) Thumb & first 2 fingers: hold laryngoscope
      2) Third (ring) finger: place on mandible
      3) Fourth (pinky) finger: apply cricoid pressure
4. After placement of tube, advance tube into trachea until insertion depth is:
   a. 6 + weight (in kg) = number of cm at the lips
   b. This translates to 7, 8 or 9 cm at lip for 1-, 2- or 3-kg neonate
5. Confirm proper tube placement
   a. Check exhaled end tidal CO_2 w/ disposable or infrared device.
   b. Observe symmetrical chest wall motion.
   c. Auscultate equal axial bilateral breath sounds w/o corresponding gastric sounds.
   d. Improvement in clinical condition (SpO_2, HR, color)
   e. Fogging of ETT during exhalation
6. If tube is to remain in place after initial resuscitation:
   a. Check leak pressure for ETT.
      1) If leak pressure >25 cm H_2O of pressure, replace ETT w/ smaller ETT to avoid compromise of laryngeal mucosal tissue circulation.
   b. Tape ETT in place.
   c. Obtain follow-up chest x-ray to confirm that position of ETT is satisfactory.
7. If intubation is unsuccessful, consider placing #1 LMA for term infants.

Observe the neonate for signs of airway compromise
- Decreased lung compliance
- Decreased oxygenation as per pulse oximeter or ABGs
- Bradycardia
- Central or peripheral cyanosis
- Hypercapnia
- Unequal expansion of chest wall
- Unequal breath sounds (can be difficult to gauge in that breath sounds are often dispersed throughout the chest cavity)
- Decreased mental status & responsiveness

Expedient correction of airway difficulty in the intubated neonate

1. Causes of airway compromise
   - The ETT position can be altered w/ neonatal head flexion/extension (ETT advanced/withdrawn)
   - The ETT can be obstructed
     - ETT kink
     - Mucus plug
     - Meconium
   - Increased intrathoracic or abdominal pressure
     - Pneumothorax
     - Gastric inflation
   - Equipment failure
2. Corrective measures
   a. Switch from mechanical ventilation to bag ventilation to confirm decreased lung compliance & rule out mechanical malfunction.
   b. Check ETT position & reposition as required.
   c. Suction airway w/ catheter to clear secretions & rule out ETT obstruction.
   d. Pass orogastric or nasogastric tube to decompress stomach, especially after prolonged bag & mask ventilation.
   e. If pneumothorax is strongly suspected, place 22- or 25-gauge needle in the second intercostal space at the midclavicular line.
   f. Obtain chest x-ray to confirm ETT position & lung expansion.

CAVEATS & PEARLS

Different types of ventilation bags have unique advantages & disadvantages

- Self-inflating bag
  - Does not require either a compressed or high-pressure oxygen source to deliver positive pressure
  - Must have a pressure release valve so that the amount of positive pressure delivered to the neonate can be regulated
  - Requires a oxygen reservoir bag & a good mask seal to deliver a high FiO_2
    - Without a oxygen reservoir bag or a good mask seal, room air can be entrained into the bag as it re-expands
- Flow inflating bags
  - Requires a compressed or high-flow oxygen source to keep the bag inflated

➤ Should have a flow control valve that allows the leakage of excess gas not delivered directly to the pt
➤ Should have a peak pressure gauge to monitor the peak inspiratory pressure administered to the neonate
➤ Flow-inflating bags have a different "feel" to operate than self-inflating bags & may require some practice before use in an emergency situation.

Continued difficulty w/ airway mgt may involve one of several congenital anomalies. Although these conditions are in general beyond the scope of this resource, brief mention is made for immediate mgt.

■ Cleft palate can make mask ventilation difficult & necessitate early endotracheal intubation.
■ Choanal atresia may exist if the neonate is pink when crying but cyanotic when quiet because the neonate is an obligate nose breather except when crying.
➤ If difficulty is encountered when gently advancing a suction catheter into each nasal passage, then place an oral airway or intubate the neonate to facilitate oxygenation & ventilation.
■ Micrognathia, as in Treacher Collins syndrome or Pierre Robin syndrome
➤ Place neonate prone to help reduce pharyngeal obstruction by the tongue.
➤ Neonate may have an airway that is exceptionally difficult to intubate.
■ Macroglossia, as in Beckwith Wiedemann syndrome
➤ Place neonate prone to help reduce pharyngeal obstruction by the tongue.
➤ Alternatively, use oral airway to stent airway open.
■ Extrinsic airway compression
➤ May include conditions such as teratomas & angiomas
➤ If anticipated from ultrasound studies, a surgical airway is indicated.
➤ If unanticipated, attempt PPV (mask & bag; if unsuccessful, endotracheal intubation) while calling for personnel for immediate surgical airway.
■ Tracheoesophageal fistula
➤ Should be suspected if bubbling secretions are noted
➤ Once suspected, discontinue bag & mask ventilation.
• Can result in gastric distention that predisposes to increased intra-abdominal pressure w/ decreased ventilation & increased risk of gastric aspiration

➤ Place neonate in reverse Trendelenburg position.
➤ Place a suction catheter in the esophageal pouch to help clear the airway of secretions.
➤ If neonate requires PPV:
  • Intubate & purposely place ETT deep past the TE fistula.
  • Slowly pull back ETT until breath sounds are confirmed bilaterally.
  • Auscultate stomach to ensure the ETT terminates distal to the fistula.
  • Tape the ETT in place.
■ If neonate has airway difficulty & a scaphoid abdomen, congenital diaphragmatic hernia (CDH) should be suspected.
  ➤ Avoid bag & mask ventilation to minimize gastric distention & decreased FRC.
  ➤ If PPV is required, intubate the neonate & carefully ventilate:
    • Use maximum airway pressures of 15 cm H2O to avoid pneumothorax in this particularly susceptible population.
    • Provide frequent ventilations (at least 60 per minute) to maintain an adequate minute ventilation.
    • Maintain high index of suspicion for pneumothorax & promptly treat if indicated. Place 22- or 25-gauge needle in the 2nd intercostal space at the midclavicular line. Obtain chest x-ray to confirm ETT position & lung expansion.
  ➤ Place orogastric tube to suction stomach.
■ Unknown airway obstruction
  ➤ Perform laryngoscopy to determine if obstruction is supraglottic or subglottic.
  ➤ Supraglottic obstruction includes
    • Meconium (see "*Meconium*")
    • Laryngeal web (carefully force ETT through web into trachea)
  ➤ Subglottic obstruction includes
    • Subglottic stenosis, tracheal agenesis, subglottic hemangioma, etc.
    • May require immediate surgical airway
Passage of orogastric tube to decompress the stomach can stimulate a vagal reaction, resulting in bradycardia or apnea.

CHECKLIST
1. Select appropriately sized mask & bag.
2. Apply PPV w/ bag & mask. Refer to "Management/Interventions" to determine the correct pressure & rate.

3. Evaluate effectiveness of bag & mask PPV during first 30 seconds of application. If effective, continue as indicated. If ineffective, prepare to intubate.
4. If intubation is indicated
   a. Select correct laryngoscope & ETTs.
   b. Intubate & place ETT.
   c. Advance ETT to appropriate depth.
   d. If ETT is to remain in place, ensure leak pressure does not exceed 25 cm H2O.
      1) Tape ETT in place.
      2) Reduce FiO2 as tolerated to avoid unnecessary oxygen-related complications
      3) Obtain chest x-ray to confirm proper placement.

NEONATAL IV ACCESS

RICHARD ARCHULETA, MD
SANDRA WEINREB, MD

FUNDAMENTAL KNOWLEDGE
Multiple routes of access to neonate are available:
■ Umbilical vein catheterization
■ Peripheral IV access
■ Interosseous access
Umbilical vein catheterization is the most reliable & quickest route of IV access in the neonate.
■ 2 techniques for umbilical vein catheterization (see the "MANAGEMENT/INTERVENTIONS" section)
■ Can be used for CVP monitoring

Umbilical anatomy
■ There are 3 apparent vessels:
   ➣ 1 relatively large umbilical vein (thin-walled) w/ end flush w/ cut end of umbilical cord
   ➣ 2 smaller umbilical arteries (thick-walled) that extend beyond the cut end of the umbilical cord
■ The umbilical vein empties into the portal vein.

STUDIES
N/A

MANAGEMENT/INTERVENTIONS

Umbilical vein catheterization

- Technique 1: applying soft catheter to proximal umbilical cord
  - ➤ Advanced technique that requires skill w/ IV access in neonates
  - ➤ Prepare umbilical catheter
    - Use sterile technique while preparing & placing umbilical catheter.
    - Catheter should have a radiopaque line.
    - Use a 3.5F or 5F catheter.
    - Flush catheter w/ heparinized saline (0.5–1 unit/cc).
    - Attach catheter to a 3-way stopcock.
  - ➤ Prepare umbilical vein.
    - The umbilical cord should be sterilely prepped.
    - At the base of the umbilical cord, apply a circumferential tie close to the base of the cord to prevent bleeding.
    - Cut the cord 1 cm distal to the skin attachment.
  - ➤ Catheterize the umbilical vein.
    - Identify the umbilical vein as the thin-walled vessel flush w/ the cut end of the umbilical cord.
    - Insert the umbilical catheter into the umbilical vein & attempt to aspirate blood.
    - Advance the catheter until good blood aspiration occurs, up to a maximum of 2 cm into the abdomen.
    - Avoid advancing the catheter more than 4 cm or the catheter may be advanced into the portal vein & either block flow or damage hepatic parenchyma.
    - Aspirate blood to clear the catheter of air bubbles & prevent venous embolism.
  - ➤ If necessary, the soft catheter can be advanced through the ductus venosus into the IVC to provide CVP. However, this technique is beyond the scope of this resource & is usually reserved for ICU care & rarely used for acute resuscitation.
- Technique 2: applying standard stiff IV to distal umbilical cord
  - ➤ More basic technique for practitioners w/ general IV access skill
  - ➤ Prepare umbilical IV.
    - Use sterile technique while preparing & placing umbilical catheter.
    - Use 20- or 22-gauge IV catheter.
    - Flush catheter w/ heparinized saline (0.5–1 unit/cc).
    - Attach catheter to a 3-way stopcock.

➤ Prepare umbilical vein.
  • The umbilical cord should be sterilely prepped.
  • Apply a circumferential tie to the cord to prevent bleeding.
  • Cut the cord at least 4 cm distal to the skin attachment (make sure the remaining umbilical cord is long enough to prevent the stiff IV catheter from entering the abdomen, where it can cause trauma).
➤ Catheterize the umbilical vein.
  • Identify the umbilical vein as the thin-walled vessel flush w/ the cut end of the umbilical cord.
  • Insert the catheter into the umbilical vein & attempt to aspirate blood to clear the catheter of air bubbles & prevent venous embolism.

Standard peripheral IV access
■ Use a 22- to 24-gauge IV catheter.

Interosseous access
■ An effective alternative technique to umbilical vein catheterization
■ Locate access site 1 cm below the tibial tuberosity & insert a 20-gauge needle.
■ An alternate method of access should be obtained immediately after acute resuscitation because the risk of infection rises w/ continued interosseous access.

CAVEATS & PEARLS
Umbilical catheterization is an advanced technique & should be attempted only by personnel skilled in IV access.

Potential side effects of access
■ Umbilical vein access
  ➤ Intra-abdominal trauma
  ➤ Hepatic injury
  ➤ Intracerebral hemorrhage
  ➤ Venous air embolism
  ➤ Hemorrhage
  ➤ Sepsis
■ Interosseous access
  ➤ Tibial fracture
  ➤ Osteomyelitis

CHECKLIST
■ Prepare umbilical catheter.
■ Sterilely prepare, tie & cut umbilical cord.

- Carefully identify umbilical vein (vs. the two umbilical arteries).
  - ➤ Insert catheter. Advance soft umbilical catheter into proximal umbilical vein just until you can aspirate blood. Do not advance the catheter too far (ie, >2 cm into abdomen). Place peripheral IV catheter into distal umbilical vein.
- Place interosseous 1 cm below tibial tuberosity.
- Avoid infusion of hyperosmolar solutions into neonate.

NEONATAL STATUS AT BIRTH

RICHARD ARCHULETA, MD
SANDRA WEINREB, MD

FUNDAMENTAL KNOWLEDGE

It is important to understand the normal physiologic changes that accompany birth to have an appreciation for the role of therapeutic measures for the neonate, as well as the expected results of a problem during the birth process.

Normal fetal circulation involves elements of parallel circulation:

- Blood travels into placenta → ductus venosus → IVC → RA → foramen ovale → LA → LV → aorta
  - ➤ Aorta → placenta
  - ➤ Preductal aorta → upper body (head, brain, right arm) → SCV → pulmonary arteries → 90% into PDA → postductal aorta → placenta

Pulmonary changes at birth

- Vaginal birth produces thoracic squeeze w/ expulsion of lung fluid.
  - ➤ Approximately 2/3 of the lung fluid is expelled when a term neonate is passed through the birth canal.
    - • At term, the lungs contain approximately 30 cc of plasma ultrafiltrate produced by the lungs.
    - • The lung fluid remaining after the thoracic squeeze is reabsorbed via lymphatics & capillaries.
  - ➤ Very small neonates (preterm) & neonates born by C-section usually experience decreased chest compression, resulting in increased residual lung fluid, which can cause transient tachypnea of the newborn.
- Lung aeration
  - ➤ The pulmonary vascular resistance (PVR) is initially high due to lack of lung aeration.

➤ Breathing
➤ First breath requires high pressure to aerate lungs.
  • Breathing should begin within 30 seconds of delivery.
  • Breathing should be regular within 90 seconds.
  • Normal respiratory rate is 30–60 per minute.
➤ With lung aeration:
  • PVR decreases
  • Surfactant is released into the alveoli if present

Cardiovascular changes at birth
■ Cord clamping increases systemic vascular resistance.
  ➤ The low-resistance placenta is removed from the vascular circuit.
■ Closure of the ductus arteriosus results from:
  ➤ Decreased pulmonary vascular resistance
  ➤ Increased SVR (exceeds the PVR) resulting in functional closure
  ➤ Increased PaO2 promotes anatomical closure
    • Usually 10–14 days in term neonates
    • Anatomical closure delayed in preterm neonates
  ➤ The neonate can revert to fetal circulation w/ a patent ductus arteriosus under conditions of stress (hypoxia, acidosis, hypothermia) until anatomical closure at 10–14 days in a term neonate.
■ Functional closure of the foramen ovale results from:
  ➤ Increased LA pressure secondary to increased pulmonary blood flow
  ➤ Decreased RA pressure secondary to decreased pulmonary vascular resistance

Normal neonatal circulation
■ Consists of series circulation as in the adult
■ Normal neonatal vital signs
  ➤ Heart rate 120–160 bpm
  ➤ Systolic BP 60–70 mm Hg
  ➤ Respiratory rate 30–60 breaths per minute
  ➤ Hgb 13–20 mg/dL
  ➤ Glucose at least 35 mg/dL

Neonatal apnea
■ Classified as primary or secondary
■ The normal peripartum respiratory course in a neonate experiencing respiratory difficulty is:
  ➤ Brief period of gasping efforts
  ➤ Brief period of apnea (primary apnea)

➤ Longer period of gasping efforts
➤ Prolonged apnea (secondary apnea)
■ Either primary or secondary apnea may be occurring in a neonate who is not breathing 90 seconds after delivery.
■ Primary apnea
➤ Typically bradycardic w/ normal BP
➤ Initiates respiratory efforts w/ tactile stimulation
➤ May have undisturbed acid-base status
■ Secondary apnea
➤ Typically bradycardic & hypotensive
➤ Usually does not initiate respiratory efforts w/ tactile stimulation
➤ Usually depressed w/ severe hypoxia & hypercapnia
■ Failure of neonate to respond to tactile stimulation w/ spontaneous respiratory efforts may signal secondary apnea & the urgent need for immediate resuscitation.

Miscellaneous information
■ The neonate is an obligate nose-breather.
■ Surfactant is present in significant amounts beginning at 34 weeks.
➤ Production can be stimulated w/ steroids.
➤ Release is stimulated by stress.

STUDIES

Heart rate determination in neonates
■ Palpate pulse at base of umbilical cord.
■ Listen to precordium w/ stethoscope if umbilical pulse is weak.
■ Palpation of pulse in brachial or femoral artery often unsuccessful
■ A cardiotachometer can be applied to the neonate to determine the heart rate.
➤ Attach two electrodes to the neonate.
➤ The cardiotachometer makes a sound w/ each heartbeat.

Apgar
■ Used to quickly assess the neonate's status
■ Definition: Score of 0–2 in 5 categories is assessed at 1 & 5 minutes after birth
➤ Heart rate
  • 0 (absent)
  • 1 (<100)
  • 2 (>100)
➤ Respirations
  • 0 (absent)
  • 1 (slow, irregular)
  • 2 (crying)
➤ Muscle tone
  • 0 (limp)
  • 1 (some tension)
  • 2 (motion)
➤ Reflex irritability
  • 0 (no response)

- 1 (grimace)
- 2 (cough, cry)
- ➤ Color
- 0 (central cyanosis)
- 1 (peripheral cyanosis)
- 2 (pink)
- Interpretation of Apgar score
  - ➤ Score of 8–10 is normal.
  - ➤ Score of 4–7 indicates moderate compromise & potential need for resuscitation.
  - ➤ Score of 0–3 signals need for immediate resuscitation.
- APGAR use
  - ➤ If the 5-minute APGAR score is <7, additional scores should be obtained every 5 minutes until the score is at least 7 or until the neonate is 20 minutes old.

Rapid initial assessment
- Clear of meconium?
- Spontaneously breathing?
- Good muscle tone?
- Color pink?
- Term gestation?

MANAGEMENT/INTERVENTIONS

Apgar
- If the 5-minute APGAR score is <7, additional scores should be obtained every 5 minutes until the score is at least 7 or until the neonate is 20 minutes old.
- Score <6, initiate neonatal resuscitation (see "*Resuscitation of the Neonate*").
- The reflex irritability of the Apgar is often determined by gently placing a suction catheter into each nasal passage. This serves two purposes:
  - ➤ Stimulates neonate for the determination of reflex irritability
  - ➤ Rules out choanal atresia, which can be lethal to the neonate w/o an oral airway or endotracheal intubation

Rapid initial assessment (Clear of meconium? Spontaneously breathing? Good muscle tone? Color pink? Term gestation?)
- If all answers are yes, then provide routine care (see "*Routine Newborn Care*").
- If there is meconium staining of the amniotic fluid, then assess the neonate's respiratory status, muscle tone & heart rate.
  - ➤ Does the neonate exhibit strong respiratory efforts (regular, respiratory rate 30 or more per minute), good muscle tone & heart rate >100 bpm?
    - If yes, proceed to routine care (see "*Routine Newborn Care*").

- If no, then pt requires resuscitation (see "*Meconium*").
- If the neonate is apneic, assume it is secondary apnea & initiate resuscitation (see "*Resuscitation of the Neonate*")
- If one or more answers are no (& are not addressed above) & there is any sign of fetal distress (irregular or ineffective respiratory effort, heart rate <100, flaccid muscle tone, central cyanosis), then proceed to resuscitation (see "*Resuscitation of the Neonate*").

CAVEATS & PEARLS

Determining heart rate
- If the pulse is weak, it may not be detectable at the base of the umbilical cord.

Listening to the precordium w/ a stethoscope is a reliable method to determine the neonate's heart rate acutely, even if pulses are weak. However, this requires an extra person during resuscitation.

Although the Apgar score is a useful evaluation in acute care of the neonate, it is a poor predictor of many neonatal parameters, such as acid-base status or long-term neurologic impairment. The APGAR score is affected by many factors other than functional status (eg, prematurity, congenital anomalies, drug exposure, compromised neurologic function).

CHECKLIST
- Be mindful of neonatal physiology changes at birth.
- Evaluate pt w/ Apgar scores & rapid initial assessment.
- Provide routine care or initiate resuscitation as appropriate.

NEUROFIBROMATOSIS

MEREDITH ALBRECHT, MD
MICHELE SZABO, MD

FUNDAMENTAL KNOWLEDGE

Definition
- Disease that entails excessive proliferation of neural crest elements (Schwann cells & melanocytes); has varied expression & can involve virtually every organ system.

Epidemiology
- NFI (neurofibromatosis 1) is an autosomal dominant disorder affecting 1/3,000 births w/ markedly variable clinical expression

- NF1 gene is located on chromosome 17 & has very high spontaneous mutation rate (50% of cases are sporadic).
- NF2, genetically distinct from NF1, has abnormality located on chromosome 22.
- NF2 rarer than NF1 (1/50,000 births)

Pathophysiology/Clinical Manifestations
- Presence of 6 or more café-au-lait spots (patches of pigmentation on the skin) that measure >1.5 cm is diagnostic.
- Diagnostic criteria: the pt should have 2 or more of the following:
  - 6 or more café-au-lait spots
  - 2 or more neurofibromas of any type or 1 or more plexiform neurofibromata
  - Axillary or groin freckling
  - Optic glioma
  - 2 or more Lisch nodules (benign melanotic iris hamartomas)
  - A distinctive bony lesion
  - A first-degree relative w/ NF1
- Broad range of severity & progression of disease
- Most commonly, disease is limited to the skin.
- Rarely, NF is associated w/ syndrome of multiple endocrine disorders, which may include medullary thyroid carcinoma & pheochromocytoma.
- Neurologic symptoms depend on location of neurofibromas.

Effects of Pregnancy on NF
- Worsening or growth of new neurofibromas of skin, CNS or visceral organs w/ regression after delivery. Greatest concern is development of increased ICP secondary to rapid expansion of intracranial lesions. If there is a marked increase in ICP, a spinal could potentially lead to herniation.
- Potential for hypertensive crisis in pts w/ undiagnosed, associated pheochromocytoma
- Mechanical disturbance if neurofibromas are in pelvis (potentially necessitating cesarean delivery) or in spinal cord (complicating regional anesthesia)

Effects of NF on pregnancy/fetus
- NF has typically been associated w/ increased risk of spontaneous abortion, intrauterine demise, IUGR & preterm labor, although a recent review did not confirm this finding.

STUDIES
- Careful history & physical focusing on pt's symptoms

- Careful airway exam (pts often have laryngeal & neck tumors)
- Consider MRI brain/spine to rule out increased ICP & lesions in the spinal cord.

MANAGEMENT/INTERVENTIONS

- Both general anesthesia & regional anesthesia have been successfully used in pts w/ NF.
- Cutaneous neurofibromas can make IV access difficult.
- For regional anesthesia
  - Severe kyphoscoliosis & presence of neurofibromas of the spine can make regional anesthetics difficult.
  - Lumbar neurofibromas are often asymptomatic & lateral, but trauma to them can have disastrous consequences.
- For general anesthesia
  - Pts w/ NF often have associated laryngeal & neck tumors that can complicate intubation.
  - In addition, if severe kyphoscoliosis is present, ventilation can be difficult.
  - Studies have shown that pts w/ NF can have increased or decreased sensitivity to depolarizing & increased sensitivity to nondepolarizing neuromuscular blockers.

CAVEATS/PEARLS

- Diagnostic criteria: the pt should have 2 or more of the following:
  - 6 or more café-au-lait spots
  - 2 or more neurofibromas of any type or one or more plexiform neurofibroma
  - Axillary or groin freckling
  - Optic glioma
  - 2 or more Lisch nodules (benign melanotic iris hamartomas)
  - A distinctive bony lesion
  - A first-degree relative w/ NF1
- Most commonly, disease is limited to the skin.
- If hypertension plus NF, rule out pheochromocytoma.
- Neurologic symptoms depend on location of neurofibromas.
- Pregnancy can cause worsening or growth of new neurofibromas of skin, CNS or visceral organs w/ regression after delivery.
- Beware of increased ICP.
- Both regional anesthesia & general anesthesia have been used successfully in pts w/ NF.
  - For regional anesthesia
    - May be difficult secondary to kyphoscoliosis

- Trauma to lumbar neurofibromas during regional anesthesia can have disastrous consequences.
➤ For general anesthesia
  - Neck/laryngeal tumors may make intubation difficult.
  - Kyphoscoliosis may make ventilation difficult.
  - Altered response to muscle relaxants (both increased & decreased sensitivity to depolarizers has been shown; expect increased sensitivity to non-depolarizers)

CHECKLIST
■ Diagnostic criteria: the pt should have 2 or more of the following:
  ➤ 6 or more café-au-lait spots
  ➤ 2 or more neurofibromas of any type or one or more plexiform neurofibroma
  ➤ Axillary or groin freckling
  ➤ Optic glioma
  ➤ 2 or more Lisch nodules (benign melanotic iris hamartomas)
  ➤ A distinctive bony lesion
  ➤ A first-degree relative w/ NF1
■ If NF & hypertension, think pheochromocytoma.
■ Assess neurologic symptoms; consider CT or MRI to rule out intracranial & paraspinal neurofibromas.
■ Both regional anesthesia & general anesthesia have been used successfully.
  ➤ If general anesthesia
    - Beware of associated head/neck tumors.
    - May be increased or decreased sensitivity to succinylcholine; expect increased sensitivity to non-depolarizers
  ➤ If regional anesthesia
■ Beware of lumbar neurofibromas.

NONINFECTIOUS FEVER W/ EPIDURALS

SISSELA PARK, MD
LAURA RILEY, MD

FUNDAMENTAL KNOWLEDGE
■ Epidural analgesia usually leads to hypothermia secondary to vasodilation.
■ Laboring women may experience hyperthermia w/ epidurals.
  ➤ May confound the diagnosis of intra-amniotic infection

- Pattern of temp increase after labor epidural placement
  - Lag of about 4–5 hours
  - Then pt's temps appear to increase about 0.1 degrees Celsius per hour
- Unclear how labor epidurals cause hyperthermia
- Pts more likely to request epidurals are more likely to have these risk factors for fever:
  - Nulliparity
  - Prolonged labor
  - Early intra-amniotic infection
  - More frequent cervical exams

Complications

- Most clinicians feel that the extent of hyperthermia in laboring women w/ epidurals is unlikely to lead to direct neonatal complications.
- Further research is needed to understand the relationship btwn epidurals & maternal/fetal temp regulation.

STUDIES

- Temp measurement
- Diagnostic tests, as needed, to determine if there is another cause for the fever
- Currently, there is no test or diagnostic sign to differentiate noninfectious epidural related fever from intra-amniotic infection.

MANAGEMENT/INTERVENTIONS

- Efforts should be made to decrease the maternal temp.
- Evaluate pt to recognize & treat a possible infection.

CAVEATS & PEARLS

- Noninfectious epidural-related fever may confound the diagnosis of intra-amniotic infection.
- Unclear how epidurals cause elevated temps during labor

CHECKLIST

- In febrile laboring pts w/ epidurals, determine if there is another cause for hyperthermia.
- Attempt to decrease temp, since maternal fever may be associated w/ increased perinatal morbidity.

NON-INITIATION OF NEONATAL RESUSCITATION

RICHARD ARCHULETA, MD
SANDRA WEINREB, MD

FUNDAMENTAL KNOWLEDGE

There are several situations in which a fetus is non-viable & neonatal resuscitation is not appropriate:

- Anencephaly
- Trisomy 13 & 18
- Extreme prematurity
  - ➤ <23 weeks of gestation
- <400 g

STUDIES

Be familiar w/ information relating to fetal viability:

- Estimated date of confinement
  - ➤ Can be determined if the last menstrual period is known
  - ➤ EDC = (LMP + 1 week) − 3 months
- Ultrasonography
- Tests for chromosomal abnormalities
  - ➤ Amniocentesis
  - ➤ Chorionic villus sampling
  - ➤ Cordocentesis

There should be an extensive discussion btwn the OB or midwife & the parents before the neonate is delivered.

MANAGEMENT/INTERVENTIONS

- Staff should be sensitive to the family's emotional needs, providing a safe & private space for the family while gently offering support.
- The neonate should be delivered as painlessly as possible for the mother.
- The neonate should be cleaned & swaddled so the family can spend time w/ the neonate.

CAVEATS & PEARLS

N/A

CHECKLIST

- Be familiar w/ information relating to fetal viability.
- Ensure there is an extensive discussion btwn the OB or midwife & the parents before the neonate is delivered.

- Ensure staff are sensitive & supportive concerning family's needs.
- Provide care so as to minimize the mother's labor discomfort.
- Allow family to spend time w/ neonate.

NONREASSURING FETAL HEART RATE TRACING

SUSANNE PAREKH, MD
ANDREA TORRI, MD

FUNDAMENTAL KNOWLEDGE

Definitions

- Nonreassuring fetal status implies that the *clinician's interpretation* of data regarding fetal status is not reassuring. This may be due to fetal heart rate (FHR) tracing abnormalities or abnormal biophysical profile, or a combination of factors.
- FHR monitoring may be:
  - ➤ Intermittent (requires 1:1 nurse-patient ratio, should be done q30min for low risk pts in active phase of labor, q15min in 2nd stage of labor. For high-risk pts, intermittent monitoring is recommended q15min in 1st stage of labor & q5min in 2nd stage).
  - ➤ Continuous (indicated when abnormalities occur w/ intermittent monitoring, or w/ high-risk pts)
- High-risk indications for continuous monitoring of FHR
  - ➤ Antepartum factors
    - Maternal age <16 or >35 years old
    - Maternal weight <50 kg
    - Maternal substance abuse, including tobacco use
    - Maternal infection
    - Lack of prenatal care
    - Maternal drug therapy (alpha blockers, beta blockers, lithium, Mg sulfate)
    - Maternal medical condition such as hypertension, diabetes mellitus, asthma, Rh negative w/ antibodies, previous cone biopsy, etc.
    - Bleeding in 2nd or 3rd trimester (either maternal or placental)
    - Pre-eclampsia or eclampsia
    - Fetal anemia or isoimmunization
    - Premature rupture of membranes (PROM)
    - Polyhydramnios

- Oligohydramnios
- IUGR
- Prior fetal or neonatal death, infant <2,500 g or premature infant <28 weeks
- Repeat pregnancy within 1 year
- Previous C-section
- Known fetal anomalies
- >1 fetus
- Post-term gestation

➤ Intrapartum factors

- Prematurity
- Fetal distress
- Prolonged labor >24 hours
- Prolonged 2nd stage of labor >4 hours
- Prolonged rupture of membranes >18 hours
- Meconium-stained fluid
- Chorioamnionitis
- Abruptio placentae or placenta previa
- Cord prolapse
- Uterine tetany
- Forceps or vacuum-assisted delivery
- Breech or other abnormal presentation
- Maternal sedatives within 4 hours of delivery
- Emergency cesarean delivery
- Use of general anesthesia

■ FHR may be monitored externally w/ a Doppler probe placed on the mother's abdomen or internally w/ a fetal scalp electrode (requires rupture of the fetal membranes & partial dilation of the cervix). A fetal scalp electrode (FSE) offers a more continuous signal that is less influenced by motion artifacts. Second-generation FHR monitors have improved FHR signal & accuracy of the recording.

■ FHR tracing may be accompanied by a tocodynamometer (external), which allows measurement of onset, duration & termination of uterine contractions. An intrauterine pressure catheter is necessary to measure strength of contractions.

■ The clinician's own judgment is paramount to optimal use of FHR tracings in order to minimize false-positive results.

■ Features of the FHR tracing & interpretations

■ **Baseline FHR**

➤ Normal baseline FHR is 120–160 bpm. Some OBs extend the lower limit of this range to 110 bpm.

➤ Baseline FHR is considered altered if the change lasts for >15 minutes.

➤ Preterm fetuses have FHR at the upper end of the normal range, while term or postdates fetuses have FHR at the lower end of the normal range.

➤ Baseline FHR may be increased by maternal anxiety, fever, hyperthyroidism, anemia or drugs administered to the mother (beta agonists such as ritodrine & terbutaline or parasympatholytic drugs such as atropine or hydroxyzine may increase FHR >160).

➤ Bradycardia
- Moderate bradycardia: 100–109 bpm
- Abnormal bradycardia: <100 bpm
- Severe prolonged bradycardia of <80 bpm lasting >3 minutes is an ominous sign indicating severe hypoxia.

➤ Tachycardia
- Mild tachycardia: 160–180 bpm
- Severe tachycardia: >180 bpm
- Tachycardia >200 bpm may be due to fetal tachyarrhythmia or congenital anomaly

■ **FHR variability**

➤ Reflects a healthy nervous system, as well as chemoreceptor, baroreceptor & cardiac responsiveness

➤ Includes short- & long-term variability
- Short-term variability (beat-to-beat variability) is the difference between 2 or 3 adjacent beats. Normal short-term variability is a change of 5–10 bpm around the baseline FHR or a change >5 bpm btwn contractions.
- Long-term variability refers to rough sine waves that occur 3–6 times per minute w/ FHR variation of at least 6 bpm.

➤ Clinically, loss of beat-to-beat variability is more ominous than loss of long-term variability.

➤ DDx of loss of variability of FHR includes:
- Fetal sleep (in which case variability should increase again after roughly 30–40 minutes)
- Fetal hypoxia (especially if associated w/ late or variable decelerations of FHR)
- Fetal neurologic abnormality
- Decreased CNS activity due to maternal administration of opioids, benzodiazepines or magnesium sulfate
- Maternal administration of parasympatholytics such as atropine or hydroxyzine, administration of centrally acting

adrenergic agents such as methyldopa, administration of beta-adrenergic agonists such as ritodrine or terbutaline in doses high enough to raise the FHR >160

➤ Increased FHR variability is present when oscillations around the baseline FHR exceed 25 bpm; this is often called a "saltatory" pattern. This may indicate acute hypoxia or umbilical cord compression. This is most often seen during the 2nd stage of labor.

■ **Periodic changes of FHR**

➤ Early decelerations: simultaneous w/ uterine contractions, onset & offset of deceleration coincides w/ onset & offset of contraction, deceleration is usually <20 bpm below baseline. May be due to fetal head compression. Not considered to be ominous.

➤ Late decelerations: begin 10–30 seconds after the onset of a uterine contraction & end 10–30 seconds after the end of a contraction. Often smooth & repetitive. Represent uteroplacental insufficiency. Late decelerations in combination w/ decreased FHR variability are thought to be an ominous sign of fetal intolerance to labor.

➤ Variable decelerations: vary in onset & offset, as well as depth, shape & duration; may look sharper in their downslope & upslope (like a V). May be due to umbilical cord compression or fetal head compression. Severe variable decelerations in combination w/ decreased FHR variability are thought to be a sign of fetal distress.

➤ Sinusoidal pattern: a smooth, wavelike pattern w/ no short-term FHR variability. May be due to fetal anemia; sometimes occurs w/ maternal opioid administration.

➤ Accelerations: Antepartum, accelerations are a sign of good fetal health. Intrapartum, their significance is less clear: they may signal the presence of umbilical cord insufficiency. Presence of FHR accelerations most likely rules out the presence of a significant metabolic acidosis.

➤ "Saltatory" pattern: excessive swings in variability (>25 bpm); may be due to acute hypoxia or mechanical compression of the umbilical cord

Nonreassuring FHR patterns that warrant further evaluation of fetal well-being using fetal scalp stimulation, fetal scalp pH, or both:

■ Tachycardia
■ Bradycardia
■ Saltatory variability
■ Variable decelerations w/ a nonreassuring pattern
■ Late decelerations w/o loss of beat-to-beat variability

Ominous FHR patterns that signal acute fetal distress; evaluation for immediate delivery is recommended:

- Persistent late decelerations w/ loss of beat-to-beat variability
- Nonreassuring variable decelerations w/ loss of beat-to-beat variability
- Prolonged severe bradycardia
- Sinusoidal pattern
- Confirmed loss of beat-to-beat variability not associated w/ fetal sleep, meds or severe prematurity

STUDIES

When FHR monitoring suggests the possibility of fetal compromise:

- Fetal scalp blood pH monitoring
  - ➤ May be indicated if decreased or absent FHR variability or if persistent late or variable FHR decelerations are present
  - ➤ Fetal scalp pH > 7.25 indicates that a pt may continue to labor.
  - ➤ Fetal scalp pH < 7.20 is consistent w/ fetal distress, & delivery should be expedited.
  - ➤ Fetal scalp pH of 7.20–7.25 may warrant a repeat measurement.
  - ➤ False-positive results may occur due to abnormal maternal pH, inadequate sample, contamination w/ amniotic fluid or sampling from the caput succedaneum).
- Fetal scalp stimulation may be used as an alternative to fetal scalp pH:
  - ➤ Fetal scalp may be digitally stimulated during vaginal exam. FHR of a healthy fetus should accelerate in response. FHR acceleration after scalp stimulation is usually associated w/ pH > 7.19.
  - ➤ If no FHR acceleration occurs after scalp stimulation, scalp sampling for pH is recommended.
- Vibroacoustic stimulation
  - ➤ Application of an acoustic generator to the maternal abdomen should result in an FHR acceleration in a healthy fetus.
- Fetal pulse oximetry
  - ➤ This is a new technology. Studies have not yet shown a correlation between fetal SaO2 & Apgar scores.
  - ➤ Mean SaO2 is 50–60%.
  - ➤ The threshold for fetal compromise has been suggested at an SaO2 of 30% for a duration of 10 minutes.
  - ➤ Multiple factors may confound measurement or impair signal quality, such as presence of meconium, thick curly fetal hair, caput succedaneum & maternal & fetal movement

MANAGEMENT/INTERVENTIONS

Presence of a nonreassuring FHR should prompt both the OB & the anesthesiologist to attempt to identify & correct the cause.

Resuscitate the fetus in utero. Possible interventions include:

- Optimize maternal position.
  - ➤ Relieve aortocaval compression or umbilical cord compression.
  - ➤ Consider left lateral, right lateral, knee-chest or Trendelenburg positions.
- Administer supplemental oxygen via tight-fitting face mask.
- Maintain maternal circulation.
  - ➤ Crystalloid bolus (avoid dextrose-containing solutions)
  - ➤ Ephedrine &/or phenylephrine if necessary for hypotension refractory to fluid resuscitation
- OB should perform a vaginal exam to check for umbilical cord prolapse & perform fetal scalp stimulation, if indicated.
  - ➤ If umbilical cord prolapse is found on vaginal exam, manual elevation of the fetal head by the OB may be indicated until operative delivery can be accomplished.
- Discontinue oxytocin.
- Consider administration of a tocolytic agent (terbutaline or other beta-adrenergic agent, magnesium, sublingual nitroglycerin spray) if there is evidence of uterine hyperactivity or uterine tetany.
- Consider saline amnioinfusion (by OB) to relieve umbilical cord compression (may infuse up to 800 cc acutely, but return of normal FHR pattern may take up to 20–30 minutes).

Urgent or emergent operative delivery may be necessary if the FHR does not improve despite the above-mentioned interventions. Optimal decision-to-delivery time should be <30 minutes.

Anesthetic preparation for urgent or emergent C-section includes the following sequence:

- Pertinent history: Do not compromise maternal safety even in an emergency. Obtain the following information if possible from every pt:
  - ➤ Previous medical & anesthetic history
  - ➤ Airway evaluation for potential difficulty of intubation
  - ➤ Allergies
- Administer an antacid (eg, 30 cc sodium citrate).
- Optimize maternal position.
  - ➤ Avoid aortocaval compression by using a roll or wedge under the pt to achieve left uterine displacement.

> Optimize head & neck position (ie, sniffing position) in anticipation of possible laryngoscopy.
- Administer supplemental oxygen.
- Apply maternal monitors.
- Monitor FHR (if possible, use fetal scalp electrode for continuous monitoring).
- Establish good IV access.
- Start IV crystalloid (not containing dextrose).
- Treat hypotension w/ IV ephedrine &/or phenylephrine if not responsive to fluids.
- If BP does not improve w/ ephedrine, start an IV phenylephrine infusion or give IV epinephrine (epinephrine should be given only in the rare case of catastrophic maternal hypotension).
- Reassure the infant's mother & father.

Choice of anesthetic technique
- See "*Anesthesia for Cesarean Delivery*" chapter.
- Emergency C-sections are divided into 3 categories: stable, urgent, stat
  > Stable: stable maternal & fetal status but C-section is necessary before decline in status occurs (eg, chronic uteroplacental insufficiency, nonreactive nonstress test, abnormal fetal presentation w/ ROM but not in labor). Epidural or spinal anesthesia is preferred.
  > Urgent: maternal or fetal status is abnormal but not imminently life-threatening (eg, cord prolapse w/out fetal distress, dystocia, variable decelerations w/ recovery & no loss of variability). Extension of pre-existing epidural or expeditious spinal anesthesia is preferred.
  > Stat: conditions that are immediately life-threatening to the mother or fetus (eg, prolonged fetal bradycardia, ruptured uterus, late decelerations w/ no FHR variability). General anesthesia is indicated unless preexisting epidural anesthesia can be extended rapidly & satisfactorily. Most FHR abnormalities do not reflect dire fetal distress; thus, few pts should require stat C-section.
- Extension of epidural anesthesia may be accomplished most rapidly w/ 15–20 cc of 3% 2-chloroprocaine. 2-chloroprocaine is the drug of choice since rapid blood metabolism limits the possibility of ion-trapping in an acidotic fetus. May also use 15–20 cc of 1.5–2% lidocaine w/ epinephrine + 2 cc of bicarbonate, but onset will

be a few minutes slower than w/ chloroprocaine. In this setting, 0.5% bupivacaine would be inappropriate due to prolonged time to onset.

- Spinal anesthesia may be considered when:
  - ➤ The spinal can be performed quickly, without delaying surgery.
  - ➤ Severe hypovolemia is ruled out.
  - ➤ Hypotension can be effectively managed.
    - Ensure good IV access & begin rapid bolus of LR or NS, but do not delay spinal for completion of fluid bolus.
    - A typical spinal dose is 12 mg of 0.75% hyperbaric bupivacaine (has rapid onset when given intrathecally). The addition of intrathecal opioids may improve the density of the spinal & provide post-op analgesia.
    - Consider prophylactic administration of ephedrine &/or phenylephrine after spinal has been placed to minimize hypotension.
    - Treat hypotension after spinal administration aggressively.
- General anesthesia is indicated when time-dependent life-threatening emergencies are present. See "*General Anesthesia & the Difficult Airway*" chapter.
  - ➤ Rapid sequence induction is standard for the parturient.
  - ➤ The standard 3–5 minutes of denitrogenation may be omitted in cases of severe fetal distress by asking the mother to take 4 vital capacity breaths of 100% oxygen.
  - ➤ Sodium thiopental, propofol or ketamine may be used for induction.
  - ➤ Consider running 100% FiO2 until fetus is delivered.
  - ➤ History or suspicion of difficult intubation or difficult mask ventilation may require performance of an awake intubation or regional anesthetic technique. The life of the mother should not be compromised to deliver a distressed fetus.
  - ➤ If there is a contraindication to rapid sequence induction or general anesthesia, local infiltration has been described as the primary anesthetic technique in rare cases.

CAVEATS & PEARLS
- The term "fetal distress" is vague & nonspecific. The character of the FHR abnormality should be a key factor in determining the urgency of delivery & the type of anesthesia to be administered.
- The OB must clearly communicate the severity of the FHR abnormality & other associated findings, such as fetal scalp pH, to help identify

pts who require urgent vs. stat C-section. Likewise, the anesthesiologist must clearly state his or her concerns.

- In high-risk pts, strongly consider early establishment of IV access & early placement of an epidural catheter to avoid the risk of emergency induction of general anesthesia. In these pts, rapid extension of the labor epidural for operative delivery can be achieved w/ 3% chloroprocaine.
- C-sections that are performed for a nonreassuring FHR pattern do not necessarily preclude the use of a regional anesthetic technique.
- If possible, FHR should be monitored continuously during administration of anesthesia for emergency C-section. Improvement of the FHR tracing at any time may allow for modification of the anesthetic or surgical plan.
- Failed intubation & aspiration of gastric contents remain the leading causes of maternal morbidity & mortality from anesthesia.

CHECKLIST
- Review indications for FHR monitoring.
- Review FHR pattern.
- Is FHR abnormality present, & is it nonreassuring or ominous?
- Communicate clearly w/ OB about the nature of the FHR abnormality, its severity & the urgency of operative intervention
- Start resuscitation of fetus in utero.
- Generate a plan for possible operative delivery as early as possible when a nonreassuring FHR tracing is present, & identify pts at high risk for complications of emergency anesthesia.

NORMAL HEMATOLOGIC CHANGES OF PREGNANCY

JEANNA VIOLA, MD
JANE BALLANTYNE, MD

FUNDAMENTAL KNOWLEDGE
- Blood volume increases by 45–55% from 6 to 36 weeks due to increase in plasma; most pts exhibit a dilutional anemia.
- Red cell mass increases approx. 20%; demand for folate and iron rises. MCV elevated to 90–102 fL; iron deficiency may be masked by high MCV.
- 25% of parturients exhibit leukocytosis (up to 15,000) due to increase in neutrophils.
- Platelet size increases; platelet count may fall.

■ Pregnant pts are considered hypercoagulable; most clotting factor levels increase:
  ➤ Factors VII, VIII, X, levels increase.
  ➤ von Willebrand factor & fibrinogen levels increase.
  ➤ Protein C levels do not change during pregnancy, but protein S levels decrease to 40–50% normal.
  ➤ AT III levels remain stable throughout pregnancy.

STUDIES
■ Changes in coagulability result in a mild decrease in PT & PTT & decrease in fibrinolytic activity.

MANAGEMENT/INTERVENTIONS
■ Routine CBC in early pregnancy is helpful to diagnose pre-existing hematologic disorders such as iron deficiency anemia, thalassemia, sickle cell disease, thrombocytopenia or leukemia.
■ Hct is repeated in third trimester to assess Hct prior to delivery.
■ Coagulation screen for suspected or documented history of bleeding disorder, anticoagulant therapy, acute peripartum complications such as pre-eclampsia & DIC.
■ Serial platelet counts may be indicated in parturients w/ thrombocytopenia prior to labor to determine safety of regional anesthesia.

CAVEATS AND PEARLS
■ Blood volume & function alters during pregnancy.
■ Routine hematologic screening is essential for identifying normal changes of pregnancy & possible derangements.

CHECKLIST
NA

NORMAL RENAL CHANGES IN PREGNANCY

JOSHUA WEBER, MD
PETER DUNN, MD

FUNDAMENTAL KNOWLEDGE
Increase in renal blood flow is due to:
■ Increased cardiac output (from increased stroke volume & heart rate)

- 30–40% expansion of blood volume (from sodium/water retention & decreased SVR)

Increased glomerular filtration rate (GFR)

- (GFR peaks at 40–50% above baseline at end of 1st trimester & returns to baseline 3 months after delivery.
- Increase in GFR is due to increased renal blood flow & increased nitric oxide synthesis, which leads to renal vasodilatation. Increased GFR causes decreased serum creatinine (Cr > 0.8 is abnormal in pregnancy), sodium, bicarbonate & osmolality.
- (Increased volume leads to dilatation of the renal pelvis & ureters, causing decreased peristalsis, which increases the risk of UTI.

STUDIES
MANAGEMENT/INTERVENTIONS
CAVEATS & PEARLS
CHECKLIST
N/A

OBESE PARTURIENT

SCOTT STREATER, MD; TIMOTHY JACKSON, MD; AND JEAN KWO, MD

FUNDAMENTAL KNOWLEDGE

Introduction

- Definition: Many definitions & indices of obesity exist. However, the best calculator of obesity is the Body Mass Index: BMI = weight (kg)/ height (m^2). BMI > 25 is, by definition, overweight; obesity is BMI > 30.
- Demographics: In the U.S., the prevalence of overweight individuals is increasing. Approx. 30.5% of adults are obese; the prevalence of overweight Americans is 64.5%. Also, there exists a corresponding increase in the prevalence of pregnant obese pts. Current estimates cite that 6–10% of parturients are obese.
- Comorbidities associated w/ obesity: Obesity increases the incidence of hypertension, coronary artery disease, cerebrovascular disease, diabetes mellitus, gallbladder disease & liver disease in nonpregnant pts. In the pregnancy of obese pts, various physiologic changes occur, potentially complicating the birthing process. These pathophysiologic changes affect anesthetic & obstetric mgt of these pts.

Physiologic Changes of Obesity

- Pulmonary changes
  - ➤ Pulmonary mechanics: In general, obese pts have decreased chest wall compliance, due to increased chest & abdominal wall weight, as well as thoracic kyphosis & lumbar lordosis. However, in morbidly obese parturients, despite an increased production of CO_2 (due to an increased metabolic demand), $PaCO_2$ is normal for pregnancy. Eucapnia is maintained by increased minute ventilation.
  - ➤ Lung volumes: In general, obese individuals have smaller tidal volumes due to a limitation in diaphragmatic excursion from increased abdominal weight. This is also manifested in a decreased pulmonary reserve: pulmonary function tests reveal decreased expiratory reserve volume (ERV), inspiratory capacity, vital capacity & functional residual capacity (FRC). Pregnancy also affects lung volumes: in both obese & non-obese parturients, ERV & FRC decline 20–25% by term.
  - ➤ Hypoxemia: Hypoxemia can result from ventilation-perfusion mismatch, intrapulmonary shunt (resulting from hypoxic pulmonary vasoconstriction) & co-existing respiratory disease. However, pulmonary diffusion often remains normal, except in pts w/ massive obesity. Also, oxygenation worsens in the supine & Trendelenburg positions. It is possible that the physiologic changes of pregnancy, such as increased ventilation & cardiac output, confer a protective effect on obese parturients by aiding in oxygen uptake & delivery.
  - ➤ Sleep apnea (OSA): The incidence of sleep apnea increases in obesity. OSA can cause episodes of apnea, snoring & daytime somnolence. In some pts, OSA can result in obesity hypoventilation syndrome, which is characterized by central apnea episodes; the sustained hypercarbia & hypoxemia can adversely affect pulmonary artery hypertension & eventually cause right heart failure.
- Cardiovascular changes
  - ➤ Cardiac output: Cardiac output & blood volume both increase in obesity & pregnancy.
  - ➤ Pulmonary hypertension: The associated increase in cardiac output & blood volume can also cause pulmonary hypertension. This effect can be exacerbated by hypoxemia & airway obstruction.

➤ Hypertension: Hypertension is the most common obesity-related health condition. BMI >30 is associated w/ a 3× increase in hypertension. Pregnancy confers no protective advantage in the consequences of obesity. Treatment is diuretic therapy to decrease the expanded blood volume.

➤ Cardiovascular mortality: In pts 25–34 years old, obese individuals have a 12× increase in mortality; cardiovascular disease was found to be the most common cause of death.

■ GI changes: Traditionally, it was thought that the morbidly obese pt is at greater risk for pulmonary aspiration of gastric contents, due to decreases in gastric pH & increased gastric volume. However, more recent evidence does not support this claim that the obese pt is at a higher risk of aspiration pneumonitis. Furthermore, it is unclear whether pregnancy increases the risk of aspiration in obese pts.

■ Endocrine changes: The incidence of diabetes is increased in obesity due to decreased insulin sensitivity. Also, the overweight & obese were found to have a relative deficiency of insulin during pregnancy.

■ Coagulation changes: Obesity increases the risk of deep venous thrombosis (DVT) & pulmonary thromboembolism (PE). It can also be extrapolated that obesity increases the risk of DVT & PE in pregnancy.

Interaction w/ Pregnancy

■ Increased risk of obstetric complications

➤ Chronic hypertension: There is an increased incidence of pre-pregnancy hypertension in pregnant, obese women. However, it is unclear whether this observation is compounded by the increased age of obese parturients.

➤ Pregnancy-induced hypertension: This condition is also significantly increased in the pregnancies of the obese compared to the non-obese.

➤ Gestational diabetes: Various studies cite a 2× to 8× increase in the incidence of diabetes during pregnancies of obese women.

➤ Thromboembolic disease: It is believed that the obese pt is at greater risk of DVT & PE. Although unproven, it can be extrapolated that this greater risk of thromboembolic complications exists for the obese parturient.

➤ Infection: In non-obstetric surgery, the obese pt is at 2× greater risk of developing post-op wound infection. The proposed mechanism is that the thick hypovascular adipose layer promotes bacterial growth. In combination w/ hyperglycemia (which obese pts are at a higher risk for developing), the risk of wound infection is increased. Again, although unproven by clinical study, it can be hypothesized that the obese, post-partum woman is at a higher risk of developing post-op wound infection relative to her non-obese counterpart.

■ Increased mortality: Current research reveals an increased risk of maternal death in obese women. In addition, other studies cite that obesity increases the likelihood of maternal death during anesthesia.

Labor & Delivery
■ Increased risk of C-section: Various studies cite increased risk of C-section in obese pts. However, the etiology is unclear. Possible causes include:
  ➤ Abnormal presentation: However, studies are equivocal as to whether malpresentation is increased in obese pregnant women.
  ➤ Prolonged labor: As many as 50% of morbidly obese pts who undergo a trial of labor eventually require C-section.
  ➤ Increased incidence of need for induction: Obese parturients have an increased incidence of induction of labor. It is possible that this observation can be explained by the increased occurrence of hypertension & diabetes in obese pregnant pts, & that the increased incidence of these elective inductions can account for the increased risk of C-section.
  ➤ Increased risk of abnormal labor: Possibly another explanation for the increased incidence of C-sections in obese parturients. It has been observed in various studies that during labor of obese pts, there is an increased incidence of meconium-stained amniotic fluid, umbilical cord accidents & late FHR decelerations.
  ➤ Increased risk of fetal macrosomia: The morbidly obese pt (+/− diabetes) is at an increased risk for fetal macrosomia. As a result, there is also an increased risk of trauma to the mother during delivery.
■ Risk of shoulder dystocia w/ vaginal delivery: It is unclear as to the etiology of the increased incidence of shoulder dystocia in the obese parturient. It is speculated that this may be due to fetal macrosomia or the altered vaginal canal of the mother. Dystocia is the most common indication for emergency C-section of the obese laboring pt.

- Perinatal outcome: The obese parturient is at a greater risk of delivering a preterm & low-birthweight infant. Her fetus is at a greater risk for fetal death.

STUDIES

N/A

MANAGEMENT/INTERVENTIONS

Preanesthetic assessment

- Room air oxygen saturation, ABGs (especially if questions exist regarding maternal ventilation & oxygenation)
- Noninvasive BP monitoring: Cuff size must exceed circumference of arm by 20%, lest overestimate systolic & diastolic BP measurement
- Pre-op labs (eg, platelet count in pre-eclampsia, serum glucose in diabetes)
- Airway assessment: The associated physiologic changes of pregnancy (eg, large breasts, increased AP diameter of the chest, airway edema, decreased chin-to-chest distance) increase the risk of difficult & failed intubation. In the obese parturient, these problems are exacerbated (eg, adipose tissue in the back limits extension of the neck). Therefore, an early & thorough exam of the airway is essential.
- IV access: Securing IV access can be problematic. An 18-gauge angiocatheter should suffice in most cases. However, if peripheral access is difficult or impossible, consider central access.

Labor & vaginal delivery

- Lumbar epidural anesthesia: Advantages include a reduction in oxygen consumption & cardiac output, while providing analgesia for the laboring pt. Due to the increased risk of difficult airway mgt, lumbar epidural analgesia must be started early & the catheter must be properly positioned, so that in the case of fetal distress, the labor epidural can be used intraoperatively for regional anesthesia.
  - ➤ Increased risk of failure/difficult placement: Studies cite a 2–20% failure rate in placement of lumbar epidural catheters. Possible explanations include increased depth of epidural space & difficulty identifying epidural space. Possible remedies for this problem include placement of epidural in sitting position. In addition, the obese pt is at a higher risk for displacement & migration of the epidural catheter from the epidural space.
  - ➤ Local anesthetic vs. opioids: In this pt subset, it is particularly important to minimize motor blockade. Addition of opioid

agonists to local anesthetic enables a total lower dose of anesthetic, possibly decreasing amount of motor blockade. However, adding opioids to epidural infusion can mask a malpositioned catheter.
- IV opioids: As w/ non-obese parturients, the potential for neonatal depression exists. Morbidly obese pts & those w/ coexistent respiratory disease are especially vulnerable to the respiratory depressive effects of parenteral opioids.
- Natural childbirth: Most obese women desire analgesia during labor & vaginal delivery.

C-section
- Increased risk of maternal mortality: In non-obese pts, C-section is associated w/ increased maternal mortality. Obesity increases the morbidity & mortality of C-section.
- Positioning: Proper positioning of the obese pt in supine position w/ left uterine displacement is essential. Hypotension has been associated w/ cephalad retraction of the pannus. It is also essential to properly position the shoulders & head as to maximize extension of the neck, in case of emergent intubation.
- Spinal anesthesia
  - Technical difficulty: Studies are equivocal as to whether obesity truly complicates placement of a spinal anesthetic.
  - Potential for exaggerated spread of anesthesia: In pregnancy, the local anesthetic dose requirement is decreased, most likely due to hormonal & mechanical factors. Obesity results in compression of the inferior vena cava, thereby increasing venous plexus blood volume & compressing the spinal space. This, in turn, appears to affect the spread of spinal anesthesia.
  - Pulmonary function after spinal anesthesia: Spinal anesthesia can cause a thoracic motor blockade. In obese parturients (who are dependent upon accessory muscles of breathing, especially in the supine position), this can result in an impairment of ventilation & oxygenation.
  - Efficacy of regional anesthesia: One study cites an increased operating duration in obese parturients in contrast to non-obese pts. Thus, it is possible that the duration of a single-shot spinal anesthetic may not be long enough. Furthermore, because emergent induction of a general anesthetic in these pts can be especially hazardous, epidural or combined spinal-epidural anesthesia may be a better choice.
- Epidural anesthesia

➤ Advantages over spinal
- Technical ease: It has been hypothesized & observed that identification of the epidural space w/ a large-gauge needle may be easier than finding the subarachnoid space w/ the smaller spinal needle.
- Ability to titrate anesthesia: The indwelling catheter permits extension of duration of the regional anesthetic. This is especially important w/ the increased operating duration of C-section in obese pts. In addition, obesity affects the spread of epidural anesthetic agents in a somewhat variable way; proper titration of epidural anesthesia limits this effect.
- Decreased hypotension: Incremental injection & slow titration of epidural anesthesia has been found to result in a decreased incidence of hypotension, especially in obese parturients who are a greater risk of hypotension, especially in the supine position and possibly w/ pannus retraction.
- Decreased potential for excess motor blockade: The ability to titrate the dose & concentration of the epidural anesthetic enables the anesthesiologist to limit the occurrence of excess motor blockade (especially to the chest wall musculature)
- Post-op analgesia: Epidural catheters may remain to provide post-op analgesia for these pts, possibly limiting post-op pulmonary complications.

■ General anesthesia
➤ Airway
- Mask ventilation: Obese pts, especially during pregnancy, manifest an increased risk of difficulty & failure in mask ventilation. Strategies to overcome this difficulty include:
  - Adequate help for induction (ie, in event of a two-handed mask placement)
  - Different sizes of masks: including disposables & non-disposables.
- Intubation
  - Increased difficult intubation/failure rate: Various studies cite an increased difficult intubation rate in morbidly obese pts. It has also been found that the incidence of difficult intubation in morbidly obese pts who received general anesthesia for C-section is as high as 33%.
  - Strategies to improve intubation outcome:
    - Additional help should be present for induction of such a pt.

- Positioning: Placement of head & neck on a ramp to facilitate maximum extension of head & neck
- Additional intubating tools (eg, short laryngoscope handles, assortment of blades, LMA, gum-elastic bougie, fiberoptic bronchoscope, transtracheal jet ventilator) should be available.
- Consider awake intubation by direct visualization or fiberoptic laryngoscopy.
- Rapid sequence induction: Do not use this technique if intubation is expected to be difficult.
- Preoxygenation: Essential; the obese parturient often has a decreased FRC; the FRC will also be decreased by general anesthesia & the supine & Trendelenburg positions.

➤ Pharmacology

- Premedication: Aspiration prophylaxis should include sodium citrate 30 cc PO (to increase pH of gastric contents) & ranitidine 50 mg IV (to decrease production of gastric acid); consider also giving metoclopramide 10 mg (to facilitate gastric emptying). For planned C-section, consider also administering ranitidine 12 hours prior, in addition to immediately pre-op.
- Induction agents: Obesity increases the volume of distribution of induction agents, prolonging the half-life of elimination & increasing the induction dose. The implication of this is that too small of an induction dose may result in a light anesthetic & one too large will result in delayed awakening. A reasonable dosage of thiopental is 4 mg/kg IV, w/ a maximum dosage of 500 mg. In addition, ketamine may be used as an adjunct or as a sole induction agent (1–2 mg IV).
- Muscle relaxation: Proper dosing of succinylcholine (for rapid sequence induction) is also unclear, based on this increased volume of distribution. Standard of practice dictates 1–1.5 mg/kg (maximum dose 200 mg), w/ dosing dependent on lean body weight. After induction, muscle relaxation is essential. It has been speculated that non-depolarizing muscle blockers that undergo hepatic metabolism (eg, vecuronium) may have prolonged action in obese pts. In contrast, agents that do not undergo hepatic metabolism (eg, cisatracurium or atracurium) are associated w/ a normal duration of action.
- Volatile anesthetics: Obesity does not increase MAC for pregnant women. However, body fat can act as a reservoir for inhalation (& IV) agents. Choice of agent: desflurane may be

a better choice over halothane or enflurane because of its decreased biotransformation in morbidly obese pts, & over isoflurane because of its lower solubility in blood & soft tissue. Titration of anesthetic must be low enough not to affect uteroplacental blood flow & high enough to limit maternal awareness & sympathetic stimulation.

- Nitrous oxide: Often nitrous is used to allow a decrease in the concentration of volatile anesthetic used. However, the obese parturient may require higher concentrations of inspired oxygen.

➤ Oxygenation: In obese parturients under general anesthesia, the FRC is decreased, possibly resulting in hypoxia. Strategies to improve oxygenation include:

- High inspired oxygen concentration
- Use of a large tidal volume
- PEEP
- Elevation of the pannus

➤ Emergence: Airway obstruction upon emergence or immediately post-opy may result in hypoxia, hypercapnia, possible pulmonary hypertension & cardiovascular decompensation.

Post-op Concerns

■ Determinants of perioperative morbidity: Unaffected by surgical incision or anesthesia method; main predictors of perioperative maternal morbidity include intraoperative blood loss & surgical duration

■ Complications

➤ Pulmonary: Acute post-op pulmonary events are twice as common in the obese relative to the non-obese. Post-op hypoxemia is more severe in obese than non-obese pts. In addition, a vertical incision has been found to also worsen post-op hypoxemia. These pts are also at a risk of atelectasis & pneumonia. All pulmonary complications may be exacerbated by the use of intraoperative general anesthesia.

➤ Infection: Obese pts also have an increased incidence of poor wound healing & wound infection (twice as common). Thus, post-op antibiotic prophylaxis is indicated in this subset of pts.

i. Post-op analgesia: Proper pain control may improve maternal outcome in this subset of pts. Different routes of analgesia administration have different advantages & disadvantages:

➤ IM Opioids: unpredictable absorption, especially in the obese pt

➤ IV Opioids: more consistent administration; however, obese pts are at a greater risk of pulmonary compromise from respiratory depression than non-obese pts. Pt-controlled analgesia may be of some utility.

➤ Thoracic Epidural Analgesia: In abdominal surgery of the obese pt there is possibly earlier ambulation, fewer pulmonary complications & shorter hospitalizations associated w/ thoracic epidural analgesia. It is possible that this observation can be extrapolated to the post-op care of the obese pt who has undergone C-section.

CAVEATS & PEARLS

Pre-op care

■ Pre-op assessment: History & physical (especially airway assessment, BP, room air oxygen saturation), indicated lab assays (eg, liver function tests & platelets in pre-eclampsia; ABGs in pts w/ pulmonary compromise; blood glucose in diabetics)

■ Equipment: large bed & NIBP cuff; longer epidural spinal/epidural needles; difficult intubation cart; central access kits

Intraoperative care

■ Vaginal delivery

➤ Lumbar epidural analgesia

• Positioning: Sitting is more effective than the lateral decubitus position for placement of epidural catheter.

• Identification of landmarks: Iliac crests; if unable to palpate, approximate a normal line from the C7 spinous processes to the belt indentation.

• Local anesthetic vs. opioids: Essential to minimize motor blockade. Thus, prudent to use opioid agonists in epidural mix. However, risk of masking a malpositioned catheter.

• Catheter placement: Obese pts are at greater risk of epidural catheter migration out of the epidural space. Thus, threading the catheter to 5–6 cm in the epidural space is recommended. As the subcutaneous tissue expands when an obese pt moves out of the flexed position, it is advisable to fix the catheter at the skin (with tape or Tegaderm) after this change in position has occurred.

➤ IV opioids: Avoid in obese pts, especially those w/ respiratory compromise, due to increased vulnerability to ventilatory depressive effects of opioids.

- C-section
  - ➤ Positioning on surgical table: Supine w/ left uterine displacement w/ special monitoring of BP when retracting pannus. In addition, it is essential to place head & neck in maximum extension (on blanket ramp) to facilitate endotracheal intubation should it become emergently necessary.
  - ➤ Spinal anesthesia
  - ➤ Exaggerated spread of anesthesia: Increase in adipose tissue further compresses the IVC, resulting in a decrease in CSF volume. Thus, local anesthesia dosing should be reduced.
  - ➤ Dosage of local anesthetics: Recommended dosing of bupivacaine is 7.5–12 mg for a primary C-section.
  - ➤ Single-shot spinal vs. combined spinal-epidural vs. continuous spinal anesthesia: Due to potential for increased duration of C-section & possible difficulty in securing the airway, a continuous neuraxial anesthetic (such as CSE or epidural or continuous spinal) may be indicated.
- Epidural anesthesia
  - ➤ Advantages: Ability to titrate anesthesia & limit excess motor blockade; decreased incidence of hypotension upon induction of the anesthetic; ability to prolong duration of anesthetic; post-op analgesia
  - ➤ Decreased risk of DVT: In hip & knee replacement surgeries, epidural anesthesia has been found to decrease incidence of DVT formation. It is possible that in C-section of obese parturients, this advantage is also conferred from the use of epidural anesthesia.

General anesthesia
- Airway
  - ➤ Positioning: Supine w/ left uterine displacement; head & neck in maximum extension on blanket/pillow/foam ramp
  - ➤ Premedication for aspiration prophylaxis: Sodium citrate 30 cc PO, ranitidine 50 mg IV, metoclopramide 10 mg IV
  - ➤ Intubation
    - Additional assistance: to aid in mask ventilation & intubation
    - Special tools: assortment of laryngoscopes including Mac 3 & 4, Miller 2 & 3, McCoy; long & short laryngoscope handles; LMA #3, 4, 5; gum-elastic bougie; fiberoptic bronchoscope; transtracheal jet ventilator

- Consider awake intubation (either by direct visualization or w/ fiberoptic bronchoscope), especially for known difficult intubations
- Rapid sequence induction: Avoid if difficult intubation is expected.
- Preoxygenation techniques: 100% oxygen for 3 minutes vs. 4 maximal inspirations of 100% oxygen

- Pharmacology
  - Recommended doses of induction agents
    - Thiopental 4 mg/kg IV (maximum dose 500 mg)
    - Ketamine 1–2 mg/kg IV
  - Recommended doses of neuromuscular blocking drugs
    - Succinylcholine: 1–1.5 mg/kg IV (maximum dose 200 mg)
    - Cisatracurium: 0.2 mg/kg IV
  - Volatile anesthetics: Desflurane may be the best choice: low blood-tissue solubility results in more rapid induction & emergence; lack of biotransformation limits hepatotoxicity.
  - Nitrous Oxide: May be used, but preexisting pulmonary disease may limit concentrations of inspired nitrous oxide.
- Oxygenation: Strategies to improve oxygenation include high FIO2, large tidal volumes, PEEP, elevation of pannus.
- Emergence: Properly assess neuromuscular & pulmonary function & mental status prior to extubation, as these pts are at a greater risk of airway obstruction vs. their non-obese counterparts.

Post-op care
- Complications
  - Prevention of pulmonary complications: Encourage pulmonary toilet, incentive spirometry & early ambulation to limit pulmonary complications.
  - Prevention of infection: Continue post-op antibiotics (cefazolin 1 g q8h) & dressing changes as indicated.
- Analgesia
  - IM opioids: Unpredictable absorption, especially in the obese parturient
  - IV opioids: Pt-controlled analgesia w/o a basal rate may be the best choice to achieve post-op analgesia w/o respiratory compromise.
  - Epidural analgesia: Consider continuation of epidural analgesia post-op. Current research cites early ambulation, fewer pulmonary complications & shorter hospitalizations when epidural analgesia is used post-op.

CHECKLIST

Preop

■ Maternal issues
➤ Pulmonary assessment: Room air oxygen saturation, ABGs
  • Cardiovascular assessment: NIBP
  • Endocrine assessment: serum blood glucose
➤ Fetal issues: FHR, biophysical profile, pelvic exam
■ Labor & delivery/C-section
➤ Monitoring/equipment
  • Assortment of cuffs
  • Longer needles for spinals/epidurals
  • Large bed
  • Intubation equipment: various laryngoscopes, handles, LMAs, fiberoptic bronchoscope, transtracheal jet ventilator
  • PEEP valve
➤ Aspiration prophylaxis: sodium citrate, ranitidine, metoclopramide
➤ Position pt for GA: supine w/ left uterine displacement; head & neck in maximum extension

Post-op care

■ CPAP for sleep apnea
■ DVT prophylaxis: SQ heparin, TED stockings, Venodyne boots
■ Pain control: IV pt-controlled analgesia vs. epidural analgesia
■ Prevention of pulmonary complications: incentive spirometry, early ambulation, pulmonary toilet
■ Prevention of infectious complications: perioperative antibiotics, wound care

OBSESSIVE-COMPULSIVE DISORDER

LATA POTTURI, MD
ADELE VIGUERA, MD

FUNDAMENTAL KNOWLEDGE

DSM IV Diagnostic criteria

A. Either obsessions or compulsions:
➤ Obsessions as defined by (1), (2), (3), & (4):
  1. Recurrent & persistent thoughts, impulses, or images that are experienced, at some time during the disturbance, as

intrusive & inappropriate & that cause marked anxiety or distress

2. The thoughts, impulses, or images are not simply excessive worries about real-life problems
3. The person attempts to ignore or suppress such thoughts, impulses, or images, or to neutralize them w/ some other thought or action
4. The person recognizes that the obsessional thoughts, impulses, or images are a product of his or her own mind (not imposed from without as in thought insertion)

➤ Compulsions as defined by (5) & (6):

5. Repetitive behaviors (e.g., hand washing, ordering, checking) or mental acts (e.g., praying, counting, repeating words silently) that the person feels driven to perform in response to an obsession, or according to rules that must be applied rigidly
6. The behaviors or mental acts are aimed at preventing or reducing distress or preventing some dreaded event or situation; however, these behaviors or mental acts either are not connected in a realistic way w/ what they are designed to neutralize or prevent, or are clearly excessive

B. At some point during the course of the disorder, the person has recognized that the obsessions or compulsions are excessive or unreasonable.

C. The obsessions or compulsions cause marked distress, are time consuming (take > 1 hour a day), or significantly interfere w/ the person's normal routine, occupational (or academic) functioning, or usual social activities or relationships.

D. If another Axis I disorder is present, the content of the obsessions or compulsions is not restricted to it (e.g., preoccupation w/ food in the presence of an Eating Disorder; hair pulling in the presence of Trichotillomania).

E. The disturbance is not due to the direct physiological effects of a substance (e.g., a drug of abuse, a medication) or a general medical condition

Course during pregnancy/postpartum

■ Pregnant & postpartum women appear to be at increased risk for the onset of OCD. Women w/ an early onset of the disorder & moderate to severe symptomatology prior to pregnancy are at higher risk for worsening of OCD during pregnancy.

■ Commonly, women experience ego-dystonic, intrusive obsessional thoughts about harming their baby. This can occur among pts w/ OCD or may occur de novo in the absence of any prior psychiatric history. Pts w/ postpartum depression may experience such thoughts as well. In general, these thoughts are transient & generally remit over time or w/ treatment of the underlying mood or anxiety disorder. These thoughts are extremely disturbing to the pt. Risk of actual harm to the baby is extremely rare in these settings since the mother has no clear intent of harming the infant. However, if psychotic symptoms are present, the risk of actual harm to the infant is elevated & merits further evaluation. Clinicians should routinely question postpartum pts about such thoughts in a non-judgmental way & provide reassurance that such thoughts are not uncommon. Typically, pts are very relieved to be able to share these thoughts w/ their clinician, & these women require careful evaluation. In rare situations, the obsessions progress to psychosis, especially in the postpartum period. Untreated OCD worsens during the postpartum period.

Meds commonly used in treatment
■ SSRIs
■ TCAs

Fetal issues & medications
The risks of treating a pregnant pt w/ psychotropic meds must be weighed against potentially harmful effects to the fetus. All psychotropic meds cross the placenta. Studies have not consistently reported an increased risk of fetal malformations or miscarriages in women taking SSRIs or TCAs.

STUDIES

History & physical
In addition to a thorough history & physical, ask pt about all prenatal psychiatric diagnoses. How has her illness been managed prior to pregnancy & during pregnancy? Ask about psychological counseling, psychiatric treatment & all meds she has taken during pregnancy. Also ask the pt regarding course of her OCD during pregnancy, symptoms encountered (onset of new obsessions and/or compulsions or any change from antepartum symptoms) & last dose of medication.

Lab tests
When applicable, check serum medication level & a full electrolyte panel.

EKG

A number of conduction abnormalities have been noted in pts on TCAs. It may be worthwhile to check an EKG or analyze the pt's rhythm on a cardiac monitor.

Barring another indication, pts w/ a history of OCD taking other psychotropic medications do not need a baseline EKG.

MANAGEMENT & INTERVENTIONS

- Psychosocial approach to the pt: Reassurance & a thorough explanation of events surrounding labor can help to alleviate any anxiety in the pt w/ OCD. Social supports & family members should be involved as deemed appropriate.
  - ➤ Tailoring anesthetic plan: Pts w/ a history of OCD who are able to give informed consent for anesthesia can safely undergo both general & regional anesthesia. Awareness of potential drug interactions will aid in developing a safe anesthetic plan.
  - ➤ Informed consent: Determine the pt's ability to give informed consent.

CAVEATS & PEARLS

- Some pregnant women w/ OCD can have obsessional, ego-dystonic thoughts about harming their baby; these pts merit careful evaluation.

CHECKLIST

- Be familiar w/ the diagnostic criteria for OCD.
- Know what meds the pt is taking & when her last dose was.
- Consider checking an EKG or analyzing cardiac rhythm in pts taking TCAs.

OSTEOGENESIS IMPERFECTA

STEPHEN PANARO, MD
EDWARD MICHNA, MD

FUNDAMENTAL KNOWLEDGE

- OI is an inherited genetic defect that affects the production of type I collagen.
- Clinical presentation can range from mild osteoporosis to the classic presentation of skeletal abnormalities, a history of multiple fractures, blue sclera & middle ear deafness.

- Accompanying abnormalities may include scoliosis, abnormal platelet function, increased thyroxin levels (increased oxygen consumption, increased basal metabolic rate), cardiovascular abnormalities (which include aortic & mitral regurgitation), cleft palate, hydrocephalus & spina bifida.
- Anticipate hyperthermia.
- Pt may be at increased risk for malignant hyperthermia, although most pts are not susceptible.
- Pt may be at increased risk for platelet dysfunction.

STUDIES
- If history reveals bleeding complications, studies of platelet function are indicated (eg, bleeding time, thromboelastography).

MANAGEMENT/INTERVENTIONS
- As pts w/ severe disease can have serious complications w/ either vaginal or cesarean delivery (increased incidence of hemorrhage, uterine rupture & pelvic fracture), relative risks/benefits must be discussed w/ the OB & the pt.
- Regional anesthesia is not contraindicated, but ligamentous landmarks may be distorted.
- General anesthesia
  - Intubation may be difficult due to limited range of motion & short neck.
  - Consider "gentle" laryngoscopy or alternatives such as fiberoptic intubation.
  - Position pt carefully, w/ all pressure points padded.
  - Consider avoiding succinylcholine, as fasciculations can cause bony injury.
  - OI may be associated w/ an increased risk of malignant hyperthermia.

CAVEATS/PEARLS
- The chest & spinal abnormalities often lead to restrictive lung disease.
- Brittle bones, fragile cervical vertebrae & dentition, short neck & large tongue can make intubation challenging.
- Position pt carefully, w/ all pressure points padded.
- The fasciculation that accompanies succinylcholine can cause injury.

- Case reports imply that OI may be associated w/ an increased risk of malignant hyperthermia, although most pts are not thought to be susceptible.

CHECKLIST
- Discuss delivery plan w/ OB.
- Pad all pressure points. All transfers & movements of the pt must be done extremely carefully.
- Avoid fasciculation & hyperextension of the neck during intubation.

OTHER CAUSES OF THROMBOCYTOPENIA

JEANNA VIOLA, MD
JANE BALLANTYNE, MD

FUNDAMENTAL KNOWLEDGE
- Cocaine-induced thrombocytopenia
  - ➤ Cocaine abuse in pregnancy is associated w/ asymptomatic thrombocytopenia, likely related to anti-platelet antibodies & bone marrow suppression.
  - ➤ Thrombocytopenia itself does not affect pregnancy much, but cocaine use is associated w/ increased risk of IUGR, abruption, fetal demise.
- HIV-associated thrombocytopenia
  - ➤ Increase in anti-platelet antibodies is common w/ HIV; pts often exhibit isolated thrombocytopenia similar to ITP.
  - ➤ Thrombocytopenia results from platelet destruction by anti-platelet antibodies & decreased production by megakaryocytes.
  - ➤ 3.2% of HIV+ parturients exhibit thrombocytopenia; 1/6 of pts will experience hemorrhagic complications.
- Bernard-Soulier disease
  - ➤ Rare, autosomal recessive bleeding disorder associated w/ low-normal platelet counts, large platelets & platelet dysfunction
  - ➤ Moderate to severe purpura
  - ➤ Platelets lack glycoproteins Ib, IX & V and do not bind readily to the subendothelium of injured vessels. Glycoprotein Ib:IX is necessary for VW factor to bind to platelet membrane.
  - ➤ Both intra- & post-partum hemorrhages may occur.
- May-Hegglin anomaly

➤ Rare autosomal dominant disorder of thrombocytopenia & platelet dysfunction
➤ Platelet levels may range from 10,000 to normal.
➤ Usually pts are asymptomatic, but they may present w/ a severe hemorrhagic episode.
➤ Fetus may be affected & sustain intracranial hemorrhage.

STUDIES
■ Cocaine-induced thrombocytopenia: history of substance abuse, toxicology screen if cocaine use is suspected
■ Thrombocytopenia in HIV+ pts attributed to the HIV disease if another cause is not found
■ Bernard-Soulier disease
➤ Characterized by prolonged bleeding time
➤ Platelet studies: normal platelet aggregation to ADP, collagen & epinephrine but not to ristocetin
■ May-Hegglin anomaly: giant platelets & blue inclusions in the cytoplasm of leukocytes on blood smear

MANAGEMENT/INTERVENTIONS
■ Cocaine-induced thrombocytopenia
➤ Discontinue cocaine use.
➤ Platelet function is usually unimpaired; regional anesthesia is considered safe if coags are normal.
➤ Fetus is at risk for thrombocytopenia; check neonatal platelet count at birth and x 72h. Monitor for signs of impaired hemostasis.
■ HIV-induced thrombocytopenia
➤ Transient response to steroids & IVIG (see "ITP")
➤ Long-term response can be achieved only w/ AZT.
➤ These parturients normally deliver via C-section to prevent neonatal trans-inoculation.
➤ Regional anesthesia is considered safe w/ evidence of adequate hemostasis, platelet count >75,000 & normal coags.
■ Bernard-Soulier disease
➤ Consider platelet transfusion: each U of platelet concentrate increases platelet count by 5–10,000.
➤ Platelet transfusions will be ineffective if the pt has developed antibodies to the GPIb:IX from prior transfusion.
➤ Pt may also suffer from immune-mediated thrombocytopenia & may be successfully treated w/ IVIG.

➤ Avoid IM injections & regional anesthesia; risk of bleeding is too great.

➤ IV opioid analgesia & N_2O useful for labor analgesia

➤ General anesthesia usually safest for C-section

➤ Aspirin & NSAIDs contraindicated

■ May-Hegglin anomaly

➤ Both spinal anesthesia & general anesthesia are safe for C-section. Risks of general anesthesia need to be weighed against the risk of spinal anesthesia.

CAVEATS AND PEARLS

■ Platelet function remains normal in most cases of cocaine- & HIV-induced thrombocytopenia, despite reduced number.

■ Consider platelet transfusion as a quick fix in pts w/ platelet count < 30,000.

■ Take universal precautions.

■ Close contact w/ a hematologist is important for pts w/ Bernard-Soulier disease & May-Hegglin anomaly.

CHECKLIST

■ Check platelet count & function prior to delivery.

■ Obtain careful history to elicit substance abuse or HIV infection.

Contact hematologist early if pt has a rare platelet disorder.

PACEMAKERS

JASMIN FIELD, MD
DWIGHT GEHA, MD

FUNDAMENTAL KNOWLEDGE

■ Information on pacemakers in the pregnant pt is exceedingly sparse. There are a handful of case reports in the literature, which note no serious complications or adverse outcomes. As more data exist on ICDs in the parturient, & most modern ICDs contain pacemakers, ICD information & results can appropriately be applied (see "*ICDs.*")

General pacemaker function & indications

■ Both anti-bradycardia (demand) & anti-tachycardia (overdrive) functions

■ Can be used w/ adjuncts such as anti-arrhythmia medications or radiofrequency ablation

- Pacing can be accomplished via both temporary & permanent methods
  - Transcutaneous
  - Transesophageal
    - There is only 1 case report of transesophageal echo confirmation of permanent pacemaker placement in a pt in her first trimester.
    - Method not ideal in parturient due to changes in gastric emptying, etc.; increased risk of aspiration
  - Transvenous
    - AV Paceport Swan-Ganz catheter
    - Transvenous pacing wire
- Temporary pacing is for emergent or transient pacing needs.
  - Pacing that is to remain for any amount of time >48 hours usually done via transvenous wires
- Permanent pacemaker components
  - Leads inserted transvenously via subclavian or cephalic veins
  - Single-chamber or dual-chamber leads
    - Atrial leads go to right atrial appendage
    - Ventricular leads go to right ventricle apex.
  - Leads attach to pulse generator.
    - Pulse generator sits in subpectoral or abdominal subcutaneous tissue.
    - Lithium batteries last for up to 10 years, depending on the modes used & the voltage required for capture.
- Pacers can also be placed for syndromes known to have the potential to cause life-threatening arrhythmias or sudden death.
- Conditions must be chronic or recurrent & in most cases must have caused symptoms such as presyncope, syncope or seizure at least once for a permanent pacer to be considered.
- Indications for permanent pacing have been established by the American College of Cardiology, American Heart Association & the North American Society for Pacing & Electrophysiology.
  - The system of categorization is quite elaborate & based on specific criteria for specific syndromes. There are 3 classes within each category:
    - Class I: benefit of permanent pacing agreed upon
    - Class II: divergence of opinion on benefit of permanent pacer placement
    - Class III: agreed that permanent pacing is not useful

- While malignant arrhythmias can be catastrophic during pregnancy, pacemakers pose little risk to mother & fetus.
    - Minimize interventions during the first 8 weeks of pregnancy if possible.
    - Women of childbearing age w/ known arrhythmias should have pacers implanted prior to becoming pregnant.

Pacemaker nomenclature

- Joint nomenclature agreed upon by the North American Society of Pacing & Electrophysiology & the British Pacing & Electrophysiology Group, called NBP Pacemaker Identification Code, classifies exact mode of function.
    - There are 5 code positions, though in practice pacemakers are often discussed in terms of the first 3 or 4 positions.
    - The abbreviations in the first 3 positions are the same throughout:
        - V = Ventricle
        - A = Atrium
        - D = Double
        - O = None
        - T = Triggers pacing
        - I = Inhibits pacing
        - S = Single chamber
    - In the fourth & fifth code positions, functions are described & abbreviations vary:
    - IV:
        Programmablefunctions
        P = Programmable rate and/or output
        M = Multi-programmable
        C =Communicating functions (i.e., telemetry)
        R = Rate response modulation (physiologic)
        O = none
    - V:
        Anti-tachyarrhythmiafunctions
        P = Anti-tachyarrhythmia
        S = Shock
        D = Dual:paces & shocks
        O = none

STUDIES
EKG
Holter monitor

Electrophysiology (EP) study
- Meds & manual stimulation are used to induce abnormal rhythms.
- Used to determine whether pt will benefit from pacemaker
  - Shows what rhythms are likely to develop & where the conduction pathways are
  - Shows cardiac cycle length & rate
  - Shows whether rhythms cause associated hemodynamic instability

MANAGEMENT/INTERVENTIONS
- During surgical procedures
  - Any high-powered electromagnetic interference device can cause malfunction, failure or resetting of the pacemaker.
  - Bipolar electrocautery is safer than unipolar.
    - All electrocautery should be minimized as able & used in short bursts only.
    - Grounding pads should be as far from leads & generator as possible.
  - Magnet application will put most pacers in asynchronous fixed rate mode.
    - **Magnet should always be available in the OR for any surgical procedures in pts w/ permanent pacemakers**.
    - Application of magnet to reset to asynchronous mode prior to any surgical procedure is not always warranted.
      - Take into consideration the nature of rhythm disturbance, nature of the surgery & knowledge of the pacer itself.
      - Pacer-dependent pts should be in an asynchronous or triggered mode during surgical procedures.
    - Rate-modulated (physiologic) modes may also be affected in the OR by meds, muscle movement, shivering, etc., & may cause rapid pacing rates, which could be harmful.
- If pacemaker program is unknown, consult EP service preoperatively for device interrogation.
- EP service should be consulted for reprogramming & evaluating pacer after operation is complete.

CAVEATS & PEARLS
- Rate-response (physiologic) modulation pacemakers use sensors such as temperature, respiratory rate, muscle activity, oxygen saturation, etc., to increase heart rate in response to physiologic demands.
  - Better choice for the changes of pregnancy than fixed-rate pacers

> There have been a few reports of fetal activity increasing maternal heart rate excessively in this mode.

■ Pacer leads are placed under fluoroscopy, which is contraindicated in pregnancy, especially in the first 8 weeks.

> Placement usually exposes the fetus to approximately 0.1 Gy (see "*ICDs*").

> Fetus can be protected w/ lead shielding to minimize exposure.

> Adverse outcomes in pregnant pts are not well documented.

CHECKLIST

■ Document device type, lead type, location of pacer leads & generator.

■ Chest x-ray can confirm location of leads & device as needed.

■ Ask about any recent syncopal episodes.

■ Document date of last interrogation.

■ Important: is pt pacer-dependent? In other words, what is the baseline rhythm disturbance without it?

PANIC DISORDER

LATA POTTURI, MD
ADELE VIGUERA, MD

FUNDAMENTAL KNOWLEDGE

DSM IV Diagnostic Criteria

The diagnostic criteria for panic disorder (w/ or w/out agoraphobia) require that the pt satisfies all of the following criteria:

1. A history of recurrent unexpected panic attacks. A panic attack is a discrete period of intense fear or discomfort, in which 4 (or more) of the following symptoms developed abruptly & reached a peak within 10 minutes:

> Palpitations, pounding heart or accelerated heart rate

> Sweating

> Trembling or shaking

> Sensation of shortness of breath or smothering

> Feeling of choking

> Chest pain or discomfort

> Nausea or abdominal distress

> Feeling dizzy, unsteady, lightheaded or faint

> Derealization (feelings of unreality) or depersonalization (feeling detached from oneself)

- ➤ Fear of losing control or going crazy
- ➤ Fear of dying
- ➤ Paresthesia (numbness or tingling sensation)
- ➤ Chills or hot flashes
2. At least one of the attacks has been followed by 1 month (or more) of one (or more) of the following: (a) persistent concern about having additional attacks, (b) worry about the implications of an attack or its consequences (eg, having a heart attack, losing control, "going crazy"), or (c) a significant change in behavior related to the attacks.

The panic attacks are not due to the direct physiological effects of a substance (e.g., drug of abuse, medication) or a general medical condition (e.g., hyperthyroidism).

Course during pregnancy/postpartum

Panic disorder affects 5% of the population & is diagnosed 2–3× as frequently in women. The course during the peripartum period is unclear. Some case reports suggest a decrease in symptoms during pregnancy, especially during the 1st trimester. Increasing levels of progesterone have been suggested to exert a protective effect. Other trials, however, have shown neither consistent improvement nor worsening of panic symptoms through pregnancy & postpartum.

Meds commonly used in treatment
- Benzodiazepines
- SSRIs
- TCAs

Fetal issues & meds

The risks of treating a pregnant pt w/ psychotropic meds must be weighed against potentially harmful effects to the fetus. All psychotropic meds cross the placenta. While there have been reports suggesting a slightly increased risk of cleft lip/palate in mothers taking benzodiazepines, particularly during the 1st trimester, these are controversial. Benzodiazepine exposure at the time of delivery can potentially lead to neonatal respiratory depression, withdrawal & agitation. In contrast, studies have not consistently reported an increased risk of fetal malformations in women taking SSRIs or TCAs.

STUDIES
- History & physical
  - ➤ In addition to a thorough history & physical, ask pt about all prenatal psychiatric diagnoses. How has her illness been managed

prior to pregnancy & during pregnancy? Ask about psychological counseling, psychiatric treatment, & all medications she has taken during pregnancy. Details regarding specific symptoms encountered during panic attacks, frequency of panic attacks, course of panic disorder during pregnancy & last dose of medication should be elicited.

■ Lab tests
  ➤ When applicable, check medication levels & a full electrolyte panel.
■ EKG
  ➤ A number of conduction abnormalities have been noted in pts on TCAs. It may be worthwhile to check an EKG or analyze the pt's rhythm on a cardiac monitor. Barring another indication, pts w/ a history of panic disorder taking other psychotropic meds do not need a baseline EKG.

MANAGEMENT & INTERVENTIONS

■ Psychosocial approach: Pts w/ panic disorder benefit from reassurance. Explaining to the pt what to expect can alleviate much of her anxiety. Social supports & family members should be involved as deemed appropriate.
■ Tailoring anesthetic plan: Pts w/ a history of panic disorder who are able to give informed consent for anesthesia can safely undergo both general & regional anesthesia. Lactated Ringer's (LR) solution has been purported to precipitate acute panic attacks. Subsequent studies have suggested that very large volumes of LR would be needed to precipitate an acute attack. LR can likely be safely used in pts w/ a history of panic disorder, but to avoid any risk of precipitating an acute attack, normal saline solution can be used as a maintenance fluid. Awareness of potential drug interactions will aid in developing a safe anesthetic plan. Pts taking benzodiazepines will have increased sensitivity to opiates & other CNS depressants.
■ Informed consent: Determine the pt's ability to give informed consent.

CAVEATS & PEARLS

■ In pts treated w/ benzodiazepines, watch for signs of neonatal respiratory depression or agitation due to withdrawal.
■ Use LR w/ caution in pts w/ panic disorder.

CHECKLIST

■ Be familiar w/ the diagnostic criteria for panic disorder.

■ Know what meds the pt is taking & when her last dose was.
■ Consider checking an EKG or analyzing cardiac rhythm in pts taking TCAs.
■ Consider using normal saline instead of LR if large-volume fluid administration is anticipated.

PARTURIENTS AFTER RENAL TRANSPLANTATION

JOSHUA WEBER, MD
PETER DUNN, MD

FUNDAMENTAL KNOWLEDGE

■ First pregnancy after renal transplant was reported in 1963.
■ Renal transplantation improves fertility from 0.12% pre-transplantation to >2% post-transplantation.
■ Allograft function increases early & decreases late in pregnancy. Women are usually advised to wait 1 year after living related donor transplant & 2 years after cadaveric transplant to avoid problems stemming from rejection.
■ Concerns about pregnancy-induced hyperfiltration having deleterious effects on transplanted kidneys have not been supported by literature.
■ Complications in pregnancy following transplantation:
  ➤ Higher risk of CMV can lead to congenital anomalies or fetal death.
  ➤ Secondary hyperparathyroidism can lead to risk of neonatal hypocalcemia.
  ➤ Spontaneous abortion (13–40%)
  ➤ IUGR (20–25%)
  ➤ Preterm delivery (45–50%)
  ➤ Hypertension/pre-eclampsia (30%)
  ➤ Persistent renal impairment (15%)
■ Adverse fetal effects from immunosuppressants are rare (see Management/Interventions" section).

STUDIES

Lab tests commonly ordered to evaluate renal function in pregnancy include:
■ Creatinine
■ BUN
■ Electrolytes

- Creatinine clearance
- CBC
- Urinalysis

In addition to labs commonly checked in pregnancy, the following tests may be performed:
- Coagulation profile
- Virology for hepatitis B/C, CMV, & HIV
- Serial ultrasound to evaluate growth & rule out anomalies
- Vaginal cultures in pts w/ lesions consistent w/ HSV

MANAGEMENT/INTERVENTIONS

Medical/OB mgt of parturients following renal transplant

- Minimize vaginal exams; use strict aseptic technique.
- Higher risk of UTI may warrant frequent urine cultures & UTI prophylaxis.
- Immunosuppressants are generally continued throughout pregnancy.
- Increased frequency of prenatal visits (q2 wks in 1st & 2nd trimesters, then q1 week)
- Monitoring: monthly measurements of serum creatinine, creatinine clearance, fetal development, BP
- Erythropoietin may be used for maternal anemia.
- Preterm delivery is considered for worsening renal function, fetal compromise or pre-eclampsia.
- Renal biopsy is considered if rapid deterioration in renal function occurs prior to 32 weeks gestation.
- See "*Parturients on Dialysis*" for dialysis mgt.

Immunosuppressants

- Steroids (prednisone, prednisolone): do not cross blood-brain barrier; considered safe in pregnancy
- Cyclosporine: associated w/ IUGR; may exacerbate hypertension; drug metabolism increased during pregnancy, so may need higher dose
- Tacrolimus: frequent monitoring of drug levels needed. Cytochrome P450 inhibited in pregnancy, which can lead to toxic levels.
- Mycophenolate mofetil (MMF): contraindicated in pregnancy; pts are usually switched to azathioprine
- Sirolimus: contraindicated in pregnancy; should be stopped 12 weeks prior to conception; pts are usually switched to cyclosporine

Anesthetic mgt for parturients following renal transplantation

- Anesthetic mgt is similar to normal parturients unless hypertension or renal dysfunction is present.
- For pts w/ abnormal renal function

  Regional anesthesia
  - Immunosuppression is not a contraindication to neuraxial anesthesia.
  - Increased toxicity from local anesthetics has been reported in pts w/ renal disease, but esters & amides can be used safely.
  - Contraindications to regional technique: pt refusal, bacteremia, significant hypovolemia, severe hemorrhage, coagulopathy, potentially preexisting neuropathy

  General anesthesia
  - Uremic pts may have hypersensitivity to CNS drugs due to increased permeability of blood-brain barrier.
  - Uremia causes delayed gastric emptying & increased acidity, leading to increased risk of aspiration pneumonitis (consider sodium citrate, H2-receptor blocker, metoclopramide).
  - Hypoalbuminemia leads to increased free drug concentration of drugs that are bound to albumin (ie, thiopental).
  - Succinylcholine is relatively contraindicated, as it causes approx. 1-mEq/L increase in serum potassium, which may precipitate cardiac dysrhythmias.
  - Use caution w/ drugs dependent on renal excretion (gallamine, vecuronium, pancuronium) & clearance (mivacurium, rocuronium).
  - Give antibiotics & stress-dose steroids for cesarean delivery.
  - Use strict aseptic technique for lines/catheters.

CAVEATS & PEARLS

- Immunosuppression is not a contraindication to neuraxial anesthesia.
- Pts are at high risk for obstetric complications such as infection, IUGR, preterm delivery, hypertension, pre-eclampsia.
- Consider antibiotics & stress-dose steroids for cesarean delivery.
- Use strict aseptic technique for lines/catheters.
- Anesthetic mgt is similar to normal parturients unless hypertension or renal dysfunction is present.

CHECKLIST

- Give antibiotics & stress-dose steroids for cesarean delivery.

- Check OB plan for pt.
- Document degree of renal dysfunction.
- Be prepared to manage hypertension.
- Consider effects of uremia, hypoalbuminemia, impaired renal excretion when choosing meds in the presence of renal dysfunction.

PARTURIENTS ON DIALYSIS

JOSHUA WEBER, MD
PETER DUNN, MD

FUNDAMENTAL KNOWLEDGE

- See "Renal Replacement Therapy." in *"ICU Care of the Parturient."*
- End-stage renal disease (ESRD) leads to decreased fertility. Incidence of pregnancy in women of childbearing age on dialysis is only 0.3–1.5% per year.
- Only 20–50% of pregnancies in dialysis pts result in delivery.
- Maternal complications of ESRD: anemia, hypertension, malnutrition
- Fetal complications of ESRD: preterm labor, IUGR, fetal demise
- Methods of dialysis: hemodialysis (HD), peritoneal dialysis (PD)
  Hemodialysis disadvantages
  ➤ Need for vascular access
  ➤ Hemodynamic instability (hypotension may disrupt uteroplacental perfusion)
  ➤ Need for anticoagulation of HD circuit
  ➤ Fluid & electrolyte shifts
  ➤ Increased incidence of infections (MRSA, VRE, hepatitis, tuberculosis, HIV)
  Peritoneal dialysis
  ➤ Advantages: less hemodynamic instability & convenience of at-home dialysis
  ➤ Complications: peritonitis, catheter problems

STUDIES

Lab tests commonly ordered to evaluate renal function in pregnancy include:

- Creatinine
- BUN
- Electrolytes
- Creatinine clearance

■ CBC
■ Urinalysis

In addition to labs commonly evaluated in pregnancy, the following tests may be performed:

■ Fetal heart rate monitoring (FHR) during dialysis
■ More intensive monitoring of BUN/creatinine & electrolytes

MANAGEMENT/INTERVENTIONS

Medical/OB mgt of parturients on dialysis

■ More intensive dialysis (4–6 times per week, to keep BUN <50)
■ Emphasis should be on hemodynamic stability during dialysis.
■ Increased erythropoietin dosage
■ Careful attention to nutrition & weight gain
■ Correction of metabolic derangements

Anesthetic mgt of parturients on dialysis

Regional anesthesia

■ Increased toxicity from local anesthetics has been reported in pts w/ renal disease, but esters & amides can be used safely.
■ Contraindications to regional technique: pt refusal, bacteremia, significant hypovolemia, severe hemorrhage, coagulopathy, potentially preexisting neuropathy

General anesthesia

■ Uremic pts may have hypersensitivity to CNS drugs due to increased permeability of blood-brain barrier.
■ Uremia causes delayed gastric emptying & increased acidity, leading to increased risk of aspiration pneumonitis (consider sodium citrate, H2-receptor blocker, metoclopramide).
■ Hypoalbuminemia leads to increased free drug concentration of drugs that are bound to albumin (ie, thiopental).
■ Succinylcholine is relatively contraindicated, as it causes approx. 1-mEq/L increase in serum potassium, which may precipitate cardiac dysrhythmias.
■ Use caution w/ drugs dependent on renal excretion (gallamine, vecuronium, pancuronium) & clearance (mivacurium, rocuronium).

CAVEATS/PEARLS

■ Beware of using dialysis ports for IV access, given risk of contamination & heparinization.
■ Consider dialysis prior to cesarean delivery.
■ Correction of metabolic derangements

- Increased toxicity from local anesthetics has been reported in pts w/ renal disease, but esters & amides can be used safely.
- Contraindications to regional technique: pt refusal, bacteremia, significant hypovolemia, severe hemorrhage, coagulopathy, potentially preexisting neuropathy
- Use caution w/ drugs dependent on renal excretion (gallamine, vecuronium, pancuronium) & clearance (mivacurium, rocuronium).
- Succinylcholine is relatively contraindicated, as it causes approx. 1-mEq/L increase in serum potassium, which may precipitate cardiac dysrhythmias.

CHECKLIST
- Determine timing of most recent dialysis.
- Anticipate pt's relative volume status based on timing of most recent dialysis.
- Check serum electrolytes.
- Check OB plan for pt.
- Document degree of renal dysfunction.
- Be prepared to manage hypertension.
- Consider effects of uremia, hypoalbuminemia, impaired renal excretion when choosing meds.

PELVIC TRAUMA

HOVIG CHITILIAN, MD
BHARGAVI KRISHNAN, MD

FUNDAMENTAL KNOWLEDGE
- Laceration of perineum, vagina or cervix; also, retroperitoneal hematoma
- Risk factors
  - ➤ Forceps or vacuum extraction
  - ➤ Prolonged labor
  - ➤ Multiple gestation
- Retroperitoneal hematoma is rare but can occur after C-section. It should be considered in a pt post C-section w/ signs of hypovolemia & a fall in Hgb in the absence of an obvious source of bleeding.

STUDIES
- Pelvic exam
- CT scan if retroperitoneal hematoma is considered

MANAGEMENT/INTERVENTIONS
- Tailored to the extent of hemorrhage & pt condition
- Repair of small lesions may be accomplished w/ local infiltration &/or parenteral opioids.
- More extensive lesions may require augmentation of epidural analgesia (ie, 3–5 cc 2% lidocaine), if present, or treatment with local anesthetic infiltration, IV ketamine (10 mg IV boluses) or spinal.
- Evacuation of a retroperitoneal hematoma may require rapid sequence induction of general anesthesia.
- If lesion is extensive, ensure the presence of large-bore IV access & the availability of blood products.

CAVEATS/PEARLS
- Pelvic trauma may be associated w/ injury to other organs.
- Risk factors include instrumented vaginal delivery, prolonged labor, multiple gestation.
- Retroperitoneal hematoma is rare but can occur after C-section.

CHECKLIST
- Large-bore IV access
- Provide analgesia or general anesthesia as dictated by the extent of surgical intervention.
- For more extensive surgical intervention, have blood products available.

PHEOCHROMOCYTOMA

GRACE C. CHANG, MD, MBA; ROBERT A. PETERFREUND, MD, PHD; AND STEPHANIE L. LEE, MD, PHD

FUNDAMENTAL KNOWLEDGE

Pathophysiology
- Tumor of chromaffin cells of neuroectodermal origin
- 90% of tumors are located in medulla of adrenal gland, remainder within abdominal cavity arising from paraaortic chromaffin cells.
- One of the tumors in multiple endocrine neoplasia (MEN) syndromes
  - ➤ Type IIa/Sipple syndrome (medullary thyroid carcinoma, hyperparathyroidism, pheochromocytoma)
  - ➤ Type IIb (medullary thyroid carcinoma, mucocutaneous neuromas, pheochromocytoma)

■ Pathophysiology is related to systemic effects of secreted products, namely norepinephrine & epinephrine.

Epidemiology
■ 0.04–0.1% of hypertensive pts; rare in pregnancy
■ Overall incidence <0.2 per 10,000 pregnancies
■ Only about 300 reported cases of pheochromocytoma in pregnancy; both malignant & benign pheochromocytomas have been described
■ May be difficult to diagnose since signs & symptoms are similar to pre-eclampsia & because so rare

Signs/Symptoms
■ Usually paroxysmal because of episodic release of hormones
  ➤ Headache
  ➤ Sweating
  ➤ Palpitations
  ➤ Pallor
  ➤ Nausea
  ➤ Tremor
  ➤ Anxiety
  ➤ Abdominal/chest pain
  ➤ Weakness
  ➤ Dyspnea
  ➤ Weight loss
  ➤ Flushing
  ➤ Visual disturbances
  ➤ Hypertension common but not universal finding (77–98% of pts)
  ➤ Orthostatic hypotension occurs in 70% of pts (due to chronic vasoconstriction w/ intravascular volume depletion & impaired reflex responses secondary to receptor downregulation or synaptic effects of circulating catecholamines).

Changes Associated w/ Pregnancy
■ Pregnancy does not accelerate growth of tumor.
■ Inverse relationship btwn BP & heart rate, increasing Hct or worsening hypertension during treatment w/ beta blocker w/ suspected pre-eclampsia are suggestive of pheochromocytoma
■ Plasma concentrations of catecholamines no different btwn pregnant & nonpregnant pts
■ Preferred method of delivery is C-section to minimize increased pressure on tumor during active labor.

Maternal Complications

■ Cases of placental abruption have been reported, likely very similar to consequences of acute cocaine intoxication.

■ Diagnosis prior to labor & delivery may reduce maternal mortality from 35% to near zero.

Fetal Complications

■ Increased incidence of fetal death & IUGR (likely due to decreased uterine blood flow from increased catecholamine secretion)

■ When diagnosed early & alpha-blockade instituted, fetal death rate declines from 50% to near zero.

STUDIES

■ Look for increased catecholamine secretion by measuring concentrations of norepinephrine, epinephrine, or their metabolites (metanephrine, normetanephrine or vanillylmandelic acid) in plasma or urine.

■ If results are equivocal, use clonidine test (clonidine fails to suppress catecholamine secretion from pheochromocytoma); glucagon test is contraindicated.

■ Imaging

➤ MRI used to locate site of tumor

➤ Nuclear medicine scan w/ MIBG (I-131-labeled metaiodobenzylguanidine) cannot be used in pregnant pts.

MANAGEMENT/INTERVENTIONS

■ Surgical mgt is definitive treatment.

➤ <24 weeks gestation, surgery should proceed as soon as pt is prepared adequately.

➤ >24 weeks gestation, gravid uterus may be mechanical obstruction for most abdominal pheochromocytomas; in this event, pt should be medically managed until term & tumor removed at time of C-section.

■ Medical mgt

➤ Only used as temporizing measure during pregnancy or in pts w/ inoperable or metastatic disease

➤ Key to mgt is BP control w/ alpha blockers.

• Phenoxybenzamine

• Most commonly used

• Greater alpha-1 selectivity than phentolamine

• Long-acting

• Crosses placenta but lacks long-term adverse effects on fetus

- Phentolamine
- Prazosin

➤ Beta blockers to treat persistent tachycardia or other cardiac dysrhythmias
  - Must be preceded by the use of alpha blockers to avoid paradoxical hypertensive response

➤ Nicardipine (calcium channel blocker)

➤ Metyrosine (however, very limited clinical experience & it is labeled a pregnancy category C drug)

➤ Nitroprusside
  - Decreases uteroplacental vascular resistance in hypertensive sheep & blocks norepinephrine-induced uterine artery vasoconstriction
  - Risk of fetal cyanide toxicity
  - Low dose, 1 mcg/kg/min, is safe during peripartum period.

■ Intravascular volume repletion
  ➤ Serially monitor Hct to evaluate adequacy of intravascular fluid volume expansion.
  ➤ Normalization of fluid status can decrease risk of intraoperative hypertension during manipulation of tumor & intraoperative hypotension after tumor is resected.

■ Echocardiogram to evaluate presence of maternal cardiomyopathy

■ Criteria for adequate pre-op alpha blockade in pts w/ pheochromocytoma:
  ➤ Preparation usually requires 10–14 days.
  ➤ All inpatient BP readings <165/90 48 hours prior to surgery
  ➤ Should have orthostatic hypotension, but BP on standing must be >80/45 mm Hg
  ➤ No ST-T wave changes on EKG
  ➤ No more than one premature ventricular contraction every 5 minutes

Anesthetic Management

■ Adequate preanesthetic alpha blockade is imperative!
  ➤ Expands intravascular volume
  ➤ Drop in Hct w/ reexpansion

■ Challenge is to prevent wide swings in hemodynamics; severe hypotension can occur after tumor excision due to abrupt decline in circulating catecholamines.

■ Standard monitors, intra-arterial catheter to monitor for rapid changes in hemodynamics, central venous line to measure right heart pressures & assess volume status

- If pt has catecholamine induced cardiomyopathy, pulmonary artery catheter or transesophageal echocardiography may be beneficial for ongoing assessments of cardiac filling pressures & volumes & cardiac contractility, especially w/ postexcision hypotension.
- Place 2 large-bore IVs for rapid infusion, if needed.
- Can use regional, general or combined (regional plus general) safely
- General anesthesia
  - ➤ Blunt hemodynamic response to laryngoscopy w/ lidocaine, labetalol or narcotic.
  - ➤ Volatile agents can be used safely, except halothane, which sensitizes the heart to catecholamine-induced arrhythmias.
- Adequate pain control is essential to prevent sympathetic response to pain.
- Meds to manage intraoperative BP: calcium channel blockers, phentolamine, trimethaphan, nitroprusside, nitroglycerin, esmolol, labetalol, propanolol, magnesium sulfate, adenosine
- Magnesium sulfate
  - ➤ Useful in controlling exaggerated BP changes due to induction, intubation & surgical incision
  - ➤ Loading dose 40–60 mg/kg
  - ➤ Infusion 2 g/hr until excision
  - ➤ Bolus 20 mg/kg to control acute changes
- Use short-acting meds because of episodic nature of catecholamine secretion.
- Hypoglycemia can occur since insulin secretion is inhibited by catecholamines & tumor removal may result in rebound insulin release.
- Perioperative meds to avoid, because of direct or indirect effects on release of catecholamines
  - ➤ Atracurium
  - ➤ Droperidol
  - ➤ Halothane
  - ➤ Metoclopramide
  - ➤ Metocurine
  - ➤ Morphine
  - ➤ Pancuronium
  - ➤ Pentazocine
  - ➤ Succinylcholine
  - ➤ Tubocurarine
  - ➤ Vancomycin
  - ➤ Ketamine

CAVEATS/PEARLS
- Use beta blockers judiciously since pts can have catecholamine-induced cardiomyopathy.
- Intubation can result in severe hypertensive reaction, leading to intracranial hemorrhage, pulmonary edema or decreased placental blood flow.

■ Magnesium sulfate impairs recovery from muscle relaxants; dose these drugs accordingly.

CHECKLIST
■ Pre-op preparation w/ alpha blockers (& beta blockers) essential
■ Aggressive volume re-expansion important
■ Large-bore IV access
■ Invasive monitoring of BP & CVP
■ Anticipate hypertension during manipulation of tumor.
■ Meds to control hemodynamic changes, preferably short-acting
■ Adequate pain control
■ Monitor for hypoglycemia.
■ Avoid perioperative meds known to increase catecholamine release.
■ Expect hypotension after removal of tumor.

PLACENTA ACCRETA

HOVIG CHITILIAN, MD
BHARGAVI KRISHNAN, MD

FUNDAMENTAL KNOWLEDGE
■ Definition: abnormally adherent placenta
  ➤ *Placenta accreta vera*: adherent to myometrium w/o invasion of uterine muscle
  ➤ *Placenta increta*: placenta invades the myometrium
  ➤ *Placenta percreta*: placenta invades the uterine serosa or beyond
■ Risk factor: prior uterine surgery or trauma. Placenta previa in a pt w/ a prior history of C-section or uterine surgery is especially concerning for placenta accreta.
■ Pts w/ placenta previa (no prior uterine surgery) are reported to have a 4–5% chance of having a placenta accreta, which may necessitate gravid hysterectomy.
■ Pts w/ placenta previa who have a history of 1 previous cesarean delivery have an increased likelihood of accreta (10–24%).
■ Pts w/ placenta previa who have a history of 2 or more previous cesarean deliveries have a 59–67% risk of accreta.

STUDIES
■ Blood, typed, cross-matched & immediately available if placenta accreta is suspected

MANAGEMENT/INTERVENTIONS
- Obstetric mgt usually consists of hysterectomy but may include uterine artery ligation or embolization.
- Ensure presence of large-bore IV access & the immediate availability of blood products.
- Be prepared to induce general anesthesia if necessary.

CAVEATS/PEARLS
- Placenta previa in a pt w/ a prior history of C-section or uterine surgery is especially concerning for placenta accreta.
- Obstetric mgt usually consists of hysterectomy but may include uterine artery ligation or embolization.
- Consider accreta in the differential diagnosis of post-partum hemorrhage in pts w/ prior uterine surgery.

CHECKLIST
- Have adequate IV access & blood products available.

PLACENTA PREVIA

HOVIG CHITILIAN, MD
BHARGAVI KRISHNAN, MD

FUNDAMENTAL KNOWLEDGE
- Definition: abnormally low-lying placenta
  - *Complete* placenta previa: placenta completely covers the cervical os
  - *Partial* placenta previa: the placenta covers only part of the cervical os
  - *Marginal* placenta previa: placenta lies close to w/o covering the cervical os
- Incidence: 1 in 200 pregnancies
- Risk factors
  - Prior placenta previa
  - Prior C-section or uterine surgery
  - Multiparity
  - Advanced maternal age
- Presentation: painless vaginal bleeding in the 2nd or 3rd trimester. First episode of bleeding is usually self-limited & rarely causes fetal distress or demise.

STUDIES

- Ultrasonography to diagnose placenta previa & provide information on the location of the placenta
- Lab studies: Hgb concentration, type & crossmatch of 2–4 units PRBCs

MANAGEMENT/INTERVENTIONS

- In the setting of active labor, persistent hemorrhage or a mature fetus, delivery by C-section is indicated. Otherwise the pt is managed expectantly w/ bed rest, vital sign monitoring & regular assessment of maternal Hgb as well as fetal well-being until the fetus is mature.
- Anesthetic evaluation should focus on airway, volume status & Hgb concentration. Check the pt's blood type. 2–4 units PRBCs should be available.
- Place two large-bore IVs & initiate fluid resuscitation w/ crystalloid.
- Anesthetic technique for C-section is dictated by the urgency of the case. Neuraxial techniques may be used in pts who are not actively bleeding or hypotensive.
    - ➤ Since pts w/ placenta previa are at greater risk for placenta accreta, it is often judicious to choose epidural anesthesia over spinal anesthesia because of possibility of gravid hysterectomy & prolonged surgical time.
- Cesarean delivery in an acutely bleeding patient is usually managed w/ a rapid sequence general anesthetic.
- Preferred induction agents for acutely bleeding patients include ketamine (0.5–1 mg/kg) & etomidate (0.3 mg/kg) to help preserve BP.
- Maintain anesthesia w/ a low concentration of a volatile agent.
- Infuse oxytocin immediately following delivery.

CAVEATS/PEARLS

- Pts w/ placenta previa (no prior uterine surgery) are reported to have a 4–5% chance of having a placenta accreta, which may necessitate gravid hysterectomy.
- Pts w/ placenta previa who have a history of 1 previous cesarean delivery have an increased likelihood of accreta (10–24%).
- Pts w/ placenta previa who have a history of 2 or more previous cesarean deliveries have a 59–67% risk of accreta.
- Where time permits, epidural may be preferred over spinal given increased likelihood of prolonged operating time and risk of gravid hysterectomy.

CHECKLIST
- Airway evaluation, hemoglobin, type & crossmatch
- Two large-bore IVs, 2–4 units PRBCs available
- Volume resuscitation w/ crystalloid if time permits
- General anesthetic w/ rapid sequence induction for emergency C-section (persistent hemorrhage, fetal distress)

PLACENTAL ABRUPTION

HOVIG CHITILIAN, MD
BHARGAVI KRISHNAN, MD

FUNDAMENTAL KNOWLEDGE
- Definition: separation of the placenta before delivery of the fetus
- Incidence: 1% of pregnancies
- Risk factors
  - History of previous abruption
  - Hypertension
  - Advanced maternal age
  - Tobacco use
  - Cocaine use
  - Trauma
  - Premature rupture of membranes
- Presentation: painful vaginal bleeding w/ increased uterine activity
- Most common cause of disseminated intravascular coagulation (DIC) in pregnancy. DIC is systemic activation of the clotting system w/ consumption of clotting factors & platelets. Manifests as diffuse bleeding from operative & venipuncture sites.

STUDIES
- Ultrasonography to diagnose abruption, determine gestational age, determine placental location & investigate presence of retroplacental hematoma
- Lab studies: Hgb concentration, type & crossmatch 2–4 units PRBCs. DIC labs: PT, PTT, fibrin degradation products (FDP), platelet, fibrinogen levels.
- Laboratory indicators of DIC are elevated PT, PTT & FDP w/ decreasing platelet count & fibrinogen levels.

MANAGEMENT/INTERVENTIONS
- Obstetric mgt is dictated by the severity of the abruption. Evidence of fetal distress or acute risk to the mother necessitates emergent

delivery in the most expeditious manner (usually by C-section, but if labor is rapidly progressing, vaginal delivery may be reasonable). If the fetus is preterm & not in distress, the pt is hospitalized & managed expectantly.

- Anesthetic evaluation should focus on the airway, volume status & Hgb concentration.
- Place two large-bore IVs & initiate fluid resuscitation w/ crystalloid.
- Cesarean delivery in an acutely bleeding patient is usually managed w/ a rapid sequence general anesthetic.
- Preferred induction agents for acutely bleeding pts include ketamine (0.5–1 mg/kg) & etomidate (0.3 mg/kg) to preserve BP.
- Maintain anesthesia w/ a low concentration of a volatile agent.
- Infuse oxytocin immediately following delivery.
- Treatment of DIC requires transfusion of platelets, FFP & cryoprecipitate.

CAVEATS/PEARLS
- Occurs in 1% of pregnancies. Risk factors include prior abruption, trauma, hypertension, advanced maternal age, cocaine & tobacco use.
- Obstetric mgt includes vaginal or cesarean delivery, depending on the status of the mother & fetus.
- Most common cause of DIC in pregnancy

CHECKLIST
- Airway evaluation, hemoglobin, type & crossmatch
- Two large-bore IVs, 2–4 units PRBCs available
- Volume resuscitation w/ crystalloid if time permits
- General anesthetic w/ rapid sequence induction for emergency C-section (persistent hemorrhage, fetal distress)
- Consider regional anesthesia if pt & fetus are stable & coagulation parameters are normal.

POLIOMYELITIS

MEREDITH ALBRECHT, MD; LISA LEFFERT, MD; AND MICHELE SZABO, MD

FUNDAMENTAL KNOWLEDGE

Definition
- Caused by a picornavirus
- Transmitted by fecal-oral route

- Affects motor neurons in the cerebral cortex, brain stem & anterior horn of the spinal cord
- Flaccid paralysis results.

Epidemiology
- Severe manifestations occur in 1% of pts w/ the disease.
- 50% of pts recover w/ no residual disabilities.
- 25% of pts are left w/ severe residual disabilities.
- Return of function mainly in first 6 months but can continue up to 2 years
- Infection more common in late summer & in the fall
- Mortality 1–4%; can approach 10% in pts w/ bulbar involvement

Pathophysiology
- Virus enters by the mouth & multiplies in lymphoid tissues.
- After secondary multiplication, the virus attacks the CNS.
- The virus attacks motor neurons specifically in the:
  - Anterior horn of the spinal cord
  - Medulla
  - Cerebellum
  - Motor cortex

Clinical Manifestations
- Incubation period of 6–20 days
- Viremia produces:
  - Fever
  - Headache
  - Malaise
  - Intestinal & respiratory symptoms
- CNS involvement presents with:
  - Neck/back soreness
  - Severe headache
  - Drowsiness
  - Irritability
- Asymmetric, flaccid paralysis within 2–5 days of onset of CNS symptoms
- Bulbar musculature involved in 15–20% of cases

Effect of Pregnancy on Poliomyelitis
- No difference in the percentage of pts w/ bulbar involvement

Effect of Poliomyelitis on Pregnancy & the Fetus
- Oral polio vaccination during pregnancy does not appear to have harmful effects on fetal development.

- During 1st trimester, acute illness: 40% pregnancy loss rate
- Maintenance of pregnancy unimpaired in later trimesters
- Respiratory function compromised by paralysis
- 1st stage of labor: normal
- 2nd stage of labor: may be facilitated by flaccidity of the pelvic floor.

STUDIES

History & Physical
- Asymmetric flaccid limb paralysis or bulbar palsies
- No sensory loss
- Acute febrile illness

Laboratory
- CSF abnormal w/ pattern of viral meningitis
- Recovery of virus present in CSF

Imaging
- None

MANAGEMENT/INTERVENTIONS

Medical Treatment
- Treatment is supportive.
- Mild cases
  - Bed rest
  - Antipyretics & analgesics
  - Physical therapy
- More severe cases require respiratory support.

Anesthesia
- Physical exam to document extent of respiratory involvement
- Respiratory support as needed
- May have increased risk for aspiration
- Avoid regional anesthesia due to risk of infectious complications.
- Avoid succinylcholine due to risk of hyperkalemia.
- Expect increased sensitivity to non-depolarizing neuromuscular blockers.

CAVEATS & PEARLS
- Caused by a picornavirus transmitted via the fecal-oral route
- Can have respiratory/bulbar involvement
- Increased risk of pregnancy loss if contracted in 1st trimester
- Avoid regional anesthesia.

- Avoid succinylcholine.
- Expect increased sensitivity to non-depolarizing neuromuscular blockers.
- If acute illness, avoid contamination of infant by maternal stool or urine.
- Collect cord blood for viral culture & antibody titers.

CHECKLIST
- Careful physical exam to document existing neurologic deficits
- Careful evaluation of respiratory function
- Respiratory support if necessary
- Avoid regional anesthesia due to possibility of viral spread.
- Avoid contamination of the infant by maternal stool or urine.
- Collect cord blood for viral culture & antibody titers.

POLYMYOSITIS/DERMATOMYOSITIS

AUGUST CHANG, MD
MIRIAM HARNETT, MD

FUNDAMENTAL KNOWLEDGE

Definition
- Polymyositis (PM) is a systemic disease of unknown etiology characterized by nonsuppurative inflammation of striated muscle, primarily proximal limbs, neck & pharynx, leading to symmetric weakness, atrophy & fibrosis
- Dermatomyositis (DM) is defined as PM w/ the addition of skin lesions
- Diagnostic criteria for PM
  1. Symmetric weakness of proximal muscles
  2. Histologic evidence of muscle inflammation & necrosis
  3. Elevation of serum skeletal muscle enzymes (the most reliable indicator of disease activity)
  4. Electromyographic evidence of myopathy
- Diagnostic criteria for DM include 3 of the above 4 plus either:
  1. Heliotrope eruption (blue-purple discoloration of the upper eyelids) or
  2. Gorton's papules (raised, scaly, violet eruptions over the knuckles)

Epidemiology
- Incidence: 0.5–8.4 per million
- Bimodal peak of onset: prepubescent & btwn 45–65 years of age
- Male:female ratio 1:2

Clinical manifestations
- GI
  - Pharyngeal involvement: dysphagia (10–15%), reflux
  - Impaired gastric & esophageal motility
- Pulmonary
  - Chronic aspiration pneumonitis (most common respiratory problem)
  - Respiratory insufficiency
  - Interstitial lung disease (5–10%)
- Cardiac
  - Arrhythmias
  - Conduction disturbances
  - Coronary vasculitis
  - Heart failure
- Arthritis: generally involves hand & finger joints

Effect on pregnancy & fetus
- Fertility is reported to be decreased via unknown mechanism
- One study reported that w/ active disease, 32% of pregnancies ended in fetal death or abortion & 26% of deliveries were premature

STUDIES

History & Physical
- Pulmonary: evaluate for evidence of chronic aspiration pneumonitis & interstitial fibrosis
- Cardiac: evaluate for evidence of arrhythmias & cardiomyopathy
- Musculoskeletal: evaluate for evidence of muscle weakness
- GI: evaluate for evidence of gastroesophageal reflux disease, dysphagia

Imaging
- Chest radiograph

Other
- ECG
- Pulmonary function testing & ABGs: consider if you suspect significant respiratory compromise

- Markers of disease activity
  - Serum creatinine kinase
  - Glutamic oxaloacetic transaminase
  - Aldolase

MANAGEMENT/INTERVENTIONS

Medical treatment

- Corticosteroids
  - First-line w/ treatment over period of months usually required for remission (until serum creatinine kinase normalizes)
  - No evidence of teratogenicity
  - Inactivation by placental 11-beta-OH-dehydrogenase results in low fetal levels of active drug
  - May precipitate gestational diabetes mellitus & hypertension
  - Longer-term adverse effects
    - Osteoporosis
    - GI ulceration
    - Impaired immunity
    - Adrenal suppression
- Cytotoxic agents may need to considered if steroids are ineffective or poorly tolerated

Anesthesia

- Regional is preferred to general, as atypical responses to both depolarizing & non-depolarizing muscle relaxants have been reported
- Stress-dose steroids during labor & delivery for pts currently on steroid therapy

CAVEATS & PEARLS

- Take care to avoid high regional block, particularly in pts w/ compromised respiratory function
- Atypical responses to both depolarizing & non-depolarizing muscle relaxants have been reported

CHECKLIST

- Document preexisting muscle weakness
- Have nerve stimulator available if muscle relaxants are used
- Stress-dose steroids during labor & delivery for pts currently on steroid therapy

PORTAL HYPERTENSION

LAWRENCE WEINSTEIN, MD
DOUG RAINES, MD

FUNDAMENTAL KNOWLEDGE

■ Normal portal venous pressures are 10–15 cm H2O; these are elevated & may be above 30 in portal hypertension.

■ Usually follows cirrhosis but can also be caused by Wilson's disease, Budd-Chiari syndrome (hepatic vein thrombosis)

➤ Women w/ Wilson's disease should continue taking chelating agents in pregnancy.

■ Most causes of portal hypertension are rare in child-bearing women.

➤ Budd-Chiari syndrome is associated w/ hypercoagulable states, including pregnancy.

■ A significant clinical consequence of portal hypertension is development of portal to systemic collateral circulation & ascites (see section on "*Ascites*").

➤ The most significant collateral shunts are those to gastric & esophageal mucosae, since they result in varices that can bleed.

■ Variceal bleeding is very dangerous & carries a significant 30% or greater mortality rate per bleeding episode.

➤ In pregnant women w/ varices, bleeding episodes are most common during the 2nd trimester.

STUDIES

■ Labs: anemia, heme in stools, altered LFTs

■ Pathologic findings include arteriovenous or venous-venous anastomoses w/ collaterals.

■ Special tests include galactose elimination capacity, antipyrine clearance.

■ Imaging studies include ultrasound of portal vein, celiac angiography.

MANAGEMENT/INTERVENTIONS

■ Treatment of variceal bleeding, which can be profuse, should be both supportive & directed toward stopping the bleeding.

➤ Supportive measures include fluid resuscitation w/ crystalloid & appropriate blood products.

• If the pt is coagulopathic, FFP, cryoprecipitate &/or platelets may be indicated.

➤ Methods to control or stop bleeding are both medical & procedural. Options include:

- Vasopressin (0.1–0.9 U/min IV): reduces rate of blood loss but in high doses may cause congestive heart failure or myocardial ischemia. This effect can be lessened w/ concomitant nitroglycerin administration.
- Somatostatin (250-mcg bolus, followed by 250-mcg/hour infusion)
- Propranolol
- Balloon tamponade w/ a Sengstaken-Blakemore esophageal tube
- Endoscopic sclerotherapy is effective in controlling or stopping bleeding in 90% of episodes.
- Transjugular intrahepatic portal-systemic shunt (TIPSS) creates a shunt between the portal & systemic circulations to relieve portal hypertension. Evidence has suggested that women w/ a TIPSS shunt prior to pregnancy have up to a 7× lower incidence of major variceal bleeding during pregnancy. Thus, prophylactic TIPSS may be beneficial for cirrhotic women desiring a pregnancy.

■ Women w/ portal hypertension planning pregnancy should undergo endoscopy w/ prophylactic sclerotherapy prior to conception, & endoscopic re-evaluation should be performed in each trimester.

■ Mode of delivery does not seem to affect risk of intrapartum variceal bleeding; delivery should be based on other OB considerations.

■ For the anesthesiologist, airway control becomes extremely important in the setting of variceal disease, as active bleeding can make intubation much more difficult.

➤ Early intubation may be preferable in cases where endoscopy is planned so that the airway can be protected & the chance of aspirating blood reduced.

■ Hemodynamic monitoring is important & an arterial line may be indicated to help w/ BP control & titration of vasopressors.

■ Large-bore IV access should be obtained in anticipation of the need for fluid resuscitation & administration of blood & blood products.

CAVEATS/PEARLS

■ Portal hypertension can be a common pathway for many forms of liver disease.

■ Where possible, treat the underlying cause.

■ Be wary of the presence of varices & potential for bleeding.

CHECKLIST
- Know history/etiology of portal hypertension.
- Know about presence of or bleeding history from existing varices.
- Be prepared to treat new-onset bleeding.
- Discuss plan for delivery w/ OBs.

POSTOPERATIVE PAIN AFTER CESAREAN SECTION

HUMAYON B. KHAN, MD
BHAVANI S. KODALI, MD

FUNDAMENTAL KNOWLEDGE
Preservative-free morphine 0.1–0.4 mg intrathecally or 3–5 mg epidurally provides analgesia for about 17–27 hours after cesarean delivery.

- Neuroaxial opioids work by binding to the opioid receptors (laminae 1, 2, 5) in the dorsal horn of the spinal cord & render analgesia by two distinct mechanisms: preventing the release of excitatory neurotransmitter from small, primary afferent fibers, & hyperpolarization of second-order neurons.

- Postop respiratory depression is a catastrophic complication of neuroaxial opioids. Postop respiratory depression is classified as early (after 1–3 hours) & delayed (after 6–12 hours of administration of neuroaxial opioids). It is rare if the aforementioned doses are used.

  - Early respiratory depression results from systemic absorption of opioids from the epidural venous plexus. It is uncommon after intrathecal administration of opioid medications.

  - Delayed respiratory depression results from the rostral spread of the opioids to the respiratory center located in the medulla & can be life-threatening.

  - Most institutions have protocols to prevent this catastrophic complication, which may include pulse oximetry, monitoring the respiratory rate, sedation scores & hourly visits by the nurse.

  - Naloxone & resuscitation equipment must always be immediately available should this occur.

  - No postop narcotics should be given to the mother for at least 24 hours after intrathecal or epidural morphine unless seen & evaluated by the physician, usually an anesthesiologist.

- Other common adverse effects after intrathecal or epidural morphine: emesis, pruritus, urinary retention

- At least 4 different receptor types are involved in the etiology of postop nausea & vomiting (PONV): dopaminergic (D2), histaminergic (H1), serotonergic (5 HT3) & cholinergic (muscarinic).
  - Antagonism against any one or more receptors perioperatively along w/ prompt treatment of intraoperative hypotension results in a decreased incidence of PONV.
  - Examples of anti-dopaminergic medications: metoclopramide (Reglan), droperidol, haloperidol (Haldol), prochlorperazine (Compazine) & promethazine (Phenergan).
  - Droperidol, although controversial, has fallen out of favor as a first-line antiemetic agent because of risk of rare fatal cardiac arrhythmias.
  - Haloperidol (1–4 mg) by IM injection has been found to be a very effective antiemetic in some recent studies.
  - Examples of antihistaminergic medications include dimenhydrinate (Dramamine) 50–100 mg I/M, hydroxyzine (Vistaril) 25–100 mg IM & cyclizine.
  - Examples of anti-serotoninergic medications include ondansetron (Zofran), granisetron, dolasetron & tropisetron. The most commonly used medication in this class is ondansetron (1–8 mg).
  - Examples of anticholinergic medications include scopolamine patch (1.5 mg), which has shown promise in preventing PONV in recent studies. It is placed behind the ear 1 hour before the scheduled C-section.
  - Other therapies that have proven effective in treating PONV include dexamethasone (8–10 mg), high-flow oxygen (0.8%), benzodiazepines, ephedrine, NK-1 receptor antagonism (GR 205171 and substance P antagonists) & nonconventional therapies (e.g., electro-acupuncture at P6 points just proximal to the wrist joint).
- Pruritus can be treated with nalbuphine (5 mg IV or IM) or naloxone (40- to 80-mcg boluses or as a continuous infusion 50–100 mcg/hr) or diphenhydramine (Benadryl, 25–50 mg IV), ondansetron 4–8 mg or subhypnotic doses of propofol (10 mg).
- Urinary retention is usually not a problem, as these pts have indwelling urinary catheters. It presumably results from inhibition of parasympathetic nervous system innervating the bladder, which results in detrusor hyporeflexia & tight closure of the internal urinary sphincter.

For pts who do not receive epidural/intrathecal morphine, postop pain can be managed by patient-controlled IV analgesia (PCIA) w/

meperidine, morphine, fentanyl or hydromorphone for the first 24–48 hours & then oral pain meds.

- Meperidine PCIA (5–15 mg; 5–15 minutes lockout) has a rapid onset & less sedation, nausea, vomiting & pruritus compared to morphine but is associated with a lower neurobehavioral score than is morphine on the third day of life. However, this should not pose a problem if meperidine is used for <24 hours. Meperidine is also not recommended in breast-feeding as a metabolite, normeperidine, can accumulate in the breast milk and cause seizures in premature & underweight infants, who cannot metabolize normeperidine as efficiently as full-term infants.

- Morphine & hydromorphone PCIA is commonly used in hospitals across the U.S. It is important to give a loading dose of these meds (morphine, 0.1–0.3 mg/kg; hydromorphone, 0.01–0.03 mg/kg) to achieve basal levels in the plasma before starting the PCIA.

- Morphine PCIA is dosed as 0.5–1 mg every 6–10 minutes (5–10 mg/hour maximum) as a starting dose. It can be increased to 3.0 mg every 5–15 minutes if pain remains uncontrolled.

- Pts may require more medication depending on their history of opioid use in the past & accompanying tolerance.

- Hydromorphone PCIA is dosed as 0.15–0.5 mg every 10 minutes (1.0–3.0 mg/hour maximum).

- Continuous infusions of either morphine or hydromorphone are not recommended because of the fear of respiratory depression unless the pt has a history of chronic pain & is monitored on a continuous basis.

- Use of nonsteroidal anti-inflammatory agents (NSAIDs), such as ibuprofen 600–800 mg q6–8h PO, diclofenac 100 mg extended-release tab once daily or 50 mg q8h suppository, or ketorolac 15 mg IV q6h, may also be prescribed to these pts if not contraindicated. Ketorolac has been found to be safe in lactating mothers.
  - ➤ It is important to give opioids & NSAIDs at the same time to have optimal pain relief via synergistic action.

- Transition to oral meds after the PCIA is stopped can be in the form of oxycodone, oxycodone w/ acetaminophen (Percocet), or hydromorphone tablets. NSAIDs can also be continued for 3–7 days postop.

- If the pt is sensitive to the potent narcotics or develops intolerable side effects such as nausea, vomiting & itching, less potent medications like acetaminophen w/ codeine or hydrocodone can be prescribed for pain mgt.

- It is reasonable for clinicians to obtain a consult from the pain mgt service for pts w/ a history of chronic pain.
  - Patient-controlled epidural analgesia (PCEA) containing bupivacaine, opiate (fentanyl, hydromorphone or morphine) & epinephrine may be a useful choice for pain mgt in these pts for the first 48 hours.

IM & SC administration of opioids is simple & economical to implement in hospital nursing protocols but offers limited flexibility in meeting variable pain needs.

A promising new agent for pain mgt is depomorphine, a long-acting epidural morphine that results is approximately 48 hours of pain relief after a single 15-mg, 20-mg or 25-mg epidural dose. It was very effective in pts undergoing hip arthroplasty in a recent study.

Fentanyl iontophoresis patient-controlled analgesia (PCA) has shown promising results in recent randomized, double-blind & placebo-controlled studies. With this method fentanyl (40 mcg q10min) is administered by electron transport technology through the intact skin without the need for an IV infusion catheter or pump.

STUDIES
- All pts receiving neuroaxial opioids should be monitored for respiratory depression.
- Monitors including pulse oximetry & apnea alarms are used in some institutions w/ some success.
- Other monitoring strategies include observing & recording the respiratory rate & sedation scores.
- None of these monitors can replace vigilant & conscientious nursing care.

MANAGEMENT/INTERVENTIONS
- Pts receiving neuroaxial opioids can develop intractable nausea, vomiting, pruritus, urinary retention & respiratory depression.
- Uncommonly, these pts may require opioid antagonism w/ naloxone & endotracheal intubation for life-threatening respiratory depression.
- It is important to manage other side effects quickly & safely w/o antagonizing opioid analgesia.
- See "Fundamental Knowledge" section for specific details.

CAVEATS/PEARLS
- Use medications that are safe & time-tested.
- Determine history of drug sensitivities or allergies.

- Anticipate potential complications & be prepared to treat them.
- Have a low threshold to call for help.
- Pts who unintentionally get a higher dose of opioid may require intensive care unit monitoring during recovery.
- Vigilant nursing care of these pts is vital.

CHECKLIST
- Confirm that the appropriate dose of opioid is being used twice & read the label carefully. Preservative-free morphine is usually dispensed as 0.5 mg/mL & 1 mg/mL.
- Always inform the pt of possible adverse effects & their treatment.
- Most bothersome side effects to the pt are pruritus, incisional pain & nausea after cesarean delivery.
- There should be good communication between the anesthesiologist & nursing staff to avoid catastrophic complications such as respiratory depression.
- Optimal pain mgt can be obtained by using a combination of different meds that prevent or treat pain by different mechanisms.

POSTPARTUM ASSESSMENT

ANJALI KAIMAL, MD
LORI BERKOWITZ, MD

FUNDAMENTAL KNOWLEDGE
See the "*Neonatal Resuscitation*" chapter for a discussion of newborn assessment & treatment.
- The Apgar score has been used to define newborn asphyxia, but this is problematic because it is subjective; it does not measure hypoxemia, hypercarbia or metabolic acidemia; & it may be affected by infection, maternal anesthesia, gestational age or congenital malformations.
- Umbilical cord blood acid-base analysis is a more objective way of evaluating a newborn's condition w/ respect to acidemia & hypoxia.

STUDIES

Cord blood sampling
- A segment of cord is double-clamped immediately after delivery; a delay of even 20 seconds can alter the arterial pH & PCO_2. Once the cord is clamped, the specimen can be collected within 60 minutes w/o significantly altering the values.

- Specimens should be obtained from the umbilical artery, as this contains blood returning from the fetus to the placenta & gives the best assessment of fetal status.
- The mean umbilical artery pH is 7.28. The critical pH cutoff to define significant acidemia is 7.00.

MANAGEMENT/INTERVENTIONS
See the "*Neonatal Resuscitation*" chapter.

CAVEATS/PEARLS
- Umbilical cord pH is an objective way to define neonatal asphyxia.
- A segment of cord is immediately clamped after delivery. An umbilical artery sample is collected within 60 minutes.
- The mean umbilical artery pH is 7.28. The critical pH cutoff to define significant acidemia is 7.00.

CHECKLIST
- Obtain a cord segment immediately if there is a question of fetal compromise.
- Send the umbilical artery sample for analysis within 60 minutes for accurate analysis.

POSTPARTUM EVALUATION & MANAGEMENT OF NEUROLOGIC COMPLICATIONS OF REGIONAL ANESTHESIA

ANDREA WAINGOLD, MD
JATINDER GILL, MD

FUNDAMENTAL KNOWLEDGE

Lower Extremity Deficits
- May present in the form of weakness, numbness, inability to ambulate
- Most often not related to the regional anesthetic, provided the local anesthetic has worn off
- Anesthetic complications (rare)
  - ➤ Injected agent (deposition of anesthetic intraneurally, rarely use of wrong drug)
  - ➤ Incorrect placement of needle or catheter resulting in direct neural injury
    - Infection or abscess

- • Ischemic or mass effect on the spinal cord
- ■ Maternal-obstetric complications can present similarly & often masquerade as "regional anesthetic complications."
  - ➣ Procedural
  - ➣ Positioning

Underlying medical condition of pt can present similarly.

Common peripheral nerve deficits: Peripheral nerve deficits in young healthy adults are uncommon. Mechanisms during labor are stretch, compression & retraction. Factors predisposing during labor include short stature, cephalopelvic disproportion (CPD), prolonged labor, use of forceps, abnormal presentation, excessive sustained hip flexion & use of surgical retractors. Electrodiagnostic studies may be done & abnormal results in the early presentation represent baseline deficit.

- ■ Femoral neuropraxia
  - ➣ Associated w/ hyperflexion of the thighs on the abdomen w/ abduction & rotation of the hips outward, or from the use of retractors
  - ➣ Frequently diagnosed mononeuropathy in diabetics
  - ➣ Usually unilateral w/ different grades of weakness of the quadriceps (extension of the leg), weak to absent knee jerk & variable pattern of numbness along the saphenous nerve below the knee
- ■ Meralgia paresthetica
  - ➣ Neuropraxia of the lateral femoral cutaneous nerve caused by compression by the inguinal ligament
  - ➣ Nerve deficits may be reproduced by palpating the inguinal ligament, w/ confirmation of diagnosis by resolution of symptoms w/ infiltration of local anesthetic in the area.
  - ➣ Presents as numbness that may be accompanied by dysesthesia
  - ➣ No motor deficits are seen; altered sensation may be noted, particularly hypesthesia in distal third of lateral thigh
  - ➣ Mechanism of injury may be stretch or trauma to the lateral femoral cutaneous nerve.
- ■ Lumbosacral plexopathy
  - ➣ Also known as postpartum foot palsy, obstetrical neurapraxia, maternal obstetrical sciatic paralysis, peroneal palsy
  - ➣ Predisposing factors are short stature, prolonged labor, CPD, abnormal presentation.
  - ➣ Non-obstetric causes include inflammatory, ischemic, hemorrhagic & metastatic insults.

- ➤ Usual presentation is unilateral foot drop, numbness of lateral leg & dorsum of foot, weakness of ankle & toe dorsiflexion, eversion & inversion & sensory impairment along L5 dermatome (lateral calf & foot).
- ➤ Variable weakness of knee flexion as well as hip extension & abduction that, if present, quickly resolves
- ➤ Possible leg pain, cramping or numbness during labor
- ➤ Lumbosacral plexopathy usually involves >1 root w/ sparing of the paraspinal muscles; as such, unlikely to be related to regional anesthesia.
- ➤ Electrodiagnostic studies after a few weeks show lumbosacral plexus involvement w/ sparing of paraspinal muscles.
- ■ Obturator neuropathy
  - ➤ Caused by fetal head or forceps
  - ➤ Usually unilateral & combined w/ femoral neuropathy
  - ➤ Weakness of hip adduction & rotation w/ diminished sensation over upper thigh
- ■ Peroneal neuropathy
  - ➤ Hypesthesia of first dorsal web space & weakness of dorsiflexion/eversion at ankle
  - ➤ More commonly seen w/ malpositioning of a pt, resulting in extrinsic compression of fibular head

Central lesions: More proximal lesions that cannot be ascribed to a peripheral nerve or lumbosacral plexus have a wide differential diagnosis, including compressive injury to nerve root (e.g., herniated disc, epidural abscess, epidural hematoma), ischemic injury to the spinal cord or cauda equina, which may be a result of diverse causes such as hypotension, compression of blood supply to the cord by the descending head, injection of a toxic substance or direct trauma to the nervous tissue. These are very rare. They may present unilaterally or bilaterally. There should be a low threshold for obtaining imaging studies in these circumstances.

- ■ Disc herniation and mechanical compression
  - ➤ Severe pain, weakness, numbness, which has a classic pattern depending on the nerve root involved
  - ➤ Prior history is extremely helpful.
  - ➤ Imaging studies are extremely helpful in diagnosis to exclude epidural hematoma & nerve root injury.
- ■ Ischemic spinal cord injury
  - ➤ Ascending iliac contribution provides a significant source of blood to the region of the cauda equina & the conus in about 15% of the pts.

➤ Prolonged labor, fetal macrosomia: arterial hypotension in these individuals may lead to a compromise of the blood supply & ischemic infarction & paraplegia. Extremely rare.

➤ Other rare causes of ischemic damage include anterior spinal artery syndrome, spinal AVMs combined with low perfusion states, increased CSF pressure leading to decreased perfusion pressure.

➤ Epinephrine has been implicated w/ vasoconstriction leading to cord ischemia, but this is unfounded.

■ Direct nerve injury: Needle placement in obstetric anesthesia is below the termination of the spinal cord.

➤ Significant variability in the level of the conus from T12 to L3 as well as the variation in the vertebral level at the intercristal line

➤ Incidence of direct neural injury w/ regional anesthesia is unknown & is probably very low.

➤ Effects of needle puncturing the neural tissue are also speculative. More damage is likely to occur from injection into the neural tissue than from a single stab by a thin needle.

➤ Many of the neurologic complications due to direct trauma have been reported in pts who had significant pain during injection.

■ Transient radicular irritation (TRI), transient neurologic symptoms (TNS)

➤ Most common w/ the use of intrathecal lidocaine but described w/ all local anesthetics

➤ Buttock & leg paresthesias after spinal anesthesia lasting up to 48 hours

➤ Unclear etiology but speculated to be local anesthetic toxicity

■ Spinal hematoma

➤ Risk factors include use of anticoagulants (especially LMWH), thrombocytopenia, difficult anatomy, spinal vascular malformations

➤ May occur in the absence of any risk factors & even spontaneously w/o spinal instrumentation

➤ Incidence of spinal hematomas may be higher than reported secondary to inadequate reporting & widespread use of anticoagulants.

➤ Presentation may be classic w/ severe back pain, radicular symptoms leading to weakness or numbness, bladder or bowel incontinence, but this is not always the case.

➤ Obtain a careful history relating to use of anticoagulants, bleeding diathesis, difficulty in placement.

> Perform neurologic exam & document it repeatedly to assess improvement or worsening of deficits.
> Contrast-enhanced MRI is the best diagnostic modality for imaging.

■ Epidural abscess
  > Risk factors include diabetes mellitus, trauma, IV drug abuse, immunosuppression, alcoholism.
  > Presentation may be delayed several days to weeks after regional anesthetic; is less dramatic than a hematoma but slowly progressive.
  > Initial presentation may be back pain (71%), unexplained fever (66%), followed by radicular symptoms, muscle weakness, numbness, sphincter dysfunction & in some pts progressing to complete paralysis (34%).
  > *S. aureus* is the most common organism.
  > MRI is the imaging method of choice.

Back Pain
■ Back pain after labor & C-section is extremely common.
■ Local tenderness at the insertion site is universal & to be expected.
■ May be a harbinger of pressure in the neuraxial space (e.g., epidural abscess, epidural hematoma)
■ Predisposing factors are young age, short stature, greater weight, prolonged/difficult labor, preexisting history of back pain.

Post-Partum Headache
Differential diagnosis
■ Post-dural puncture headache
■ Nonspecific muscle tension headache
■ Pregnancy-induced hypertension, pre-eclampsia, eclampsia
■ Migraine
■ Meningitis
■ Intracranial pathology including cerebral tumor, subarachnoid hemorrhage, subdural hematoma, cortical vein thrombosis

Symptoms
■ Postural component: resolves when recumbent, returns on upright posture
■ Bifrontal or occipital
■ Throbbing
■ May be accompanied by nausea, vomiting, neck stiffness, blurring of vision, photophobia, diplopia
■ Most pts will develop headache in 24–48 hours.

Incidence of inadvertent dural puncture in the obstetric population according to recent meta-analysis: 1.5% (95% CI); about half (52.1%, 95% CI) of those will result in PDPH.

Risk factors
- Young age
- Previous history of PDPH
- Cutting needles (Quincke) vs. non-cutting (Whitacre, Sprotte, Atraucan)
- Inadvertent dural puncture w/ epidural needle

Pathophysiology
- First theory of CSF loss through the puncture, leading to sagging of the brain & traction on the pain-sensitive structures, with possible involvement of CN III, IV, VI
- Second theory of CSF outflow leading to cerebral vasodilation, which leads to the headache

With conservative mgt most patients improve in 1–2 weeks, but an occasional patient will continue to be symptomatic for months or years.

STUDIES

Lower Extremity Deficits
- Signs & symptoms can be attributable to preexisting deficits, neurapraxia of a nerve, or central neuraxial process.
- Obtain a careful history relating to use of anticoagulants, bleeding diathesis, difficulty in placement.
- A basic understanding of the innervation of the lower extremity & a good neurologic exam are critical in localizing the site of injury & further mgt.

Innervation:
- Motor function:
- Hip flexion: L2/3 (femoral nerve) to assess iliopsoas muscle
- Hip adduction: L2/3/4 to assess hip adductors
- Hip abduction: L4/5S1 to assess gluteus maximus & minimus
- Hip extension: L4/5 (gluteal nerve) to assess gluteus minimus
- Knee extension: L3/4 (femoral nerve) to assess quadriceps
- Knee flexion: L5/S1 (sciatic nerve) to assess hamstrings
- Ankle dorsiflexion: L4/5 (peroneal nerve) to assess anterior compartment muscles of LE
- Ankle plantar flexion: S1/2 (tibial nerve) to assess gastrocnemius & soleus
- Long toe extensors: L5 to hallucis longus
- Sensory function (localized by dermatomes):

- T10: level of umbilicus
- L1: level of groin/inguinal ligament
- L2: upper thigh
- L3: lower thigh
- L4: medial anterior calf/foot
- L5: lateral calf/foot
- S1: medial posterior calf/heel
- S2: posterior thigh
- S3: medial buttocks
- S4–5: perineum

Imaging studies are extremely helpful in diagnosis to exclude epidural hematoma/abscess. Contrast-enhanced MRI is the best diagnostic modality for imaging. EMG & nerve conduction studies are not useful w/ acute presentations.

Back Pain

- Good history & exam to exclude radicular symptoms, weakness, numbness of extremities
- Guided by concomitant signs & symptoms
- See "Lower Extremity Deficits" and "Post-Partum Headache."

Post-Partum Headache

- Exam is normal. Neck & back tenderness, scalp tenderness, cranial nerve palsy may be detected. Other focal neurologic deficits should prompt a review of the differential diagnosis.
- MRI findings in intracranial hypotension include pachymeningeal thickening, enhancing w/ gadolinium. Subdural hygromas & hematomas may be seen in long-standing cases. Imaging studies are not needed in straightforward presentations.

MANAGEMENT/INTERVENTIONS

Lower Extremity Deficits

Peripheral nerve deficits

- Most of the neurapraxias are expected to resolve within a period of weeks to months.
- Usually demyelinating injuries, accounting for the excellent prognosis
- Treatment is expectant; risk factors are identified & modified if possible.

Central lesions

- Herniated disc/mechanical compression is managed conservatively unless there is the presence of severe pain, motor loss, cauda equina syndrome or a large disc fragment causing severe compression that is unlikely to improve w/o surgical intervention.

■ Direct nerve injury can be lessened by stopping the injection & redirecting the needle in the face of reports of pain by the pt.

■ The possibility of transient radicular irritation or transient neurologic symptoms may guide the choice of local anesthetic used.

Spinal hematoma

■ High index of suspicion is important in vague presentation, as the consequences of delay can be devastating.

■ Obtain emergent neurosurgical consult & imaging studies.

■ Treatment for compressive hematoma producing neurologic deficits is emergent surgical decompression. High-dose steroid protocol is also initiated. Time btwn presentation & decompression is critical for good outcomes.

Epidural abscess: Treatment is urgent decompression, depending on location & size, & antibiotic therapy for several weeks

Back Pain

■ Symptomatic treatment w/ oral analgesics, heat, brief bed rest

■ See "Lower Extremity Deficits" and "Post-Partum Headache."

Post-Partum Headache

Mgt is initially conservative & continued if successful

■ Bed rest

■ Oral or intravenous caffeine

■ Analgesics, including NSAIDs, butalbital (Fioricet), or low-dose opioids

■ Liberal intake of fluids

Epidural blood patch is offered when conservative measures fail or are poorly tolerated.

■ This is an invasive procedure, exposing the patient to possibility of another wet tap.

■ Although very rare, complications such as subdural hematomas have been associated w/ intracranial hypotension, so the headache is not entirely benign.

■ Obtain informed consent, mentioning failure to relieve pain as well as the risk of another dural puncture.

■ Consider all contraindications as for regional anesthesia.

■ Make a case-by-case decision.

➤ Minor headache w/ a small-bore needle that seems to be resolving can be managed conservatively; severe headache after a

large-bore needle that is not improving should be managed w/ an epidural blood patch.
➤ Prophylactic blood patches are usually not done.
■ Mechanism
➤ Initial pain relief secondary to restoring the pressure in the intrathecal space by tamponade effect
• Prolonged effect by sealing the dural tear
■ Efficacy rates from 70% to more than 90% are reported.
■ Possible return of symptoms after initial resolution
➤ Take a careful history before repeating the injection.
➤ Second injection may provide permanent relief.
➤ Use caution in proceeding further after 3 injections.

Subarachnoid catheter threaded at the time of dural puncture may actually reduce the incidence of PDPH.
■ Decrease in loss of CSF
■ Increased fibrin deposition at dural puncture secondary to irritation of the dura by the catheter

CAVEATS/PEARLS

Lower Extremity Deficits
■ Maternal-obstetric complications can present similarly & often masquerade as "regional anesthetic complications."
■ Maintain a high index of suspicion for a central process when neurologic deficits are difficult to explain, as the window of opportunity for decompression in compressive processes is very small

Back Pain
■ Back pain that is more pronounced on maneuvers increasing the pressure inside the space, such as coughing & Valsalva, sometimes represents increased neuraxial pressure such as in epidural hematoma.
■ Pts w/ difficult & prolonged labor are more likely to receive epidural analgesia, and these patients may as such have a higher incidence of back pain. Back pain is extremely common after labor & delivery, whether or not the pt has had a neuraxial anesthetic.
■ Epidural analgesia itself does not increase the incidence of long-term back pain.

Post-Partum Headache
■ Incidence of migraine & nonspecific headache in the first postpartum week has been reported to be as high as 39%.

- The level of the previous puncture is chosen for epidural blood patch, but since there is good spread in the epidural space for 3–4 levels, a level above or below may also be chosen.
- Volume to be injected for an epidural blood patch is often determined by how the pt tolerates the injection.

CHECKLIST

Lower Extremity Deficits
- Obtain a thorough history & physical exam prior to induction of regional anesthesia as well as once a nerve deficit is noted.
- Pay careful attention to pt's coagulation status, reports of pain during placement of regional anesthetic & asepsis during administration.
- Pay careful attention to pt positioning to minimize incidence of neurapraxia.
- Close follow-up during & after regional anesthetic
- Maintain a high index of suspicion for nerve deficits w/ prompt evaluation, appropriate consultation & treatment & explanation of prognosis.

Back Pain
- Rule out radicular symptoms, weakness, numbness of extremities, severe progressive pain exacerbated w/ cough.
- Treat symptomatically.
- Reassure pt & advise about prognosis. Consider neurologic consult for long-term follow-up.

Post-Partum Headache
- Rule out other causes of headache.
- Treatment depends on severity of symptoms, pt's functionality & response to conservative measures.
- Review risks & benefits of epidural blood patch w/ pt prior to placement.
- Seek appropriate consultation & studies should epidural blood patch prove unsuccessful.

POSTPARTUM HEMORRHAGE

HOVIG CHITILIAN, MD
BHARGAVI KRISHNAN, MD

FUNDAMENTAL KNOWLEDGE
Definition: >500 mL blood loss following delivery

Incidence: 10% of pregnancies
Etiology
- Uterine atony
- Retained placenta
- Pelvic trauma
- Placenta accreta
- Uterine inversion

For all postpartum hemorrhage cases, ensure presence of adequate large-bore IV access & an adequate blood bank sample.

STUDIES
MANAGEMENT/INTERVENTIONS
CAVEATS/PEARLS
CHECKLIST
N/A

POSTPARTUM INFECTION

SISSELA PARK, MD
LAURA RILEY, MD

FUNDAMENTAL KNOWLEDGE
- Definition: temp > 100.4 degrees F after first 24 hours after delivery
  - May be associated w/ virulent pelvic infection caused by group A or group B streptococci
- Most fevers in the puerperium are caused by genital tract infections.
- DDx for extragenital causes of postpartum fever includes:
  - Respiratory complications
  - Pyelonephritis
  - Severe breast engorgement
  - Thrombophlebitis
  - Mastitis
  - Incisional wound infection
  - Epidural abscess

Uterine infection
- Infection involving the decidua, myometrium, parametrial tissue
- Relatively rare after uncomplicated vaginal delivery
- More common after cesarean delivery
- Risk factors
  - Long labor
  - Prolonged duration of rupture of membranes

- ➤ Multiple cervical exams
- ➤ Internal fetal monitoring
- ➤ Low socioeconomic status
- ■ Common bacteria include:
  - ➤ Group A, B, D streptococci
  - ➤ *Staphylococcus aureus*
  - ➤ Gram-negative bacteria
  - ➤ *Clostridium* species
  - ➤ *Peptococcus* species
  - ➤ *Fusobacterium* species
  - ➤ *Mycoplasma hominis*
  - ➤ *Chlamydia trachomatis*
- ■ Symptoms
  - ➤ Abdominal pain
  - ➤ Parametrial tenderness w/ bimanual exam
  - ➤ Malodorous lochia
- ■ Diagnosis is usually clinical.

Complications
- ■ Wound infection
- ■ Pelvic abscess
- ■ Septic pelvic thrombophlebitis
- ■ Peritonitis

STUDIES
- ■ Temp measurement
- ■ Blood count
- ■ Consider blood cultures.
- ■ Ultrasound or CT scan may reveal a pelvic mass.

MANAGEMENT/INTERVENTIONS
- ■ With supportive therapy & antibiotics, most pts improve in 1–3 days.
- ■ Treatment of endomyometritis after vaginal delivery should include good anaerobic coverage.
  - ➤ Broad-spectrum penicillin or cephalosporin
  - ➤ Penicillin combined w/ beta-lactamase inhibitor
- ■ Endomyometritis after cesarean delivery
  - ➤ Initial therapy: broad-spectrum antibiotics that cover anaerobes, gram-positive aerobes & gram-negative aerobes
  - ➤ Treatment regimens
    - • Clindamycin w/ gentamicin
    - • Cephalosporin

- Ampicillin-sulbactam
- Ticarcillin-clavulanic acid
- Piperacillin
- Clindamycin w/ aztreonam
- Metronidazole w/ gentamicin

■ Parenteral antibiotics should be continued for 24–48 hours after the pt becomes afebrile & asymptomatic.

■ Some pts do not respond after 48–72 hours of antibiotics. Consider:
  ➤ Abscess or infected hematoma of incision site or in pelvis
  ➤ Extensive pelvic cellulitis
  ➤ Septic pelvic thrombophlebitis
  ➤ Retained placenta
  ➤ Resistant organism
  ➤ Nongenital source of infection
  ➤ Noninfectious fever
  ➤ Inadequate dosage of correct antibiotic

■ Change in antibiotic therapy is effective in about 80% of unresponsive pts.

Prevention

■ Prophylactic antibiotics decrease the frequency of infection after C-section.

■ Most appropriate agent is a limited-spectrum cephalosporin.
  ➤ Cefazolin 1 g IV immediately after clamping of umbilical cord

■ Alternative treatments for pts w/ allergy to cephalosporin
  ➤ Metronidazole 500 mg IV
  ➤ Clindamycin 900 mg IV w/ gentamicin 1.5 mg/kg IV

CAVEATS & PEARLS

■ Postpartum infection = temp > 100.4 degrees F, 24 hours after delivery

■ Postpartum uterine infection is most common after C section.
  ➤ Diagnosis is usually clinical.
  ➤ Treatment: supportive therapy & antibiotics
  ➤ Frequency of infection decreased by prophylactic antibiotics

CHECKLIST

■ With postpartum fever, determine & treat the cause.

■ Most common cause of fever postpartum is genital tract infections.

POSTPARTUM TUBAL LIGATION

JAMES WILLIAMS, MD
RODGER WHITE, MD

FUNDAMENTAL KNOWLEDGE

Elective procedure but w/ advantages in postpartum period
- Convenience for pt & OB, possibly decreased cost
- Technical ease for OB, as uterine fundus remains near umbilicus
- Rates of serious complications (bowel laceration, vascular injury) are lower w/ minilaparotomy than laparoscopy.
- If any contraindications, pt can return at 6 weeks for elective laparoscopic procedure.

Potential disadvantages
- Typical concerns for pregnant pt, including full stomach & potential for difficult airway
- Immediate surgery precludes complete assessment of newborn.

Timing
- "Immediate" postpartum within 8 hours
- Many prefer to wait at least 8 hours after delivery to allow increased gastric emptying.

STUDIES

- Hct after delivery (allowing several hours for equilibration), as blood loss is often underestimated
- Other studies as indicated by clinical scenario & medical comorbidities

MANAGEMENT/INTERVENTIONS

General considerations
- Typical concerns of pregnant pt balanced w/ physiologic/ pharmacologic changes of postpartum period
- Assessment of intravascular volume & uterine tone
- Intense stimulation w/ ligation of tubes can be comparable to cesarean delivery.
- Continued concerns about delay in gastric emptying
  - Aspiration prophylaxis reasonable for every pt
  - Intrapartum opioids (including neuraxial) associated w/ increased risk of delayed gastric emptying

Local/MAC
- Not approved by ASA guidelines
- Concerns for level of sedation required & protection of airway

General anesthesia (controversial since elective procedure)
- Rapid sequence induction
- Avoid high concentrations of volatile anesthetics (>0.5 MAC) to prevent uterine atony.

Epidural (T4 level)
- Reactivation of labor epidural
  - ➤ Success related to interval from delivery; the longer the interval from delivery, the lower the likelihood of success
  - ➤ Overall costs may be higher for reactivation vs. spinal anesthetic (especially when reactivation unsuccessful), but balance w/ increased risk of post dural puncture headache w/ additional spinal anesthetic.
- Lidocaine 2% w/ epinephrine or chloroprocaine 3% 15–20 mL administered incrementally in lumbar catheter +/− fentanyl 50–100 mcg. If catheter has been out of use, it is prudent to give an initial dose test dose (3 cc 1.5% lidocaine w/ epinephrine) to rule out intravascular/intrathecal/intraneural catheter & a small additional dose (5–7 cc) to document that the catheter appears to be working.

Spinal (T4 level)
- Concern for transient neurologic symptoms has led to decreased use of intrathecal lidocaine.
- Local anesthetic requirements may be increased compared to pregnant pt.
  - ➤ Return to normal by 36 hours post-partum
- Typical dosing hyperbaric 0.75% bupivacaine 12–15 mg, +/− fentanyl 10–25 mcg (can alternatively use 45–60 mg hyperbaric mepivacaine)
- Intrathecal meperidine reported to compare favorably to local anesthetics
- Typical dose 1 mg/kg (50–80 mg) of preservative-free preparation

Post-op analgesia
- Typically single dose of parenteral opioids followed by oral analgesics
- Intrathecal morphine 100 mcg provides superior pain relief, but use cautiously since it carries an increased risk of delayed respiratory depression & requires 24 hours of pt monitoring.
- Intrathecal meperidine: 6–8 hours of post-op analgesia

CAVEATS AND PEARLS

■ Elective procedure, so should be reserved for those w/ uncomplicated deliveries & no serious medical comorbidities

■ Activity of both depolarizing & nondepolarizing muscle relaxants is altered in the postpartum period.

■ Controversy in pts w/ hypertension
> If pt has preeclampsia, consider postponing procedure until at least 24 hours post-partum.
> Spinal anesthesia has been performed safely in hypertensive pts undergoing elective surgery.
> Compared to normotensive controls, pts w/ hypertension may experience a greater net decrease in MAP w/ the sympathectomy that accompanies spinal anesthesia.
> Avoid in pts w/ refractory disease or cases complicated by oliguria, pulmonary edema or MgSO4 therapy.
> Post-partum tubal ligation may be technically more difficult in obese pts. A supraumbilical incision is often necessary, which may be difficult to cover w/ regional anesthesia. Discuss plan w/ surgeon, as such pts may be better served by having a laparoscopic procedure 6 weeks postpartum under general anesthesia.

CHECKLIST

■ Full pre-op evaluation

■ Consult w/ OB. Consider deferring this elective procedure if any complicating comorbidities (eg, pre-eclampsia, hemodynamic instability, morbid obesity) are present.

POSTPOLIOMYELITIS MUSCULAR ATROPHY (POSTPOLIO SYNDROME)

MEREDITH ALBRECHT, MD; LISA LEFFERT, MD; AND MICHELE SZABO, MD

FUNDAMENTAL KNOWLEDGE

Definition

■ New onset of progressive muscle weakness & fatigue in skeletal or bulbar muscles unrelated to any other known cause

■ Develops 25–30 years after acute polio attack

Epidemiology

■ Postpolio pts suffer small decrement in muscle strength per year.

Pathophysiology

- Reactivation of the virus
- Late death of additional motor neurons
- Late denervation of the previously reinnervated muscle fibers

Clinical Manifestations

- Fatigue
- Myalgia
- Fasciculations
- Weakness of skeletal & bulbar muscles
- Development of new respiratory difficulties
- Sleep apnea

Effect of Pregnancy on Postpolio Syndrome

- None known

Effect of Postpolio Syndrome on Pregnancy & the Fetus

- Paralysis can affect respiratory status of mother.
- Pelvic asymmetry, if present, can affect vaginal delivery.
- Can cause inability to push effectively during 2nd stage of labor

STUDIES

History & Physical

- Muscle atrophy
- Decreased reflexes
- Abnormal swallowing function
- Vocal cord paralysis

Laboratory

- None

Imaging

- None

MANAGEMENT/INTERVENTIONS

Medical Treatment

- Supportive
- Physical therapy

Anesthesia

- Increased incidence of respiratory problems
- May have:
  - ➤ Laryngeal dysfunction due to muscle weakness
  - ➤ Unilateral or bilateral vocal cord paralysis
  - ➤ Increased risk of postanesthetic apnea

➤ Increased risk of aspiration
- Succinylcholine can cause severe hyperkalemia.
- Increased sensitivity to non-depolarizing muscle relaxants
- Regional anesthesia is not associated w/ reactivation of virus.

CAVEATS & PEARLS
- Progressive bulbar & skeletal muscle weakness 25–30 years after acute polio
- Increased incidence of respiratory problems, laryngeal dysfunction & vocal cord paralysis
- Increased risk of postanesthetic apnea
- Increased risk of aspiration
- Avoid succinylcholine.
- Expect increased sensitivity to nondepolarizing muscle relaxants.
- Regional anesthesia acceptable

CHECKLIST
- Careful physical exam documenting preexisting neurologic/muscle deficits
- Careful assessment of pulmonary function
- Pretreat w/ H2 antagonists, sodium citrate & metoclopramide due to risk of aspiration.
- Regional anesthesia acceptable
- Avoid succinylcholine.

POST-RESUSCITATION CARE

RICHARD ARCHULETA, MD
SANDRA WEINREB, MD

FUNDAMENTAL KNOWLEDGE
- The neonatal airway is a major source of morbidity & mortality in the post-resuscitative period. Continuous monitoring is needed for maintenance of the airway & effective oxygenation.
- Post-resuscitation, the neonate should be cared for in an ICU by personnel trained & experienced in caring for sick neonates.
- The goal of post-resuscitation care is to normalize the neonate's physiologic parameters in preparation for either a less acute level of care or further corrective measures.

STUDIES
Observe the neonate for indications of possible airway difficulty:

- Decreased lung compliance
- Decreased oxygenation as per pulse oximeter or ABGs
- Bradycardia
- Central or peripheral cyanosis
- Hypercapnia
- Unequal expansion of chest wall
- Unequal breath sounds (can be difficult to gauge in that breath sounds are often dispersed throughout the chest cavity)
- Decreased mental status & responsiveness

MANAGEMENT/INTERVENTIONS

Concentrate on a smooth transfer from the OR to the ICU.

- Qualified personnel should accompany the neonate throughout the transfer
- Required resuscitative measures must be continued through the transfer period.
- Comprehensive transfer of maternal & neonatal information to the neonatal ICU team.

Ensure good oxygenation & ventilation of the neonate (see "*Neonatal Airway Management*").

- Factors that can degrade the airway
  - ➤ The ETT position can be altered w/ neonatal head flexion/extension (ETT advanced/withdrawn)
  - ➤ The ETT can be obstructed
    - ETT kink
    - Mucus plug
    - Meconium
  - ➤ Increased intrathoracic or abdominal pressure
    - Pneumothorax
    - Gastric inflation
  - ➤ Equipment failure
- Corrective measures
  - ➤ Switch from mechanical ventilation to bag ventilation to confirm decreased lung compliance & rule out mechanical malfunction.
  - ➤ Check ETT position & reposition as required.
  - ➤ Suction airway w/ catheter to clear secretions & rule out ETT obstruction.
  - ➤ Pass orogastric or nasogastric tube to decompress stomach, especially after prolonged bag & mask ventilation.
  - ➤ Obtain chest x-ray to confirm ETT position & rule out pneumothorax.
- Ensure heart rate >100 bpm (see "*Resuscitation of the Neonate*").

- Ensure adequate BP.
  - ➤ Preterm neonates: usually systolic BP of 45–60 mm Hg
  - ➤ Term neonates: usually systolic BP of 60–70 mm Hg
- Provide neonatal warming w/ continued temperature monitoring.
- Provide continuous monitoring & required corrective measures:
  - ➤ Respiratory rate, arterial oxygenation
  - ➤ BP
  - ➤ Heart rate
  - ➤ Temp
  - ➤ Fluid balance
  - ➤ Blood glucose
  - ➤ ABGs
- Imaging studies
  - ➤ Check position of ETT & lines.
  - ➤ Check pulmonary status.
- Family support
  - ➤ Multidisciplinary
  - ➤ Regular meetings w/ medical team for updates & care discussions

Provide complete notification of family pediatrician for long-term integrated care.

CAVEATS & PEARLS
N/A

CHECKLIST
- Careful transfer of information & neonate to ICU setting
- Continued assessment of oxygenation, BP & heart rate & interventions as needed
- Provide supportive environment for neonate:
  - ➤ Warmth
  - ➤ Personnel trained & experienced in the care of sick neonates
  - ➤ Continuous monitoring of vital signs & physiologic parameters
- Provide support for family.
- Notify family pediatrician of situation & developments.

PRE-ECLAMPSIA AND HELLP SYNDROME

JEANNA VIOLA, MD
JANE BALLANTYNE, MD

FUNDAMENTAL KNOWLEDGE
- See "*Severe Pre-eclampsia.*"

- Pre-eclampsia: HTN >140/90; proteinuria after 20 weeks
- HELLP syndrome: subsegment of pts w/ pre-eclampsia develop hemolysis, elevated liver enzymes, thrombocytopenia.
  - ➤ Usually present preterm w/ RUQ pain, nausea/vomiting, malaise
- Hypertension & proteinuria are not always pronounced. Post-partum presentation of the disease is associated w/ a higher incidence of pulmonary edema & renal failure.
- Thrombocytopenia may be pronounced (<20,000); nadir usually occurs post-partum.
- Recovery of platelet count to >100,000 may take 10 days.
- Morbidity from HELLP is attributed to DIC, placental abruption, acute renal failure, pulmonary edema, liver hematoma, retinal detachment.
- Associated w/ a high rate of both maternal & fetal mortality; therefore, delivery is always indicated.

STUDIES

- Platelet count, serum creatinine concentration, urine protein level
- Presence of risk factors strongly associated w/ the disease
  - ➤ Nulliparity
  - ➤ Prior history of pre-eclampsia
  - ➤ Age >35
  - ➤ Black race
  - ➤ Chronic HTN or chronic renal insufficiency
  - ➤ Antiphospholipid Ab syndrome
  - ➤ Diabetes mellitus
  - ➤ Vascular or connective tissue disease
  - ➤ Multiple gestations
  - ➤ High BMI
  - ➤ Angiotensin geneT235 mutation
- Decreased platelets, increased fibrin split products, possible elevated PTT
- Bleeding time (BT) may be elevated w/ normal platelet count.
- Consider thromboelastogram.
- High-risk pts get an angiotensin II challenge test: AT II is infused & the amount required to raise the diastolic BP by 20 mm Hg is recorded.
  - ➤ Healthy pregnant women require a higher dose of AT II than non-pregnant women.
  - ➤ Those w/ HELLP syndrome develop increasing responsiveness to the AT II.
- Rollover test: pt lies in left lateral decubitus for 15 min & diastolic BP is measured. Pt then rolls onto back & diastolic BP is remeasured.

An increase in diastolic BP >15–20 mm Hg is considered a positive test.

MANAGEMENT/INTERVENTIONS

- ■ >50% of these pts require blood, FFP or platelet transfusion.
- ■ Treatment is delivery of the fetus.
- ■ Thromboxane >> prostacyclin
- ■ Magnesium sulfate therapy
- ■ In general, in pts w/ >80,000 platelets & no evidence of bleeding, regional anesthesia may be performed.
  - ➤ Spinal for C-section: 0.75% bupivacaine w/ dextrose 1.4–1.6 cc + fentanyl 10–20 mcg + preservative-free morphine sulfate 200 mcg
  - ➤ Epidural for labor or C-section: bicarbonated 2% lidocaine +/− epinephrine 1:200K, or 3% chloroprocaine, depending on urgency of delivery & acidosis of fetus
- ■ Trend of the platelet count is more important than absolute number.
- ■ Advantages of regional anesthesia in pts w/ HELLP syndrome include improvement in uteroplacental & renal blood flow & avoidance of a difficult airway.
- ■ GETA may be unavoidable; use caution w/ edematous airway.

CAVEATS AND PEARLS

- ■ HELLP syndrome is an emergency, requiring rapid delivery of the fetus.
- ■ DIC is a major cause of morbidity in these pts; careful attention to signs of DIC (liver involvement) & rapid treatment are necessary
- ■ Lab values may appear elevated due to intravascular volume constriction.
- ■ Regional anesthesia decreases circulating catecholamines.
- ■ Epidural can be initiated early in anticipation of further platelet drop.
- ■ Aggressive volume expansion can cause pulmonary or cerebral edema.
- ■ Magnesium sulfate may inhibit clotting & potentiate the effects of GETA.

CHECKLIST

- ■ Obtain a careful history regarding severity of pre-eclampsia (BP, platelets, liver function tests, uric acid, urine output).
- ■ Know obstetric plan.
- ■ Follow platelet trend; consider early epidural placement.

- Evaluate airway; prepare for GETA.
- Obtain type & cross of blood sample & arrange for blood products in case of an emergency.

Recheck platelet count prior to removal of epidural.

PRENATAL DIAGNOSIS

ANJALI KAIMAL, MD
LORI BERKOWITZ, MD

FUNDAMENTAL KNOWLEDGE

- Clinically significant chromosomal defects occur in 0.65% of all births; congenital malformations are found in about 3–4% of all births.
- Prenatal diagnosis provides reassurance to couples at high risk for abnormalities, allows for directed testing & planning for postnatal care of the infant & offers the opportunity for termination of an affected pregnancy.
- Screening generally begins w/ low-risk, noninvasive testing such as ultrasound & maternal serum screening, w/ the option of progression to higher-risk interventions such as amniocentesis based on risk assessment & pt desires.
- Indications for prenatal diagnosis include routine screening, advanced maternal age, previous child or fetus w/ a genetic disorder, a parent w/ a genetic disorder, consanguinity or environmental exposures that threaten fetal health.

STUDIES

First-trimester screening for Down syndrome & trisomy 18

- Two maternal serum markers in combination w/ an ultrasound marker are used in first-trimester screening for trisomy 21 & 18.
- Free beta hCG is increased & PAPP-A is decreased on average in fetuses w/ Down syndrome; both markers are low in fetuses w/ trisomy 18.
- In combination w/ maternal age & a nuchal translucency, a detection rate of 85% w/ a false-positive rate of 5% is achieved.
- This is a risk assessment; the screening test is considered positive if the risk of Down syndrome is equal to the age-related risk for a pregnancy in a 35-year-old woman (1 in 380 term births).

Second-trimester screening for aneuploidy

■ The triple screen involves measuring alpha-fetoprotein, hCG & unconjugated estriol in the maternal serum during the 15–20th week of pregnancy.

■ The quadruple screen involves the addition of inhibin-A to this panel.

■ Risk assessment is based on maternal age & modified based on the results of these markers.

■ By convention, the cutoff for a positive screen is the level of risk of having an affected fetus in a 35-year-old woman (1 in 380 at term).

■ A detection rate of 80% w/ a false-positive rate of 6% is achieved.

■ An ultrasound showing normal anatomy & the absence of any markers associated w/ chromosomal abnormalities decreases the risk by 50%.

■ Measurement of AFP also serves as a screening test for neural tube defects or abdominal wall defects.

Diagnostic ultrasound

■ Many chromosomally abnormal fetuses have structural defects or anomalies.

■ In the first trimester, increased nuchal translucency can be associated w/ fetal trisomies, especially trisomy 21.

■ Nuchal translucency will also be increased in some other genetic syndromes & structural anomalies such as heart defects.

■ Measurement of the nuchal translucency is technically difficult & requires extensive training.

■ In the second trimester, a genetic ultrasound assessing multiple markers for Down syndrome & other aneuploidies as well as a detailed structural survey is performed.

Amniocentesis

■ Amniocentesis refers to withdrawal of amniotic fluid for diagnostic or therapeutic purposes.

■ Diagnostic indications include genetic testing, fetal lung maturity & evaluation for infection; therapeutic indications include polyhydramnios or twin-twin transfusion syndrome.

■ Amniocentesis for genetic testing is generally performed in the 15th to 17th week of pregnancy; early amniocentesis can be performed at 11 to 14 weeks but is generally not recommended due to increased complications.

■ Risks: membrane rupture, fetal injury, fetal loss, fetomaternal hemorrhage, infection & abruption.

■ Risk of complications: approximately 1 in 200.

CVS

- Chorionic villus sampling refers to obtaining a small piece of placenta transcervically or transabdominally for genetic analysis.
- Can generally be done safely after 10 weeks
- Risks: bleeding, infection, miscarriage, fetomaternal hemorrhage & misdiagnosis
- While second-trimester amniocentesis is the safest invasive form of fetal diagnosis, CVS is safer than first-trimester amniocentesis.

Fetal blood sampling

- Fetal blood can be obtained by percutaneous umbilical blood sampling, cardiocentesis or intrahepatic blood sampling.
- Percutaneous umbilical blood sampling is considered the safest technique.
- Indications: fetal karyotype, diagnosis of immunodeficiencies, coagulopathies, platelet abnormalities, acid-base status & hematocrit differential in the setting of twin-twin transfusion syndrome
- Complications: bleeding, infection, cord hematoma, bradycardia, fetomaternal hemorrhage, fetal loss

MANAGEMENT/INTERVENTIONS

First-trimester screening for Down syndrome & trisomy 21

- A positive screen indicates that a woman's risk for having an affected fetus is greater than or equal to that of a 35-year-old woman.
- Women who are screen positive are offered definitive karyotype analysis w/ amniocentesis or CVS.
- If the screen is negative, it is not necessary to perform second-trimester screening for Down syndrome such as the triple screen, but an ultrasound for assessment of fetal anatomy is usually offered at 18–20 weeks.

Second-trimester screening for aneuploidy

- A positive screen indicates that a woman's risk for having an affected fetus is greater than or equal to that of a 35-year-old woman.
- Women who are screen positive are offered definitive karyotype analysis w/ amniocentesis.

Diagnostic ultrasound

- Ultrasound is generally used in combination w/ serum screening to assess for chromosomal & structural anomalies.
- In an abnormal fetus, karyotype analysis and termination are options, depending on extent of findings & pt's wishes.

Amniocentesis, CVS, fetal blood sampling
Mgt is dictated by the clinical scenario, the specific findings & the pt's wishes on a case-by-case basis.

CAVEATS/PEARLS
■ Clinically significant chromosomal defects occur in 0.65% of all births.
■ Congenital malformations are found in 3–4% of all births.
■ First- or second-trimester maternal serum screens in combination w/ diagnostic ultrasound provide an assessment of risk of aneuploidy or genetic disorder.
■ If the risk of aneuploidy is found to exceed that of a 35-year-old woman, invasive testing by CVS or amniocentesis is offered to provide a definitive diagnosis.

CHECKLIST
■ Assess risk factors for genetic or chromosomal abnormalities.
■ Offer serum screening and ultrasound in the first or second trimester.
■ Offer amniocentesis or CVS if risk is elevated based on results.
■ Discuss options for continuing or terminating the pregnancy depending on the clinical scenario & pt's wishes.

PREPARATION FOR NEWBORN RESUSCITATION

RICHARD ARCHULETA, MD
SANDRA WEINREB, MD

FUNDAMENTAL KNOWLEDGE
Personnel designated for neonatal care
■ 1 person skilled in neonatal routine care & capable of initiating neonatal resuscitation should be available for each fetus delivered.
■ In addition, at least 1 person equipped & skilled in administering neonatal resuscitation (other than the anesthesiologist attending the mother) should be available for each fetus delivered. This person should be immediately available for normal low-risk deliveries & present for high-risk deliveries.

"The primary responsibility of the anesthesiologist is to provide care to the mother. If the anesthesiologist is also requested to provide brief assistance in the care of the newborn, the benefit to the child must be compared to the risk of the mother." (ASA guideline)

- The anesthesiologist caring for the mother should not be expected to simultaneously care for both the mother & neonate & should contemplate doing so only in unexpected emergency situations.

How often are newborn care measures beyond routine care required?
- 5–10% of neonates require some assistance beyond routine care.
- 1% of neonates require major resuscitative efforts.

Equipment required for newborn resuscitation includes, at minimum:
- Airway equipment
  - Oxygen source, flowmeter, tubing
  - Oral airways & neonatal face masks, both preterm & term sizes
  - Ventilation bags, 250–500 ml, w/ pressure release valve set at 35 cm H2O or pressure manometer, either:
    - Flow-inflating (has flow control valve & requires compressed gas source providing 5–10 L/min) or
    - Self-inflating (fills spontaneously, should have reservoir bag, can provide positive-pressure ventilation w/o a compressed gas source)
  - Bulb syringe, suction catheters (5F or 6F, 8F, 10F or 12F), meconium aspirator
  - Endotracheal tubes (2.5–4.0 mm ID), stylet, Miller 0 (premature neonate) & Miller 1 (term neonate) laryngoscope/blades ready & checked for good function
  - LMA (size 1.0)
- Umbilical vessel catheterization
  - Sterile gloves, scalpel or scissors, umbilical catheters (3.5F, 5F), 3-way stopcock, umbilical tape, Povidone-Iodine solution
- Medications
  - Epinephrine (1:10,000 concentration), naloxone (0.4 mg/mL), NaHCO3 (0.5 mEq/mL, 4.2% solution)
  - Isotonic NaCl or LR, dextrose (10%)
- Other equipment
  - Warmed blankets, gloves, tape (0.5 or 0.75 inch), syringes (1, 3, 5, 10, 20, 50 mL), stethoscope, alcohol sponges, needles (25, 21, 18 gauge)
  - 5F orogastric tube to administer tracheal medications
  - 8F orogastric tube to empty stomach after prolonged PPV

STUDIES

Assess relevant fetal studies for evidence of fetal compromise, including:
- Fetal heart monitoring
  - Bradycardic or tachycardic patterns consistent w/ fetal distress

- Ultrasonography
  - May reveal risk factors for high-risk delivery, examples include:
    - Fetal anomalies, oligohydramnios, hydramnios, multiple gestations, placentae previa, breech presentation
- Fetal scalp blood pH monitoring
  - Fetal scalp pH < 7.20 is consistent w/ fetal distress.

MANAGEMENT/INTERVENTIONS
Discuss likelihood of high-risk delivery w/ personnel caring for mother & neonate, including consideration of the following risk factors:

- Antepartum factors
  - Maternal age <16 or >35 years old
  - Maternal substance abuse
  - Maternal infection
  - Maternal drug therapy (alpha blockers, beta blockers, lithium, Mg sulfate)
  - Chronic maternal disease such as hypertension or diabetes mellitus
  - Bleeding in 2nd or 3rd trimester (could be maternal or placental)
  - Pre-eclampsia or eclampsia
  - Fetal anemia or isoimmunization
  - PROM
  - Hydramnios
  - Oligohydramnios
  - IUGR
  - Prior fetal or neonatal death
  - Fetal anomalies
  - >1 fetus (should have a pediatric team for each fetus)
  - Post-term gestation
- Intrapartum factors
  - Prematurity
  - Fetal distress
  - Prolonged labor >24 hours
  - Prolonged 2nd stage of labor >4 hours
  - Prolonged rupture of membranes >18 hours
  - Meconium-stained fluid
  - Chorioamnionitis
  - Abruptio placentae or placentae previa
  - Cord prolapse
  - Uterine tetany
  - Forceps or vacuum-assisted delivery

➤ Breech or other abnormal presentation
➤ Maternal sedatives within 4 hours of delivery
➤ Emergency C-section
➤ Use of general anesthesia

Ensure at least 1 person certified for neonatal resuscitation is assigned to each fetus.

CAVEATS & PEARLS

■ Always use Universal Precautions.
■ The need for neonatal resuscitation is often unanticipated until the baby is born.

CHECKLIST

■ Review fetal studies.
■ Review neonatal risk factors.
■ Ensure appropriate personnel are assigned to care for neonate during birthing process.
■ Discuss high-risk cases w/ personnel caring for mother & neonate.
■ Always be ready for unanticipated neonatal resuscitation.
■ Always care for the mother.

PSYCHOTIC DISORDERS & BIPOLAR DISORDER

LATA POTTURI, MD
ADELE VIGUERA, MD

FUNDAMENTAL KNOWLEDGE

Schizophrenia & Schizoaffective Disorder

DSM IV Diagnostic Criteria for Schizophrenia

A. Two (or more) of the following, each present for a significant portion of time during a 1-month period (or less if successfully treated):
   1. Delusions
   2. Hallucinations
   3. Disorganized speech (e.g., frequent derailment or incoherence)
   4. Grossly disorganized or catatonic behavior
   5. Negative symptoms, i.e., affective flattening, alogia, or avolition
B. For a significant portion of the time since the onset of the disturbance, one or more major areas of functioning such as work, interpersonal relations, or self-care are markedly below the level achieved prior to the onset (or when the onset is in childhood or adolescence,

failure to achieve expected level of interpersonal, academic, or occupational achievement)

C. Continuous signs of the disturbance persist for at least 6 months. This 6-month period must include at least 1 month of symptoms (or less if successfully treated) that meet Criterion A (i.e., active-phase symptoms) & may include periods of prodromal or residual symptoms. During these prodromal or residual periods, the signs of the disturbance may be manifested by only negative symptoms or two or more symptoms listed in Criterion A present in an attenuated form (e.g., odd beliefs, unusual perceptual experiences).

D. Schizoaffective Disorder & Mood Disorder w/ Psychotic Features have been ruled out because either (1) no Major Depressive, Manic, or Mixed Episodes have occurred concurrently w/ the active-phase symptoms; or (2) if mood episodes have occurred during active-phase symptoms, their total duration has been brief relative to the duration of the active & residual periods.

E. The disturbance is not due to the direct physiological effects of a substance (e.g., a drug of abuse, a medication) or a general medical condition.

F. If there is a history of Autistic Disorder or another Pervasive Developmental Disorder, the additional diagnosis of Schizophrenia is made only if prominent delusions or hallucinations are also present for at least a month (or less if successfully treated).

DSM IV Diagnostic Criteria of Schizophrenia Subtypes
Criteria for Manic Episode

■ A distinct period of abnormally & persistently elevated, expansive, or irritable mood, lasting at least 1 week (or any duration if hospitalization is necessary).

■ During the period of mood disturbance, 3 (or more) of the following symptoms have persisted (4 if the mood is only irritable) & have been present to a significant degree:
  ➤ Inflated self-esteem or grandiosity
  ➤ Decreased need for sleep (e.g., feels rested after only 3 hours of sleep)
  ➤ More talkative than usual or pressure to keep talking
  ➤ Insomnia or hypersomnia nearly every day
  ➤ Psychomotor agitation or retardation nearly every day (observable by others, not merely subjective feelings of restlessness or being slowed down)
  ➤ Flight of ideas or subjective experience that thoughts are racing

➤ Distractibility (i.e., attention too easily drawn to unimportant or irrelevant external stimuli)

➤ Increase in goal-directed activity (either socially, at work or school, or sexually) or psychomotor agitation

➤ Excessive involvement in pleasurable activities that have a high potential for painful consequences (e.g., engaging in unrestrained buying sprees, sexual indiscretions, or foolish business investments)

■ The symptoms do not meet criteria for a Mixed Episode.

■ The mood disturbance is sufficiently severe to cause marked impairment in occupational functioning or in usual social activities or relationships w/ others, or to necessitate hospitalization to prevent harm to self or others, or there are psychotic features.

■ The symptoms are not due to the direct physiological effects of a substance (e.g., a drug of abuse, a medication, or other treatment) or a general medical condition (e.g., hyperthyroidism).

Criteria for Mixed Episode

■ The criteria are met both for a Manic Episode & for a Major Depressive Episode (except for duration) nearly every day during at least a 1-week period.

■ The mood disturbance is sufficiently severe to cause marked impairment in occupational functioning or in usual social activities or relationships w/ others, or to necessitate hospitalization to prevent harm to self or others, or there are psychotic features.

■ The symptoms are not due to the direct physiological effects of a substance (e.g., a drug of abuse, a medication, or other treatment) or a general medical condition (e.g., hyperthyroidism).

Course during pregnancy/postpartum

The perinatal period does not appear to be a high-risk period for new-onset psychoses. In contrast, the postpartum period represents one of the highest risk periods for developing a psychotic illness. The course of psychotic illness during pregnancy usually reflects the pt's course of illness prior to pregnancy.

Meds commonly used in treatment

■ Antipsychotics

Fetal issues & medications

The risks of treating a pregnant pt w/ psychotropic meds must be weighed against potentially harmful effects to the fetus. All psychotropic meds cross the placenta. Studies have shown that conventional antipsychotics, such as phenothiazines, do not increase the risk for congenital birth defects. Reproductive safety data on the newer antipsychotics known as "atypicals" (ie, clozapine, risperidone, olanzapine, quetiapine, aripiprazole) are limited. In addition, it has been shown that untreated schizophrenia increases the risk for birth defects & intrauterine fetal demise independent of medication exposure. Neonates exposed to antipsychotics have been reported to have transient effects such as hypotension, extrapyramidal symptoms, sedation, tachycardia, restlessness, dystonic & and parkinsonian movements.

Bipolar disorder

DSM IV Diagnostic criteria

- Bipolar I is a disorder involving one or more manic episodes (see section entitled "Schizoaffective Disorder" for diagnostic criteria) or mixed episodes. Often individuals have had at least one major depressive episode (see section entitled "Depression" for diagnostic criteria). The symptomatology cannot be accounted for by substance abuse, medication effect, mood disorder due to a general medical condition, schizophrenia, schizophreniform disorder, delusional disorder or psychotic disorder not otherwise specified.
- Bipolar II is a disorder characterized by the presence of one or more major depressive episodes accompanied by one or more hypomanic episodes. As above, other disorders should not account for the pt's symptomatology. The symptoms also should not count toward a diagnosis of Bipolar I disorder.

Hypomanic Episode

A. A distinct period of persistently elevated, expansive, or irritable mood, lasting throughout at least 4 days, that is clearly different from the usual nondepressed mood

B. During the period of mood disturbance, 3 (or more) of the following symptoms have persisted (4 if the mood is only irritable) & have been present to a significant degree:
   1. Inflated self-esteem or grandiosity
   2. Decreased need for sleep (e.g., feels rested after only 3 hours of sleep)
   3. More talkative than usual or pressure to keep talking
   4. Flight of ideas or subjective experience that thoughts are racing
   5. Distractibility (i.e., attention too easily drawn to unimportant or irrelevant external stimuli)
   6. Increase in goal-directed activity (either socially, at work or school, or sexually) or psychomotor agitation

7. Excessive involvement in pleasurable activities that have a high potential for painful consequences (e.g., the person engages in unrestrained buying sprees, sexual indiscretions, or foolish business investments)

C. The episode is associated w/ an unequivocal change in functioning that is uncharacteristic of the person when not symptomatic.

D. The disturbance in mood & the change in functioning are observable by others.

E. The episode is not severe enough to cause marked impairment in social or occupational functioning, or to necessitate hospitalization, & there are no psychotic features.

F. The symptoms are not due to the direct physiological effects of a substance (e.g., a drug of abuse, a medication, or other treatment) or a general medical condition (e.g., hyperthyroidism).

Course during pregnancy/postpartum

- The prevalence of bipolar disorder in the U.S. is estimated to be around 3.4%, affecting men & women equally. Women w/ bipolar disorder are often in their teens & 20s at the onset of the illness, which places them at risk for episodes through their reproductive years. The issue of whether bipolar illness improves during pregnancy is controversial. However, for the majority of pts w/ bipolar disorder, pregnancy does not appear to be protective, & these pts are at high risk for relapse if their maintenance meds are discontinued. Risk for recurrence of depression or mania is even higher if maintenance mood stabilizers are discontinued abruptly (ie, within 24 hours to up to 2 weeks) compared to a gradual tapering of medications (>2-week taper).

- Women w/ bipolar disorder are at high risk for symptom exacerbation during the immediate postpartum period. The risk for recurrence of a mood episode in the immediate postpartum period is around 50–70% if pts are off their mood stabilizer.

- Symptoms often arise rapidly & can commence a few weeks before or within the first few days to weeks following delivery. The current standard of care is to recommend postpartum prophylaxis for this high-risk pt population, which is to reintroduce the mood stabilizer (atypical antipsychotics, lithium, or anticonvulsants) several weeks to months prior to delivery or within 24–48 hours after delivery. Since the highest-risk period for recurrence of illness is during the first 6 weeks postpartum, many researchers recommend that prophylaxis begin well before delivery.

■ Women w/ bipolar disorder are also at a 20–30% risk for postpartum psychosis, which is characterized by rapid onset of manic &/or psychotic symptoms within the first 24–48 hours after delivery & is considered a psychiatric emergency. These pts typically require inpatient psychiatric hospitalization & acute treatment w/ neuroleptics & other mood stabilizers. Electroconvulsive therapy (ECT) is another first-line option for acute treatment. Postpartum prophylaxis w/ a mood stabilizer prior to delivery can significantly reduce the risk for postpartum psychosis as well.

Meds commonly used in treatment
■ Lithium
■ Anticonvulsants

Fetal issues & medications
The risks of treating a pregnant pt w/ psychotropic meds must be weighed against potentially harmful effects to the fetus. All psychotropic meds cross the placenta. Lithium use in the first trimester has been linked to an increased risk of cardiac malformations in the fetus, particularly Ebstein's anomaly. The current estimated risk for Ebstein's anomaly w/ 1st-trimester exposure to lithium is around 1/1,000–1/2,000 births. The most recent risk estimated is substantially lower than previous risk estimates of 1/50 births. In the 2nd & 3rd trimesters, lithium use has been linked to fetal thyroid goiter, although this is an exceedingly rare event. The risk for polyhydramnios is also increased w/ the use of lithium during pregnancy & requires close monitoring. Neonates exposed to lithium at delivery can experience hypotonia & lethargy, also known as "floppy baby syndrome." The incidence of these symptoms is low & usually self-limited. Carbamazepine & valproate use in the 1st trimester has been linked to an increased risk of multiple malformations, including neural tube defects, cardiac anomalies, low birthweight, craniofacial abnormalities, microcephaly & other congenital anomalies. Use of carbamazepine & valproate in the 3rd trimester has been associated w/ coagulopathy in the infant.

STUDIES

History & physical
■ In addition to a thorough history & physical, ask pt about all prenatal psychiatric diagnoses. How has her illness been managed prior to pregnancy & during pregnancy? Ask about psychological counseling, psychiatric treatment & all meds she has taken during pregnancy.

- Also ask the pt regarding course of her bipolar disorder, schizophrenia or schizoaffective disorder during pregnancy, symptoms encountered (relapses, recent episodes of mania, hypomania or depression, change in symptomatology during pregnancy) & last dose of medication.

Lab tests

- When applicable, check serum medication level & a full electrolyte panel.

EKG

- Barring another indication, pts w/ a history of schizophrenia, schizoaffective disorder or bipolar disorder do not need a baseline EKG.

MANAGEMENT & INTERVENTIONS

- Psychosocial approach to the pt: Pts w/ a history of bipolar disorder benefit from reassurance of their safety & the safety of their baby. Keeping pts as calm & comfortable as possible can prevent manic or psychotic episodes during the stressful period of labor. Prolonged sleep deprivation secondary to an arduous labor can also precipitate an episode. Ensuring that the mother remains relaxed & does not get overly exhausted is important in the clinical care of these pts. Social supports & family members should be involved as deemed appropriate.
- Tailoring anesthetic plan: Pts w/ a history of schizophrenia, schizoaffective disorder or bipolar disorder who are able to give informed consent for anesthesia can safely undergo both general & regional anesthesia. Awareness of potential drug interactions will aid in developing a safe anesthetic plan.
- Informed consent: Determine the pt's ability to give informed consent.

CAVEATS & PEARLS

- Antipsychotics, both conventional & newer, can cause numerous effects in the neonate, including hypotension, extrapyramidal symptoms, sedation, tachycardia, restlessness, dystonia, parkinsonian movements & agranulocytosis. The incidence of these adverse events is low compared to the high risk for recurrence of illness in the mother if such meds are discontinued around the time of labor & delivery.
- Pregnancy is not protective against bipolar disorder, & women w/ bipolar disorder are at a very high risk for relapse during pregnancy if maintenance psychotropic meds are discontinued. Recent estimates

of risk for relapse among women w/ bipolar disorder during pregnancy range from 50–75%.

■ The postpartum period is a particularly high-risk period compared to pregnancy for new-onset psychoses and/or exacerbation of bipolar disorder.

■ Mood stabilizers such as lithium, carbamazepine & valproate are known teratogens. Recent reproductive safety data on valproic acid suggest an overall risk of major malformations of close to 9%. Some of the newer mood stabilizers, in particular lamotrigine, may not increase the risk for major malformations. Recent risk estimates for malformations w/ lamotrigine exposure during the 1st trimester are around 3%.

CHECKLIST

■ Be familiar w/ the diagnostic criteria for schizophrenia, schizoaffective disorder & bipolar disorder.

■ Know what meds the pt is taking & when her last dose was.

PULMONARY ARTERY (PA) CATHETER

KRISTOPHER DAVIGNON, MD
HARISH LECAMWASAM, MD

FUNDAMENTAL KNOWLEDGE

Indications

■ Evaluation of a pt's intravascular volume status & response to a positive or negative volume challenge

■ Assessment of adequacy of cardiac output (oximetric PA catheters)

■ Conduit for transvenous pacing

■ See also "Caveats & Pearls" section.

Sites

■ A flow-directed PA catheter can be inserted through any 9F introducer placed in a large vein.

■ Common sites for PA catheter introduction: internal jugular veins, subclavian veins, femoral veins

Waveforms

■ Presence of the PA catheter tip in a central vein & ultimately the right atrium is indicated by the presence of a CVP tracing when transducing the PA port.

- Passage across the tricuspid valve & into the right ventricle is indicated by a systolic "step-up" in pressure w/ a mean diastolic pressure equal to the previous CVP. The diastolic pressure is also up-sloping, indicating ventricular placement, as opposed to the down-sloping diastolic pressure seen w/ arterial placement.
- Passage across the pulmonic valve into the pulmonary artery is indicated by a down-sloping diastolic "step-up" in pressure w/ a systolic pressure equal to the right ventricular systolic pressure.
- Placement of the catheter in "wedge" is indicated by the appearance of a, c, v, x & y waveforms similar to that seen w/ a CVP tracing.

Normal values
- Right ventricular systolic/diastolic pressure: 15–25/0–5 mm Hg
- Pulmonary artery systolic/diastolic pressure: 15–25/5–12 mm Hg
- Pulmonary artery occlusive ("wedge") pressure: 5–12 mm Hg

STUDIES
- In addition to pressure transduction, a chest radiograph should be obtained to evaluate placement of the PA catheter tip. In general, placement of catheter tip beyond the mediastinal contour indicates a too-distal placement of the PA catheter.

MANAGEMENT & INTERVENTIONS
- Technique
  - A PA catheter should always be placed under sterile conditions.
  - Prior to insertion, a sterile sheath should be placed over the PA catheter & the integrity of all ports & balloon & appropriate transducer calibration should be confirmed.
  - Once placed in a central vein (typically inserted to 20 cm w/ an internal jugular approach), the PA balloon should be gradually inflated. If resistance is encountered, the position of the catheter & introducer should be verified.
  - The PA catheter w/ balloon fully inflated should then be gradually inserted until a right ventricular pressure waveform & then pulmonary arterial waveform are encountered. Typically the catheter should be inserted approximately 10 cm between the RV & PA. If insertion of a greater length results in continued RV pressure tracing, it is likely that the catheter is coiling in the RV. The catheter will then have to be withdrawn w/ balloon deflated & reinserted.
  - Once in the PA, the catheter should be inserted w/ balloon inflated until a PA occlusion ("wedge") tracing is obtained. The

balloon should then be deflated to ensure the presence of a PA tracing (with balloon completely deflated) & re-inflated to ensure that a full 1.5 mL of air is required to obtain an occlusive tracing. The latter 2 steps are important to ensure that the PA catheter has not been inserted too far, a risk factor for PA rupture & pulmonary infarction.

➢ Once appropriately placed, the sterile sheath should be pulled over the entire catheter length & locked into the introducer hub.

■ Interpretation of data
➢ All "filling pressures" (CVP, PAOP) should be measured at end-expiration.
➢ Great care should be exercised in simply relating a single filling pressure to a volume, since their relationship is dynamic & can be affected by multiple extrinsic factors in the critically ill pt (eg, positive-pressure ventilation, inotropic agents, intra-abdominal pressure).
➢ The optimal method to assess a pt's intravascular volume status is to generate a Starling curve (stroke volume vs. PAOP curve) & assess the pt's position on the Starling curve over time using a positive or negative volume challenge.
➢ A rise in the PAOP w/ a rise in stroke volume w/ a positive volume challenge indicates volume responsiveness. A rise in the PAOP without a significant change in stroke volume indicates that the pt's intravascular volume is optimized. A low stroke volume w/ hypotension in this instance is consistent w/ cardiogenic shock. A high stroke volume w/ hypotension in this instance is consistent w/ vasodilatory shock.

CAVEATS & PEARLS
■ Choice of PA catheter: Multiple varieties of PA catheters exist; choice should be based on clinical indication.
➢ Need for transvenous pacing requires placement of a PA catheter containing ports for pacing wires. Both atrial & ventricular wires may be placed. If atrioventricular conduction is aberrant, ventricular pacing is mandatory.
➢ A need for multiple infusions indicates the use of a VIP+ (4 ports for infusions) over a VIP (3 ports for infusions) PA catheter.
➢ A need for continuous assessment of cardiac output adequacy requires placement of a oximetric PA catheter.
■ Placement of a PA catheter through the right ventricle is associated w/ a 3% incidence of new right bundle branch block. Therefore, when

placing a PA catheter in a pt w/ a pre-existing left bundle branch block, a mode of pacing should always be available prior to catheter insertion.

■ Since PA catheters are flow-directed, their placement is assisted by placing the pt in a neutral position (as opposed to the Trendelenburg position for access of the great veins) & maintaining the catheter's natural curvature in the direction of blood flow.

■ Since the thermistor of a PA catheter contains metal, a PA catheter should be removed prior to obtaining any MR study.

■ Anticipate dysrhythmias during placement.

■ PA rupture or pulmonary infarction may result from too-distal placement. Appropriate positioning should be confirmed by chest radiography & ensuring that balloon inflation w/ a full 1.5 mL of air is needed to obtain an occlusive tracing.

■ Thrombosis

➤ Infection & thrombosis rates are reduced by the use of heparin- & antibiotic-coated catheters. However, since their rates are still finite, all PA catheters should be removed as soon as they are not clinically required.

➤ A heparin-coated PA catheter should be removed in a pt w/ the heparin-induced thrombocytopenia (HIT) syndrome.

CHECKLIST

■ Confirm appropriate placement.

■ Secure PA catheter sheath onto introducer & suture introducer in place.

■ Appropriately dress introducer insertion site.

■ Monitor for adequate function & appropriate catheter tip position; monitor insertion site for infection.

PULMONARY EDEMA

WILTON C. LEVINE, MD
TONG-YAN CHEN, MD

FUNDAMENTAL KNOWLEDGE

■ Pulmonary edema during pregnancy can be divided into cardiogenic & non-cardiogenic. During pregnancy this distinction can be difficult due to disease states that exacerbate the hypotonic state of pregnancy.

➤ Cardiogenic: results from high intravascular pressure creating a hydrostatic pressure gradient leading to extravasation of fluid into the lung tissues despite normal lung integrity

➤ Non-cardiogenic: results from leaky pulmonary capillary bed despite normal pulmonary capillary wedge pressure

■ Causes of pulmonary edema in pregnancy

➤ Hypertension

➤ Tocolytic therapy

  • Related to IV beta-mimetics

  • Magnesium sulfate

  • Corticosteroids

➤ Amniotic fluid embolism

➤ Gastric acid aspiration

➤ Massive transfusion after hemorrhage

➤ Increased risk w/ multiple gestation & subclinical infection

➤ Primary pulmonary hypertension

STUDIES

■ Determine etiology of pulmonary edema or pulmonary hypertension.

■ Monitor SaO_2, EKG, BP.

■ Echocardiogram

■ Invasive hemodynamic monitoring as clinically indicated

MANAGEMENT/INTERVENTIONS

■ Treatment depends on the etiology.

■ Intubation & mechanical ventilation may be required in hypoxic pts unresponsive to therapy w/ diuretics & increased FiO_2.

■ Selective pulmonary vasodilators, including nitric oxide, may be useful.

■ Non-cardiogenic pulmonary edema unresponsive to the above measures may represent ARDS.

■ If primary pulmonary hypertension, consider epoprostenol.

■ Mgt for delivery

➤ Avoid increase in pulmonary vascular resistance (PVR).

➤ Invasive monitoring, including arterial catheter & pulmonary artery catheter, during labor & delivery

➤ Maintain R ventricular preload.

➤ Maintain L ventricular afterload.

➤ Maintain R ventricular contractility.

➤ Consider epidural analgesia to avoid pain, increased oxygen consumption & hemodynamic consequences of labor.

➤ Avoid Valsalva maneuver.
➤ Pt should be monitored & treated in an ICU setting.
■ Avoid PGF2a, as it is a pulmonary vasoconstrictor.

CAVEATS / PEARLS
■ Pulmonary hypertension is defined as mean PAP > 25 mm Hg.
■ Pulmonary edema results from cardiogenic & non-cardiogenic causes.
■ Causes of pulmonary edema in pregnancy are multiple.
■ Appropriate mgt of pulmonary edema requires determination of the etiology.
■ Pts need appropriate physiologic monitoring & intensive care during labor, delivery & post-partum.
■ If primary pulmonary hypertension, consider epoprostenol & inhaled nitric oxide.
■ Avoid PGF2a, as it is a pulmonary vasoconstrictor.

CHECKLIST
■ Does the pt have underlying pulmonary hypertension? What is the etiology?
■ Does the pt have pulmonary edema? What is the etiology?
■ Do you have adequate monitoring & access to care for the pt?
■ Does the pt need to be transferred to an ICU?

PULMONARY EMBOLUS (PE)

JASON JENKINS, MD
LEE WESNER, MD

FUNDAMENTAL KNOWLEDGE

Incidence, morbidity, mortality
■ Deep venous thrombosis (DVT) 0.02–0.36% of all pregnancies. Untreated, 15–25% progress to pulmonary embolus (0.05% of all pregnancies).
■ Hypoxic & ischemic injury to mother & fetus common in survivors
■ 15% mortality, 2/3 within first hour. PE accounts for up to 25% of direct maternal deaths due to all causes.

Risk factors
■ Current or past history of thromboembolic disease
■ Labor & delivery, especially C-section
■ Surgical procedures (eg, C-section, tubal ligation)

- Maternal age >35 years
- Obesity
- Prolonged bed rest
- Concomitant malignancy
- Disordered hemostasis (eg, protein C/S & antithrombin deficiencies, lupus)

Etiology
- Virchow's triad
  - Hypercoagulability, present in pregnancy but generally compensated by increase in fibrinolysis
  - Turbulent blood flow or venous stasis. The gravid uterus compresses the inferior vena cava & pelvic vessels, resulting in pelvic & lower extremity venous stasis.
  - Vascular endothelial damage, which occurs during normal vaginal delivery. Surgical trauma greatly increases the amount of damage & thus the risk of thromboembolic events.

Clinical presentation
- General: May occur throughout pregnancy & labor. Up to 2/3 of PE occur post-partum. Symptoms similar to AFE but usually less dramatic.
- Cardiovascular: tachycardia & dysrhythmia, may progress to cardiac arrest. Pulmonary artery hypertension & mechanical obstruction, followed by RV failure & eventual LV failure from impaired filling & perfusion. Low cardiac output.
- Pulmonary: dyspnea, hypoxia, tachypnea, ventilation-perfusion mismatch due to redistribution of blood flow, wheezing or bronchospasm, pulmonary edema, rales, cough, chest pain (may be pleuritic)
- Neurologic: anxiety, restlessness, headache, apprehension, unconsciousness
- Hematologic: predominantly hypercoagulable state
- Fetal: fetal distress may result from profound hypoxemia or hypotension

STUDIES

Lab tests
- Hematologic
  - Elevated d-dimer or fibrinogen split products, though d-dimer is often falsely elevated to the "diagnostic" or abnormal range near term

- ABGs may show hypoxemia &/or significant A-a gradient.

Imaging
- Ultrasound
  - ➤ Cardiac: Transthoracic echocardiography may show RV dysfunction & pulmonary hypertension. Transesophageal ultrasonography may show larger clots but is more invasive.
  - ➤ Vascular: Ultrasound studies are useful to locate thromboses, but pelvic imaging is limited by the gravid uterus.
- Radiographic: Most modalities can be performed w/o excessive radiation exposure to fetus.
  - ➤ Chest x-ray often displays atelectasis, consolidation & effusions.
  - ➤ Pulmonary angiography remains the benchmark for diagnosis but exposes fetus to higher radiation. Avoid femoral route if possible (6× the radiation exposure compared to brachial approach).
  - ➤ Helical contrast CT is becoming popular, but sensitivity is highly variable. Not recommended as sole screening tool, but useful in confirming higher suspicion.
  - ➤ V-Q scanning is most helpful if high clinical suspicion for PE, where a high-probability scan has a positive predictive value of 96%. Utility decreases w/ lower clinical suspicion.
  - ➤ Magnetic resonance angiography & venography show future promise but are not widely available.

Monitoring
- Noninvasive
  - ➤ ECG w/ evidence of RV strain, possibly left axis deviation. ST-T changes & tachycardia are common but nonspecific.
  - ➤ End-tidal CO2 decreases acutely due to V/Q mismatching.
- Invasive
  - ➤ PA line: Increased pulmonary vascular resistance, CVP & mean pulmonary arterial pressure. PA wedge pressure near normal or low.
  - ➤ Arterial line: useful for pressure monitoring & frequent blood sampling

MANAGEMENT/INTERVENTIONS
- General principles: Manage & treat hemodynamic instability first. Massive PE requires medical or surgical thromboembolectomy.
- Cardiovascular: see "*Amniotic Fluid Embolus*" section.
- Pulmonary: see "*Amniotic Fluid Embolus*" section.
- Hematologic

➤ Prevention of PE by treating diagnosed DVT: see "*Hematologic Changes*" chapter.

➤ Unfractionated IV heparin, loaded at 100–150 U/kg (5,000–10,000 U), then continuous infusion (15–25 U/kg/hr or 1,000–1,500 U/hr) to maintain aPTT at 2x normal.

➤ Consider thrombolytic (eg, t-PA, urokinase, streptokinase) therapy. Recombinant t-PA reported useful in pregnancy to avoid systemic fibrinolysis.

➤ Surgical embolectomy has high mortality & is reserved for catastrophic cases.

■ Neurologic: "*Amniotic Fluid Embolus*" section.

■ Fetal

➤ Maintain adequate perfusion & oxygenation.

➤ Consider delivery when fetus is mature, possible perimortem cesarean.

CAVEATS/PEARLS

■ Cardiopulmonary bypass uncommon but successful cases reported

■ Absence of hypoxia or large A-a gradient does not rule out PE.

■ Symptoms mimic other disorders.

■ Routine reversal of anticoagulation for regional anesthesia is not recommended.

CHECKLIST

■ High index of suspicion

■ Prevention by treating diagnosed DVT through & after delivery

■ Cardiovascular support

■ Pulmonary support

■ Anticoagulation, possible thromboembolysis

PULMONARY HYPERTENSION

WILTON C. LEVINE, MD
TONG-YAN CHEN, MD

FUNDAMENTAL KNOWLEDGE

■ Pulmonary hypertension is defined as mean PAP > 25 mm Hg.

■ Pulmonary hypertension may be primary or secondary due to cardiac or pulmonary disease.

- Increase in pulmonary vascular resistance can markedly increase pulmonary artery pressure. Pain, hypoxemia, acidosis & hypercarbia must all be avoided as they may lead to pulmonary edema.

STUDIES
- Determine etiology of pulmonary hypertension.
- Monitor SaO_2, EKG and arterial BP.
- Echocardiogram
- Invasive hemodynamic monitoring as clinically indicated.

MANAGEMENT/INTERVENTIONS
- Avoid physiologic changes that increase pulmonary vascular resistance:
  - Pain
  - Hypoxemia
  - Acidosis
  - Hypercarbia
- Maintain intravascular volume
  - Maintain venous return & avoid aortocaval compression.
  - Blood loss should be replaced w/ blood.
- Avoid myocardial depression & take great care w/ general anesthesia.
- Provide supplemental oxygen to the mother throughout labor & delivery.
- Epidural anesthesia has been used safely & w/ success.
  - Induce the epidural level slowly & w/ caution.
  - First treat hypotension w/ increased fluids.
  - Vasopressors such as ephedrine may increase pulmonary artery pressure.
  - Avoid epidural anesthesia if there is evidence of R heart failure.
- Use general anesthesia w/ caution, as myocardial depression & increase in PVR must be avoided.
- Consider epoprostenol & inhaled nitric oxide.
- Avoid PGF2a, as it is a pulmonary vasoconstrictor.
- See "*Pulmonary Edema.*"

CAVEATS AND PEARLS
- Pulmonary hypertension is defined as mean PAP > 25 mm Hg.
- Pulmonary edema results from cardiogenic & non-cardiogenic causes.
- Causes of pulmonary edema in pregnancy are multiple.
- Appropriate mgt of pulmonary edema requires determination of the etiology.

- Pts need appropriate physiologic monitoring & intensive care during labor, delivery & post-partum.
- If primary pulmonary hypertension, consider epoprostenol & inhaled nitric oxide.
- Avoid PGF2a, as it is a pulmonary vasoconstrictor.

CHECKLIST
- Does the pt have underlying pulmonary hypertension? What is the etiology?
- Does the pt have pulmonary edema? What is the etiology?
- Do you have adequate monitoring & access to care for the pt?
- Does the pt need to be transferred to an ICU?

PULMONARY PHYSIOLOGIC CHANGES OF PREGNANCY

WILTON C. LEVINE, MD
TONG-YAN CHEN, MD

FUNDAMENTAL KNOWLEDGE
- Pregnancy is associated w/ changes in maternal respiratory physiology that are of notable concern to the anesthesiologist.
- Changes at term
  - 15–20% decrease in functional residual capacity (FRC) due to changes in expiratory reserve volume & residual volume
  - Total lung capacity (TLC) decreases by about 5%.
  - Transverse & anterior-posterior diameters of the chest increase to compensate for diaphragm elevation.
  - Closing volume is unchanged, yet in the supine position nearly one third of parturients have airway closure w/ normal tidal ventilation. This increases the risk for developing atelectasis & an increased oxygen alveolar-arteriolar gradient.
  - Dead space is unchanged.
  - Vital capacity (VC) remains essentially unchanged throughout pregnancy.
  - Minute ventilation (MV) is increased 50%.
  - Alveolar ventilation is increased 70%.
  - Oxygen uptake is increased 20% due to the increased maternal metabolism, work of breathing & fetal metabolism.
    - The increase in minute ventilation is most directly related to an increase in tidal volume (40%), as respiratory rate increases only 15%.

- The result of the increased minute ventilation is a decrease in arterial carbon dioxide tension to about 32 mm Hg w/ preserved arterial pH as a result of decreased serum bicarbonate.
- ➤ The oxyhemoglobin curve is shifted to the right (increased p50) as a result of increased 2,3-DPG.
- ➤ This allows greater unloading of oxygen to the fetus.
- ➤ Total pulmonary resistance is decreased by 50%.
- ➤ Total lung compliance is decreased by 30% as a result of a 45% decrease in chest wall compliance & no significant change in isolated lung compliance.
- ■ Pain of labor can increase the minute ventilation as much as 300% over non-pregnant minute ventilation w/ significant increase in oxygen consumption.
- ■ Epidural anesthesia reduces this increase in minute ventilation & oxygen consumption.
- ■ Capillary engorgement of the entire respiratory tract is common during pregnancy. This leads to edema of the oro- & nasopharynx, larynx & trachea.
- ➤ Airway manipulation may lead to easy bleeding of the engorged mucosa.
- ➤ Airway mgt may be more difficult than predicted.

STUDIES
- ■ Flow volume loops in pregnant women compared with non-pregnant women are essentially unchanged.
- ■ FEV_1 is unchanged.
- ■ Vd/Vt is unchanged.

MANAGEMENT/INTERVENTIONS
- ■ Induction of anesthesia must be preceded by preoxygenation w/ 100% oxygen.
- ■ Intubation may be unpredictably difficult & airway manipulation may cause bleeding from friable & edematous mucosa.
- ➤ Extreme care must therefore be taken when suctioning the oropharynx, using oral or nasal airways & using laryngoscopes, endotracheal & nasotracheal tubes.
- ■ Induction of anesthesia w/ volatile anesthetics is more rapid in the pregnant pt.
- ➤ This is a result of decreased MAC during pregnancy, a decrease in FRC & an increase in MV.

> ➤ The increased MV/FRC ratio increases induction of anesthesia w/ volatile anesthetics.

CAVEATS AND PEARLS
- Pregnancy is associated w/ numerous changes in pulmonary physiology.
- Flow-volume loops in pregnant women are unchanged from non-pregnant women.
- The oxyhemoglobin curve is shifted to the right at term.
- Induction of general anesthesia must be preceded by preoxygenation.
- Airway mgt may be more difficult than anticipated.
- Capillary engorgement of the entire respiratory tract is common during pregnancy.
- Care must be taken before manipulating the airway to avoid bleeding from friable mucosa.

CHECKLIST
- Careful airway evaluation
- Check pt positioning
- Ensure proper equipment for airway & difficult airway mgt
- Ensure availability to provide a backup surgical airway
- Assess for comorbid pulmonary disease.

RELIEF OF LABOR PAIN WITH SYSTEMIC MEDICATION

MICHAEL KAUFMAN, MD
PHILIP E. HESS, MD

FUNDAMENTAL KNOWLEDGE
Most women, no matter their age, race or culture, describe childbirth as painful. Observations of both primitive human cultures as well as various animal species attest to labor being a natural yet tormenting process. The pain of parturition has an anatomic source, a neurologic transmission & a proportional physiologic response. Thus, previous claims that childbirth should be painless for all women & that the pain of labor is the result of culturally derived fear are not supported by the literature.

A recent opinion published by the American College of Obstetricians & Gynecologists (ACOG) states, "Labor results in severe pain for many women. There is no other circumstance in which it is considered acceptable for a person to experience untreated severe pain, amenable to safe intervention, while under a physician's care."

Severity of Labor Pain

Labor pain has been described as one of the worst forms of pain experienced by women. The ancient Romans referred to it as the *poena magna*, the "great pain" or "great punishment." In the extreme, the pain that some women feel can taint an otherwise miraculous experience of childbirth, leading to posttraumatic stress disorder. Fortunately, most women do not experience this degree of pain, but the experience of each woman's labor is unpredictable. Several observational studies have documented women's experiences during labor. For example:

- Melzack et al. observed that 60% of primiparas rated their pain as severe or extremely severe during parturition, while 30% described their pain as moderate. Among multiparas 75% had at least moderate pain, w/ the majority describing extremely severe pain.
- Ranta et al. found that 89% of primiparous & 84% of multiparous women rated their pain as severe or even intolerable.
- Nettlebladt et al. reported that 35% of parturients described their pain as intolerable, 37% as severe & 28% as moderate.

Anatomy of Labor Pain

The pain of parturition parallels the process of labor. The stimulus for pain occurs primarily in the first 2 stages of labor.

- The first stage of labor is characterized by cervical dilation & effacement & ends w/ full cervical dilation. It comprises a latent phase, in which the closed cervical os dilates slowly, & an active phase, in which the rate of cervical dilation is much more rapid. Within this first stage, the severity of pain correlates to the dilation of the cervical canal. The pain is mostly visceral, diffuse & poorly characterized, & generally felt in the abdomen btwn the pubis & umbilicus or in the back. Anatomic bases for the pain during the first stage of labor are such that this pain is amenable to blockade of peripheral afferents from the T10-L1 nerve roots.
- The second stage of labor lasts from the full dilation of cervix to the birth of the infant. Uterine contractions, along w/ maternal pushing, now force the fetus through the bony pelvic outlet. The pain of the second stage of labor is mostly due to the presenting part of the fetus distending the perineum, causing stretching & tearing of the skin, subcutaneous tissues & fascia. This leads to somatic pain in the vaginal & rectal areas, which can often be referred to the thighs.

This pain reflects the activation of the same afferents involved in the transmission of the visceral pain as well as additional afferents coursing from the S2–4 nerve roots.

Physiologic Response to Labor Pain
The intense stress of labor results in several physiologic changes.

■ Respiratory system
Pain is a stimulus for ventilation. Minute ventilation increases by 75–150% of normal during the first stage of labor. Further increases are noted during the second stage of labor, w/ a peak increase of up to 300% of normal ventilation during expulsion of the fetus. Hypocapnia causes uterine artery vasoconstriction, compromising fetal gas exchange & resulting in a progressive fetal acidosis throughout labor. The hyperventilatory response to pain results in compensatory periods of hypoventilation & causes transient hypoxemia of both mother & fetus.

Maternal oxygen demand increases through the course of labor. This is primarily a result of the high demands of the uterus, which increases oxygen consumption by 40% during the first stage of labor. Maternal pushing further increases oxygen consumption by 75% above normal.

■ Cardiovascular system
Pain increases sympathetic nervous system output & thus increases the plasma circulation of catecholamines, which are tocolytic. Increases in concentrations of epinephrine & norepinephrine both cause increases in cardiac output & peripheral vascular resistance; both are also responsible for decrease in the uteroplacental blood flow.

■ Hormonal changes
Pain during parturition results in the release of several hormones, including ACTH, beta-endorphins & cortisol. The plasma levels of these hormones increase as labor progresses & parallel the degree of pain reported by parturients. Plasma beta-endorphins at the levels found during labor are of only a mild analgesic quality & probably provide no more than minimal modulation of pain. The correlation between reported pain & beta-endorphin levels suggests that these hormones are a response to, not a modifier of, maternal pain & anxiety. Maternal anxiety, such as that found before elective cesarean delivery, can also be a cause of increased plasma beta-endorphins. Although the levels of beta-endorphins are increased in plasma, they remain similar to pre-labor values in the CSF.

Anesthesia & Analgesia for Labor Pain

Obstetric anesthesia practice has evolved greatly in the past 20 years. A survey of obstetric anesthetists published in 1997 shed light on the evolving practice. A few observations included:

■ More parturients are requesting & receiving some form of pain relief during labor. Compared w/ the previous decade, fewer pts received no analgesic medications.

■ Despite the greatly increased number of regional anesthetics in 1992, systemic medications remained the most frequently used form of pain relief for labor.

A recent survey of obstetric anesthetic practice in U.S. hospitals showed that the use of parenteral opioids for labor anesthesia was 39–56%, depending on the number of births per year.

➤ 39% if the hospital had >1,500 births

➤ 56% if the hospital had 500–1,500 births

➤ 50% if the hospital had <500 births

The use of systemic medications for relief of labor pain remains popular for many reasons:

■ Contraindications to the regional techniques (hemorrhage, coagulopathy, unsuitable back anatomy, infection)

■ Fear of neuraxial analgesia

■ Patient preference for systemic medication

■ Physician preference (both anesthesiologist & obstetrician)

■ Belief that regional techniques (epidural) slow the progression of labor

■ Lack of resources

➤ Some community medical centers & small regional hospitals lack 24-hour anesthesia availability & hence cannot offer around-the-clock regional anesthesia to all parturients.

➤ Lack of 24-hour in-house coverage by an obstetrician, which is required for pts desiring a regional analgesic

Parenteral Medications Used for Relief of Labor Pain

Opioids

■ Most widely used systemic medications for labor analgesia, allowing the parturient to better tolerate the pain of labor

■ Multiple choices available to practitioners & little scientific evidence to prejudice use of one over another. The efficacy & the incidence of side effects depend on the dose rather than the drug.

■ Multiple modes of administration are available to practitioners, including IV, IM, SC & PO.

- Easily cross the placenta & are associated w/ a risk of neonatal respiratory depression & neurobehavioral changes such as abnormal sleep patterns & poor adaptation to suckling
- May result in decreased beat-to-beat variability of the fetal heart tracing, which may interfere w/ interpretation
- Can be used in pt-controlled analgesia mode (PCA)
- Despite a multitude of choices, parenteral opioids appear useful for the treatment of mild to moderate pain that occurs during early labor; when given parenterally, they fail in the treatment of high-intensity pain of the later stages of labor.
- Commonly used opioids: meperidine (Demerol, Pethidine), morphine, fentanyl, remifentanil (Ultiva), nalbuphine (Nubain), butorphanol (Stadol). See the Management/Interventions section for details about each drug.

NSAIDs
- Rarely used for relief of labor pain due to their tocolytic effects & potential to cause closure of fetal ductus arteriosus
- Several randomized control trials looking at addition of NSAIDs to opioids did not show any benefit.

Adjunctive Medications
- Multiple classes of drugs used in adjunct w/ narcotics to provide comfort, relieve anxiety & reduce unpleasant effects of labor. Classes include anxiolytics, sedatives, antiemetics, etc.

Parenteral Adjuncts to Management of Labor Pain
- Phenothiazines
  - Often used in combination w/ opioids to reduce nausea & vomiting & produce sedation; possibly potentiate the analgesic effects of the opioids
  - Rapidly crosses the placenta & may result in decreased beat-to-beat variability; however, clinical doses do not seem to cause neonatal respiratory depression.
    - Promethazine (Phenergan)
      - IV dose of 25–50 mg rapidly produces effective sedation.
      - Moderate respiratory stimulant resulting in an increase in minute ventilation & ventilatory response to CO_2, thus counteracting the respiratory depressant qualities of narcotics
    - Propiomazine (Largon)

- Mild respiratory depressant, thus potentiating ventilatory depression by narcotics; however, it has no effect on neonatal respiratory drive
- Benzodiazepines
  - A class of anxiolytic medications that has never achieved widespread use during labor because of significant side effects
  - Occasionally used for the treatment of prolonged latent phase, to provide maternal rest prior to the onset of active labor
  - Readily cross the placenta & accumulate in the fetus w/ a long elimination half-life, causing neonatal neurobehavioral changes & decreased muscle tone
  - Not welcomed by mothers due to amnestic properties
- Barbiturates
  - Anxiolytics that can be effectively used in early labor
  - Can provide therapeutic rest for women having prodromal labor
  - Readily cross the placenta. However, when given in early labor, they result in minimal, if any, neonatal depression.
  - Pentobarbital (Nembutal) & secobarbital (Seconal) are both approved in the U.S.
- Other options
  - Hydroxyzine (Vistaril)
    - An antihistamine used to provide sedation & prevent maternal nausea & vomiting
    - Often administered w/ a narcotic
    - Standard dose is 25–50 mg IM (IV administration is irritating to veins)
    - Combination of meperidine & hydroxyzine results in better analgesia than meperidine alone
    - Does not cause neonatal respiratory depression
  - Scopolamine
    - Anticholinergic used in combination w/ narcotics to provide "twilight sleep"
    - Associated w/ a high incidence of maternal amnesia
    - Rapidly crosses the placenta & has been shown to increase the FHR & decrease beat-to-beat variability
    - Maternal sedation & decreased FHR variability are reversed by maternal administration of physostigmine.
  - Metoclopramide
    - Often used to treat maternal nausea & vomiting
    - Some studies note possible analgesic effects. Has been shown to decrease narcotic requirements in labor. When given in

combination w/ narcotics, results in better pain scores reported by parturients.

➤ Ketamine
- Administration of ketamine IV or IM in small doses provides dissociative state of analgesia, w/ or w/out amnesia; large doses are used to induce general anesthesia.
- IV ketamine has a rapid onset & short duration of action; therefore, it is not very useful for analgesia during the first stage of labor. However, ketamine may provide effective analgesia just before vaginal delivery.
- Best avoided in preeclamptic pts because of the activation of the sympathetic nervous system (SNS)
- Small doses do not result in neonatal depression. High doses have been associated w/ low Apgar scores & abnormal neonatal muscle tone.

■ Inhalation agents

Although many inhalation anesthetic agents have been tried for pain relief during childbirth, only nitrous oxide has been regularly used throughout the world.

➤ Nitrous oxide
- Entonox is a 50% oxygen/50% nitrous oxide mixture.
- Intermittent inhalation of nitrous oxide can provide analgesia for labor but does not eliminate the pain of contractions.
- Requires substantial maternal cooperation. The pt is encouraged to breathe the Entonox mixture from the very beginning of the contraction & to continue until the end.
- Does not interfere w/ uterine activity
- With intermittent inhalation, accumulation over time is negligible. The neonate eliminates most of the gas within minutes of birth. No notable effects on neonatal respiration or neurobehavior.

■ Volatile agents
➤ Uncommonly used in the U.S.
➤ All volatile agents cause a dose-dependent relaxation of the uterine smooth muscle & decrease the responsiveness of the uterus to oxytocin.
➤ Provide superior pain relief compared to oxygen/nitrous oxide mixture alone
➤ When compared to nitrous oxide, no significant difference in Apgar scores, umbilical cord blood gases & neurobehavioral scores

➤ Routine use is limited by need for special equipment, potential for maternal amnesia, potential for the loss of protective airway reflexes & aspiration of gastric contents by the mother.

STUDIES
- Usually no further studies are required beyond the typical history, physical exam & routine lab work performed for women admitted in labor.
- History should include questions about previous sensitivities or adverse reactions to medications.

MANAGEMENT/INTERVENTIONS

Opioids
- Meperidine (Demerol, Pethidine)
  ➤ Most widely used opioid worldwide due to its familiarity, availability & low cost
  ➤ Often used in combination w/ phenothiazines to diminish nausea & vomiting
  ➤ Usual dose is 25–50 mg IV or 50–100 mg IM q2–4h, w/ the onset of analgesia within 5 minutes of IV administration & 45 minutes after IM injection. The half-life is 2.5–3 hours in the mother & 18–23 hours in the neonate. A major metabolite is normeperidine, which acts as a potent respiratory depressant in both mother & neonate.
  ➤ Easily crosses the placenta by passive diffusion & equilibrates btwn the maternal & fetal compartment. Maximal fetal uptake of meperidine occurs within 2–3 hours of maternal administration; therefore, the best time for delivery of the fetus is within 1 hour of last administered dose or >4 hours after the single IV dose.
  ➤ Administration of both a single dose as well as multiple doses was shown to have subtle effects on the neonate. Single dose was thought to account for altered infant breast-feeding behavior; multiple doses, as would be administered during a prolonged labor, were thought to contribute to various neurobehavioral changes (decreased duration of wakefulness, decreased attentiveness & decreased duration of non-REM sleep).
- Morphine
  ➤ Oldest anesthetic used for treatment of labor pain
  ➤ Usual dose for maternal analgesia is 2–5 mg IV or 5–10 mg IM. The onset of analgesia is 3–5 minutes after IV administration & within 20–40 minutes after the IM dose.

➤ Rapidly crosses the placenta & equilibrates btwn the maternal & fetal plasma

➤ As w/ other opioids, morphine causes a decrease in the FHR & beat-to-beat variability.

➤ Neonatal side effects are related to the neonatal plasma concentration of morphine & mostly manifest as respiratory depression.

➤ Olofsson et al assessed the efficacy of morphine in relief of labor pain: although fewer women reported back pain, the decrease in overall pain intensity was clinically insignificant. The investigators concluded that systematically administered morphine does not relieve the visceral pain of labor.

■ Fentanyl

➤ Highly lipid-soluble synthetic anesthetic that is 800x more potent than meperidine. It has a rapid onset of action, short half-life & no active metabolites.

➤ Doses vary from 25–100 mcg & are administered every hour based on maternal request. Peak effect is seen about 3–5 minutes after IV administration

➤ Randomized control trials comparing fentanyl & meperidine did not show improved pain scores in pts receiving fentanyl, but maternal nausea, vomiting, & prolonged sedation were less common in pts receiving fentanyl.

➤ In studies assessing the effects of fentanyl on neonates, the Apgar scores, umbilical blood gases & neurobehavioral scores of neonates exposed to fentanyl were not different from controls.

■ Remifentanil (Ultiva)

➤ Ultrashort-acting synthetic opioid receptor agonist w/ rapid onset

➤ Rapidly metabolized by plasma & tissue esterases & thus is cleared independently of liver or kidneys; the context-sensitive half-life is 3.5 minutes independent of the mode of administration. Rapid transplacental transfer, but similar metabolism by the fetus ensures rapid drug clearance.

➤ Theoretically ideal for PCA administration for labor pts. Multiple studies have evaluated its use for labor PCA at various doses. No consensus exists on whether it should be used as a standard drug for PCA in labor. There is concern regarding the need for an initial large bolus, which results in significant maternal respiratory depression. Studies have shown large individual variation in the dose required, as well as an incremental increase that is required as labor progresses. The best dosing regimen remains undiscovered.

■ Nalbuphine (Nubain)
➤ Mixed agonist-antagonist opioid analgesic w/ similar effects of respiratory depression as morphine at equianalgesic doses. However, nalbuphine has a ceiling effect w/ increasing doses & results in no further respiratory depression w/ doses >30 mg.
➤ Usual dose is 10–20 mg q4–6h given IV, SC or IM. The onset of analgesia is within 2–3 minutes of IV dose & within 15 minutes of SC/IM dose. Duration of effect is 3–6 hours.
➤ RCTs comparing nalbuphine w/ meperidine found no difference in efficacy of analgesia, but nalbuphine accounted for less nausea & vomiting.
➤ High degree of transplacental transfer, resulting in increased incidence of decreased FHR variability compared to meperidine

■ Butorphanol (Stadol)
➤ An opioid w/ agonist-antagonist properties (40x more potent than meperidine). Similar to nalbuphine, it has a ceiling effect on respiratory depression.
➤ Typical dose is 1–2 mg IV or IM & can be given as frequently as 1–2 hrs.
➤ RCTs showed that butorphanol offers analgesia that is similar to meperidine/phenothiazine combination.

CAVEATS/PEARLS
■ Analgesic approach depends on what is available & what nursing, obstetric & anesthetic resources are readily available at the hospital.
■ Be wary of potential effects that parenteral medications have on FHR patterns; interpretation of FHR patterns may become more complicated.
■ When medications can affect the clinical status of the parturient or the newborn, this information needs to be relayed to the obstetrician & pediatrician.
■ Pts on methadone may experience "withdrawal" symptoms when given opiate partial agonist-antagonists.
■ Appropriate "reversal agents" or antidotes for mother & newborn should be considered.

CHECKLIST
■ Does pt have a history of allergies & sensitivities?

■ Is the choice of analgesic regimen consistent w/ level of nursing, obstetric & anesthesia care available?
■ Have potential complications of medicines been relayed to other disciplines caring for parturient & newborn?
■ Are protocols & medications available for treatment of adverse reactions?

RENAL REPLACEMENT THERAPY

KRISTOPHER DAVIGNON, MD
HARISH LECAMWASAM, MD

FUNDAMENTAL KNOWLEDGE
■ Definition of renal failure
  ➤ Characterized by an acute decrease in glomerular filtration rate (GFR) in the setting of either previously normal renal function or stable chronic renal insufficiency
  ➤ A consensus on the definition of ARF using an elevation in creatinine (Cr) does not exist. Most studies have used an absolute increase of 0.5–1.0 mg/dL or a relative increase of 25–100% in the Cr over 24 hrs as criteria for ARF.
■ Manifestations
  ➤ Accumulation of nitrogenous waste, primarily Cr & urea nitrogen (BUN)
  ➤ Remember that the relationship between Cr & GFR & the BUN/Cr ratio & the GFR can be affected by a variety of factors, including muscle mass, presence of chromophores, GI bleeding, liver disease, nutrition & steroid use.
  ➤ Can be associated w/ oliguria (urine output <400–500 mL/24 hr) or non-oliguria
■ Classification
  ➤ Divided into prerenal, intrinsic renal & postrenal etiologies
    • Prerenal ARF
      • Caused by decreased renal perfusion in the setting of decreased effective circulating volume, or altered intrarenal hemodynamics
      • Characterized by a fractional excretion of sodium (FENa) <1%, urinary sodium <20 mEq/L & urinary osmolarity >500 mOsm/L

- If the duration of hypoperfusion is brief, prerenal azotemia is typically reversible. However, w/ a sustained insult, prerenal azotemia can progress to acute tubular necrosis.
- Postrenal ARF
  - Caused by obstruction of urinary flow, either bilateral ureteral or infra-vesicular obstruction w/ normal kidneys; or unilateral obstruction anywhere along the path of urine flow w/ a solitary kidney
  - Diagnosis can be made by ultrasonography or CT (more sensitive) by evaluating for hydronephrosis.
  - Treatment involves relief of obstruction.
  - Recovery of renal function is dependent on the duration of obstruction.
- Intrinsic renal ARF
  - Divided into tubular disease (ATN), interstitial disease, glomerular injury & vascular injury; ATN is the most common form

STUDIES
- Urinary indices
  - A determination of the fractional excretion of sodium (FENa), urine sodium concentration & urine osmolarity is useful in distinguishing prerenal etiologies from others, as discussed above.
  - A urine dip-stick assessment is useful in the diagnosis of myoglobinuric or hemoglobinuric renal failure (heme positive dipstick w/ no blood cells seen in the sediment).
  - Evaluation of the urine sediment: epithelial cells w/ ATN, crystals w/ crystal nephropathy, fragmented RBCs w/ glomerulonephritis, WBC casts w/ allergic interstitial nephritis
  - Renal ultrasound or abdominal CT can be used to look for evidence of obstructive uropathy.

MANAGEMENT & INTERVENTIONS
- Pharmacologic
  - Prevention
    - Volume repletion: Hypovolemia is a major risk factor for ARF under almost every circumstance.
      - While there is some evidence suggesting a benefit of normal saline (0.9) over hypotonic (0.45) saline & sodium bicarbonate over normal saline in specific instances such as in the prevention of radiocontrast nephropathy, there is no

evidence overwhelmingly supporting one fluid choice over another.

- Discontinuation of nephrotoxic agents (eg, aminoglycoside antibiotics, NSAIDs)
- Use of non-ionic, low-osmolality radiocontrast agents.
- Other than the use of peri-procedure acetylcysteine in pts at high risk for contrast nephropathy, current evidence does not support the routine use of pharmacologic agents in the prevention of ARF (including dopamine, fenoldopam, mannitol & atrial natriuretic peptide).

➤ Treatment
  - There is no evidence supporting the use of any agent in the treatment of ARF.
    - Dopamine
      - Dopamine, when infused at low rates (0.5–2 ug/kg/min), increases renal plasma flow, GFR & renal sodium excretion.
      - While some anecdotal evidence supports the use of dopamine w/ ARF, all randomized prospective trials to date have shown no benefit in terms of disease progression, need for renal replacement or mortality.
    - Fenoldopam
      - Fenoldopam, a selective agonist of the dopamine type I receptor, is currently FDA approved in the U.S. only for the treatment of hypertensive emergencies.
      - When infused at low doses (0.03–0.1 ug/kg/min), fenoldopam has been shown to increase renal plasma flow & reduce the aberrant renal hemodynamics seen w/ aortic cross-clamping without significantly affecting systemic hemodynamics.
      - However, definitive evidence supporting the use of this agent in the treatment of ARF is not available.
    - Diuretics
      - Non-oliguric renal failure is associated w/ a better prognosis than oliguric renal failure.
      - However, there is no evidence showing that conversion of oliguric renal failure to a non-oliguric form by the use of diuretics has any beneficial impact in terms of mortality, disease progression or need for renal replacement therapy.
      - Conversely, a recent retrospective analysis suggested that high-dose loop diuretics may in fact worsen outcome w/

ARF. This same study showed that impaired responsiveness to loop diuretics is a poor prognostic indicator w/ ARF.

■ Renal replacement therapy

➤ Renal replacement therapy is often indicated in the mgt of the critically ill pt w/ ARF.

➤ Controversy exists regarding the timing of dialysis, but the trend has been toward earlier initiation.

➤ Several modes of renal replacement therapy are available.

- Acute peritoneal dialysis (PD)
  - PD has been largely replaced by continuous venovenous therapy.
  - PD catheter insertion can be associated w/ leakage of PD fluid, infection, catheter malfunction & rarely perforation of a viscus.
- Hemodialysis (HD)
  - Suitable for pts who are hemodynamically stable
  - Some studies have suggested that daily hemodialysis is associated w/ better prognosis.
  - HD requires the establishment of vascular access in the femoral, internal jugular or subclavian vein.
  - Complications include hypotension, arrhythmias, bleeding & infection.
- Continuous renal replacement therapy
  - The preferred modality in an unstable pt
  - Access is the same as for HD.
  - Anticoagulation can be w/ heparin, citrate (serving as a regional anticoagulant & base replacement) & prostacyclin.
  - The most commonly used therapy is venovenous hemofiltration (CVVH).
  - Ultrafiltration rates are generally 1.6–3.2 L/hr w/ replacement fluid calculated to achieve the desired body balance & containing bicarbonate, citrate or lactate.
  - Pts w/ hepatic dysfunction are at risk for citrate toxicity when a citrate buffer is used. The features of citrate toxicity include normal to high serum calcium, a low ionized calcium & a metabolic acidosis w/ an elevated anion gap.
  - Other complications include infection, bleeding, metabolic alkalosis & hypophosphatemia, especially w/ prolonged therapy.

CHECKLIST

■ Optimize intravascular volume status & discontinue all nephrotoxic agents as possible.

■ Assess need for dialysis & consider whether hemodialysis or CVVH is required.

■ Obtain a nephrology consult.

■ Monitor need for ongoing intervention, adequacy of dialysis & its complications.

RESTRICTIVE LUNG DISEASE

WILTON C. LEVINE, MD
TONG-YAN CHEN, MD

FUNDAMENTAL KNOWLEDGE

■ Restrictive lung disease encompasses a wide spectrum of pulmonary diseases characterized by an increased ratio of FEV_1/FVC & can involve lung parenchyma, pleura, chest wall & neuromuscular apparatus.

➤ These alterations are a result of limited lung expansion due to
  - Lung parenchyma disease
  - Abnormal pleura
  - Abnormal chest wall
  - Abnormal neuromuscular apparatus

■ General examples

➤ Interstitial lung disease (idiopathic pulmonary fibrosis [IPF], sarcoidosis, hypersensitivity pneumonitis, pneumoconiosis, connective tissue disease)

➤ Pleural disease (pleural effusion, empyema, pneumothorax, hemothorax, fibrothorax)

➤ Chest wall disease (kyphoscoliosis, neuromuscular disease, thoracoplasty)

➤ Extrathoracic conditions (obesity, peritonitis, ascites, pregnancy)

■ Specific examples

➤ Sarcoidosis
  - Clinical course of sarcoid is not altered by pregnancy.
  - Pregnancy has no adverse effect on sarcoid.

➤ Hypersensitivity pneumonitis

- There are no data related to the effects of hypersensitivity pneumonitis & pregnancy outcome.
- Idiopathic pulmonary fibrosis
  - Case reports of young pts w/ IPF note progression of disease during pregnancy.
  - Pts w/ IPF should be able to increase oxygen consumption at least 300% from resting values in order to tolerate pregnancy safely.
- Kyphoscoliosis
  - Associated w/ increased premature birth rate
  - Data are conflicting regarding the stability of scoliosis & progression during pregnancy.
  - Associated w/ increased shortness of breath during pregnancy
  - May cause difficulty w/ pt positioning during labor or C-section
- Restrictive lung diseases have a decreased DLCO/VA.
- Pts tend to have normal or hypoxic resting ABGs that become hypoxic w/ exercise.
- Pts w/ restrictive lung disease & VC < 1 L should avoid pregnancy.
- Specific mgt depends on the underlying disease.
- Restrictive lung disease is characterized by a reduction in lung volume & increase in ratio of FEV_1/FVC.
- Airway flow rates are generally maintained.

STUDIES
- Restrictive lung disease is associated w/
  - Decreased DLCO/VA due to effacement of the alveolar capillary units
  - Normal or hypoxic resting ABGs (secondary to V/Q mismatch)
  - Abnormal ABGs w/ exercise

MANAGEMENT/INTERVENTIONS
- Most restrictive lung disorders are only a relative contraindication to pregnancy.
- Pts w/ severe restrictive lung disease (VC < 1 L) should avoid pregnancy.

CAVEATS AND PEARLS
- Restrictive lung disease encompasses a wide spectrum of pulmonary diseases characterized by an increased ratio of FEV_1/FVC & can

involve lung parenchyma, pleura, chest wall & neuromuscular apparatus.
- Restrictive lung diseases have a decreased DLCO/VA.
- Pts tend to have normal or hypoxic resting ABGs that become hypoxic w/ exercise.
- Pts w/ restrictive lung disease & VC < 1 L should avoid pregnancy.
- Specific mgt depends on the underlying disease.
- Restrictive lung disease is characterized by a reduction in lung volume & increase in ratio of FEV_1/FVC.

CHECKLIST
- Assess underlying disease.
- Understand specific physiologic changes related to underlying disease.
- Assess pt's functional status.

RESUSCITATION OF THE NEONATE

RICHARD ARCHULETA, MD
SANDRA WEINREB, MD

FUNDAMENTAL KNOWLEDGE
Neonatal resuscitation is a dynamic process that requires repeated rapid assessment.
- Interventions should be performed in 30-second cycles w/ simultaneous rapid assessment.

Most neonates requiring intervention beyond routine care respond to positive-pressure ventilation alone.

Sequential steps in resuscitation
- Positive-pressure ventilation w/ 100% oxygen
- Chest compressions w/ endotracheal intubation & ventilation
- Epinephrine administration
- Treatment of hypovolemia
- Treatment of hypoglycemia
- Treatment of severe metabolic acidosis

Routes of medication administration
- Tracheal route
  - ➤ Usually the most rapidly available route for initial administration of epinephrine
- IV route

➤ Usually through umbilical vein catheterization (see "**Neonatal IV Access**")
➤ Direct venous access
■ Intraosseous route
  ➤ Less commonly used because:
    • Small size & fragility of neonatal bones
    • More easily obtained access via umbilical or peripheral veins

STUDIES

Rapid assessment
■ Should begin immediately after birth & continue throughout resuscitative process
  ➤ Start initially w/ rapid initial assessment if not previously accessed (see "**Neonatal Status at Birth**").
    • Clear of meconium?
    • Spontaneously breathing?
    • Good muscle tone?
    • Color pink?
    • Term gestation?
  ➤ After initial assessment, evaluate neonate's respiration, heart rate & color every 30 seconds until resuscitation is complete.
    • These determinants are most predictive of neonate's status after the initial assessment.
■ Respiration is sufficient if:
  ➤ It is regular
  ➤ Neonate retains good color (no central cyanosis)
  ➤ Neonate maintains heart rate >100 bpm.
■ Heart rate
  ➤ Should be consistently >100 bpm
  ➤ Determined by:
  ➤ Palpation of the base of the umbilical cord, or
  ➤ Auscultation of cardiac precordium w/ stethoscope
■ Perform assessment & intervention simultaneously in 30-second cycles.
  ➤ Based on heart rate, respirations & color as explained above
■ Color
  ➤ Most neonates have some degree of cyanosis at birth because the fetal PO2 is low.
    • Acrocyanosis (cyanosis of hands & feet) is common & is not a reliable indication of hypoxemia.
  ➤ Effective respirations should quickly improve color.

MANAGEMENT/INTERVENTIONS

After providing routine care, assess neonate for respirations, heart rate & color.

1. If neonate is spontaneously breathing, heart rate >100 bpm & pink (acrocyanosis is ok), continue supportive care. If any of the following exist, then proceed to step 2 below:
   - ➤ Respirations are weak (apnea or gasping respirations)
   - ➤ Heart rate <100 bpm
   - ➤ Color poor (central cyanosis after administration of 100% oxygen)

2. Provide PPV (see "*Neonatal Airway Management*").
   - ➤ Briefly, first assisted breath should provide 30–40 cm H2O w/ recruitment maneuver (held for several seconds). Subsequent breaths should be delivered at pressures up to 20–30 cm H2O at a rate of 40–60 breaths per minute assuming no chest compressions; 30 breaths per minute w/ chest compressions. Continue for 30 seconds while assessing neonate's respirations, heart rate & color. After 30 seconds:
     - If neonate is spontaneously breathing, heart rate >100 bpm & pink (except acrocyanosis), provide supportive care.
     - If neonate exhibits apnea, gasping respirations or heart rate <100, repeat step 2 above.
     - If neonate has heart rate <60, proceed to step 3 below.

3. Continue PPV & administer chest compressions (see "*Chest Compressions*").
   - ➤ Apply 3 chest compressions for every positive-pressure breath delivered. Neonate should be intubated for PPV during chest compressions. Ideally, 90 chest compressions & 30 breaths should be delivered per minute in a 3:1 ratio. Continue for 30 seconds while assessing neonate's respirations, heart rate & color. After 30 seconds:
     - If neonate is spontaneously breathing, heart rate >100 bpm & pink (except acrocyanosis), provide supportive care.
     - If neonate exhibits apnea, gasping respirations, heart rate <100 but >60 bpm, then repeat step 2.
     - If neonate continues to have heart rate < 60, then proceed to step 4 below.

4. Continue PPV & chest compressions & administer epinephrine. Epinephrine route is usually tracheal for the first dose, IV via umbilical (see "*Neonatal IV Access*") or peripheral veins for subsequent doses, rarely via interosseous access. Dose is 0.01–0.03 mg/kg via tracheal or IV route. Equivalent to 0.1–0.3 mL/kg of 1:10,000

epinephrine solution. If delivered tracheally, first dilute w/ normal saline to 1–2 cc. If first dose is administered via trachea & neonate fails to respond, then establish vascular access to administer further doses. May be repeated every 3 to 5 minutes if needed. Continue PPV & chest compressions for 30 seconds while assessing neonate's respirations, heart rate & color. After 30 seconds:

> If neonate is spontaneously breathing, heart rate >100 bpm & pink (except acrocyanosis), provide supportive care.

> If neonate exhibits apnea, gasping respirations, heart rate <100 but >60, then repeat step 2.

> If neonate continues to have heart rate <60 & <3–5 minutes has passed since last epinephrine dose, then repeat step 3 above while obtaining vascular access.

> If neonate continues to have heart rate <60 & 3–5 minutes has passed since last epinephrine dose, then repeat step 4 after establishing vascular access.

5. If neonate displays poor response to resuscitation, consider:

> Treatment of hypovolemia
  • If acute bleeding occurred before delivery of the fetus & the neonate exhibits pallor despite good oxygenation, faint pulses w/ heart rate >100 or poor response to resuscitation, then provide volume expanders (see "*Volume Expansion for the Neonate*").

> Treatment of hypoglycemia
  • Test bedside blood glucose.
  • Neonatal hypoglycemia exists if blood glucose is <35 mg/dL.
  • Administer dextrose 200 mg/kg (or 2 mL/kg of 10% dextrose solution) *slow IV push* for hypoglycemia

> Treatment of severe metabolic acidosis
  • Do not administer NaHCO3 for brief neonatal resuscitations. Consider NaHCO3 only for prolonged resuscitation where the neonate has failed to respond to other measures. NaHCO3 is hyperosmolar & can cause hepatic injury & cerebral hemorrhage.
  • If appropriate, administer 1–2 mEq/kg of NaHCO3 by *slow IV push* while ensuring good ventilation.
    • Usually available as a 0.5-mEq/cc (4.2%) solution; therefore, administer 2–4 cc/kg *over 1–2 minutes*. Do not administer faster than 1 mEq/kg/min.

> Treatment of opioid-related apnea w/ naloxone
  • Dose: 0.1 mg/kg IV

- Suspect when mother has received opioids within 4 hours prior to delivery & neonate continues to be apneic despite adequate oxygenation & heart rate.
- Avoid if there is chronic maternal opioid abuse to avoid acute withdrawal in neonate.
- Administer cautiously because naloxone can worsen hypoxia-related neurologic damage.
- After administration, neonate should be observed for apnea for 24 hours.

CAVEATS & PEARLS

The neonatal dose for epinephrine administered though the tracheal route is the same as for IV or IO route.

- This is different than the algorithm described in PALS (for children beyond the neonatal stage), where the IV & IO doses are the same as neonatal resuscitation but the tracheal dose is different.

Medication administration is not benign.

- Epinephrine poses the potential for intracranial hemorrhage due to hypertension. The risk is highest in preterm neonates.
- Bicarbonate
  - ➢ Can cause hepatic injury & cerebral hemorrhage due to hyper-osmolar effects
  - ➢ Must not be administered via ETT because bicarbonate is caustic to the lungs
- Naloxone can cause acute withdrawal in neonates where there has been chronic maternal opioid abuse. Naloxone can also worsen hypoxia-related neurologic damage.

Neonatal umbilical vein blood gases may be more indicative of utero-placental gas exchange & the mother's acid-base status than of the neonate's acid-base status.

- Neonatal arterial blood is indicative of the neonate's true acid-base status.
- The normal neonatal arterial pH is controversial & dependent on several factors, including route of birth, duration of labor & gestational age (beyond the scope of this resource). However, it is safe to assume a neonatal arterial pH <7.00 is abnormal.

CHECKLIST

Repeated rapid assessment

- Initially w/ questions to assess at birth
  1) Clear of meconium?
  2) Spontaneously breathing?

3) Good muscle tone?
4) Color pink?
5) Term gestation?
■ Subsequently w/ each intervention
6) Neonatal respiration?
7) Heart rate?
8) Color?

Perform sequential steps in resuscitation in 30-second cycles:
■ PPV w/ 100% oxygen
■ Chest compressions & endotracheal intubation for PPV
■ Epinephrine administration q3–5min (0.01–0.03 mg/kg)
  ➣ Tracheal route initially; IV route (umbilical or direct venous access) for subsequent doses
■ Treatment of hypovolemia
■ Treatment of hypoglycemia
■ Treatment of severe metabolic acidosis

Continue resuscitation until neonate has stabilized w/
■ Adequate oxygenation (no central cyanosis, acceptable PaO2)
■ Heart rate > 100

Transfer care to a unit capable of providing post-resuscitation support (see "*Post-resuscitation Care*").

RETAINED PLACENTA

HOVIG CHITILIAN, MD
BHARGAVI KRISHNAN, MD

FUNDAMENTAL KNOWLEDGE
■ Occurs in up to 1% of all vaginal deliveries
■ Requires manual exploration and extraction by obstetrician

STUDIES
N/A

MANAGEMENT/INTERVENTIONS
■ Analgesia for manual extraction can be provided w/ augmentation of the epidural if one is in place. Otherwise, give small doses of ketamine (10 mg IV) or fentanyl (50 mcg IV). Analgesia can also be provided with a spinal.
■ If necessary, uterine relaxation can be provided w/ nitroglycerin (50- to 100-mcg IV boluses) or the induction of general anesthesia.
■ D& C may be necessary in OR setting (see "*Dilation & Curettage/Evacuation*" chapter).

CAVEATS/PEARLS

- Consider using epidural, spinal or small doses of IV medication for analgesia.
- Consider using IV nitroglycerin (50- to 100-mcg bolus) or induction of general anesthesia if additional uterine relaxation is needed.

CHECKLIST

- Large-bore IV access
- Provide analgesia w/ augmentation of preexisting epidural, or, in the absence of an epidural, IV analgesics or a spinal.

RHEUMATOID ARTHRITIS: AUTOIMMUNE DISEASE

AUGUST CHANG, MD
MIRIAM HARNETT, MD

FUNDAMENTAL KNOWLEDGE

Definition

- Chronic, systemic inflammatory disease characterized by synovial proliferation that leads to symmetric polyarthritis

Epidemiology

- Prevalence 1–2% general population
- 1 in 1,000–2,000 in pregnant population
- Male:female 1:3

Pathophysiology

- Etiology & mechanism unclear
- Autoantibody rheumatoid factor detectable in 80–90% of pts

Clinical manifestations

- Most commonly affected joints: proximal interphalangeal, metacarpophalangeal, wrists
- Pt may also have cervical spine involvement, usually manifested by limited range of motion
- Extra-articular involvement
  - ➤ Airway
    - Mandibular hypoplasia
    - Cricoarytenoid arthritis
    - TMJ dysfunction
    - Laryngeal deviation & rotation
  - ➤ Cardiovascular

- Arteritis/vasculitis
- Pericarditis
- Pericardial effusion
- Endocardial vegetations
- Conduction disturbances
- ➤ Pulmonary
  - Pleural effusion
  - Interstitial fibrosis
  - Granulomas (cavitation may lead to pneumothorax or bronchopleural fistula)
- ➤ Chest wall
  - Costochondritis
- ➤ Neurologic
  - Peripheral neuropathies
  - Cervical nerve root neuropathies
- ➤ Hematologic
  - Anemia
  - Felty syndrome
- ➤ Ophthalmic
  - Keratoconjunctivitis

Effect of pregnancy on RA
- Studies indicate 75–90% of women report improvement of symptoms during pregnancy
- Relapse often 2–3 weeks postpartum

Effect on pregnancy & fetus
- Typically does not complicate pregnancy
- No increase in premature labor
- Some evidence of association btwn rheumatoid vasculitis (extremely rare) & IUGR

STUDIES

History & Physical
- Airway: examine for indicators of potentially difficult intubation
  - ➤ TMJ may be ankylosed w/ limited mouth opening
  - ➤ Cervical spine
    - Flexion deformity & atlantoaxial instability
    - Possible spinal cord injury w/ neck extension
  - ➤ Cricoarytenoid joint
  - ➤ Mandibular hypoplasia
  - ➤ Laryngeal deviation

- Pulmonary: evaluate for evidence of pleural effusions & restrictive lung disease secondary to kyphosis
- Cardiac: evaluate for evidence of pericarditis, pericardial effusion, valvular or conduction defects, cardiomyopathy
- Musculoskeletal: involvement of hip, knee & lumbar intervertebral joints may make optimal positioning for regional techniques challenging
- Neurologic: examine for evidence of peripheral neuropathies
- Skin: examine mouth & skin for skin eruptions & oral ulcers if pt is on gold therapy

Imaging
- Chest radiograph
- Lateral cervical spine radiographs in full flexion & extension; consider, depending on severity & duration of disease or neck symptoms

Other
- Pulmonary function testing: consider if markedly reduced FRC suspected
- Thromboelastography (TEG): consider if pt is on aspirin to evaluate platelet function
- CBC & BUN/creatinine: obtain if pt is on gold therapy to rule out aplastic anemia & evaluate renal function

MANAGEMENT/INTERVENTIONS

Medical treatment: 3 main categories of medications
- Aspirin/NSAIDs
  - First-line therapy
  - No evidence of teratogenicity
  - No need for prophylactic cessation, but pregnancy should be closely monitored
  - Recommend discontinuation during 3rd trimester because of:
    - Inhibitory effect on platelets & hemostasis
    - Increased risk of fetal CNS hemorrhage
    - Possible premature closure of ductus arteriosus
    - Possible compromised fetal renal perfusion & abnormal amniotic fluid dynamics
    - Possible factor in necrotizing enterocolitis (NEC)
- Corticosteroids
  - Second-line therapy
  - No evidence of teratogenicity

➤ Inactivation by placental 11-beta-OH-dehydrogenase results in low fetal levels of active drug
➤ May precipitate gestational diabetes mellitus & hypertension
➤ Longer-term adverse effects
- Osteoporosis
- GI ulceration
- Impaired immunity
- Adrenal suppression

■ Disease-modifying antirheumatic drugs (DMARD): insufficient data regarding need for prophylactic withdrawal during pregnancy
■ Gold salts
➤ • Transplacental transfer limited due to high protein-binding
- Recommend discontinuation as soon as pregnancy is recognized
➤ Antimalarials
- Generally considered safe
- Case reports of possible ocular & ototoxicity
➤ D-Penicillamine
- Case reports of fetal connective tissue disorders
- Fetal risks are probably not high enough to warrant discontinuing during pregnancy
➤ Sulfasalazine & azathioprine
- Considered safe during pregnancy & breast-feeding
➤ Cytostatic drugs
- Methotrexate, cyclophosphamide & chlorambucil are teratogenic & should be discontinued at least 3 months prior to conception

Anesthesia
■ General anesthesia
➤ Increased likelihood of difficult airway
➤ Avoid excessive manipulation of neck
■ Regional anesthesia
➤ Strongly preferred because it avoids the potential hazards of intubation
➤ Epidural: may be difficult to position pt optimally if hip & knee joints are affected
➤ Spinal: in severe disease, perhaps best avoided due to unpredictable spread of anesthetic
■ Stress-dose steroids during labor & delivery for pts currently on steroid therapy

■ Invasive monitoring may be required in pts w/ extensive cardiopulmonary involvement

CAVEATS & PEARLS
■ Anticipate potentially difficult airway due to possible TMJ, cricoarytenoid & cervical spine involvement
■ Optimal positioning for regional techniques may be difficult if hip & knee joints are affected
■ Take care to avoid a high regional block, particularly in pts w/ restrictive lung disease
■ Possible unpredictable spread of regional anesthetics in pts w/ severe disease

CHECKLIST
■ Thorough airway exam
■ Immediate availability of special airway equipment: laryngeal mask airway, fiberoptic laryngoscope, transtracheal jet ventilation, emergency cricothyrotomy kit
■ Document preexisting peripheral neuropathies prior to general or regional anesthesia
■ Stress-dose steroids during labor & delivery for pts currently on steroid therapy

---

RHEUMATOID ARTHRITIS: BACK PROBLEMS

STEPHEN PANARO, MD
EDWARD MICHNA, MD

FUNDAMENTAL KNOWLEDGE
See also "*Autoimmune Disease.*"
■ Inflammatory in etiology & characterized by symmetric inflammation of the peripheral joints, often progressing to distortion & destruction of the articular & periarticular surfaces
■ Prevalent in 0.35% to 1% of the population
■ Women are affected 2 to 3x more often than men.
■ May be accompanied by systemic manifestations
■ Systemic involvement can include, but is not limited to, pericarditis, pericardial effusions, myocardial nodules, conduction disturbances, pneumonitis, pleural effusions, pulmonary nodules & airway abnormalities such as cricoarytenoid arthritis, laryngeal deviation, small mandible & temporomandibular joint (TMJ) dysfunction.

- Pregnancy rarely complicates RA.
  - 75% of women experience an amelioration of their symptoms during pregnancy & a relapse post-partum.
- The lumbosacral spine is involved in 5% of cases.
- 20–40% of pts demonstrate involvement of the cervical spine w/ anterior atlantoaxial subluxation.
- Surgery is traditionally reserved for those who are symptomatic.
  - Symptoms are usually secondary to a weakness or disruption of the transverse ligament.
- The necessity of screening asymptomatic pts has been debated, although one report noted a 5.5% incidence of unsuspected C1-C2 subluxation.

STUDIES
- Radiographically, atlantoaxial subluxation is best seen on a lateral cervical spine film w/ the neck in flexion.
- Laboratory data as directed by medication profile
- Echocardiography/ECG if suspicion of cardiac involvement

MANAGEMENT/INTERVENTIONS
- See "*Autoimmune Disease.*"
- General anesthesia
  - TMJ compromise can create extremely difficult intubating conditions.
  - Avoid direct laryngoscopy in pts w/ known vertical & posterior atlantoaxial subluxations.
  - Pts w/ anterior & rotary subluxations can tolerate careful laryngoscopy w/ little risk of neurologic compromise.
  - Regional anesthetic may be preferable in pts w/ cervical involvement.
- Regional anesthesia
  - The lumbosacral spine is involved in 5% of cases.
  - Positioning the pt for placement of a regional anesthetic may be challenging if knee & hip joints are affected.

CAVEATS/PEARLS
- Carefully evaluate all pts w/ RA, not only for spinal involvement but also for other systemic manifestations.
- RA is not a contraindication to the placement of a regional anesthetic.
- TMJ compromise can create extremely difficult intubating conditions.

- Avoid direct laryngoscopy in pts w/ known vertical & posterior atlantoaxial subluxations.
- Pts w/ anterior & rotary subluxations can tolerate careful laryngoscopy w/ little risk of neurologic compromise.
- Take a careful medication history w/ attention to NSAIDs & immunosuppressants, including steroids.

CHECKLIST
- Careful airway exam; plan for potential difficult intubation
- Look for other system manifestations of RA.

RISK MANAGEMENT

JOSEPH MELTZER, MD
LISA LEFFERT, MD

FUNDAMENTAL KNOWLEDGE

A Note to the user: THIS DOCUMENT HAS BEEN PREPARED BY A PHYSICIAN & THE SECTION SHOULD NOT BE CONSTRUED AS PROVIDING LEGAL ADVICE, WHICH CAN ONLY BE GIVEN BY AN ATTORNEY.

- *Informed consent* is the provision & exchange of necessary information (potential risks & benefits & available alternatives) to enable the pt to make a reasoned decision about a course of treatment. It is a process & should not be limited to a document.
  - ➤ Documentation of informed consent is critical as it provides a record of the informed consent process that can help providers defend their actions.
  - ➤ Standardized forms provide uniform documentation within a practice or institution.
    - Most publications recommend separate anesthesia consent forms.
    - Forms serve as a guide for what types of information to convey.
    - Provides tangible evidence of discussion/exchange
  - ➤ "Negligible" risks are not "material" & need not be discussed.
  - ➤ Tailor explanations to the individual pt's competency, comprehension, need & desire for detail.
  - ➤ Always also document informed consent processes in the pt's chart:
    - Discussions w/ pts
    - Discussions w/ families
    - Specific questions asked & answered

- Anesthesia treatment option & risks separate from surgical risks
➤ See ASA statement, "Documentation of Anesthesia Care"
  - Capacity/competence
    - Pt must be able to make an informed decision.
    - Understand risks & benefits
    - If deemed incompetent, then
      - Guardian
      - Durable Power of Attorney for Health Care
      - Spouse
      - Adult children
      - Parents
      - Adult siblings
    - Minor pts
      - In most states, minors can consent to treatment of STDs at 14 years of age & mental health treatment at 13 years of age.
      - In most states, case law expands this to contraception & abortion.
      - In most states, minors have the right to privacy & autonomy for some medical decisions.
      - Consistent w/ the above 3 points, a minor is typically able to consent for obstetric care.
    - Emancipated minor/Mature minor doctrine
      - Allows healthcare providers to determine whether a minor is able to give consent
        - Maturity
        - Intelligence
        - Training
        - Economic independence
        - Freedom from parental control
      - When a minor is deemed emancipated for medical consent, document the objective facts that led to this determination.
      - Emancipation does not alter the requirement for consent.
➤ Labor analgesia: Obtain separate consent for labor analgesia/anesthesia.
  - Provides opportunity for pt to ask questions
  - Additional documentation that consent was obtained
  - Consent best obtained early in labor
  - Ideally, should be obtained prior to severe pain & distress

- May tailor consent process due to severe maternal pain
- Pain does not obviate need for frank discussion of risks.
- Surveys show women prefer informed consent process despite labor pain.
➤ Refusal to sign consent
  - If potential medical interventions are leading to refusal to sign the form, more dialogue about the pt's preferences regarding medical judgment is indicated.
  - If trust issues are involved, consider referral to another practitioner. This may be difficult during labor.
  - Document in the medical record the substance of the dialogue that occurred.
  - Note verbal consent in the medical record.
■ Refusal of care
➤ Adult pts may refuse medical treatment, even if life-saving.
  - Assess pt's capacity to provide informed consent.
  - Consider psychiatry consultation
  - Document objective facts that support determination of capacity.
➤ Pregnant patient w/ viable fetus
  - ACOG emphasized that maternal-fetal relationship is unique & requires balance btwn maternal health & autonomy & fetal needs.
    - "Obstetricians should refrain from performing procedures that are unwanted by a pregnant woman."
    - "Every reasonable effort should be made to protect the fetus, but the pregnant woman's autonomy should be respected."
    - "The use of courts to resolve these conflicts is almost never warranted."
  - If a competent pregnant pt refuses recommended care, document your recommendations & the pt's decision not to follow the recommended care.
    - Honor the competent pregnant person:
      - Document competency.
      - Document every attempt made to counsel the pt.
      - Document how, why & what information was provided to the pt & her family.
      - Reevaluate treatment options at frequent intervals w/ the pt.
    - Judicial review: Conflicts regarding maternal vs. fetal rights have yielded inconsistent results in the courts.

- Claims against healthcare providers
  - ➤ Liability: A physician is liable for a mistake or misjudgment when it occurred through a failure to act w/ the care of a prudent practitioner.
    - Every physician has a duty to provide professional services that are consistent w/ the average level of competence based on qualifications, expertise & circumstances.
    - Standard of care is changing & dynamic. Standards change w/ the adoption of new treatments & approaches.
      - Laws vary from state to state, but often pts may sue for injuries resulting from the provision of healthcare using medical malpractice, breach of contract or lack of informed consent.
      - To prevail, the plaintiff must prove that injury resulted from the provider's failure to follow accepted standards.
  - ➤ Establishing medical malpractice
    - Duty: It must be shown that a duty to provide care existed.
      - The anesthesiologist's duty is usually easy to establish.
      - When an anesthesiologist performs a service for a pt, duty is established.
    - Breach of duty: It must be shown that a provider failed to meet his or her duty.
    - Injury/Damage: It must be shown that a pt experienced injury.
    - Proximate cause/Causation: It must be shown that negligence caused the pt's injury.
    - The more devastating the injury, the more likely the pt is to decide to file suit & be able to find a competent plaintiff's attorney to represent her.
  - ➤ Establishing lack of informed consent
    - Medical ethics & law recognize the concepts of pt self-determination & autonomy.
    - Establishing a lack of informed consent:
      - The physician failed to inform the pt of material facts related to the treatment.
      - Pt consented without being fully aware or informed.
      - A reasonably prudent pt would not have consented, if informed.
      - Treatment was the proximate cause of injury.
    - State laws generally provide for "implied consent" for emergency treatment when the pt cannot provide consent & no surrogate is immediately available.

- Documentation in the chart should contain a description of the presenting condition, immediacy, magnitude & nature of immediate threat.
- Two healthcare providers should chart this information.
- A reasonable attempt must be undertaken to find a surrogate.

- Litigation process
  - Legal authority is derived from multiple sources.
    - Constitutions: These are fundamental laws of nations or states, which act as philosophical touchstones for society.
    - Statutes: These are laws written & enacted by elected officials.
    - Regulations: These are written by governmental agencies.
    - Case law: These are written opinions or decisions of judges that arise from individual lawsuits.
    - Courts give strong weight to healthcare standards as set forth from bodies such as JCAHO or ASA.
      - In some jurisdictions, guidelines & practice parameters may be used as an affirmative defense.
      - In some jurisdictions, physicians are immunized if their practices were consistent w/ professional standards.
  - Initiation of lawsuit
    - Complaint: Filed by plaintiff
    - Summons: Notice of legal action
    - Answer: Required of physician in a timely manner
  - Discovery is the early phase of a lawsuit where the strengths & weaknesses of a case are reviewed by examining medical records & medical literature & interviewing witnesses (plaintiff, healthcare providers, experts).
    - Interrogatories are written questions that are served from one party to another, answered under oath.
    - Depositions involve testimony under oath, recorded by a court reporter.
    - Purposes of discovery:
      - Obtain facts
      - Encourage one side to commit to a position
      - Discover names of potential witnesses
      - Assess witnesses
      - Limit facts or issues for the lawsuit
      - Encourage admissions
      - Evaluate case for it value & potential settlement
  - Trial
    - Jury selection

- Opening statements
- Plaintiff's trial testimony
- Defendant's trial testimony
- Closing arguments
- Jury instructions
- Delivery of jury verdict

➤ Most cases never go to trial.
- Approx. 10% of medical malpractice claims go to trial.
- Settlement negotiations result in disposal of many cases.
- Many of the cases that proceed to trial are decided in favor of the defendant.

■ ASA Obstetric Closed Claims Project
➤ What is it?
- A claim is a demand for financial compensation by an individual who has sustained an injury from medical care.
- A closed claim file contains a broad assortment of documents, including medical records, narrative statements, expert & peer reviews, deposition summaries, outcome & follow-up reports & the cost of settlement or jury award.
- Closed claims database contains detailed information about adverse events.
  - Recovered from 35 insurance carriers
  - 50% of U.S. anesthesiologists covered by these carriers
  - Currently >5,000 cases in database
  - Claims for dental injuries not included
- Most cases involve healthy adults undergoing non-emergent surgery w/ general anesthesia
  - 91% age >16
  - 76% non-emergent
  - 69% ASA I or II
  - 59% female
- Closed claims database is an important source of information for the study of the genesis of adverse events.
- Claims are organized according to 2 features: damaging events or adverse outcomes.
  - Damaging event is a specific incident or mechanism that leads to an adverse outcome.
    - Respiratory system: 24%
    - Cardiovascular-related: 13%
    - Equipment-related: 10%
    - Other: 53%

- Adverse outcome is the injury sustained by the patient
  - Death: 30%
  - Nerve damage: 18%
  - Brain damage: 12%
  - Airway trauma: 6%
  - Eye injury, pneumothorax: 4% each
  - Fetal/newborn injury, stroke, aspiration, back pain, headache: 3% each
  - Other: 6%
- ➤ Limitations
  - Cannot be used to determine incidence
    - "Denominator" is unknown
    - Not all injuries result in claims.
    - Anesthesiologist may not be named in anesthesia-related injury.
    - Anesthesiologist may be named in non-anesthesia-related injury.
    - Not a random sampling of data
- ➤ What injuries are most common in obstetrical anesthesia claims?
  - No anesthetic technique for cesarean delivery is more or less likely to result in a malpractice suit.
  - Maternal death, 19%: greater proportion of GA & C-section may represent higher-risk pts
  - Neonatal brain damage, 19%: no difference w/ type of anesthetic
  - Headache, 15%: associated w/ regional anesthetic & vaginal delivery
  - Maternal nerve damage, 10%: associated w/ regional anesthesia
  - Pain during anesthesia, 9%: associated w/ regional anesthetic & C-section
  - Back pain, 8%: associated w/ regional anesthetic & vaginal delivery
  - Maternal brain damage, 7%
  - Emotional distress, 7%
  - Neonatal death, 6%
  - Aspiration pneumonitis, 5%: associated w/ GA
  - Wrong drug/dose, 1%
  - Equipment failure, 1%
- ➤ What is the relationship between type of anesthesia & presumed injury?

- Maternal files have greater proportion of relatively minor injuries.
- Maternal/patient death, OB < non-OB
- Headache, OB > non-OB
- Maternal/patient nerve damage, OB < non-OB
- Pain during anesthesia, OB > non-OB
- Back pain, OB > non-OB
- Maternal/patient brain damage, OB < non-OB
- Emotional distress, OB > non-OB
- Aspiration pneumonitis, OB > non-OB

➤ What events lead to injuries?

- Respiratory system (see "*General Anesthesia & the Difficult Airway*")
- Obesity (see "*Obese Parturient*")
- Seizures
  - Eclampsia (see "*Severe Preeclampsia*")
  - Local anesthetic toxicity (see "*Local Anesthetic Pharmacology*")
- Equipment problems
- Cardiovascular system (see "*Mitral Stenosis*," "*Mitral Regurgitation*," "*Mitral Valve Prolapse Syndrome*," "*Aortic Stenosis*," "*Aortic Regurgitation*," "*Cardiomyopathy*," "*Arrhythmias*," "*Pacemakers*," "*ICDs*," "*Ischemia & MI in Pregnancy*," "*Cardiac Arrest*," "*Pulmonary Physiologic Changes of Pregnancy*," "*Asthma*," "*Aspiration*," "*Cystic Fibrosis*," "*Restrictive Lung Disease*," "*Pulmonary Hypertension*," "*Pulmonary Edema*," "*ARDS*")
- Wrong drug/dose

➤ How do payment rates compare btwn obstetric & non-obstetric claims?

- No payment: OB 39%, non-OB 33%
- Payments made: OB 52%, non-OB 59%
- Median payment: OB $200,000, non-OB $100,00
- Range of payment: OB $675-$6,800,00, non-OB, $15-$23,200,000

■ Risk mgt: minimizing the number of pt injuries

➤ Resist "production pressure." Safe, reasonable care must prevail.

➤ Continuing medical education

➤ Believe your monitors!

➤ Familiarize yourself w/ ASA standards & guidelines (e.g., difficult airway, transfusion practices).

➤ Know departmental policies & procedures.
➤ Preanesthetic evaluation is the most important tool
  • Ask yourself, "How urgent is the surgery & need for analgesia?"
  • Honest & realistic preanesthetic counseling will prevent pt disappointment.
  • Review of medical & anesthetic history, vital signs
  • Careful exam of maternal airway, heart & lungs
  • Exam of maternal back
  • Assessment of fetal condition
  • Review of labor course & understanding of obstetric plans for delivery
  • Presentation of anesthetic plan, procedures, risks & choices as appropriate
  • Intravascular volume status
  • Non-particulate antacid
➤ Epidural placement for labor
  • See "*Relief of Labor Pain With Regional Anesthesia.*"
➤ Preventing respiratory injury
  • Most deaths or CNS injuries result from respiratory failure.
  • 50% of respiratory failures occur in the postop period
    • OB recovery areas should be of the same quality as the general PACU area, w/ pulse oximetry & continual visual monitoring w/ qualified nursing personnel.
    • No attorney will accept a standard of care different from that rendered to other patients in the same hospital.
  • 50% of respiratory failures occur during anesthesia, most often on induction.
    • Airway mgt is the single largest problem.
      • Use rapid sequence intubation.
      • Cricoid pressure until endotracheal tube cuff is inflated & end-tidal CO_2 is confirmed
    • Aspiration of gastric contents is more common in pregnancy & may complicate airway mgt (see "*General Anesthesia & the Difficult Airway*").
      • Use non-particulate oral antacid.
        • Consider metoclopramide.
        • Consider ranitidine.
        • Consider orogastric tube while anesthetized.
    • Visualization of the airway is more difficult during pregnancy. If difficult airway is anticipated, consider awake intubation.

- Follow difficult airway algorithm & consider a regional blockade.
- Recognize need for cricothyrotomy or tracheotomy.
- Extubate pt when fully awake & following commands.
- Neuraxial blockade (see "*Postpartum Evaluation & Management of Neurologic Complications of Regional Anesthesia*")
  - Pt must recognize failure rate & all potential complications.
  - Higher incidence of claims w/ epidural than subarachnoid block
  - High-severity injuries
    - Neuraxial cardiac arrest (vast majority resulting in brain damage or death)
    - Intravascular injection
    - High spinal/epidural blockade
    - Permanent nerve injury
  - Low-severity injuries
  - Headache
  - Back pain
  - Temporary nerve damage
  - Inadequate analgesia
  - Emotional distress
- OB pts should receive the same standard of care, including monitors & equipment, as general surgical pts.
  - Correct, preventative maintenance & servicing
  - Performance checks every 4–6 months
  - Annual safety inspection
  - Pre-service & in-service training for new equipment & new providers
  - Faulty medical devices must be reported to the FDA at www.fda.gov.
- Multiple, carefully drawn-up policies & procedures, although often perceived as bureaucratic, lead to good pt care.
  - JCAHO Standards
  - ASA Statements & Guidelines
  - Procedural protocols
  - Staff responsibilities & duties
- Risk mgt: minimizing pt's motivation to sue
  - Pts are less likely to sue physicians they know well & believe to be truly interested in their health.
  - Bedside arguments btwn physicians undermine both physicians' credibility.

➤ Nurses spend the majority of time at the bedside; including their input & expertise in labor plans solidifies plans & reinforces pt confidence.

➤ Fastidious record keeping is a must!

- For example, for neuraxial blockade, record the size & type of needle used, the number of attempts, the occurrence of paresthesias, the use of a test dose & the anesthetic level achieved.
- "If you didn't write it down, it didn't happen" in the legal sense

➤ Perform exams & answer questions w/ kindness.

➤ To address patient dissatisfaction, an anesthesiologist must visit ALL pts postop to answer questions & initiate treatment of any complication that becomes evident.

➤ Anesthesiologists, not OBs, should address pt complaints regarding potential anesthetic complications.

➤ Effective intra-OR communication is a must!

➤ Anesthesiologists should meet w/ patient educators in their hospitals to ensure that accurate information about anesthesia is being taught to pts.

➤ Limitations of anesthesia should be discussed w/ pts & OBs.

■ Adverse events

➤ Sincere sympathy & compassion to the pt and/or family is often the most important response to diffuse a volatile situation.

➤ Refrain from infighting & castigation.

➤ Assign the most knowledgeable staff members to meticulously document relevant information in the medical record.

- State only facts.
- Make no judgments.
- Never change any existing entries in the chart.
- Avoid "chart wars" & any information unrelated to the care of the pt.

➤ Make your own detailed set of notes on the event.

- Will prove useful 2–5 years later if legal action is taken
- Place these notes in the hands of your attorney "in anticipation of litigation"
  - These notes are "attorney-client work product."
  - Difficult to discover
  - It is best if these notes are hand-written.
- There is no protection of conversations among colleagues to discovery unless it is in a "peer review" context.

➤ Maintain contact w/ patient/family to answer questions.

➤ Organize family meeting as needed.

> Seek counseling & support from family, colleagues, medical experts.
> - Note: These are potentially discoverable conversations.
> Seek counseling from lawyers & risk managers.
> - Note: These are undiscoverable conversations.
> Empathize w/ patient & offer emotional support.
> Analyze the event, the outcome & the causes for the problem.
> Attempt to reconcile opposing perceptions of what has occurred.
> Basic outline of appropriate immediate response at www.apsf.org

STUDIES
MANAGEMENT/INTERVENTIONS
CAVEATS/PEARLS
CHECKLIST
N/A

ROUTINE NEWBORN CARE

RICHARD ARCHULETA, MD
SANDRA WEINREB, MD

FUNDAMENTAL KNOWLEDGE

Neonatal Suctioning

■ Suction neonate's oropharynx & nose.
> Performed by obstetrician or midwife during delivery (after delivery of the shoulder, but before delivery of the chest)
> Performed again after delivery

■ Neck flexion or hyperextension can produce airway obstruction & is prevented w/ proper neonatal positioning (see "Management/Interventions" section).

Routine neonatal stimulation

■ Mild stimulation consists of airway suctioning & gentle drying.
■ Stimulates spontaneous ventilation in most neonates

Need for routine neonatal temperature maintenance

■ Neonates are especially susceptible to heat loss due to large surface area to volume ratio.
■ Hypothermia increases oxygen consumption & impedes resolution of acidosis.
> Cold stress induces catecholamine release, which stimulates brown fat metabolism for non-shivering thermogenesis, which results in significant oxygen consumption.

➤ Cold stress is particularly difficult for infants w/ low fat stores (preterm & IUGR).

STUDIES

Continuously monitor neonatal respirations, heart rate & color for signs of deterioration (apnea or slow & irregular respirations, heart rate <100, central cyanosis).

MANAGEMENT/INTERVENTIONS

Routine neonatal airway mgt

■ The neonatal airway is normally filled w/ amniotic fluid & secretions upon birth & suctioning is needed to clear the airway.
  ➤ The nose, mouth & superficial oropharynx are suctioned w/ a bulb suction, 8F or 10F catheter.
  ➤ Avoid negative pressure >100 mm Hg (135 cm H2O).
  ➤ Avoid deep oropharyngeal suction, which may cause a vagal response (bradycardia &/or apnea).
  ➤ If the infant is crying vigorously w/ minimal secretions, may only require gentle wiping of mouth & nose
■ Position neonate to maintain slight neck extension.
  ➤ Place neonate supine w/ a rolled blanket or towel under the back/shoulders to compensate for large occiput & caput succedaneum.
  ➤ If copious secretions are present, place neonate on side w/ neck slightly extended.
■ If neonate is breathing spontaneously but has central cyanosis or acrocyanosis w/ Apgar < 8, free-flowing 100% oxygen (at least 5 L/min) should be administered via:
  ➤ Simple face mask
  ➤ Hand cupped over face w/ O2 tubing
  ➤ Face mask attached to flow-inflating bag

Routine neonatal stimulation

■ Gently dry neonate.
■ Gently stimulate neonate to breath. Avoid rigorous stimulation.
  ➤ May advance to flicking the soles of the feet & rubbing the back to stimulate spontaneous ventilation.
  ➤ The neonate is especially susceptible to stimulation, so avoid more vigorous forms of stimulation.
  ➤ Neonates w/ poor respiratory efforts after routine care should receive resuscitative measures (see "*Resuscitation of the Neonate*").

Routine neonatal heating
- Keep neonate warm.
  - Neonatal environment should be 34–35 degrees C.
  - Usually use radiant heater
  - May use skin-to-skin contact w/ mother covered by blanket

CAVEATS & PEARLS
- Continue to monitor & care for the mother as your pt. Make sure that the neonate's care does not distract you from this primary responsibility.
- Self-inflating bags do not reliably provide free-flowing O2 because they may entrain room air when bag is re-expanding.

CHECKLIST
- Constantly observe neonate for deterioration in:
  - Respirations (should be regular & 30 or more breaths per minute)
  - Heart rate (should be >100 bpm)
  - Color (should not have central cyanosis)
- Ensure airway has been suctioned.
  - Do not suction deeply w/ routine care.
  - Do not use negative pressure >100 mm Hg.
- Position neonate w/ mild neck extension.
- Gently dry neonate.
- Keep neonate warm & avoid inadvertent hypothermia.
- Provide free-flowing oxygen if necessary (ie, central cyanosis in spontaneously breathing neonate).

SCLERODERMA

AUGUST CHANG, MD
MIRIAM HARNETT, MD

FUNDAMENTAL KNOWLEDGE

Definition
- Chronic progressive disease of unknown etiology characterized by overproduction of connective tissue by fibroblasts, resulting in microvascular obliteration & fibrosis of the skin & visceral organs
- Also known as systemic sclerosis; characterized by the presence of antinuclear & anticentromere antibodies

- Diagnostic triad
  - Raynaud's phenomenon
  - Nonpitting edema
  - Hidebound skin

Epidemiology
- Prevalence of 28–130 per million
- Incidence of 2–10 per million per year
- Male:female 1:3–5; limited cutaneous, diffuse equal predilection
- Peak onset during 4th decade of life

Clinical manifestations: heterogenous disorder separated into 2 entities
- CREST syndrome: limited cutaneous scleroderma
  - Calcinosis
  - Raynaud's
  - Esophageal dysfunction
  - Sclerodactyly
  - Telangiectasia
- Diffuse cutaneous scleroderma
  - Skin
    - Raynaud's phenomenon
    - Nonpitting edema
    - Hidebound skin
  - GI
    - Dysphagia
    - Reflux esophagitis
    - Hypomotility/constipation/ileus
    - Postprandial fullness
    - Abdominal pain
    - Intermittent diarrhea
    - Malnutrition
  - Pulmonary
    - Pleuritis
    - Interstitial fibrosis
    - Pleural effusion
    - Pulmonary hypertension
    - Chest wall restriction
  - Renal
    - Proteinuria
    - Renal insufficiency & failure
    - Malignant hypertension

- ➤ Cardiac
  - Myocardial ischemia & infarction
  - Chronic pericardial effusion
  - Conduction disturbances
  - Heart failure
- ➤ Musculoskeletal
  - Arthritis
  - Myopathy
  - Muscle wasting
- ➤ Other
  - Peripheral or central neuropathies
  - Trigeminal neuralgia
  - Keratoconjunctivitis sicca
  - Xerostomia
  - Coagulopathy secondary to vitamin K deficiency
  - Absence of ANA antibodies

Effect on pregnancy

- ■ Renal crisis
  - ➤ May be precipitated by sclerodermal flare during 3rd trimester
  - ➤ Presentation can mimic preeclampsia w/ acute onset of hypertension, microangiopathic hemolysis, thrombocytopenia, proteinuria, increased creatinine
  - ➤ Differentiation is usually made on clinical grounds but can be difficult
    - Sclerodermal renal crisis: transaminase levels usually normal, renin levels high, typically occurs during 1st half of pregnancy
    - Pre-eclampsia: transaminase levels may be elevated, renin levels low, rarely occurs before 3rd trimester
  - ➤ ACE inhibitors are the only meds that control the hypertension in renal crisis
    - Their use should be considered if needed, despite association w/ fetal renal defects
  - ➤ Encourage pt to delay pregnancy 3–5 years after onset of symptoms, because disease process usually stabilizes & risk of renal crisis is reduced

Effect on pregnancy & fetus

- ■ Preterm delivery more likely
- ■ No increase in spontaneous abortion
- ■ More likely to have small full-term infants

STUDIES

History & Physical
- Airway: evaluate for indicators of potentially difficult intubation & be wary of the presence of oral &/or nasal telangiectasias
- Cardiac: evaluate for evidence of pericarditis or pericardial effusions
- Pulmonary: evaluate for evidence of pulmonary hypertension

Imaging
- Chest radiograph
- Echocardiography: consider if pulmonary hypertension is suspected

Other
- ECG
- Coagulation studies
- CBC
- Electrolytes
- BUN/creatinine, urinalysis, 24-h urine protein & creatinine
- Resting renin levels
- Pulmonary function testing: consider if significant lung disease is suspected
- BP measurement at home several times per week

MANAGEMENT/INTERVENTIONS

Medical treatment
- *D*-Penicillamine
  - Interferes w/ collagen cross-linking
  - Used to modulate skin, renal, pulmonary involvement
  - Case reports of fetal connective tissue disorders
  - Fetal risks are probably not high enough to warrant discontinuing during pregnancy
- Glucocorticoids
  - Used to reduce inflammatory myositis
  - Reportedly linked to induction of renal crisis
  - No evidence of teratogenicity
  - Inactivation by placental 11-beta-OH-dehydrogenase results in low fetal levels of active drug
  - May precipitate gestational diabetes mellitus & hypertension
  - Longer-term adverse effects
    - Osteoporosis
    - GI ulceration
    - Impaired immunity
    - Adrenal suppression

- Immunosuppressive agents
  - Chlorambucil & azathioprine
    - No demonstrated benefit
- Stanozolol & prostacyclin analogs
  - Help w/ vasospastic component of Raynaud's
- ACE inhibitors
  - Agents of choice for hypertensive crisis of scleroderma in pregnancy, even though they are associated w/ fetal renal defects
- NSAIDs
  - No evidence of teratogenicity
  - No need for prophylactic cessation, but pregnancy should be closely monitored
  - Recommend discontinuation during 3rd trimester because of:
    - Inhibitory effect on platelets & hemostasis
    - Increased risk of fetal CNS hemorrhage
    - Possible premature closure of ductus arteriosus
    - Possible compromised fetal renal perfusion & abnormal amniotic fluid dynamics
    - Possible factor in necrotizing enterocolitis (NEC)

Anesthesia
- General anesthesia
  - Significantly increased risk of difficult intubation & aspiration vs. that associated w/ pregnancy alone
  - Antacids, histamine-2 blockers, head-up position if possible
  - Awake fiberoptic intubation recommended
- Regional anesthesia
  - Epidural is preferred over spinal because you are better able to titrate & avoid high regional blockade
  - Start w/ significantly lower doses of local anesthetic, as unpredictable spread & longer than normal duration have been reported
  - Use small intermittent boluses as needed instead of continuous epidural infusion
  - Use of short-acting (2-chloroprocaine) local anesthetics is preferred, but this can still result in markedly prolonged block
- NIBP measurement may be difficult & invasive BP monitoring may be required
- Pulmonary artery catheter may be indicated if significant pulmonary hypertension is present

- Pay special attention to preserving body warmth in pts w/ Raynaud's:
  - ➤ Warm delivery room
  - ➤ Warm IV fluids
  - ➤ Thermal socks
- Stress-dose steroids during labor & delivery for pts currently on steroid therapy

CAVEATS & PEARLS
- Significantly increased risk of difficult intubation & mask fit as well as aspiration over that associated w/ pregnancy alone
- Increased incidence of unpredictable spread of local anesthetic & longer than normal duration of block
- ACE inhibitors are the agent of choice for hypertensive crisis of scleroderma in pregnancy, even though they are associated w/ fetal renal defects
- Venous access should be obtained early; may be difficult
- NIBP measurement may be difficult & invasive BP monitoring may be required
  - ➤ Radial artery catheterization is contraindicated in pts w/ Raynaud's because of risk of hand ischemia
  - ➤ Brachial artery catheterization may be considered instead
- Pulse oximetry readings may be difficult on extremities
- Avoid vasoconstrictors
- Anticipate vaginal delivery, but pt may have dysfunctional labor or cervical dystocia due to uterine & cervical wall thickening
- Pt has increased vulnerability to corneal abrasions due to decreased tear production

CHECKLIST
- Thorough airway exam
- Immediate availability of special airway equipment: laryngeal mask airway, fiberoptic laryngoscope, transtracheal jet ventilation, emergency cricothyrotomy kit
- Document preexisting peripheral neuropathies prior to general or regional anesthesia
- Establish early IV access & epidural
- Immediate availability of ACE inhibitor for treatment of sclerodermal renal crisis
- Stress-dose steroids during labor & delivery for pts currently on steroid therapy

SCOLIOSIS

STEPHEN PANARO, MD
EDWARD MICHNA, MD

FUNDAMENTAL KNOWLEDGE

- Scoliosis is defined as a lateral deviation of the vertical axis of the spine.
- The severity of the scoliosis is defined quantitatively by measuring the Cobb angle, the angle btwn the intersection of the lines that are drawn perpendicularly to the parallel lines btwn the superior & inferior cortical plates.
- Pts w/ large Cobb angles have an axial component that angles the spinous processes away from the convexity & toward the midline.
- The pedicles are shorter & thinner on the concave side in severe cases (Cobb angle > 40 degrees).
- Prevalence of scoliosis w/ Cobb angle >10 degrees is 2–3%.
- In curvatures <20 degrees, rotary deviation of the vertebrae is not common.
- Severe scoliosis affects 0.03% of pregnancies.
- Obtain a comprehensive history & physical exam of any pt w/ scoliosis to determine whether further testing is necessary.
  - ➤ Review any concomitant medical conditions for their particular peri-anesthetic implications.
- Although usually idiopathic, scoliosis may be associated w/ congenital conditions such as spina bifida, cerebral palsy, neurofibromatosis, muscular dystrophy, Marfan's, osteogenesis imperfecta & rheumatoid arthritis.
- Pregnancy alone can compromise respiratory function secondary to the obligatory decrease in functional residual capacity (FRC) that occurs as the uterus enlarges.
- Pulmonary architectural changes include a reduction in alveoli, less developed pulmonary vasculature & the potential for pulmonary hypertension & subsequent cor pulmonale in the most severe cases.
- Pregnancy may exacerbate the curvature & the associated cardiopulmonary comorbidities.
- Severe scoliosis can cause a restrictive breathing pattern w/ a resultant decrease in vital capacity, total lung capacity, pulmonary compliance & functional residual capacity. Pts may require higher respiratory rates to increase ventilation.
- **Physiologic** dyspnea is common & usually begins early in pregnancy.

- **Pathologic** dyspnea tends to present between the 2nd & 3rd trimester & is generally progressive. In extreme cases it can herald an evolving cardiopulmonary decompensation
- Pre-pregnancy functional status gives an initial indication of how the pt will tolerate pregnancy.

STUDIES
- Evaluate the pt for cardiopulmonary functional status, including an echocardiogram if right heart dysfunction is suspected.
- Pulmonary function tests if indicated (there is an inverse relationship between the severity of the curvature & PFTs, including VC & FEV1)
- Review radiographic studies & operative reports (if surgical correction has been undertaken).

MANAGEMENT/INTERVENTIONS
- Epidurals are not contraindicated, although there may be an increased incidence of inadvertent dural puncture (if the pt has had prior surgery) or one-sided or patchy block in the case of severe scoliosis.
- Epidural blood patch may not be feasible in pts who have had an inadvertent dural puncture because of tethering of the dura to the ligamentum flavum.
- Patients w/ large Cobb angles will have axial rotation toward the midline. Therefore, direct the epidural or spinal needle toward the convexity.
- Consider alternative means of anesthesia/analgesia (GA or spinal or cesarean delivery & IV medication or labor spinal for vaginal delivery) if the epidural space is thought to be disrupted.
- Scoliosis surgery may extend below L4 & may result in significant distortion in the landmarks that are usually employed for neuraxial anesthetic techniques.
- Pts w/ severe right heart failure may need a pulmonary arterial catheter during delivery.

CAVEATS & PEARLS
- Pre-pregnancy functional status gives an initial indication of how the pt will tolerate pregnancy.
- Pregnancy may exacerbate the curvature & the associated cardiopulmonary comorbidities.
- Patients w/ large Cobb angles will have axial rotation toward the midline. Direct the epidural or spinal needle toward the convexity.

- Pts who have had back surgery have a slightly increased incidence of failed epidural blocks & complications, including dural puncture.
  - ➤ Pts w/ myotonic or neurologic disease may have distorted anatomy that impedes access to the epidural or subarachnoid space.
- Be particularly cautious in pts who have had spinal surgery because adhesions can increase the rate of an inadvertent dural puncture.
- Epidural blood patch may not be feasible in pts who have had an inadvertent dural puncture because of tethering of the dura to the ligamentum flavum.

CHECKLIST
- Compile relevant information concerning pt's scoliosis & respiratory/cardiovascular status, w/ particular attention to prior surgical interventions.
- Informed consent detailing anesthetic options (GA & IV sedation as well as regional anesthesia) & potential increased risk of inadvertent dural puncture & inadequate block

---

SEVERE PRE-ECLAMPSIA

TIMOTHY OLSON, MD
RICHARD PINO, MD

FUNDAMENTAL KNOWLEDGE

Introduction
- Pre-eclampsia is traditionally known as the triad of hypertension, proteinuria & edema, usually beginning in the 2nd half of gestation. More recent definitions no longer require edema as a component.
  - ➤ Present in 5–8% of all pregnancies
  - ➤ Accounts for approx. 15% of maternal deaths in U.S., up to 80% of maternal deaths in countries w/ inadequate prenatal care

Pathophysiology
- Immunologic: some evidence suggests that pre-eclampsia develops in part as a result of a maternal response to paternal antigens
  - ➤ Risk decreases w/ increased duration of unprotected preconception sex w/ the father of the child.
  - ➤ Risk in subsequent pregnancies returns to primiparity levels if woman has changed partners.

- Genetic: increased incidence w/ positive family history
- Endothelial: damage to the vascular endothelium represents the final common pathway to the onset of pre-eclampsia
  - Normal pregnancy is characterized by trophoblast invasion of the myometrium & development of a high-flow, low-resistance placental perfusion system.
  - Failure of appropriate invasion of the myometrium & the spiral arteries results in the high-resistance, low-flow state of pre-eclampsia.
  - This state is likely exacerbated & maintained by an imbalance btwn thromboxane-mediated vasoconstriction & prostaglandin GI2-mediated vasodilation.

Risk Factors
- Chronic hypertension
- Renal disease
- Diabetes mellitus
- Obesity
- Vascular disease (lupus anticoagulant, protein S deficiency, APC resistance)
- African-American race
- Family history of pre-eclampsia or pre-eclampsia w/ previous pregnancy
- Nulliparity
- Multiple gestation
- Age > 40

Differential Diagnosis
- Pregnancy-induced hypertension (PIH)
  - Pre-eclampsia
    - Mild
      - SBP > 140 mm Hg or DBP > 90 mm Hg on 2 occasions
      - Urine protein > 0.3 g/day
    - Severe
      - SBP > 160 mm Hg or DBP > 110 mm Hg
      - Urine protein > 5 g/day
  - Eclampsia
    - New onset of seizures in the pre-eclamptic pt
    - Seizure cannot be explained by other disease process
  - HELLP (hemolysis, elevated liver enzymes & low platelets)
    - Hemolysis: abnormal peripheral smear; bilirubin > 1.2 mg/dL or LDH > 600

- Elevated liver enzymes: AST > 2× normal
- Thrombocytopenia: platelets < 100,000
- Chronic hypertension
  - Hypertension prior to pregnancy, <20 weeks gestation or >12 weeks postpartum
  - Present in 3–5% of all pregnancies
- Chronic hypertension w/ PIH
  - Occurs in approx. 20–25% of women w/ chronic hypertension

STUDIES

Lab studies & pre-op evaluation are critical to the optimal mgt of the pre-eclamptic pt. Important aspects of the history, physical exam & lab findings include:

- BP monitoring
- Lab studies
  - Urine protein (24-hour collection & spot urine protein), microalbuminuria
  - CBC (thrombocytopenia)
  - Liver function tests
  - Electrolytes (including $Ca++$, $Mg++$ if on $MgSO_4$ therapy)
- History/physical exam findings
  - CNS: headache, visual disturbances
  - Cardiovascular: hypertension
  - Hepatic: RUQ pain secondary to liver capsule distention
  - Hematologic: hemolysis, low platelets (HELLP syndrome)
  - Pulmonary: pulmonary edema
  - Renal: oliguria, peripheral edema
  - Placenta: IUGR, oligohydramnios

MANAGEMENT/INTERVENTIONS

Appropriate mgt of the pre-eclamptic pt is dependent on many factors, including the severity of the pre-eclampsia, the gestational age of the pregnancy & the fetal well-being. The only definitive cure for pre-eclampsia is delivery, & mgt is a shared responsibility between the OB & the anesthesiologist.

- Peri-op considerations
  - Volume status
    - Fluid resuscitation
      - Pre-eclamptic pts are typically intravascularly depleted.
      - An initial fluid bolus of about 500 mL crystalloid is usually appropriate.

- Urine output
  - Placement of Foley catheter
  - Watch carefully for oliguria (<400 mL urine/24 hours).
- Invasive hemodynamic monitoring
  - Severe pre-eclampsia
  - Oliguria that fails to respond to fluid bolus
  - Volume resuscitation to CVP 5–8
  - Monitoring of PCWP usually reserved for severe pre-eclampsia w/ pulmonary edema, intractable hypertension or oliguria. PCWP & CVP fail to correlate in approx. 50% of pre-eclamptic pts.
- Control of hypertension
  - Goals of anti-hypertension therapy
  - Hydralazine
    - Historical first-line agent
    - Small arteriole vasodilator, via increase in intracellular cGMP
    - Increased heart rate due to reflex tachycardia, also increases cardiac output, SVR w/ little documented effect on uterine blood flow
    - Slower-acting than labetalol
    - Dosing: 5 mg IV q20min; recommended max dose 20 mg
  - Labetalol
    - Combined alpha- & beta-adrenergic antagonist (ratio 1:7 when delivered IV)
    - Decreases maternal SVR w/o decreasing uterine blood flow. Case reports have suggested fetal bradycardia & hypotension w/ the use of labetalol, but no study has demonstrated increased risk to the fetus using labetalol for control of hypertension.
    - Faster onset than hydralazine
    - Dosing: 5 mg IV q5min, max dose up to 1 mg/kg or 300 mg
    - Combination therapy w/ hydralazine has been advocated by some providers.
  - Other agents
    - Sodium nitroprusside
    - Nitroglycerin
    - Esmolol
- Seizure prophylaxis/therapy
  - $MgSO_4$ therapy

- Treatment of choice for seizure prophylaxis in the pre-eclamptic pt
- In addition to role in seizure prophylaxis, also has a beneficial hemodynamic effect, w/ small increase in cardiac index & decrease in SVR
- Treatment is typically continued 24 hours after delivery.
- Long history of safe use
- Normal lab values: approximately 1.5–2.5 mg/dL
- Therapeutic range: 5–9 mg/dL
- Watch carefully for signs of magnesium overdose:
  - Loss of reflexes (patellar) begins around 12 mg/dL.
  - Respiratory arrest around 15 mg/dL
  - More common in pts w/ renal dysfunction
  - Treatment
    - Discontinue infusion.
    - Administer $CaCl_2$ or Ca gluconate.
- Dosing: 4–6 mg IV bolus, followed by infusion of 1–2 mg/hour
- $MgSO_4$ promotes uterine relaxation, which can result in failure to progress in labor &/or postpartum uterine atony.
- Treatment of the eclamptic pt
  - Seizures may be terminated w/ benzodiazepines or thiopental.
  - Goal is to prevent aspiration & maternal hypoxemia.
- Intra-operative considerations
  - Airway evaluation
  - Monitoring
    - Standard monitors (EKG, pulse oximetry, NIBP) are adequate for most cases.
    - A-line is indicated for severe pre-eclampsia (accurate BP monitoring, serial blood sampling).
    - Consider need for invasive hemodynamic monitoring.
  - Regional anesthesia
    - Helps avoid the need to secure a potentially difficult airway
    - Epidural anesthesia
      - Provides excellent pain relief during labor
      - Decreases serum catecholamine levels & improves uterine blood flow & intervillous blood flow in the fetus
      - Typically performed w/ a dilute local anesthetic w/ small amount of narcotic (eg, 0.08–0.1% bupivacaine w/ 2 mcg fentanyl/cc)

- Can be converted to anesthesia for C-section (goal approx. T4 level)
- Induce block slowly if possible to reduce risk of hypotension (which can be treated w/ IV fluids &/or ephedrine 2.5–5 mg).
- Prehydration w/ approx. 500 mL crystalloid can be beneficial.
- Left uterine displacement also important after induction to maintain optimal maternal & fetal hemodynamics
  - Spinal anesthesia
    Has been shown to be safe in the setting of severe pre-eclampsia in the literature
  - Combined spinal-epidural
- General anesthesia
  - ➤ $MgSO_4$ may potentiate the effects of anesthetics & muscle relaxants.
  - ➤ $MgSO_4$ may contribute to uterine atony & increased blood loss intra-operatively.

CAVEATS & PEARLS
- General vs. regional
  - ➤ The pt w/ worsening thrombocytopenia may have a narrow window in which a regional technique may be considered. Consider leaving epidural catheter in situ post-partum until platelet count returns to normal.
  - ➤ The literature supports the use of either general or regional anesthesia
- $MgSO_4$ prolongs effect of non-depolarizing muscle relaxants.
- $MgSO_4$ can prolong the effects of other anesthetics & delay emergence.
- $MgSO_4$ can contribute to uterine atony.

CHECKLIST
- Pre-op assessment of pt
  - ➤ ABCs
  - ➤ Past medical history, including comorbid illness, severity of pre-eclampsia, gestational age of fetus
  - ➤ Airway evaluation
  - ➤ Lab results
- Discuss plan regarding expectant mgt, labor induction or cesarean delivery w/ OB.

SPINA BIFIDA

STEPHEN PANARO, MD
EDWARD MICHNA, MD

FUNDAMENTAL KNOWLEDGE

■ Heterogeneous group of disorders that result from a failure of the vertebrae to completely enclose the neural elements in a bony canal

■ Spectrum of disease

➤ *Spina bifida occulta* does not involve any herniation of the meninges or neural elements.

- Most frequently there are no outward signs (isolated arch deformity & normal cord). May be present in 5–30% of overall population.
- Signs can include a dimple, tuft of hair on the skin or a cutaneous angioma
- Diagnosis can be made incidentally based on spine radiographs

➤ *Spina bifida cystica* is less common & can have devastating neurologic manifestations.

- Defined as a failed closure of the neural arch w/ herniation of the meninges (meningocele) or meninges & neural elements (myelomeningocele)
- Potential for devastating neurologic consequences most often associated w/ deficits of the lower extremities & sphincter function
- Usually associated w/ hydrocephalus; pts often have ventriculoperitoneal shunts
- Scoliosis common

➤ *Occult spinal dysraphism* lies between the two ends of the spectrum.

- There is no frank herniation, but there are bony defects associated w/ cord abnormalities such as dermal sinus tracts, split cord, intraspinal lipomas & fibrous bands.
- About half of affected pts have cutaneous stigmata of the underlying process.
- Some of these pts are asymptomatic, but others have minor neurologic issues of motor or sensory deficits & bowel or bladder compromise.

- Tethered cord: the spinal cord may be attached abnormally to structures in the lumbar spine, often marked by a low-lying (L2–L3) conus
  - ➤ MRI studies suggest that nearly all pts w/ spina bifida cystica have some degree of tethering, & it may be common in pts w/ *occult spinal dysraphism*. Probably uncommon in spina bifida occulta.

STUDIES
- Detailed history & physical
- MRI

MANAGEMENT/INTERVENTIONS
- Epidurals are not always contraindicated, but keep in mind several facts:
  - ➤ Spina bifida occulta
    - Pt may have an epidural space that is discontinuous or absent at the level of the lesion & formation of the lamina can be variable, suggesting a theoretical increase in the risk of an unintentional dural puncture.
    - This potential risk is mitigated by:
      - The level of the lesion is most commonly at L5-S1, below the level of placement of the epidural.
      - The most common defect is a midline split in the lamina.
    - There may also be uneven spread of medication in the epidural space, resulting in a patchy block.
  - ➤ Cystica
    - Assess & document pulmonary & neurologic function.
    - Note the presence of a ventriculoperitoneal shunt. Enlist the aid of neurosurgeons if appropriate.
    - Pts w/ a level above T11 may experience painless labor.
    - Pts w/ higher thoracic level involvement (particularly btwn T5–T8) are at risk for autonomic hyperreflexia.
    - Not much is known about epidural anesthesia in pts w/ spina bifida cystica.
    - For pts who already have severe compromise of extremity & sphincter function, the presence of a low-lying or tethered cord should not interfere w/ spinal placement.

CAVEATS/PEARLS
- Successful placement of a spinal or epidural block has been described in the literature, although it is important to recognize that the cord may terminate lower than normal and may be tethered.

■ Spinals & epidurals (with risk of inadvertent dural puncture) are usually contraindicated in pts w/ tethered cord & preserved neurologic function.

■ Inadequate epidural anesthesia & inadvertent dural puncture are more likely in pts w/ discontinuous epidural spaces.

CHECKLIST

■ Complete & thorough understanding of the pt's anatomy, function & comorbidities

■ Neurology or neurosurgical consultation is appropriate in many cases.

SPINAL ANALGESIA

KRISTEN STADTLANDER, MD; MAY PIAN-SMITH, MD; AND LISA LEFFERT, MD

FUNDAMENTAL KNOWLEDGE

See "*Basics of Regional Anesthesia.*"

■ Determinants of the spread of spinal anesthesia

➤ Drug dose

• The larger the dose, the higher the dermatomal level of the block

• Pregnant pts require a 20–30% lower dose of local anesthetic to achieve the same anesthetic level as a non-pregnant patient. Proposed explanations for this observation include:
  • Increased progesterone levels
  • Pregnancy-related changes in diffusion barriers
  • Endogenous analgesia systems

• Drug volume: All things being equal, a larger volume of injectate produces a greater spread of blockade.

• Increased intra-abdominal pressure caused by pregnancy, obesity or ascites impedes venous return in the lower part of the body & forces more blood through the epidural venous system, engorging these vessels. This, in turn, compresses the CSF in the subarachnoid space & forces injected local anesthetic to travel farther.

• Baricity of injectate/position of pt
  • Injected local anesthetics can be hypo-, hyper- or isobaric relative to the specific gravity of CSF (1.003–1.008).
  • To make a hypobaric solution, the anesthetic is mixed w/ sterile water.

- To make a hyperbaric solution, the anesthetic is mixed w/ dextrose.
- The lumbar lordosis (approx. L3,4) & the thoracic kyphosis (approx. T5–6), the baricity of the local anesthetic solution & the pt position interplay to determine the height of the subarachnoid block. There is some variation in the spinal curvature due to the weight of the gravid uterus on the spine.

STUDIES

■ CBC: The literature is insufficient to assess the predictive value of a platelet count for anesthesia complications in parturients w/out comorbid illness or in those w/ pregnancy-induced hypertension.
■ ACOG 1999 Practice Bulletin recommends, "Although limited, data support the safety of epidural anesthesia in patients with platelet counts greater than 100K. In women with gestational thrombocytopenia with platelet counts less than 99K but greater than 50K, epidural anesthesia also may be safe, but its use in such patients will require a consensus among the obstetrician, anesthesiologist, and patient. When platelet counts are less than 50K, epidural anesthesia should not be given."
■ Normal coagulation profile
■ Exam of the area where the spinal will be administered
■ Thorough informed consent w/ full explanation of the procedure & possible complications
■ Detailed history & physical highlighting bleeding abnormalities or pre-anesthetic neurologic deficits
■ Access to FHR monitoring

MANAGEMENT/INTERVENTIONS

■ Equipment necessary to perform spinal anesthesia includes:
  ➤ Monitoring equipment, including BP, pulse oximetry, EKG
  ➤ A functioning IV to facilitate administration of IV fluids & resuscitative medications
  ➤ Airway equipment including a face mask, Ambu bag, oxygen source & emergency intubation equipment & medications
  ➤ Suction device
  ➤ A bed capable of Trendelenburg position
  ➤ A commercial sterile spinal kit & sterile gloves
  ➤ A code cart should be readily available
■ Types of spinal needles

➤ Spinal needles come w/ more rounded tips (pencil point) or sharper tips (cutting needle).

➤ Pencil point needles (e.g., Whitacre/Sprotte) have a blunter tip than the traditional cutting-tip needles. Data suggest that by separating rather than slicing dural fibers, these needles are associated w/ a lower incidence of post-dural puncture headache.

➤ The Quincke is a traditional cutting-tip needle.

➤ Spinal needles come in different lengths & gauges (16–30). The higher the gauge of the spinal needle, the lower the incidence of post-dural puncture headache.

■ Approaches to the subarachnoid space

➤ The lumbar spinous processes project more horizontally than those of the thoracic spine, facilitating access to the subarachnoid space through a midline approach.

➤ In pts w/ prior spinal surgery, scoliosis, osteoporosis or spinal stenosis, a paramedian approach may be useful.

➤ To perform the paramedian approach, palpate the spinous process at the desired level & then direct the needle 2 cm laterally from midline & at a 10- to 20-degree angle toward midline until CSF is obtained. If lamina is encountered, redirect the needle in increments until the needle enters the subarachnoid space.

➤ Pt position for spinal or epidural anesthesia

• Sitting: This position can sometimes facilitate palpation of the midline. It is important to have something for the pt to lean on as she flexes her head & rounds her back ("cooked shrimp"/"cannonball" position).

• Lateral: Some patients cannot sit upright due to pain, instability, obstetric reasons or comorbidities or are simply better able to position themselves laterally. For the lateral position, the pt's knees should be drawn up & her head flexed down onto her chest ("cannonball" position/"fetal" position).

■ Procedure for placing a single-shot spinal anesthetic for labor

➤ Check w/ nurse & OB staff to ensure readiness.

➤ Infuse 250–500 cc LR though functioning IV.

➤ Ensure that monitoring & emergency equipment & medications are available as described above.

➤ Administer 30 cc sodium citrate (Bicitra) orally to the pt.

➤ Have pt assume lateral or sitting position.

➤ Palpate the pt's back to find optimal interspace.

➤ Apply sterile prep & drape (make sure that the Betadine does not contaminate the contents of the spinal kit).

➤ Make sure the spinal needle stylet is fixed properly into the spinal needle.

➤ Use the small-gauge needle to anesthetize the skin & to locate bony landmarks.

➤ Place the large-bore introducer in the desired space.

➤ Place the spinal needle through the introducer & advance until either bone or a gentle pop is felt.

➤ Remove the stylet to confirm the free flow of clear CSF. After bracing one hand against the pt's back & grasping the hub of the spinal needle, use your other hand to gently attach a syringe (most prefer non-Luer-locking type) containing the spinal anesthetic of choice to the spinal needle hub. Confirm proper placement by aspirating CSF into the syringe.

➤ The syringe should fill w/ liquid as more CSF is drawn back into the syringe. If there is difficulty aspirating CSF, recheck your spinal needle positioning. If aspiration is easily accomplished, slowly inject the local anesthetic. Recheck your ability to aspirate CSF once the contents of the syringe are emptied. Many practitioners also advocate checking the ability to aspirate CSF once half of the contents of the syringe have been injected, so that the spinal needle can be repositioned if needed. Next, remove the introducer & spinal needle as a single unit.

➤ Check the BP every 2 minutes for the first 10 minutes. If systolic BP drops by >30%, if the parturient becomes symptomatic or if the FHR becomes non-reassuring in the setting of hypotension, administer IV fluids & 5- to 10-mg doses of ephedrine as needed.

➤ If BP continues to drop, place the pt in Trendelenburg position & establish even more left lateral decubitus displacement, & lift the pt's legs to increase venous return.

➤ If the pt becomes bradycardic, treat w/ ephedrine or atropine or glycopyrrolate if necessary.

➤ Check the level in 2–5 minutes to assess the block's success, keeping in mind that a full level may not be yet apparent.

■ Spinal catheters

➤ Continuous spinal anesthesia (CSA) allows small volumes of local anesthesia to be continuously administered into the subarachnoid space. At one time, small microbore spinal catheters (26–32 gauge) were used for CSA, but they were associated w/ an increased incidence of cauda equina syndrome in the setting of 5% lidocaine use. The FDA has since banned the use of these microbore catheters in the U.S.

➤ Benefits of this technique include titration to the desired level of anesthesia, minimizing significant changes in BP & the potential high block that a single bolus might yield. This technique also allows redosing of the spinal through the catheter should a longer duration of action be needed.

➤ The disadvantages of CSA include a high incidence of spinal headache (with a large-gauge dural hole), the potential for the catheter to act as a route of subarachnoid infection & the potential for nerve trauma, which may be more common than w/ a single-dose spinal anesthetic.

➤ Procedure for placing a spinal catheter
- Enter the subarachnoid space as described using a hollow, large-bore needle (e.g., the epidural needle).
- When free-flowing CSF is confirmed, advance a spinal catheter (i.e., catheter manufactured for epidural use) through the epidural needle 2–4 cm into the space.
- Do not advance further, as knotting of the catheter or passage of the catheter into a dural sleeve has been reported.
- If the catheter cannot be threaded, remove the catheter & epidural needle together. Removing only the catheter can result in the epidural needle bevel shearing off the catheter's tip.
- Aspirate CSF from the catheter to ensure proper placement.
- Place special warning labels on catheter itself & in patient's chart to ensure that epidural doses are not inadvertently administered.

CAVEATS & PEARLS
1. Contraindications to regional anesthesia:
   ➤ Absolute: Pt refusal, uncorrected coagulation disorder, localized infection at proposed injection site, generalized sepsis, increased intracranial pressure, extreme hypovolemia
   ➤ Relative: Demyelinating disease, chronic back pain or lumbar surgery, skin infection close to proposed site, mild hypovolemia, severe aortic or mitral stenosis. Spinals & epidurals have been used safely in some pts w/ demyelinating disease (e.g., multiple sclerosis) & some pts who have undergone back surgery (e.g., laminectomy).
2. Use only preservative-free medications for injection into the subarachnoid space.
3. Always aspirate before injecting local anesthetic to test for presence of blood or CSF.

4. Always carefully monitor for hypotension, bradycardia & impending respiratory or cardiac arrest (in the pt receiving a spinal anesthetic). The ability to flex the elbow indicates that the block has not reached the high cervical dermatomes.

5. Nausea in a pt who has just received a spinal anesthetic can be an early sign of hypotension.

6. If an epidural wet tap occurs, a spinal catheter can be threaded through the epidural needle & CSA used. The spinal catheter can be infused w/ a standard epidural mix (e.g., 0.08–0.125% bupivacaine w/ 2 mcg/mL fentanyl) at 1–3 mL/hr. Special warning labels should be placed on catheter itself & in patient's chart to ensure that epidural doses are not inadvertently administered.

7. If bone is encountered shallowly when attempting to enter the subarachnoid space, it is probably the lower spinous process as it projects out. If bone is encountered deeply, it may be the upper spinous process where it attaches to lamina, or the lamina itself. This information can help guide your spinal needle angle for the next pass.

8. When using a small-gauge spinal needle (e.g., 25 or 26G), the characteristic "pop" may not be felt when the needle passes into the subarachnoid space. If this is the case, withdraw the stylet at regular intervals to check for CSF. It is possible to go through the space & out the dura on the other side.

9. The complications of spinal anesthesia are addressed in "*Troubleshooting/Managing Inadequate Regional Anesthesia.*"

CHECKLIST

1. Before placing a spinal anesthetic, review the contraindications w/ special attention to bleeding disorders/coagulopathies & pre-existing neurologic deficits.

2. Make sure the parturient is monitored using, at minimum, BP & pulse oximetry, & make sure that fetal monitoring is available.

3. Make sure the patient has a functioning IV & is well hydrated. Emergency airway & cardiovascular resuscitation supplies (including pressors & a defibrillator) must be accessible.

4. Aspirate before injecting local anesthetic.

5. Obtain informed consent, including all possible complications of spinal anesthesia (headache; bleeding; infection; nerve, neck, back injury) & the risk of a failed block.

6. Monitor closely for hypotension, high spinal & cardiovascular problems; prompt treatment w/ pressors, hydration & ventilatory support can prevent disastrous complications.

SPINAL CORD INJURY

MEREDITH ALBRECHT, MD
MICHELE SZABO, MD

FUNDAMENTAL KNOWLEDGE

Definition

- Spinal cord injury (SCI) is an insult to the spinal cord resulting in a change, either temporary or permanent, in its normal motor, sensory, or autonomic function.

Epidemiology

- 1,000 new SCIs per year in women age 16 to 30 years
- 50% of SCI in pregnant population are due to motor vehicle accidents.

Pathophysiology

- Caused by primary mechanical or ischemic injury
  - Motor vehicle accidents
  - Falls
  - Gunshot wounds
  - Transverse myelitis
  - Spinal cord hematomas due to spinal vascular abnormalities
- Quadriplegia: injury at or above T1 level
- Paraplegia: injury below T1

Clinical Manifestations of *Acute* Spinal Cord Injury

- Cardiovascular
  - Sympathetic outflow: disrupted below level of lesion
  - Result: generalized vasodilation below lesion leads to hemodynamic shock secondary to SCI
  - Higher spinal lesion has more significant hypotension.
  - BP: very sensitive to hypovolemia & changes in position
  - Lesions above T4 interrupt sympathetic cardio-accelerator nerves.
    - Bradycardia in all pts
    - Reflex tachycardia is absent.
    - 15% of pts w/ cervical lesions experience an asystolic arrest caused by maneuvers that increase unopposed vagal tone.
  - Thermoregulation is impaired.
    - Pts are at increased risk for both hypothermia & hyperthermia.

- Respiratory
  - ➤ SCI produces flaccid paralysis in respiratory muscles below lesion.
  - ➤ Respiratory impairment depends on the level of the lesion.
  - ➤ Lesion above C5 leads to phrenic nerve dysfunction, diaphragmatic paralysis & life-threatening airway emergency.
  - ➤ Flaccid paralysis of the rib cage results in paradoxic chest wall motion & frequently necessitates ventilatory support.
  - ➤ Flaccid paralysis of the abdominal muscles results in impaired cough & inability to clear secretions.
  - ➤ SCI pts have an increased risk of pneumonia; it is the #1 cause of death.
- GI
  - ➤ SCI produces gastric atony.
  - ➤ Consider all pts to have a full stomach.
- Other
  - ➤ Pts are hypercoagulable for 8 weeks following SCI.
  - ➤ Pts are at increased risk for DVT & pulmonary embolism.

Clinical Manifestations of *Chronic* Spinal Cord Injury
- Cardiovascular
  - ➤ Following spinal shock, SCI pts develop compensatory enhancement of renin-angiotensin-aldosterone system, which leads to improved BP.
  - ➤ Therefore, chronic SCI pt is very sensitive to ACE inhibitors.
  - ➤ Some orthostatic hypotension remains; compensation is incomplete.
  - ➤ Thermoregulation remains impaired & pts are at risk for both hypothermia & hyperthermia.
  - ➤ Autonomic dysreflexia (ADR)
    - Occurs in 85% of pts w/ lesion above T6
    - Can produce severe hypertension w/ life-threatening complications
    - Mechanism: SCI disrupts the brain's inhibition of spinal cord sympathetic ganglions
    - Result: exaggerated sympathetic activity in response to noxious stimuli below the level of the spinal cord lesion
    - BP response is variable & degree of variability depends on level of lesion.
    - Symptoms of mild ADR: nausea, nasal congestion, tinnitus

- • Symptoms of severe ADR: headache, blurry vision, profuse sweating & flushing of the face, muscle twitching
- • ADR triggers: any pelvic manipulation, including exam & uterine contractions, urinary catheter manipulation, constipation, decubitus ulcers, abrupt temp changes
- ■ Pulmonary
  - ➤ Pulmonary function improves w/ onset of spastic muscle paralysis.
  - ➤ Pts w/ lesions above T5 continue to have moderate to severe respiratory impairment (vital capacity < 13 mL/kg) & may require ventilatory support during labor.
  - ➤ Most pts continue to have some difficulty clearing secretions & thus remain at increased risk for respiratory infections.
- ■ GU/GI
  - ➤ High incidence of bacteriuria & infection in setting of neurogenic bladder requiring catheterization
  - ➤ Increased incidence of constipation; can lead to ADR
- ■ Dermatologic
  - ➤ Decubitus ulcers occur frequently in pts w/ SCI.
  - ➤ Can result in sepsis & trigger ADR

Effect of pregnancy on SCI
- ■ Cardiovascular
  - ➤ Possible increased risk for ADR w/ increased uterine stimulation, decubitus ulcers & UTIs
- ■ Pulmonary
  - ➤ Further decrease in respiratory reserve
  - ➤ Increased atelectasis
  - ➤ Increased risk for pneumonia
  - ➤ Reserve may not be sufficient to keep up w/ increased demands of labor.
- ■ Dermatologic
  - ➤ Increased risk for decubitus ulcer w/ increased weight & poorly fit wheelchair
- ■ Hematologic
  - ➤ Increased risk for anemia
  - ➤ Anemia contributes to development of decubitus ulcers.
  - ➤ Debate whether chronic SCI pt is at increased risk for thromboembolic complications
  - ➤ Most agree that *acute* SCI pregnant pt is at greatly increased risk for thromboembolic complications; pts protected w/ either

anticoagulation or IVC filter (as uterus enlarges, risk of complication from procedure to place IVC filter increases)
- Urogenital
  - ➤ Increased risk for UTI; bladder catheterization becomes more difficult as pregnancy progresses

Effect on pregnancy & fetus
- Spinal cord injury antecedent to pregnancy
  - ➤ No increased risk of congenital malformations
  - ➤ No increased risk of intrauterine fetal death
  - ➤ Lesion above T11: possible risk of preterm labor
  - ➤ At risk for unattended delivery because nociceptive pathway for uterine contractions is absent
- Traumatic spinal cord injury during pregnancy
  - ➤ Increased risk for spontaneous abortion
  - ➤ Increased risk for fetal malformation
  - ➤ Increased risk for fetal injury
  - ➤ Increased risk for abruptio placentae
  - ➤ At risk for unattended delivery because nociceptive pathway for uterine contractions is absent
- During labor, ADR can result in:
  - ➤ Uteroplacental vasoconstriction
  - ➤ Fetal hypoxia & bradycardia

STUDIES
History & Physical
- Airway: determine neck safety & mobility if cervical lesion present
- Cardiac: evaluate for symptoms & history of ADR, presence of spinal shock in setting of acute injury
- Pulmonary: evaluate respiratory reserve & evidence of pneumonia
- Skin: exam for evidence of decubiti
- Neurologic: take a complete history of the neurologic injury, do physical exam & determine sensory & motor level of injury

Imaging
- Chest radiograph
- If history incomplete, consider spine radiograph to determine anatomy & location of instrumentation.
  - ➤ Shield fetus for cervical x-ray.
  - ➤ PA to decrease fetal radiation exposure for lumbar film

Other

- Obtain baseline & serial pulmonary function tests in pts w/ spinal lesion above T5.
- Obtain baseline ABGs in pts w/ spinal lesion above T5.
- CBC to detect or determine level of anemia
- Urinalysis to rule out UTI
- Cr: determine CRI due to recurrent UTIs

MANAGEMENT/INTERVENTIONS

Acute SCI During Pregnancy

- Immobilization of the spinal cord is the overriding principle!
- CPR key to prevent secondary spinal neurologic injury
  - ➤ Aggressive fluid resuscitation
  - ➤ Pressor support to keep SBP ≥ 90–100 mm Hg to maintain spinal cord blood flow
  - ➤ Consider direct measurement of pulmonary capillary wedge pressure for cervical lesions; pts at increased risk for pulmonary edema
  - ➤ Maintain oxygenation.
  - ➤ Maintain high index of suspicion for internal hemorrhage.
- High-dose steroids are ideally given within 3 hours of injury & up to 8 hours following injury; evidence exists this improves long-term neurologic outcome.
  - ➤ Bolus methylprednisolone 30 mg/kg over 15 minutes
  - ➤ Administer methylprednisolone 5.4 mg/kg over the next 23 hours.
- Consider anticoagulation for 8 weeks once pt stabilized or place IVC filter.

Chronic Spinal Cord Injury

- Mgt w/ spinal or epidural primarily aimed at preventing ADR in susceptible pts
- Prophylactic antibiotics for UTIs, frequent cultures
- Topical anesthesia for bladder catheterization
- Stool softeners & high-fiber diet to prevent constipation & ADR
- Prophylactic administration of nifedipine or terazosin to reduce incidence of ADR
- Uterine activity monitoring as per OB

Acute mgt of ADR

- First step: remove offending stimulus if possible
  - ➤ Regional dose anesthetic if in place

➤ May need to expedite delivery w/ forceps

➤ C-section if medical therapy ineffective

■ Antihypertensives

➤ IV nitroprusside or hydralazine

➤ Sublingual nitroglycerin 0.3–0.6 mg or nifedipine 10–20 mg

➤ Terazosin 1–10 mg orally

Anesthesia

■ Consider continuous hemodynamic monitoring w/ EKG, pulse oximetry & arterial line in acute injuries & in injuries at or above T5 level.

■ Adequate hydration key to hemodynamic stability for all pts w/ SCI; highly susceptible to hypotension

■ Closely monitor body temp.

■ Foley catheter: insertion during labor under epidural to avoid bladder distention

■ Change pt position q2h to prevent decubiti.

■ Consider ventilatory assistance during labor for pts w/ VC <13 mL/kg.

■ General anesthesia

➤ May be preferable or required in pts w/ significantly reduced respiratory reserve

➤ Alternative for pts where regional anesthesia is technically difficult to establish

➤ Increased likelihood of difficult airway w/ fused cervical spine or if pt is in halo apparatus; use fiberoptic scope to intubate

➤ Avoid succinylcholine if spinal cord injury >24 hours, as its use can produce profound hyperkalemia & cardiac arrest.

■ Regional anesthesia

➤ Preferred for the prevention or treatment of ARD

➤ Epidural anesthesia should be instituted at the onset of labor.

➤ Ideally, maintain sensory level of at least T10 (although dense surgical level is not necessarily required).

➤ Motor/sensory level difficult to assess unless it is cephalad to level of lesion

➤ Choice of volume/dose of local anesthetic & insertion of block may be technically challenging due to anatomic distortion by injury or fusion.

CAVEATS & PEARLS

■ SCI, either acute or chronic, has the potential to produce profound cardiovascular & respiratory effects.

- ADR is the most significant complication; prevent & treat aggressively.
- May be difficult to distinguish ADR from preeclampsia
  - Reported that w/ ADR, hypertension develops rapidly w/ uterine contraction & dissipates during diastole
- Multidisciplinary team should develop an intrapartum care plan aimed at prevention & treatment of ADR; for example:
  - Epidural anesthesia T10 sensory level or higher should be established at onset of labor to prevent ADR in susceptible pts
  - Foley insertion to prevent bladder distention
  - Change position & examine skin q2h.
  - Avoid exposure to cold stirrups.
- Meticulously monitor hemodynamic & respiratory parameters.
- Do not use succinylcholine.
- Pts have fixed flexion contractures that often make IV access difficult to establish.
- Pts may be unaware of painful stimuli such as labor or abruption.

CHECKLIST
- Immediate availability of appropriate pressors & antihypertensive agents at bedside
- Immediate availability of airway equipment & mechanical ventilation in pts w/ cervical or high thoracic lesions
- Anticipate more difficult airway, so have intubating aids available: gum elastic bougie, various direct laryngoscopy blades & tube sizes & fiberoptic scope.
- Adequate hydration is key to hemodynamic stability.
- Monitor body temp.
- Do not use succinylcholine.
- Consider spinal/epidural if spinal cord injury level higher than T6 to avoid ADR.

STROKE

MEREDITH ALBRECHT, MD
MICHELE SZABO, MD

FUNDAMENTAL KNOWLEDGE

Definition
- Sudden disruption of blood flow to the brain

■ Subtypes: ischemic stroke, hemorrhagic stroke & cortical venous sinus thrombosis

Epidemiology
■ Not well understood
■ Estimate: 5–15 per 100,000 deliveries
■ General risk factors
  ➤ Smoking history
  ➤ Higher parity
  ➤ Advanced maternal age
  ➤ Non-white race
  ➤ Presence of other medical problems: infections, hypertension, pre-eclampsia & acid-base abnormalities
■ Specific risk factors & causes of stroke (similar to causes of stroke in the young)
  ➤ Vasculopathy
    • Intracranial aneurysm (see section on "Intracranial Aneurysms")
    • Arteriovenous malformations (see section on "Arteriovenous Malformations")
    • Venous thrombosis (see section on "Central Venous Thrombosis")
    • Arterial dissection
    • Atherosclerosis
    • Vasculitis
    • SLE
    • Arterial dissection
    • Tay-Sachs disease
    • Moya-moya
    • Migraine
  ➤ Embolism
    • Fat or air embolism, paradoxical embolus
    • Peripartum cardiomyopathy
    • Atrial fibrillation
    • Endocarditis
  ➤ Hematologic disorders
    • Sickle cell anemia
    • Anticardiolipin & lupus anticoagulant
    • Polycythemia
    • Factor V Leiden mutation
    • Protein S, C or antithrombin III deficiency

- Antiphospholipid antibodies
- Thrombotic thrombocytopenic purpura
➤ Cocaine use

Clinical Manifestations

■ Symptoms vary & depend on the type & location of stroke in the brain. Symptoms, usually of abrupt onset, include:
➤ Headache
➤ Nausea & vomiting
➤ Focal neurologic deficit
➤ Blurred vision
➤ Altered sensorium, including unconsciousness
➤ Seizure

Effect of pregnancy on stroke

■ Widely believed that pregnancy increases risk for stroke
■ Few data available to quantify the risk
■ Highest occurrence around time of delivery & post-partum
■ Similar time distribution to pregnancy-induced hypercoagulable state
■ Rare pregnancy-specific causes of stroke include:
➤ Eclampsia
➤ Choriocarcinoma
➤ Amniotic fluid embolism
➤ Peripartum cardiomyopathy
■ Maternal mortality reported 5–38%
■ 42–63% of pts will have residual neurologic deficit.

Effect on pregnancy & fetus

■ Increased risk of fetal mortality
■ Possible teratogenic & carcinogenic effects of radiation during diagnostic testing
■ Possible teratogenic effects of drug therapy

STUDIES

History & Physical

■ Obtain neurologic history & presenting symptoms of the stroke.
■ Determine history of risk factors: smoking, hypertension, drug use.
■ Determine seizure history.
■ Neurologic
➤ Mental status exam
➤ Examine for focal neurologic deficits.

- Cardiac
  - Assess for signs of cardiac failure, presence of patent foramen ovale.
  - Rhythm or rate disturbance
- Ophthalmologic
  - Papilledema (sign of increased ICP)
  - Vascular irregularities, resulting from vasculitis
- Skin
  - Examine for evidence for emboli.
  - Livido reticularis
  - Signs of connective tissue disorder

Imaging
- Do not avoid appropriate diagnostic testing because of perceived risk to fetus, as stroke can be life-threatening or produce significant neurologic deficit.
- CT scan
  - Usually initial diagnostic procedure of choice for pregnant pt
  - Appropriately shielded fetus, safe radiation exposure
- CT angiography
  - Ideal method to identify suspected vascular lesions
  - Avoids complications of invasive angiography
  - Contrast dye does not cross placenta, physiologically inert; considered safe for fetus
  - Contrast dye is a diuretic, so hydrate pt well.
  - Shield fetus from radiation exposure.
- Cerebral angiography
  - Shielded fetus, safe radiation exposure
  - Contrast agents pose little risk for fetus.
  - Hydrate well to prevent maternal & fetal dehydration; contrast dye is a diuretic.
- MRI
  - No long-term data on fetal outcome
  - MRI generally avoided during 1st trimester
  - MRI contrast agent, gadolinium, crosses the placenta.
  - No reported adverse effects of fetal exposure to gadolinium
  - Nevertheless, most advise against contrast use during pregnancy unless clinically necessary (its use is not FDA approved for this purpose).
- Cardiac echo: Assess LV function, intracardiac thrombosis, valvular disease; rule out patent foramen ovale

Other
- Guided by history & physical
- May include other diagnostic studies for potential etiology, such as screen for hypercoagulable disorders, ANA, cardiac echo
- PT/PTT or anti-factor Xa assay for anticoagulated pts
- Platelets for pt on heparin, HIT antibody if heparin-induced thrombocytopenia is suspected
- Serum anticonvulsant level

MANAGEMENT/INTERVENTIONS
- Stabilize pt.
- Treat hypotension & hypoxia aggressively.
  - Even mild hypotension &/or hypoxia dramatically worsen neurologic outcome.
- Determine stroke type & etiology.
- Goal of stroke treatment is to minimize neural damage w/o excessive maternal or fetal risk.
- Thrombolytics/endovascular procedures: for acute ischemic stroke care
  - IV tPA
    - Used for treatment of pt within 3 hours of symptom onset
    - Pregnancy is considered a contraindication to IV tPa, but there are case reports of therapeutic success w/o adverse fetal outcomes w/ IV or intra-arterial thrombolysis.
    - Maternal bleeding complication rate 1–6%; no different from non-pregnant population
- Anticoagulants & anti-thrombotics are mainstay of ischemic stroke prevention
  - Unfractionated heparin
    - Titrated to target a therapeutic PTT
    - Increased risk of osteoporosis after long-term (>1 month) administration
    - Can produce heparin-induced thrombocytopenia
    - No teratogenic effects have been reported, but no direct studies have been performed.
    - Not excreted in breast milk
  - Low-molecular-weight heparin
    - Anti-factor Xa assays used for dosage adjustment
    - Animal studies: no teratogenicity
    - Not excreted in breast milk
    - Less risk of osteoporosis

- Time to peak & half-life shorter in pregnancy, so BID dose is recommended
- Often used throughout pregnancy.
- Consider converting from low-molecular-weight heparin to dose-adjusted, subQ unfractionated heparin at 36 weeks or earlier in the event of preterm labor.

➤ Coumadin
  - Readily crosses the placenta
    - Potential to cause bleeding in the fetus
    - Established teratogenicity
    - Not recommended for use during pregnancy

➤ Aspirin
  - No known teratogenicity
  - Adverse effects limit its use during later part of gestation.
    - Associated w/ decreased birthweight
    - Increased rate of stillbirth
    - Platelet dysfunction described in newborns, resulting in CNS hemorrhage
    - Possible premature closure of PDA
  - Low dose (81 mg) sometimes used

➤ Clopidogrel
  - Inhibits platelet aggregation
  - Thought to be a safe & effective alternative to aspirin

■ Neurosurgical treatment as indicated for aneurysms, AVMs & intracerebral hemorrhage

■ Endovascular treatment as indicated for aneurysms, AVMs & for treatment of venous thrombosis

Anesthesia

■ Discussion regarding pts w/ thrombotic or embolic strokes below

■ Anesthesia for pts w/ intracranial vascular disease discussed elsewhere

■ Balance btwn sufficient coagulation for regional anesthesia & delivery vs. re-thrombosis

■ Regional anesthesia is often appropriate if pt is not coagulopathic.
  ➤ Many centers advocate changing to dose0adjusted unfractionated subQ heparin at 36 weeks or in the event of threatened preterm delivery.
  ➤ Hold morning dose of unfractionated heparin when induction of labor or C-section is planned. Check coagulation studies (PTT).

➤ Hold LMWH for 24 hours prior to regional technique.
  • If uncertainty exists, measure anti-factor Xa activity. If present, most would advocate not doing regional anesthetic.
➤ Frequent neurologic exams are required for early detection of epidural hematoma following regional technique.
■ General anesthesia is indicated for C-section in the presence of increased ICP.
➤ Succinylcholine is contraindicated in presence of motor neurologic deficits >24 hours' duration as it can cause significant hyperkalemia & cardiac arrest.
➤ If pt has upper extremity motor deficit, monitor TOF on unaffected side as affected side will show resistance to neuromuscular blockade.
➤ Pts on anticonvulsants will have accelerated metabolism of nondepolarizing relaxants.
➤ If ICP is elevated, maintain adequate CPP by increasing MAP & lowering ICP.
➤ Arterial line for blood pressure monitoring
➤ "Modified" rapid sequence induction w/ rocuronium & pentothal or propofol
➤ Hyperventilate pt prior to delivery of fetus only if ICP elevation is life-threatening.
  • Adverse fetal effects can be minimized w/ adequate maternal hydration & minimizing increases in maternal airway pressure.
➤ Mannitol
  • Indicated if ICP elevation is severe
  • Effective for mother; can cause fetal hypovolemia
  • Be prepared for fluid resuscitation of the newborn.
➤ Plan anesthetic for a prompt emergence that permits early neurologic exam
➤ Treat narcotic-induced depression in fetus w/ naloxone or respiratory support.
■ In setting of an acute ischemic stroke, hypotension may worsen neurologic injury. Treat aggressively during both regional or general anesthesia.

CAVEATS & PEARLS
■ Stroke is rare but contributes significantly to maternal & fetal mortality.
■ Acute stroke is a medical emergency.
  ➤ Thrombolysis ASAP ("Time is Brain")

➤ Concurrent w/ resuscitation
■ Do not delay diagnosis or therapy.
■ Differentiate from eclampsia.
  ➤ Different treatment
  ➤ Presumption of eclampsia delays diagnosis of stroke in 41% of pts.
  ➤ MRI w/ diffusion-weighted imaging can be used to identify a stroke if present.
■ Obtain thorough neurologic history & document baseline neurologic exam.
■ Perform frequent neurologic assessment as indicated.
  ➤ During labor & delivery
  ➤ Following C-section
  ➤ If change in neurologic status, contact neurologist.
  ➤ Change in neurologic status may indicate development of new thrombosis.
■ Check for normalization of coagulation status prior to regional technique.
■ Identify & inform the pt's neurologist of your anesthetic plans. Determine most efficient means of emergency communication.

CHECKLIST
■ Identify pt's neurologist & mechanism of contact.
■ Hold anticoagulants & check for normalization of coagulation studies prior to regional technique or C-section.
■ Perform frequent neurologic exams to detect worsening neurologic status.
■ Have pressors readily available to treat hypotension in the setting of acute stroke.

STURGE-WEBER SYNDROME

MEREDITH ALBRECHT, MD
MICHELE SZABO, MD

FUNDAMENTAL KNOWLEDGE
Definition/Epidemiology:
■ Rare, congenital vascular disorder of unknown etiology

Clinical Manifestations

- Characteristic features: facial port-wine stain & leptomeningeal angioma. Only a small percentage of children w/ port-wine stains have Sturge-Weber syndrome.
- Neurologic features of Sturge-Weber are variable in severity & include seizures, focal neurologic deficits & mental retardation.

Pathophysiology

- Ipsilateral leptomeningeal angioma occurs in 10–20% of cases when a typical face lesion is present. The parietal & occipital areas are affected most commonly (typically on the same side as the facial lesion). Rarely does leptomeningeal angiomatosis occur w/o the facial angioma.

Effects of Pregnancy on Sturge-Weber:

- Parturients w/ Sturge-Weber are rare.

Effects of Sturge-Weber on Pregnancy:

- Parturients w/ Sturge-Weber are rare.

STUDIES

- MRI w/ gadolinium is preferred modality to demonstrate the extent of involvement of the brain.

MANAGEMENT/INTERVENTIONS

- Prognosis depends on the extent of the leptomeningeal angioma as well as the severity of ocular involvement, the age of onset of seizures & whether they can be controlled.
- Neurologic function may deteriorate w/ age.

CAVEATS/PEARLS

- Rare, congenital vascular disorder of unknown etiology
- Neurologic features of Sturge-Weber are variable in severity & include seizures, focal neurologic deficits & mental retardation.
- Parturients w/ Sturge-Weber are rare. Few published data exist.

CHECKLIST

- MRI w/ gadolinium is preferred modality to demonstrate the extent of involvement of the brain.

SUBSTANCE ABUSE

HUMAYON KHAN, MD
JYOTSNA NAGDA, MD

FUNDAMENTAL KNOWLEDGE

- Incidence of substance abuse during pregnancy has been steadily increasing over the past decade.
- Nearly 90% of substance-abusing women are of child-bearing age.
- Illicit substances most commonly abused in pregnancy: alcohol, tobacco, cocaine, marijuana, opioids, caffeine, amphetamines, hallucinogens, solvents
- Identifying these pts is extremely important because they can present a host of challenges to obstetricians, obstetric anesthesiologists & neonatologists.
- One of the most important characteristics of these pts is that they may not have any antenatal care, may appear rather cavalier to their state of health & are frequently in the state of denial of the substance abuse. Hence a high index of suspicion is necessary.
- This chapter reviews commonly abused drugs & substances during pregnancy & their effect on anesthetic mgt.

Cigarette Smoking

- 20–30% of pregnant females continue to smoke during pregnancy. Low cigarette consumption before pregnancy is the best predictor of smoking cessation during pregnancy.
- Smoking during pregnancy has been associated w/ spontaneous abortion, ectopic pregnancy, IUGR, increased risk of PROM, placenta previa, abruptio placentae, preterm delivery, sudden infant death syndrome, bronchitis, pneumonia, chronic middle ear infections & asthma.
- Nicotine causes vasoconstriction & hence decreases in placental blood flow, oxygen delivery leading to fetal distress.
- Several longitudinal studies have shown 4–5× increased risk of conduct disorder in boys & adolescent-onset drug dependence in girls whose mothers smoked 10 or more cigarettes a day.
- Smoking cessation interventions include counseling sessions & behavioral interventions. Self-help groups have been shown to be effective in 60–70% of pregnant pts. Pharmacotherapy is used for heavy smokers. First-line agents: bupropion, nicotine gum, nicotine inhaler, nasal spray & patch. Second-line medication: clonidine.

Safety & efficacy of these treatments for pregnant smokers remain unknown.

Anesthetic Management

- Neuroaxial anesthesia is preferred in active smokers unless contraindicated.
- These pts are at increased risk of laryngospasm & post-op pulmonary complications if general anesthesia is used.
- 4–6 weeks of abstinence from smoking is recommended to decrease post-op respiratory morbidity if general anesthesia becomes the only choice.
- Even 2 days of smoking cessation will decrease levels of carboxyhemoglobin levels in blood. Carbon monoxide has 200x affinity for oxygen compared to hemoglobin.
- Chronic smoking can also lead to alteration in the hepatic microsomal enzymes system, which may affect the dose of induction agents & the maintenance infusions.

Alcohol

- 15 million people in the U.S. are addicted to alcohol & women make up 25% of this number.
- In a pregnant female, heavy alcohol consumption can lead to poor nutrition, liver disease, coagulopathy, pancreatitis, cardiomyopathy, esophageal varices, altered drug metabolism.
- Alcohol has been linked to fetal alcohol syndrome, first described in France in 1968. The prevalence of FAS is 10–50% among the offspring of moderate to heavy drinkers (1–2 oz of absolute alcohol per day). The diagnosis is based on following 4 criteria, all of which must be present:
  - ➤ Prenatal alcohol consumption
  - ➤ Growth restriction
  - ➤ Facial malformation (ie, short palpebral fissures, thin upper lip, abnormal philtrum, hypoplastic midface)
  - ➤ Neurodevelopmental disorder
- Long-term problems include dental misalignment, malocclusion, myopia, eustachian tube dysfunction, deficits in language, decreased IQ, hyperactivity & attention deficit disorder. Cardiovascular, GU & musculoskeletal abnormalities can also be present.

Anesthetic management

- Neuroaxial anesthesia can be safely used unless contraindicated (eg, coagulopathy, neuropathy, infection, pt refusal).

- Pts are at increased risk of aspiration, so aspiration precautions (eg, metoclopramide, sodium citrate, cricoid pressure) must be used for general anesthesia.
- Presence of hepatic dysfunction, hypoalbuminemia & cardiac failure will require appropriate dose adjustments of induction agents & need for invasive monitoring.
- Acute alcohol withdrawal usually presents within 6–48 hours of abstinence but can be delayed for as long as 10 days. Signs & symptoms of withdrawal are nausea, vomiting, hypertension, tachycardia, dysrhythmias, delirium, hallucinations, seizures & cardiac failure.

Opioids

- Opioid abuse & addiction in a pregnant pt can have multiple implications for both mother & fetus. Numerous medical problems such as cellulitis, skin abscesses, septic thrombophlebitis, AIDS, hepatitis, endocarditis & malnutrition are encountered in an opioid-addicted pt. Abuse of other substances, absence of prenatal care & HIV-positive status has high predictive value.
- Opioid-abusing pts may present w/ dysphoria, bizarre behavior, slow breathing & meiotic pupils. The ability to protect the airway may be compromised & risk of aspiration is greatly increased. These pts can also present w/ opioid withdrawal symptoms, including lacrimation, rhinorrhea, sweating, tachycardia, diarrhea, tachypnea, hypertension, restlessness, dehydration & insomnia.

Perinatal outcome

- Opiate-dependent pregnant women experience significant increases in obstetrical complications, such as:
  - ➤ Preeclampsia
  - ➤ 3rd-trimester bleeding
  - ➤ Fetal distress
  - ➤ Malpresentation
  - ➤ Passage of meconium
  - ➤ Low birthweight
  - ➤ Perinatal mortality
  - ➤ Puerperal morbidity
  - ➤ Neonatal opioid withdrawal

Methadone maintenance

- Methadone maintenance has been used to treat pregnant opiate addicts for nearly 30 years. It is usually given once daily. It offers a unique opportunity to bring women into the medical & obstetric care systems. It offers overwhelming advantages (eg, oral administration, known dose & purity, safe & steady availability) when compared to medical detoxification. It provides a stable nutritional & social environment, decreases the risk of infectious complications in the mother & fetus & reduces the problems of cyclic intrauterine fetal withdrawal, chronic fetal hypoxia & intrauterine death.

■ Methadone maintenance does not prevent neonatal abstinence syndrome, which must be treated diligently if signs & symptoms of withdrawal develop. Buprenophine, a partial agonist, may offer an advantage over methadone maintenance as it may decrease the risk of neonatal abstinence syndrome.

Anesthetic management

■ Treat symptoms of withdrawal w/ clonidine (alpha agonist), doxepin or diphenhydramine.

■ Opioids should be continued throughout labor to prevent acute withdrawal. These pts may have increased opioid requirements, manifesting tolerance.

■ If increased doses of opioids are used, monitor respiratory status.

■ Neuroaxial anesthesia is safe in these pts, but they are at increased risk of spinal, epidural & disc space infections.

■ If general anesthesia becomes unavoidable, use of NMDA antagonists (eg, methadone, ketamine) is warranted to decrease opioid tolerance & obtain optimal pain control during C-section.

■ Recent studies indicate that naltrexone implants are safe in pregnant pts who abuse heroin.

■ Rapid opioid detoxification under general anesthesia, which is becoming a popular technique to suppress withdrawal symptoms, has not been tried in pregnant pts.

Marijuana

■ Marijuana is the most commonly used illicit substance taken during pregnancy. It is a naturally occurring substance obtained from the plant *Cannabis sativa*. Marijuana is smoked for its hallucinogenic properties. Of 61 known cannabinoids, delta-9-tetrahydrocannabinol (THC) is the most potent psychoactive agent & is extremely important in the recreational use of cannabis.

■ The effects of acute marijuana use include euphoria, tachycardia, conjunctival congestion & anxiety. The pt may present a host of symptoms as the pharmacologic effects of marijuana are complex & include a unique blend of effects of alcohol, opioids, tranquilizers &

hallucinogens. Therefore, the clinical picture can be unpredictable & the diagnosis is often difficult. A high level of suspicion is necessary.

■ THC freely crosses the placenta & directly affects the fetus. Chronic use of marijuana during pregnancy can lead to following complications:

➤ IUGR

➤ Decreased uteroplacental perfusion

➤ Alteration in pituitary-adrenal axis & hormone production, adversely affecting fertility & pregnancy

➤ Increased incidence of bronchitis, squamous metaplasia, emphysema, oropharyngitis & uvular edema, leading to airway obstruction during general anesthesia

➤ Delayed cognitive development in infants

➤ Preterm labor

➤ Sudden infant death syndrome

➤ Smaller head circumferences

Anesthetic management

➤ Neuroaxial anesthesia is preferred.

➤ Marijuana can be a cardiovascular stimulant at moderate doses & myocardial depressant at high doses, so induction & maintenance anesthetic agents should be carefully titrated.

➤ If possible, avoid agents such as atropine, pancuronium, ketamine, epinephrine, propanolol & physostigmine because the risk of extreme tachycardia & bradycardia & reversible ST-segment & T-wave abnormalities.

➤ Airway exam should also document the presence of oropharyngitis & uvular edema to avoid airway catastrophe. Backup airway equipment should always be available, including cricothyroidotomy kits.

Cocaine

■ Cocaine, a local anesthetic, was introduced to modern medicine in 1884. It is derived from the *Erythroxylum coca* plant, a small tree native to the mountainous regions of Bolivia, Peru, Ecuador & Brazil. Crack cocaine is an alkalinized form of cocaine that is widely smoked throughout the world.

■ Cocaine produces prolonged adrenergic stimulation by blocking the presynaptic uptake of norepinephrine, dopamine & serotonin. This can lead to life-threatening hypertension, tachycardia & vasoconstriction. Myocardial ischemia &/or infarction, malignant arrhythmias & rupture of aorta can also occur, although these are less frequent. Other signs & symptoms of cocaine abuse include tremors, seizures, hyperreflexia, fever, dilated pupils, emotional instability, proteinuria & edema. These symptoms may suggest pre-eclampsia, which can be differentiated by the absence of liver abnormalities, normal kidney function & the presence of positive urine toxicology for cocaine.

■ There is some evidence that chronic cocaine use during pregnancy can lead to thrombocytopenia, so obtaining a platelet count before performing regional anesthesia may be advisable.

■ Cocaine is rapidly transferred across the placenta by simple diffusion. It has the following deleterious effects on the fetus & the pregnant woman:

➤ IUGR
➤ Fetal distress
➤ Placental abruption presenting as hemodynamic instability & tender uterus
➤ Uterine rupture
➤ Preterm labor
➤ Cardiac arrhythmias
➤ Cerebral infarction
➤ Hepatic rupture
➤ Learning & language difficulties & decreased IQ scores in children
➤ Congenital anomalies in urogenital tract

Anesthetic Management

■ Both regional & general anesthesia can be associated w/ serious complications during pregnancy.

■ If regional anesthesia is used, issues such as combative behavior, altered pain perception, cocaine-induced thrombocytopenia & ephedrine-resistant hypotension may be encountered. Obtaining a platelet count is advisable before neuroaxial anesthesia is attempted. Use of epinephrine is recommended early if high spinal anesthesia is threatened.

■ A slow, controlled epidural anesthesia may be the best option for a pt w/ a history of cocaine abuse. It would avoid the complications of both spinal anesthesia (high spinal) & general anesthesia (myocardial ischemia, infarction, cardiac arrhythmias, hypotension & hypertension).

■ Before any operative procedure, obtain type & cross-matched blood, as these pts can have underlying placental abruption or partial uterine rupture, necessitating aggressive blood transfusion.

- Treat hypotension w/ phenylephrine, as these pts may be resistant to indirect-acting vasopressor, ephedrine.
- Manage hypertension w/ either hydralazine or labetalol. Avoid pure beta-blockers like propanolol to reduce the risk of unopposed alpha-mediated vasoconstriction.
- Avoid halothane & isoflurane. Use sevoflurane if general anesthesia is required.
- Avoid ketamine, as it will act synergistically w/ cocaine, potentiating the cardiac side affects.
- Prolonged block from succinylcholine in a pt w/ a history of cocaine abuse has been reported.
- Nitroglycerin has been reported safe & effective for chest pain associated w/ cocaine ingestion.
- Invasive monitoring w/ arterial line & Swan-Ganz catheter may be warranted.

Amphetamines

- Amphetamines are a group of noncatecolamine sympathomimetic drugs that resemble norepinephrine. They can be abused individually or in conjunction w/ other CNS stimulants such as cocaine. They can be used orally or IV (methamphetamine) or smoked (crystal metamphetamine).
- Ecstasy or MDMA (3,4 methylene-dioxymethamphetamine) is an analog of methamphetamine that shares properties w/ amphetamines & hallucinogenic drugs. It has become tremendously popular in young adults.
- Ecstasy users tend to be young & single, w/ a higher rate of unplanned pregnancies & therapeutic abortions. They report frequent psychological morbidity combined w/ heavy alcohol consumption, binge drinking, cigarette use & concurrent illicit drug use.
- Amphetamine ingestion leads to increased release of norepinephrine from presynaptic terminals, which can present as hypertension, tachycardia, arrhythmias, dilated pupils, hyperreflexia, fever, proteinuria, agitation, confusion & seizures. Signs & symptoms closely resemble those of cocaine.
- Fetal & infant deaths have been associated w/ methamphetamine abuse, as well as strokes in pregnant females. Profound disturbances of thermoregulation (heat stroke) leading to death may result from MDMA use.
- Amphetamines taken during pregnancy can have the following adverse outcomes for the mother & baby:

➤ Cleft lip & palate
➤ Cardiac anomalies
➤ IUGR
➤ Biliary atresia
➤ Intrauterine fetal demise
➤ Cerebral hemorrhage
➤ Placental abruption & fetal distress can be secondary to an IV injection of amphetamines.

Anesthetic management

■ Regional anesthesia is preferred.
■ If general anesthesia becomes unavoidable because of placental abruption or fetal distress, avoid halothane.
■ Typed & cross-matched blood should be available immediately.
■ Acute intake of amphetamines increases the MAC of volatile inhalational agents.
■ Chronic ingestion of amphetamines decreases the dose of anesthetic agents.
■ Use of direct cardiovascular stimulants is recommended for intraoperative hypotension, such as epinephrine, phenylephrine or isoproterenol.

Solvents

■ Inhalants are the most easily obtainable substances for illicit use. They include a chemically diverse group of substances, including organic solvents & volatile agents that affect the CNS.
■ Solvents may be used orally or sniffed from open containers, bags or soaked rags. Toluene, an industrial solvent, is a major component in many household paints & cleaning agents. Chronic inhalation of toluene-based solvents can result in cerebellar degeneration & diffuse brain atrophy. Disturbances in cardiac function, ventricular fibrillation & myocardial infarction have been reported w/ toluene sniffing. Acute respiratory distress syndrome, increased airway resistance, pulmonary hypertension & liver toxicity have also been described in parturients exposed to solvents. Glue sniffing can cause distal & proximal tubular acidosis.
■ Abuse of solvents can lead to following complications during pregnancy:
➤ IUGR
➤ Preterm labor
➤ Prenatal death
➤ Augmentation of fetal alcohol syndrome

➤ Inconclusive evidence of toluene embryopathy & fetal solvent syndrome

Anesthetic management

■ A complete neurologic exam is mandatory before performing neuroaxial anesthesia, as these pts may have motor or sensory deficits.

■ Manage any hemodynamic instability expeditiously. Take it seriously.

Hallucinogens

■ These include substances taken orally such as lysergic acid diethylamide (LSD), phencyclidine (PCP), psilocybin & mescaline. They cause visual, auditory & tactile hallucinations w/ distortion of surroundings & body image. Despite high psychological dependence, there appears to be no evidence of physical dependence or withdrawal symptoms when these substances are discontinued acutely.

■ Clinical presentation
➤ Activation of sympathetic nervous system w/ increase in body temp, tachycardia, hypertension, mydriasis
➤ Psychological symptoms like anxiety, panic attacks & hallucinations
➤ Seizures & apnea may occur rarely w/ LSD.

■ Prenatal exposure is associated w/ following complications:
➤ IUGR
➤ Preterm labor & delivery
➤ Meconium staining
➤ Fetal heat-induced neurologic injury

Anesthetic management

■ Important issues
➤ Precipitation of panic response w/ anesthesia & surgery
➤ Exaggerated response to symapthomimetic agents
➤ Analgesic & ventilatory effects of the opioid may be prolonged
➤ Action of succinylcholine may be prolonged in some cases w/ PCP & LSD.

Other substances

■ **Caffeine**, although it has the theoretical disadvantage of causing vasoconstriction, uteroplacental insufficiency & IUGR, has not been found to have a significant effect on birthweight. >600 mg (>5 cups of coffee per day) can lead to small infants. Regional anesthesia can be safely used in parturients w/ high caffeine intake. Withdrawal headaches respond well to acetaminophen.

Benzodiazepines

- Benzodiazepines are the most commonly prescribed sedative-hypnotic meds in the world. Their use in pregnancy have raised concerns that they may be associated w/ a high incidence of cleft lip & palate, but in reality it is very unlikely to occur because most of the studies involved experiments in which animals were exposed to very high doses of benzodiazepines during pregnancy. There is some evidence that their use may increase the incidence of anal atresia, but again more studies are needed to evaluate the effects of benzodiazepines during pregnancy.
- Regional anesthesia can be safely used in pts w/ a history of benzodiazepine abuse, but withdrawal symptoms including delirium, seizures & tremors should be managed expeditiously.

STUDIES

- **Ontrak TesTcup**
  A very simple test; costs only $20. An anesthesiologist can complete it in <5 minutes. This test has high sensitivity & specificity & can be used in any hospital setting. It is quick & reliable & gives a qualitative assay of various illicit substances.
- **Maternal & fetal urine toxicology**
  Gas chromatography or mass spectrometry can be performed on maternal or fetal urine to determine the presence of illicit substances. This is also done as a confirmatory test after the TesTcup test becomes positive. Marijuana can be detected in the urine for a long time because of its long half-life.
- **Fetal hair analysis**
  Fetal hair analysis is another method to determine drug abuse during pregnancy. Cocaine can be detected in fetal hair even when used few months ago.
- **Meconium analysis**
  Meconium is usually positive for 3 days after delivery for cocaine, compared to 12–24 hours for neonatal urine.

MANAGEMENT/INTERVENTIONS

- See each individual drug section in "Fundamental Knowledge."
- In general, women who test positive during pregnancy should be evaluated, educated & treated. The assessment itself & counseling & support provided by a nonjudgmental clinician can be highly

salutary in motivating some women to abstain. Others require referral for in-depth counseling & treatment regimens.

CAVEATS & PEARLS
- Establish a rapport w/ your pt; she will not speak if she does not trust you.
- Always start by asking about legal substances like alcohol & cigarettes & then move on to illicit drugs.
- Be aware of the presence of HIV, STDs, hepatitis B & TB.
- Most women abuse multiple substances, so the clinical picture might be confusing.
- Assemble a multidisciplinary team of health care & social service providers to comprehensively assess these gravida & their offspring.
- Review antenatal record if available.

CHECKLIST
- Always have a high index of suspicion.
- Perform a complete history & detailed physical exam. Needle marks, vital signs & neurologic status can provide a clue to drug abuse & withdrawal symptoms.
- Be prepared to treat any catastrophe.
- Always communicate your concerns & be a team player.
- Be nonjudgmental & thorough.

SUICIDE/HOMICIDE/DOMESTIC VIOLENCE

LATA POTTURI, MD
ADELE VIGUERA, MD

FUNDAMENTAL KNOWLEDGE
- Pregnant women have a significantly lower risk of suicide than women of childbearing age who are not pregnant. Even when thoughts of suicide are frequent, pregnant & postpartum women rarely commit suicide. The two exceptions to this are women who experience stillbirth & adolescents, in whom the suicide risk is significantly elevated.
- Pregnant or recently pregnant women are more likely to be the victims of homicide than to die from any other cause.
- Pregnant women are more likely than nonpregnant women to be victims of domestic violence. Women suffer both physical & psychological effects from the abuse. Complications include blunt trauma

to the abdomen, hemorrhage (including placental separation), uterine rupture, miscarriage, stillbirth, preterm labor & PROM. There has been a suggestion that a history of sexual abuse can prolong the 2nd stage of labor by delaying the baby from descending into the pelvis. In addition, many women who are battered during pregnancy participate in unhealthy behaviors to cope w/ stress. These include cigarette smoking, drug & alcohol use & poor nutritional habits.

STUDIES
- History & physical: In addition to a thorough history & physical, ask pt about any prenatal psychiatric diagnoses. Ask about psychological counseling, psychiatric treatment & any meds she has taken during pregnancy. With regard to suicide, ask about frequency of ideations, prior suicide attempts, current feelings about suicide & whether she has a plan. Along w/ the pt's obstetrician it is important to identify the pt's feelings about her pregnancy & the baby. Depression often worsens in the postpartum period, which may lead a pt to act on suicidal ideations. Social supports, family members, psychiatry & social services should be involved as deemed appropriate. In contrast to most pts w/ psychiatric illness, women who are victims of domestic violence may benefit from being managed w/out intimate partners or family members involved in their care. Many pts will not be forthcoming about intimate partner abuse when others are present for fear of escalating violence or even homicide if they speak up. They may additionally worry about the dissolution of the family at home if they speak out against the partner. It is critical to screen pts for domestic violence. Involving social services & psychiatry may help provide options to the abused pregnant pt.
- These pts are also prone to negative coping behaviors (ie, alcohol abuse, drug use, cigarette smoking) to cope w/ the stresses of the abuse. Education regarding these behaviors & their effects on the fetus along w/ recommendations for alternative coping strategies should be part of the pt interview.
- Lab studies: When applicable, check serum medication level & a full electrolyte panel.
- EKG
  - ➤ Barring another indication, pts w/ a history of suicidality or who are victims of abuse do not need a baseline EKG. However, if drug (ie, cocaine) or alcohol abuse is suspected, the clinician may be justified in checking an EKG to evaluate for arrhythmias or cardiac conduction defects.

MANAGEMENT & INTERVENTIONS

■ Psychosocial approach to the pt: The suicidal pt w/ a plan poses a mgt challenge to clinicians. Reassuring the pt, keeping her from harming herself & her fetus & treating depressive symptoms are critical. Suicidal ideations & actions may worsen in the postpartum period as depressive symptoms acutely worsen. Discuss the need for social services & psychiatry earlier rather than later w/ the actively suicidal pt. Ensure that the pt understands that clinicians are working to help the pt & keep her safe. The pt may need inpatient hospitalization in the postpartum period if she is actively suicidal.

■ The pt who is a victim of domestic violence poses another challenge. Be familiar w/ the symptoms & signs of family violence. Look for domestic violence when these symptoms & signs are present & know what to do when you learn that a pt is a victim of domestic violence. Appropriate actions include documenting the abuse, making sure that the pt receives appropriate treatment for injuries & psychological problems & giving the pt information about protective services. Asking the pt about this issue during future office visits would also be appropriate. Reporting child & elder abuse is mandatory in all states & some states require reporting of domestic partner violence.

■ Tailoring anesthetic plan: Pts w/ a history of suicidal ideation who are able to give informed consent for anesthesia can safely undergo both general & regional anesthesia. Pts who are victims of domestic violence & face the threat of homicide can also undergo both general & regional anesthesia. An important consideration among abused women is that they may have chronically elevated levels of catchecolamines from living in a stressful environment. In extreme circumstances, direct-acting vasopressors should be used over indirect-acting agents for hypotension. Appropriate precautions should be taken in the pt suspected of abusing drugs or alcohol. Awareness of potential drug interactions will aid in developing a safe anesthetic plan.

■ Informed consent: Determine the pt's ability to give informed consent. If the pt does not speak English, avoid having the partner of the pt be the interpreter.

CAVEATS & PEARLS

■ Pregnancy is a low-risk period for suicide. The exceptions to this are women who experience stillbirth & pregnant adolescents.

■ Pregnant women are more likely to be the victims of homicide than to die of any other cause.

- Pregnant women are at higher risk for domestic violence than nonpregnant women. All pregnant women should be screened for domestic violence apart from family members or intimate partners.
- Abused pts are prone to undertake negative coping behaviors such as drug & alcohol abuse.
- Involving a psychiatrist & social services earlier rather than later may be prudent.

CHECKLIST
- Screen all pts for suicidal ideation, domestic violence & safety in their living environment.
- Identify negative coping behaviors.
- Consider consulting psychiatry & involving social services.
- Know what meds the pt is taking & when her last dose was.
- Consider checking an EKG or analyzing cardiac rhythm in pts taking TCAs.

SYSTEMIC LUPUS ERYTHEMATOSUS

AUGUST CHANG, MD
MIRIAM HARNETT, MD

FUNDAMENTAL KNOWLEDGE

Definition
- Systemic, chronic inflammatory disease characterized by production of autoantibodies against nuclear, cytoplasmic & cell membrane antigens

Epidemiology
- Prevalence
  - 15–50 per 100,000 population
  - 1 in 700 women of child-bearing age
- Male:female 1:10
- Most commonly affects those btwn 15–50 years of age, w/ peak incidence at 30 years of age

Pathophysiology
- Autoantibodies
  - Antinuclear (ANA), particularly anti-dsDNA
  - RNA-protein conjugates: antiphospholipid, nRNP, Sm, Ro/SSA, La/SSB

- Antigen-antibody complexes w/ secondary inflammatory response
  - Deposition in renal glomeruli lead to irreversible damage
  - Deposition in skin, choroid plexus & other endothelial surfaces

Clinical manifestations
- Characterized by periods of remission & relapse
- Most common clinical signs & symptoms during pregnancy
  - Arthralgias: >90% of pts, often the presenting complaint
  - Fever
  - Skin lesions
  - Renal disease
- Diagnostic criteria for SLE (4 or more criteria):
  1. Malar rash: butterfly rash over malar region
  2. Discoid rash: erythematous, raised patches w/ scaling
  3. Photosensitivity: rash as a result of sun exposure
  4. Oral ulceration: oral or nasopharyngeal, usually painless
  5. Arthritis: nonerosive arthritis, generally of 2 or more peripheral joints
  6. Serositis: pleuritis, pericarditis
  7. Renal: persistent proteinuria or urinary casts
  8. Neurologic: seizures, psychosis in the absence of offending drugs or metabolic disturbances
  9. Hematologic: hemolytic anemia, leukopenia, lymphopenia, thrombocytopenia
  10. Immunologic: positive LE cell preparation, anti-DNA, anti-Sm, false-positive VDRL syphilis test
  11. Antinuclear antibody: in the absence of drugs associated w/ "drug-induced lupus" syndrome

Effect of pregnancy on SLE
- Flares of lupus nephritis during pregnancy may lead to renal dysfunction.
  - 30% incidence of transient renal dysfunction
  - 7% incidence of permanent renal dysfunction
- May be difficult to distinguish btwn lupus nephritis flare & pre-eclampsia
  - Both may present w/ hypertension, proteinuria, edema.
  - However, renal flare usually does not include hypertension & responds to prednisone, whereas pre-eclampsia does not
  - Increasing levels of SLE autoantibodies & typical SLE symptoms (polyarthritis, rash, mucosal ulcers, urinary casts)

➤ Abnormal levels of alternative pathway complement activation products

➤ Definitive diagnosis of lupus nephritis requires renal biopsy, but this is rarely done because of the increased risk for biopsy-related hematoma

Effect on pregnancy & fetus

- Increased incidence of pre-eclampsia
- Increased risk of pregnancy loss
  - ➤ Spontaneous abortion: 5–28%
  - ➤ Intrauterine fetal demise: 1–18%
  - ➤ Most important increased risk factor is presence of antiphospholipid (lupus anticoagulant, anticardiolipin) antibodies
- Increased risk of IUGR; reported in up to 32% pts w/ SLE
- Preterm delivery: 6–47% of pts w/ SLE
  - ➤ Most common causes are pre-eclampsia, fetal compromise & preterm premature rupture of membranes (PPROM)
- Neonatal SLE: linked to transplacental passage of anti-Ro & anti-La antibodies
  - ➤ Transient lupus dermatitis: usually resolves w/in first 6 months of life
  - ➤ Complete congenital heart block
    - Irreversible because cardiac conductive tissue has been destroyed & replaced by fibrosis
    - Treatment consists of antepartum maternal administration of steroids, digitalis, early delivery & newborn cardiac pacing

STUDIES

History & Physical

- Cardiac: evaluate for evidence of pericarditis, pericardial effusion & cardiomyopathy
- Pulmonary: evaluate for evidence of pleural effusion, pulmonary hypertension, pulmonary infarct, pulmonary vasculitis
- Neurologic: examine for evidence of peripheral neuropathies (15%) & evaluate for history of seizures & psychiatric disorders (depression, mania, schizophrenia)

Imaging

- Fetal ultrasound: accurate gestational age is important because of increased risk for preterm delivery & IUGR
- Echocardiogram: consider if valvular disease suspected: thickening (52%), vegetations (43%), regurgitation (25%), stenosis (4%)

■ Fetal echocardiography at week 18–20 of gestation to evaluate for early signs of congenital heart block, if anti-Ro/La antibody is present or fetal heart rate is approx. 60 bpm w/ no beat-to-beat variability during 2nd trimester

Other
■ Monitor for pre-eclampsia
■ Non-stress tests: weekly after 32 weeks gestation
■ CBC: assess for anemia &/or thrombocytopenia
■ Coagulation studies
  ➢ aPTT not corrected by 1:1 control plasma mix suggests presence of either lupus anticoagulant or autoantibodies against coagulant factors.
■ Baseline values for BUN/creatinine, creatinine clearance, 24-h urinary protein
■ Antiphospholipid antibodies
■ Serial complement levels (C3 or C4) are of controversial utility
■ Pulmonary function testing & ABGs: consider if there is evidence of a restrictive pattern w/ decreased vital capacity & diffusion capacity

MANAGEMENT/INTERVENTIONS

Medical treatment
■ Corticosteroids
  ➢ Mainstay of treatment
  ➢ No evidence of teratogenicity
  ➢ Inactivation by placental 11-beta-OH-dehydrogenase results in low fetal levels of active drug
  ➢ May precipitate gestational diabetes mellitus & hypertension
  ➢ Longer-term adverse effects
    • Osteoporosis
    • GI ulceration
    • Impaired immunity
    • Adrenal suppression
■ Aspirin/NSAIDs
  ➢ No evidence of teratogenicity
  ➢ No need for prophylactic cessation, but pregnancy should be closely monitored
  ➢ Recommend discontinuation during 3rd trimester because of:
    • Inhibitory effect on platelets & hemostasis

- Increased risk of fetal CNS hemorrhage
- Possible premature closure of ductus arteriosus
- Possible compromised fetal renal perfusion & abnormal amniotic fluid dynamics
- Possible factor in necrotizing enterocolitis (NEC)

■ Azathioprine
  ➤ No evidence of teratogenicity, but has been associated w/ reversible neonatal lymphopenia, decreased serum immunoglobulin levels, decreased thymic size
■ Hydroxychloroquine
  ➤ Generally considered safe, but there are case reports of possible ocular toxicity & ototoxicity
■ Cyclosporine A
  ➤ Has been used safely under close obstetric supervision
■ Cyclophosphamide
  ➤ Teratogenic & thus contraindicated

Anesthesia
■ Regional anesthesia
  ➤ Check for coagulopathy & thrombocytopenia prior to administering regional anesthetic.
■ Antibiotic prophylaxis for pts w/ known valvular involvement
■ Stress-dose steroids during labor & delivery for pts currently on steroid therapy

CAVEATS & PEARLS
■ Coagulopathy &/or thrombocytopenia may contraindicate regional anesthetic until corrected
■ Blood cross-matching may be difficult & time-consuming due to the presence of multiple additional antibodies

CHECKLIST
■ Check for coagulopathy & thrombocytopenia prior to administering regional anesthetic
■ Document preexisting peripheral neuropathies prior to general or regional anesthesia
■ Stress-dose steroids during labor & delivery for pts on steroid therapy
■ Antibiotic prophylaxis for pts w/ known valvular involvement
■ Request blood cross-matching early if need for blood products anticipated

THALASSEMIA

JEANNA VIOLA, MD
JANE BALLANTYNE, MD

FUNDAMENTAL KNOWLEDGE

- Inherited abnormality in rate of synthesis of hemoglobin chains
- Exists in many forms, ranging from mild to severe
- Most pts have a mild heterozygous form of thalassemia that is manifested as anemia & is well compensated.
- Most pts experience a lower-than-normal drop in their Hbg level due to the dilutional anemia of pregnancy; however, most pts are able to compensate well.
- Two types of thalassemia major
  - ➤ Beta-thalassemia: decreased production of beta globin chains
    - Pts w/ homozygous beta-thalassemia usually develop hemosiderosis by their child-bearing years, which is associated w/ endocrinopathy & cardiomyopathy.
    - Cardiac dysrhythmias & CHF may be exaggerated by pregnancy.
  - ➤ Alpha-thalassemia: decreased production of alpha chains
    - A 3-gene deletion state of alpha-thalassemia is known as hemoglobin H disease
    - Associated w/ chronic anemia & splenomegaly
    - Pts usually progress to a symptomatic anemia by the third trimester.
- Monitor closely for IUGR, preterm labor & fetal symptoms of anemia (any of these factors would indicate the need for transfusion).
- Rarely, spinal cord compression occurs from extramedullary hematopoiesis.

STUDIES

- Hgb electrophoresis
  - ➤ Elevated levels of Hgb A2 are present in beta-thalassemia minor.
  - ➤ In alpha-thalassemia minor, no abnormal hemoglobins are present.
- Associated clinical symptoms include "chipmunk facies" and "hair on end" pattern on skull radiographs.

MANAGEMENT/INTERVENTIONS

- No specific treatment needed, except PRBC transfusion in certain circumstances:
  - ➤ IUGR

- ➤ Preterm labor
- ➤ Fetal symptoms of anemia
- ■ Focus on mgt of pt's hemodynamic status & monitoring for any amount of hemodynamic or cardiac compromise.
- ■ In pts w/ severe anemia, opioids are relatively contraindicated, as these drugs may depress their respiratory function.
- ■ Application of supplemental oxygen & monitoring of oxygen saturation are necessary regardless of anesthetic technique.
- ■ Careful attention to fluid balance is required.
- ■ Regional anesthesia is not contraindicated unless there is evidence of a coexisting thrombocytopenia or coagulopathy.

CAVEATS AND PEARLS
- ■ Thalassemia disease ranges from mild to severe; most parturients present w/ anemia that is well compensated.
- ■ Severe thalassemia major can be associated w/ cardiomyopathy, endocrinopathy, CHF, dysrhythmias & a severe chronic anemia, all of which may lead to hemodynamic compromise.
- ■ Regional anesthesia is not contraindicated except in cases of concomitant thrombocytopenia or coagulopathy.

CHECKLIST
- ■ Obtain Hct, Hgb to assess severity of anemia prior to delivery.
- ■ Carefully evaluate pt's hemodynamic status & oxygen saturation.
- ■ Send type & cross if transfusion may be necessary.

Obtain consult w/ hematologist as early in pregnancy as possible.

THROMBOTIC MICROANGIOPATHY

JOSHUA WEBER, MD
PETER DUNN, MD

FUNDAMENTAL KNOWLEDGE
Characterized by acute renal failure late in pregnancy, associated w/ thrombocytopenia & hemolytic anemia

Two principal causes
- ■ Thrombotic thrombocytopenic purpura-hemolytic uremic syndrome (TTP-HUS)
- ■ Severe pre-eclampsia/HELLP syndrome

TTP-HUS

- Time of onset is variable, from mid-pregnancy to postpartum.
- Average onset is 4 weeks after delivery.
- TTP is characterized by predominant neurologic symptoms w/ minimal renal failure.
- HUS is characterized by predominant renal failure, minimal neurologic symptoms.

Severe pre-eclampsia, usually w/ HELLP syndrome

- Typically occurs late in 3rd trimester
- Pre-eclampsia/eclampsia may cause up to 1/5 of ARF cases during pregnancy.
- Many causes of ARF mimic pre-eclampsia.
- Usually preceded by hypertension, edema, proteinuria
- HELLP = hemolysis, elevated LFTs, low platelets
- Severe pre-eclampsia/HELLP are indications for urgent delivery, as symptoms generally resolve spontaneously postpartum.

STUDIES

- Creatinine
- BUN
- Electrolytes
- Creatinine clearance
- CBC
- Urinalysis

TTP-HUS

- CBC typically shows hemolytic anemia & thrombocytopenia.
- Chemistries show elevated BUN/creatinine.
- Coagulation profile may show coagulopathy w/ low clotting factors.

Severe preeclampsia/HELLP syndrome

- CBC shows hemolytic anemia & thrombocytopenia.
- Chemistries show elevated LFTs & mildly elevated BUN/creatinine.

MANAGEMENT/INTERVENTIONS

Medical/OB mgt of TTP-HUS

- Plasma infusion +/− plasma exchange
- For decreased renal function
  - ➤ Increased frequency of prenatal visits (q2 wks in 1st & 2nd trimesters, then q1 week)
  - ➤ Monitoring: monthly measurements of serum creatinine, creatinine clearance, fetal development, BP
  - ➤ Erythropoietin may be used for maternal anemia.
  - ➤ Preterm delivery is considered for worsening renal function, fetal compromise or worsening signs of pre-eclampsia.

Medical/OB mgt of severe pre-eclampsia/HELLP syndrome

- Urgent delivery
- Steroids have been used successfully in some cases (but no randomized, controlled trials).
- Supportive therapy following delivery

Anesthetic mgt of pts w/ thrombotic microangiopathy

- Monitor coagulation parameters, electrolytes, LFTs.
- Seizure prophylaxis w/ MgSO4

Anesthetic mgt for pts w/ pre-existing renal dysfunction

Pre-op

- Evaluate degree of renal dysfunction & hypertension.
- Evaluate for anemia & electrolyte abnormalities.

Intraoperative mgt

- Monitors: standard monitoring +/− arterial line +/− CVP
- Limit fluids in pts w/ marginal renal function to prevent volume overload.
- Use strict aseptic technique, as uremic pts are more prone to infection.

Regional anesthesia

- Uremia-induced platelet dysfunction leads to increased bleeding time.
- Pts may have thrombocytopenia from peripheral destruction of platelets.
- Increased toxicity from local anesthetics has been reported in pts w/ renal disease, but amides & esters can be used safely.
- Contraindications to regional technique: pt refusal, bacteremia, hypovolemia, hemorrhage, coagulopathy, neuropathy

General anesthesia

- Uremic pts may have hypersensitivity to CNS drugs due to increased permeability of blood-brain barrier.
- Uremia causes delayed gastric emptying & increased acidity, leading to increased risk of aspiration pneumonitis (consider sodium citrate, H2-receptor blocker, metoclopramide).
- Succinylcholine is relatively contraindicated, as it causes approx. 1-mEq/L increase in serum potassium, which may precipitate cardiac dysrhythmias.
  - ➤ Use caution w/ drugs dependent on renal excretion (gallamine, vecuronium, pancuronium) & clearance (mivacurium, rocuronium).

CAVEATS/PEARLS

■ Succinylcholine is relatively contraindicated, as it causes approx. 1-mEq/L increase in serum potassium, which may precipitate cardiac dysrhythmias.

■ Use caution w/ drugs dependent on renal excretion (gallamine, vecuronium, pancuronium) & clearance (mivacurium, rocuronium).

➢ Cisatracurium is a good muscle relaxant for pts w/ renal dysfunction, as its clearance is independent of renal function (Hoffman degradation).

➢ Standard doses of anticholinesterases are used for reversal of neuromuscular blockade.

➢ Consider whether pt is likely to have platelet dysfunction (secondary to uremia or pre-eclampsia) or significant peripheral neuropathy before doing regional anesthetic.

CHECKLIST

■ Check OB plan for pt.

■ Document degree of renal dysfunction.

■ Be prepared to manage hypertension.

■ Consider effects of uremia, hypoalbuminemia, impaired renal excretion when choosing meds.

THROMBOTIC THROMBOCYTOPENIC PURPURA/ HEMOLYTIC UREMIC SYNDROME

JEANNA VIOLA, MD
JANE BALLANTYNE, MD

FUNDAMENTAL KNOWLEDGE

■ A rare disorder that occurs primarily in young women

■ Thrombotic thrombocytopenic purpura (TTP) affects 1/25,000 parturients.

■ 58% of parturients who develop TTP present before 24 weeks gestation.

■ TTP is caused by 12 mutations in the AdamTS13 gene, which encourages the accumulation of multimers of von Willebrand factor.

■ Unknown pathophysiology, but may involve several different mechanisms, all of which result in microvasculature thrombi formation

■ Classic pentad of TTP

➢ Fever

➤ Neurologic changes (persistent memory loss, hemiparesis)
➤ Microangiopathic hemolytic anemia
➤ Severe thrombocytopenia
➤ Renal dysfunction

▦ Differentiation between HELLP syndrome & TTP is difficult, but the distinction is important, as the treatments are different.
▦ Pts in active TTP at delivery may experience severe thrombocytopenia, leading to hemorrhage.
▦ Occasionally, TTP also presents post-partum.
▦ Hemolytic uremic syndrome (HUS) associated w/ pregnancy occurs post-partum as opposed to TTP, which usually is early in pregnancy.
▦ HUS & TTP share many features, but HUS is associated w/ severe renal failure, thrombocytopenia w/ fewer neurologic sequelae than TTP.
▦ TTP & HUS can also be induced by endothelial damage or by drugs such as clopidogrel & ticlopidine, as well as pneumococcal infection.

STUDIES

▦ Hyaline thrombi are found on pathology; otherwise, the diagnosis is clinical.
▦ Because the disease is severe, the dyad of thrombocytopenia & microangiopathic hemolytic anemia alone requires treatment.

MANAGEMENT/INTERVENTIONS

▦ Aggressively treat TTP w/ transfusions to exchange plasma for FFP.
▦ Avoid platelet transfusion: it can exacerbate the underlying disease.
▦ Any transfusion of FFP or PRBCs needs to be given through a large-bore catheter to prevent hemolysis.
▦ Neurologic function is often tentative:
➤ Sedatives are relatively contraindicated w/ altered mental status
➤ Pts are prone to seizures & may require pharmacologic measures to break the seizure.
▦ Regional anesthesia & IM injections are contraindicated in pts w/ a bleeding diathesis.
▦ Maintain adequate fluid volume & urine output: these pts are prone to renal damage.
▦ IV PCA opioids & N2O are commonly used for labor analgesia.
▦ General anesthesia is recommended for C-sections.
▦ Smooth induction & intubation are important in pts w/ plt counts <10,000, as hypertension on intubation may cause intracranial hemorrhage.

CAVEATS AND PEARLS

- The diagnosis of TTP and HUS is mainly clinical.
- Avoid transfusion of platelets, as this can exacerbate the disease.
- Blood products need to be transfused through a large-bore catheter to prevent hemolysis.
- Adequate hydration is necessary to prevent further renal failure.
- Most pts w/ TTP or HUS who require C-section will need GETA.

CHECKLIST

- If TTP is suspected, look for the pentad of fever, neurologic changes, hemolytic anemia, severe thrombocytopenia & renal dysfunction
- Begin treatment for TTP if thrombocytopenia & hemolytic anemia are present.
- Careful airway exam to prepare for GETA for C-section
- Have appropriate monitors (pulse oximetry, EKG, BP cuff), emergency airway equipment & anti-epileptic meds ready in case of seizure.

THYROID NODULAR DISEASE

GRACE C. CHANG, MD, MBA; ROBERT A. PETERFREUND, MD, PhD; AND STEPHANIE L. LEE, MD, PhD

FUNDAMENTAL KNOWLEDGE

Epidemiology

- Relatively common; affects 17–40% of adult population, predominantly women
- Incidence in pregnant women was 15.3% in one study.
- Incidence of malignancy in solitary thyroid nodule is 5%.

Etiology

- Benign
  - ➤ Multinodular goiter
  - ➤ Hashimoto's thyroiditis
  - ➤ Cysts
  - ➤ Follicular adenomas
- Malignant
  - ➤ Papillary carcinoma
  - ➤ Follicular carcinoma
  - ➤ Medullary carcinoma
  - ➤ Anaplastic carcinoma
  - ➤ Primary thyroid lymphoma
  - ➤ Metastatic carcinoma

Risk Factors
- Living in area of iodine deficiency
- Family history of goiter or autoimmune thyroid disease
- Radiation exposure
- Parity

Pathophysiology
- Classical thought is that elevation of TSH levels stimulates thyrocyte proliferation & goiter formation.
- New evidence shows growth of nodules has multiple causes.
  - Chronic stimulation of TSH receptor (ie, iodine deficiency)
  - Stimulation by IGF-I & epidermal growth factor
  - hCG stimulation

Effect of Pregnancy
- Prospective ultrasonographic study showed that pregnancy is associated w/ increased incidence of thyroid nodular disease (15.3% at 1st trimester to 24.4% at 3 months postpartum) & increase in number & size of thyroid nodules.
- Reasons for these associations are unclear but include increased thyroid blood flow & iodine deficiency from increased urinary iodine loss.

STUDIES
- Fine-needle aspiration biopsy
  - Determines characteristics of nodule (solid, cystic or mixed)
  - Provides cytology to rule out malignancy
  - Many thyroid experts recommend routine thyroid biopsy be performed postpartum; studies show outcome is not different in women whose nodule evaluation & thyroidectomy is postponed until postpartum.
- High-resolution ultrasound
  - Determines characteristics of nodule
- Ultrasound-guided biopsy
  - Records nodule size for monitoring growth & detection of other nodules
  - Improves sampling accuracy if results are equivocal from fine-needle aspiration biopsy
- Thyroid scintigraphy: contraindicated in pregnancy
- Thyroid CT scan: not recommended in pregnancy
- Thyroid MRI scan: if there is concern about significant tracheal compression or extensive metastatic disease

MANAGEMENT/INTERVENTIONS

■ Fine-needle aspiration biopsy positive for thyroid cancer
  ➤ Total thyroidectomy should be performed in 2nd trimester, plus thyroid suppression therapy.
  ➤ If pt declines surgery, can use L-thyroxine suppression therapy, monitoring of nodule size by palpation & ultrasound
  ➤ If diagnosis is made in 3rd trimester, delay surgery until postpartum to reduce risk of premature delivery.
  ➤ If cancer is aggressive (undifferentiated carcinoma or lymphoma) or distant metastases are found, may require therapeutic abortion & surgery and/or radiation & chemotherapy
  ➤ Routine serum thyroglobulin measurements not recommended
■ Fine-needle aspiration biopsy suspicious for malignancy
  ➤ Cellular aspirate without atypia has 20–25% risk of carcinoma in hypofunctional nodule.
  ➤ Cannot differentiate btwn hyperfunctional & hypofunctional nodule since thyroid scintigraphy is contraindicated unless TSH level is suppressed
  ➤ Administer thyroid suppression therapy w/ L-thyroxine & carefully monitor growth of nodule.
  ➤ If pt is unwilling to wait until postpartum for further workup, can proceed w/ partial thyroidectomy w/ intraoperative pathology results & total thyroidectomy if results are positive for malignancy
■ Fine-needle aspiration biopsy w/ benign cytology or nondiagnostic
  ➤ Monitor for growth.
  ➤ Can defer L-thyroxine treatment unless TSH level is elevated

CAVEATS/PEARLS

■ Goiter associated w/ hyperthyroidism may compromise airway.

CHECKLIST

■ Thorough airway exam

TOLAC AND VBAC

CHARLES DOBBS, MD; JASMIN FIELD, MD; LISA LEFFERT, MD; AND MAY PIAN-SMITH, MD

FUNDAMENTAL KNOWLEDGE

Historically, there have been changing concepts about the safety of VBAC vs. repeat C-section. For most of the 1900s, general obstetric philosophy was "once a cesarean, always a cesarean." Btwn 1970 & 1990, the C-section rate in the U.S. increased from 5% to 25%. With improvements in obstetric care over the past 30 years, VBAC was embraced as a way to slow the increasing C-section rate. As VBAC rates rose, so did reports of complications, such as uterine rupture.

- Current trends show the rate of VBAC decreasing (from 55% to 12.6%) and the C-section rate increasing.

Candidates for VBAC should meet the following ACOG selection criteria:

- No more than one previous low-transverse incision cesarean
- Clinically adequate pelvis
- No other uterine scars or history of previous rupture
- Physicians immediately available for labor monitoring & for performance of emergent cesarean delivery if necessary
- Anesthesia personnel immediately available for emergent cesarean delivery

ACOG suggests it may also be reasonable to consider a spontaneous trial of labor after C-section (TOLAC) in pts under the following circumstances:

- History of 2 prior low-transverse incision cesarean deliveries w/ prior successful vaginal delivery
- Fetal macrosomia
  - ➤ Rate of uterine rupture is not increased if pt has had a previous vaginal delivery
  - ➤ Chance of successful VBAC delivery decreases
- Post-dates gestation
  - ➤ Does not significantly increase risk of uterine rupture
  - ➤ Without spontaneous labor prior to 40 weeks' gestation, successful VBAC is less likely.
- Previous low vertical incision
  - ➤ No increase in maternal or fetal morbidity
  - ➤ Rate of successful VBAC equal to previous low-transverse incision
- Unknown uterine scar
  - ➤ Type of scar may be inferred from indication for previous C-section
- Twin gestations
  - ➤ Rate of successful VBAC & uterine rupture does not appear to differ btwn twin & singleton pregnancies.

Success rates for TOLAC

- Most studies indicate 60–80% will have successful vaginal births.
- Women w/ 1 prior vaginal delivery are 9–28% more likely to have successful TOL than those who have not delivered vaginally.

- Generally, success rate is higher if circumstances causing prior C-section are not present in current pregnancy.
- If previous C-section was performed for dystocia, VBAC success decreases slightly to 50–80%.
  - Without complete cervical dilation, subsequent VBAC success rate is higher (67–73%).
  - With complete cervical dilation, success rate decreases to 13%.
- Success rates for VBAC are equivocal, irrespective of epidural analgesia or other forms of pain relief.
- Factors that negatively affect successful VBAC
  - Labor induction or augmentation
  - Maternal obesity
  - Gestational age >40 weeks
  - Birthweight >4,000 g
  - Inter-delivery interval <19 months

Benefits of VBAC vs. repeat C-section
- Shorter maternal hospital stay
- Less blood loss w/ fewer transfusions
- Fewer surgical infections
- Fewer thromboembolic events
- Decreased risk of placenta previa & accreta (which increases w/ each additional C-section)

Risks associated w/ VBAC, including complications associated w/ failed TOL
- Uterine rupture
- Operative injury during emergency C-section (higher than for elective C-section)
- Hysterectomy
- Increased incidence of maternal infection such as endometritis
- Increased need for transfusion
- Increased neonatal morbidity
  - Increased incidence of arterial umbilical cord blood pH < 7.0
  - Increased incidence of 5-minute Apgar scores < 7
  - Increased incidence of neonatal infection
- Low incidence of maternal & perinatal death
  - 3 maternal deaths reported in one major meta-analysis of >27,000 attempted VBACs
  - Though perinatal death rate is <1%, it is significantly more likely to occur during TOL than during elective repeat cesarean delivery.

VBAC contraindications according to current ACOG practice guidelines (July 2004)

- Previous classic or T-shaped uterine incision or extensive transfundal uterine surgery
- History of uterine rupture
- Other contraindication to vaginal delivery
- Inability to perform emergent cesarean delivery (surgeon, nursing, anesthesia staff must be immediately available)
- History of 2 prior uterine scars w/ no prior successful vaginal deliveries

STUDIES
- Standard studies for laboring pts
  - CBC, type, screen
  - Other tests as indicated
- Review maternal health history, w/ particular attention to risk factors for VBAC complications or contraindications
- Careful airway assessment in preparation for potential general anesthetic in event of emergent C-section

MANAGEMENT/INTERVENTIONS
- Standard monitors during labor: FHR, uterine contraction, maternal BP, pulse, SpO_2
- Personnel familiar w/ potential complications of VBAC present to identify non-reassuring FHR tracing, inadequate progress of labor, signs of uterine rupture
- Current blood bank sample sent for type & screen
- Epidural analgesia
  - Several large retrospective studies show that epidural anesthesia is safe for VBAC & does not adversely affect success rates.
  - Concerns that epidural anesthesia will mask the pain of uterine rupture are not supported by data; rupture presents with pain <10% of the time, but it is constant in nature (unlike contractions) & often significant enough to break through epidural analgesia for labor.
  - A functioning epidural catheter can facilitate the transition to surgical anesthesia should C-section become necessary.
  - Labor epidural may be used effectively with 3% chloroprocaine in the event of emergency C-section for uterine rupture.
- Successful VBAC increases likelihood of need for uterine exploration:
  - Particularly important if excessive vaginal bleeding, maternal hypovolemia or hemodynamic instability is present
  - Consider leaving epidural catheter in place to facilitate postpartum exam.

CAVEATS AND PEARLS

1. Overall VBAC success rate is 60–80%.
2. Epidural anesthesia is safe & effective for VBAC.
3. Use of prostaglandins for cervical ripening or induction of labor should be discouraged in most VBACs.
4. Oxytocin augmentation of labor may or may not increase likelihood of uterine rupture in TOL by a clinically insignificant degree.

CHECKLIST

1. Maternal history, reason for prior C-section, risk factors for failed TOLAC, potential VBAC contraindications
2. Careful airway assessment
3. Blood bank sample for type & screen
4. Obstetric & anesthesia personnel immediately available for emergent C-section
5. Early epidural placement can help avoid emergent general anesthetic.
6. Watch for signs/symptoms of uterine rupture.

TROUBLESHOOTING/MANAGING INADEQUATE REGIONAL ANESTHESIA

KRISTEN STADTLANDER, MD; MAY PIAN-SMITH, MD; AND LISA LEFFERT, MD

FUNDAMENTAL KNOWLEDGE

■ While obtaining consent for regional anesthesia, discuss the risk of a failed regional anesthetic & the potential need for repeated spinal or epidural placement should the first attempt fail.

■ Spinal: If a spinal anesthetic fails to achieve the desired pain relief, ask yourself 3 questions:

➤ Was the local anesthetic placed in the right location? The presence of free-flowing CSF usually confirms that the needle is in the correct place. If care is not taken to stabilize the spinal needle & to repeatedly aspirate as the drug is incrementally injected, it is possible to deliver the local anesthetic outside of the intrathecal space (e.g., into the subdural space). This is the most common reason for a failed spinal anesthetic.

➤ Did I inject the correct medication? It is possible to inadvertently inject saline or the 1% local anesthetic for subcutaneous injection.

➤ Has this pt or any other member of the pt's family had a similar occurrence? Although extremely rare, there are case reports of pts who are genetically resistant to local anesthetics.

Remedies for failed spinal depend on the assumed cause & on the clinical situation. Potential next steps include:

➤ Activation of epidural catheter (in CSE)
➤ Placement of epidural catheter de novo
➤ Repeat labor spinal. If pt already has a partial block, then there is a risk of getting a high spinal or total spinal if additional medication is given intrathecally.
➤ Parenteral medication
➤ Local blocks by obstetricians (including pudendal block)

Inadequate epidural block

■ Do a careful sensory/motor exam (when dilute labor mixes are used, objective motor/sensory changes may be very subtle).

■ Check the skin site. Make sure the tape is intact & the catheter does not appear to have moved in or out of the space.

■ Confer w/ obstetricians, midwives & labor nurses as to relevant changes in the pt's labor or for the presence of a full bladder. Any of these conditions can precipitate changes in the pt's level of comfort.

■ One-sided block: This is more likely if the catheter is threaded slightly lateral to midline or if the catheter is threaded into the space more than the recommended 3–5 cm. A unilateral block can also develop if the pt lies on one side for a prolonged period. If a one-sided block develops, position the pt w/ the uncomfortable side down & administer a bolus dose of medication. Reasonable possibilities include 5 cc 0.25% bupivacaine, 10 cc 0.125% bupivacaine or 10 cc 0.75% lidocaine w/ epinephrine, or 10 cc of a mix of dilute bupivacaine & dilute lidocaine. Examine for signs of intravascular catheter placement. If no improvement is noted & the catheter is threaded at least 4 cm in the space, the catheter can be pulled back 1 cm & the drug rebolused. Ultimately the catheter may need to be replaced.

■ Patchy block: Pts may report areas that are spared by their epidural analgesia. This often occurs in the sacral area, where nerve roots are large & more impervious to blockade. There are also reports of this occurring more commonly when air loss of resistance is used, possibly because the injected air acts as a barrier to dispersion of the liquid anesthetic. If this occurs, position the pt w/ the uncomfortable side down & administer an epidural bolus (e.g., 5 cc of 0.25% bupivacaine or 10 cc of 0.125% bupivacaine). There is some evidence to suggest that injecting a larger volume of dilute local anesthetic, rather than a small volume of concentrated anesthetic, is more efficacious in covering a patchy block. If the pt reports pain in her perineum, tailbone or back, it may be the fetal head descending. This occurs more commonly in occiput-posterior fetal position. This pain is often not adequately covered by local anesthetic alone. In this case, a small dose of fentanyl (25–50 mcg) through the epidural is often beneficial.

■ Progressively denser block: If a pt receiving an epidural infusion reports progressively denser anesthesia, carefully evaluate the catheter for intrathecal migration. If the catheter proves to be intrathecal, the decision should be made to either replace it or to dose it according to CSA (continuous spinal anesthesia) guidelines.

■ Progressively lighter block: If the pt reports diminishing anesthesia, carefully examine the delivery equipment & then evaluate the catheter for potential migration. There are numerous points in the infusion system that can become disconnected. Examine the skin site. If the visible markings on the catheter have not changed, re-administer a test dose; if negative, rebolus the epidural. If repeated boluses fail to achieve adequate analgesia, replace the catheter or administer parenteral pain relief. As stated above, take care not to mistake the increasing pain of progressing labor or a full bladder w/ the diminishing analgesia of a failed epidural.

■ Subdural block: If a pt reports a patchy, unilateral or unusually high epidural block, a subdural insertion may have occurred. The subdural space is located between the dura & arachnoid mater. The onset time to a subdural block is btwn that of an epidural & intrathecal blockade. The block typically extends in the cephalad direction & sacral anesthesia is often spared. A "high spinal" can result from an epidural dose inadvertently given through a subdural catheter. If a catheter is thought to be subdural, it should be removed immediately & replaced.

CAVEATS/PEARLS

■ Regional anesthesia is a valuable tool & is becoming progressively safer. However, if mismanaged, it can lead to deleterious results

■ An epidural catheter should be monitored carefully. The pt's feedback gives the practitioner valuable information & should never be discounted.

- Before bolusing any epidural, a test dose should be administered to evaluate for intravascular or intrathecal migration.
- Intravascular & intrathecal complications can be avoided by dosing incrementally.

CHECKLIST

1. Before placing a regional anesthetic, review contraindications to regional anesthesia, w/ special attention to bleeding disorders/coagulopathies & pre-existing neurologic deficits.
2. Make sure the parturient has full monitoring, including fetal monitoring (if applicable) & a working IV.
3. Make sure the pt is prehydrated, pressors are readily available & emergency airway & cardiovascular supplies are accessible.
4. Always aspirate before injecting local anesthetic.
5. Obtain informed consent, including all possible complications of a regional anesthetic & the possibility of a failed block or need for a second anesthetic.
6. Monitor closely for hypotension & intravascular or intrathecal placement. Catheter removal & prompt treatment w/ pressors, hydration & ventilatory support can prevent disastrous complications
7. Always take the pt's feedback under careful consideration, as she can give you valuable clues when there are problems w/ a spinal/epidural.

TUBULOINTERSTITIAL DISEASE

JOSHUA WEBER, MD
PETER DUNN, MD

FUNDAMENTAL KNOWLEDGE

- Tubulointerstitial diseases are characterized by abnormal tubular function.
- Tubulointerstitial diseases account for 1/3 of pts w/ chronic renal failure.
- Causes of tubulointerstitial disease: renal cystic disease, interstitial nephritis, renal neoplasia, functional tubular defects
- Pts typically have abnormal urine composition, but GFR is not decreased until late in disease.
- Pts w/ parenchymal disease may be asymptomatic for years or may have progressive renal insufficiency & hypertension.

- Severe renal dysfunction before pregnancy is associated w/:
  - ➤ Higher likelihood of worsened renal function during pregnancy. The pathophysiology of how pregnancy worsens renal disease is unknown.
  - ➤ Higher incidence of obstetric complications (prematurity, fetal death)

STUDIES

Lab tests commonly ordered to evaluate renal function in pregnancy include:
- Creatinine
- BUN
- Electrolytes
- Creatinine clearance
- CBC
- Urinalysis

In addition to labs commonly evaluated in pregnancy the following tests may be performed:
- Urinalysis to identify renal casts &/or bacteria
- Serial BP monitoring
- Fetal ultrasound at 20 weeks to monitor growth
- Renal biopsy: generally not performed after 32 weeks gestation
- Renal ultrasound: generally useful in renal cystic disease or reflux nephropathy

MANAGEMENT & INTERVENTIONS

Medical/OB mgt of pts w/ tubulointerstitial disease
- Increased frequency of prenatal visits (q2 wks in 1st & 2nd trimesters, then q1 week)
- Monitoring: monthly measurements of serum creatinine, creatinine clearance, fetal development, BP
- Erythropoietin may be used for maternal anemia.
- Preterm delivery considered for worsening renal function, fetal compromise, pre-eclampsia
- Renal biopsy considered if rapid deterioration in renal function prior to 32 weeks gestation
- See "*Parturients on Dialysis*" for dialysis mgt.

Anesthetic mgt of pts w/ tubulointerstitial disease
Pre-op
- Evaluate degree of renal dysfunction & hypertension.
- Evaluate for anemia & electrolyte abnormalities.

- If pre-existing peripheral neuropathy, consider avoiding regional techniques.

Intraoperative mgt
- Monitors: standard monitoring + fetal heart rate monitoring (FHR) +/− arterial line +/− CVP
- Limit fluids in pts w/ marginal renal function to prevent volume overload.
- Use strict aseptic technique, as uremic pts are more prone to infection.
- Careful padding/protection of dialysis access is important.
- Consider promotility agents, as uremic pts may have impaired GI motility.

Regional anesthesia
- Uremia-induced platelet dysfunction leads to increased bleeding time.
- Pts may have thrombocytopenia from peripheral destruction of platelets.
- Increased toxicity from local anesthetics has been reported in pts w/ renal disease, but conflicting literature exists.
- Contraindications to regional technique: pt refusal, bacteremia, significant hypovolemia, severe hemorrhage, coagulopathy, potential preexisting neuropathy

General anesthesia
- Uremic pts may have hypersensitivity to CNS drugs due to increased permeability of blood-brain barrier.
- Uremia causes delayed gastric emptying & increased acidity, leading to increased risk of aspiration pneumonitis (consider sodium citrate, H2-receptor blocker, metoclopramide).
- Hypoalbuminemia leads to increased free drug concentration of drugs that are bound to albumin (ie, thiopental).
- Succinylcholine is relatively contraindicated, as it causes approx. 1-mEq/L increase in serum potassium, which may precipitate cardiac dysrhythmias.
- Use caution w/ drugs dependent on renal excretion (gallamine, vecuronium, pancuronium) & clearance (mivacurium, rocuronium).

CAVEATS & PEARLS
- Serum Cr of 2.0 or greater prior to pregnancy implies a 33% chance of developing dialysis-dependent end-stage renal disease during or shortly after pregnancy.

- Cisatracurium is a good muscle relaxant for pts w/ renal dysfunction, as its clearance is independent of renal function (Hoffman degradation).
- Standard doses of anticholinesterases are used for reversal of neuromuscular blockade.
- Consider whether pt is likely to have platelet dysfunction (secondary to uremia) or significant peripheral neuropathy before doing regional anesthetic.

CHECKLIST
- Check OB plan for pt.
- Document degree of renal dysfunction.
- Be prepared to manage hypertension.
- Consider effects of uremia, hypoalbuminemia, impaired renal excretion when choosing meds.

UMBILICAL CORD PROLAPSE

SUSANNE PAREKH, MD
ANDREA TORRI, MD

FUNDAMENTAL KNOWLEDGE
- Umbilical cord prolapse (UCP) occurs when the umbilical cord precedes the presenting fetal part.
- It can be *overt* (umbilical cord is protruding from the cervix) or *occult* (umbilical cord becomes entrapped between the presenting fetal part and the utero-vaginal birth canal). Some authors define UCP as palpation of the umbilical cord below the presenting fetal parts after rupture of the membranes.
- UCP is an infrequent complication of labor: it is observed in 0.2–0.6% of all labors. It is more frequent when the fetal presenting part has abnormal shape or volume, as in the abnormal fetal presentations, in the low-weight singleton, in the twin pregnancy, in the premature delivery & when the fetus has malformations. It is also more frequent when the membranes rupture before the presenting fetal part is engaged in the birth canal. Most cases are seen in the vertex presentation, w/ breech & shoulder presentations accounting together for close to 50%.
- The perinatal mortality rate of UCP has fallen in recent decades from close to 400 per 1,000 in the 1920s to 36 per 1,000 in the 1990s.
- Unrelenting mechanical compression on the prolapsed umbilical cord causes a reduction in umbilical blood flow & as a consequence

abnormal heart rate & hypoxia in the fetus. In some instances of overt prolapse the fetus is not in immediate danger: the fetal heart rate (FHR) is normal & the cord is prolapsed but not compressed; this is occasionally observed in complete & incomplete breech or shoulder presentation, as the fetal presenting part incompletely fills the birth canal.

STUDIES
- FHR monitor may show an abnormal tracing at first w/ an evolution toward severe fetal bradycardia & cardiac arrest as the umbilical cord flow of blood becomes insufficient to sustain fetal oxygen exchange & transport.
- The role of obstetrical interventions as a cause of UCP is controversial: one study showed that cervical ripening, labor induction, amnioinfusion & amniotomy did not increase the likelihood of UCP. Another study concluded that obstetrical interventions like scalp electrode placement, expectant mgt of PROM & attempted cephalic version contributed to about half of the observed cases of UCP.

MANAGEMENT AND INTERVENTIONS
Obstetric Mgt & Interventions
- UCP in the presence of FHR changes typical or suggestive of fetal hypoxia is an obstetric emergency requiring immediate transfer to the obstetric OR & stat cesarean delivery. Depending on the OB's preference, a manual attempt to elevate the fetal presenting part might be attempted while on the way to the OR. This is controversial, as any manual intervention has the potential to worsen umbilical cord compression, further reducing umbilical blood flow.
- When the prolapse is not associated with FHR changes & the cord is visibly not compressed, the pt is immediately taken to the OR, where preparations for stat cesarean delivery are made and a vaginal exam is performed to decide on the best delivery method for the fetus.

Anesthesia Mgt
- Key to effective & successful mgt is quick induction of anesthesia to allow a rapid delivery of the hypoxic fetus.
- It is important to formulate individual anesthesia plans for urgent & stat C-sections when the fetal presentation is non-cephalic, the fetus is small & premature, fetal malformations are present or the pregnancy is multiple.
- When the obstetrician calls for a stat cesarean delivery, the first-choice anesthetic may be a rapid sequence induction of general anesthesia.

■ In selected cases, when the FHR abnormality is mild or has eased or resolved, the pt might have an expeditious spinal anesthetic for the urgent cesarean delivery. The pt should be placed in the lateral decubitus position to minimize recurrence or worsening of the umbilical cord compression.

■ When a prolonged surgical operative time is expected, an epidural catheter placement might be indicated.

■ With a preexisting tested & functioning epidural catheter, the anesthesiologist should judge the best anesthetic mgt on a case-by-case basis. Dosing the epidural with 20 mL of 3-chloroprocaine requires a few minutes. A stat general anesthetic w/ rapid sequence induction is usually faster but requires intubation of the trachea.

■ The time required for patient transport to the OR, transfer to the OR bed, skin preparation & sterile draping & for the OB to be scrubbed, gowned & gloved should be estimated & considered in the clinical decision making.

CAVEATS AND PEARLS

■ Not all UCPs are indications for a stat C-section. A pulsatile umbilical cord & a normal or mildly abnormal FHR may leave some time for regional anesthesia.

■ Always plan for stat general anesthesia when the fetal presentation is other than cephalic.

■ Consider the time required to secure the airway in the plans for stat cesarean delivery.

CHECKLIST

■ FHR monitoring type (ultrasound or fetal scalp electrode): data from a scalp electrode are less influenced by movement and position.

■ FHR tracing: Is a palpable pulse present in the prolapsed umbilical cord? Does the FHR tracing show effects of hypoxia?

■ Repeat FHR evaluation in the operating room: If it normalizes, it may be feasible to proceed w/ a spinal instead of a general anesthetic.

UROLITHIASIS

JOSHUA WEBER, MD
PETER DUNN, MD

FUNDAMENTAL KNOWLEDGE

■ Urolithiasis is caused by formation of calculi in renal calyces or pelvis.

■ Most kidney stones (70%) are composed of calcium oxalate.

- Incidence is of urolithiasis is 1–5% & is not affected by pregnancy.
- Caused by hypersaturation of urine due to:
  - Low urinary pH
  - Increased excretion of minerals
  - Decreased urine output

Symptoms
- Flank pain
- Abdominal pain
- Fever
- Nausea
- Dysuria
- Urgency

Complications
- UTI
- Preterm labor
- Ureteral rupture (rare)
- Obstructed labor (rare)

STUDIES
Lab tests commonly ordered to evaluate renal function in pregnancy include:
- Creatinine
- BUN
- Electrolytes
- Creatinine clearance
- CBC
- Urinalysis

In addition to labs commonly checked in pregnancy, the following tests may be performed:
- Renal ultrasound
- Excretory urography is typically 2nd-line imaging due to the use of small amount of radiation.

MANAGEMENT/INTERVENTIONS
Medical/OB mgt of kidney stones
- Conservative treatment (rest, fluids, analgesia +/- antibiotics)
- Cystoscopy
- Percutaneous nephrostomy
- Open stone removal & nephrectomy are rare.
- Shock wave lithotripsy is contraindicated in pregnancy.

■ Be judicious w/ calcium supplementation in women w/ history of urolithiasis.
■ For decreased renal function:
➤ Increased frequency of prenatal visits (q2 wks in 1st & 2nd trimesters, then q1 week)
➤ Monitoring: monthly measurements of serum creatinine, creatinine clearance, fetal development, BP
➤ Erythropoietin may be used for maternal anemia.
➤ Preterm delivery is considered for worsening renal function, fetal compromise or pre-eclampsia.
➤ Renal biopsy is considered if rapid deterioration in renal function occurs prior to 32 weeks gestation.
➤ See *"Parturients on Dialysis"* for dialysis mgt.

Anesthetic mgt of parturients w/ kidney stones
■ Epidural analgesia facilitates passage of stones.
■ Shock-wave lithotripsy is contraindicated in pregnancy.
■ Narcotics may be used to treat associated pain, realizing that narcotics decrease peristalsis (& thus may delay passage of the stone) & can cross the placenta.
■ For pts w/ compromise of renal function
➤ Evaluate degree of renal dysfunction & hypertension.
➤ Evaluate for anemia & electrolyte abnormalities.
➤ Succinylcholine is relatively contraindicated, as it causes approx. 1-mEq/L increase in serum potassium, which may precipitate cardiac dysrhythmias.
➤ Use caution w/ drugs dependent on renal excretion (gallamine, vecuronium, pancuronium) & clearance (mivacurium, rocuronium).

CAVEATS & PEARLS
■ Open stone removal & nephrectomy are rare.
■ Shock wave lithotripsy is contraindicated in pregnancy.
■ Epidural analgesia facilitates passage of stones.
■ Narcotics may be used to treat associated pain, realizing that narcotics decrease peristalsis (& thus may delay passage of the stone) & can cross the placenta.
■ If pt has compromised renal function, consider avoiding succinylcholine & use caution w/ drugs dependent on renal excretion (gallamine, vecuronium, pancuronium) & clearance (mivacurium, rocuronium).

CHECKLIST
- Check OB plan for pt.
- Document degree of renal dysfunction.
- In severe cases of urolithiasis, consider effects of uremia, hypoalbuminemia, impaired renal excretion when choosing meds.

UTERINE ATONY

HOVIG CHITILIAN, MD
BHARGAVI KRISHNAN, MD

FUNDAMENTAL KNOWLEDGE
- Most common cause of postpartum hemorrhage
- Risk factors
  - Prolonged labor
  - Augmented labor
  - Precipitous labor
  - Multiple gestation
  - Polyhydramnios
  - High parity
  - Tocolytic agents
  - Macrosomia
  - Chorioamnionitis
- Diagnosis: vaginal bleeding, soft uterus

STUDIES
Lab studies: Hgb concentration, blood type & screen

MANAGEMENT/INTERVENTIONS
In the following order:
- Uterine massage
- Oxytocin infusion of 20 U/L in normal saline or Ringer's lactate
  - Onset is immediate.
  - May cause hypotension if infused at too high a rate
  - May have a mild antidiuretic effect
- Ergot alkaloids (ie, methylergonovine)
  - Second-line agent for treatment of uterine atony
  - Administer 0.2 mg IM.
  - Onset in a few minutes; duration 2–3 hours
  - May repeat dose q3min as long as pt is not hypertensive
  - Avoid in pts w/ hypertension, preeclampsia.

- 15 methyl-prostaglandin F2-alpha
  - Administer 0.25 mg IM.
  - May repeat q15min to a maximum dose of 2 mg
  - May cause bronchospasm & hypoxemia. Do not use in pts w/ reactive airwaydisease.
- If uterine atony persists, embolization or ligation of uterine arteries or hysterectomy
- Monitor blood loss & replace w/ fluid and/or blood products as required.

CAVEATS AND PEARLS
- Avoid ergot alkaloids in pts w/ preeclampsia or baseline hypertension.
- Avoid prostaglandins in pts w/ reactive airway disease.
- If pt has an epidural in place, delay removal until hemorrhage has completely resolved; it can be used if surgical measures are required to control the hemorrhage.

CHECKLIST
- Have adequate IV access & blood products available.
- Have oxytocin, ergot alkaloids & 15 methyl F2-alpha available.
- Replace blood products as necessary.

UTERINE INVERSION

HOVIG CHITILIAN, MD
BHARGAVI KRISHNAN, MD

FUNDAMENTAL KNOWLEDGE
- Definition: turning inside out of uterus
- Risk factors
  - Umbilical cord traction
  - Uterine atony
  - Inappropriate fundal pressure
- Diagnosis: vaginal bleeding & a mass in the vagina

STUDIES
- Lab studies: Hgb concentration, blood type & screen
- Ultrasound imaging

MANAGEMENT/INTERVENTIONS

- Replacement of the uterus by obstetrician
- Replacement can be facilitated by administration of terbutaline (0.25 mg IV), nitroglycerin (50–200 mcg IV) or general anesthesia w/ a volatile anesthetic to promote uterine relaxation.
- Administer analgesic (parenteral or neuraxial, depending on the circumstances) for pain associated w/ uterine replacement.

CAVEATS AND PEARLS

- Administer uterotonic agent following repositioning of uterus.
- Endotracheal intubation is necessary if general anesthesia is induced.
- Be prepared to treat hypotension associated w/ the administration of uterine relaxants.

CHECKLIST

- Large-bore IV access
- Analgesia for uterine replacement (parenteral or neuraxial, as appropriate)
- Be prepared to assist w/ pharmacologic uterine relaxation w/ IV nitroglycerin or the induction of general endotracheal anesthesia.

UTERINE RUPTURE

CHARLES DOBBS, MD; LISA LEFFERT, MD; JASMIN FIELD, MD; AND MAY PIAN-SMITH, MD

FUNDAMENTAL KNOWLEDGE

- Uterine rupture is most commonly associated w/ separation of a uterine scar.
- Can result in significant fetal & maternal morbidity & mortality
- Requires immediate cesarean delivery or post-partum laparotomy
- Variable presentations
  - ➤ Fetal heart rate decelerations, bradycardia &/or loss of heart rate trace (70%)
  - ➤ Uterine or abdominal pain (10%)
  - ➤ Maternal hemodynamic instability; hypovolemia (10%)
  - ➤ Vaginal bleeding (5%)
  - ➤ Recession of the presenting part; loss of station (5%)
  - ➤ Asymptomatic

Rate depends on type of previous incision.

- Classic incisions & T-shaped incisions: 4–9% risk
  - ➤ Rate increased from overall rate of 5/1,000 w/ spontaneous labor to 24/1,000 for labor induced w/ prostaglandin cervical-ripening agents
    - 4× increase in rate w/ single-layer closure of hysterotomy compared to double-layer closure
    - Rate increased by shorter interval btwn deliveries: interval <24 months has 2–3× increased chance of uterine rupture compared to VBAC after 24 months since last delivery
  - ➤ Rate not increased (above spontaneous labor rates) by oxytocin augmentation/induction
    - Rate decreased by any previous vaginal birth

Uterine rupture is often followed by uterine atony, w/ increased potential for substantial blood loss after delivery.

STUDIES
- Continuous fetal heart rate & uterine contraction monitoring
- Personnel familiar w/ possible presentations of uterine rupture, as delayed diagnosis can lead to significant morbidity

MANAGEMENT/INTERVENTIONS
- Uterine rupture requires immediate C-section via laparotomy.
- The emergent nature of uterine rupture often requires general anesthesia.
- If a functioning epidural is in place & mother & fetus are stable, then the epidural can be used for C-section (using 10–20 cc of 3%, 2-chloroprocaine for a T4 surgical level).
- Despite the presence of adequate regional anesthesia, prolonged surgical time, large-volume resuscitation & massive fluid shifts may dictate conversion to general anesthesia. The airway may become more edematous & difficult to secure in this situation.

CAVEATS AND PEARLS
- Delayed diagnosis of uterine rupture causes significant maternal & fetal morbidity.
- Regional anesthesia is acceptable provided that it does not cause surgical delay & mother & fetus are stable.
- Be prepared for the possibility of massive bleeding, gravid hysterectomy.

- Conversion to general anesthesia after extended operative time and/or large-volume fluid resuscitation may cause increasing difficulty w/ airway mgt.

CHECKLIST

- Ensure that all personnel involved in patient care for attempted TOLAC must be knowledgeable & vigilant about the signs & symptoms of uterine rupture.
- Review pt's history for risk factors & contraindications.
- Careful, early airway assessment w/ anticipation of increasingly adverse airway changes
- If rupture is suspected, immediately assess maternal & fetal hemodynamics.
- Be prepared for & proceed to emergent C-section.
- Have blood products readily available.
- Consider early conversion to general anesthesia during long cases w/ substantial volume loss.

UTI/ACUTE PYELONEPHRITIS

JOSHUA WEBER, MD
PETER DUNN, MD

FUNDAMENTAL KNOWLEDGE

- UTIs are among the most common infections in pregnancy.
- In most cases renal function is maintained, but acute renal failure can develop.
- Pregnancy has been associated w/ increased progression from pyelonephritis to acute renal failure.

STUDIES

Lab tests commonly ordered to evaluate renal function in pregnancy include:

- Creatinine
- BUN
- Electrolytes
- Creatinine clearance
- CBC
- Urinalysis will typically show increased WBC, nitrites &/or leukocytes.

In addition:
- Renal biopsy may show microabscesses (rarely performed).

MANAGEMENT/INTERVENTIONS

Medical/OB mgt of acute renal failure
- Rapid recognition of derangement in renal function
- Rule out reversible causes.
- Optimize fluid status, electrolytes, acid-base status, BP.
- Rule out DIC.
- Dialysis should keep BUN < 30 & minimize fluid shifts.
- Delivery once fetus is mature, w/ pediatric follow-up.
- See *"Parturients on Dialysis"* for dialysis mgt.

Anesthetic mgt in pts w/ acute renal failure
- Optimize maternal condition prior to delivery or C-section.
- Consider CVP monitoring for volume assessment.
- Assess BUN/Cr, electrolytes, CBC.
- Regional anesthesia: evaluate for coagulopathy, thrombocytopenia, hypovolemia.
- When time permits, epidural is preferred over spinal in cases of uncertain volume status because onset of blockade is more gradual.

CAVEATS & PEARLS
- Pregnancy is associated w/ an increased progression from pyelonephritis to acute renal failure.
- Optimize maternal condition prior to vaginal or cesarean delivery.
- Consider CVP monitoring for volume assessment.
- Regional anesthesia: evaluate for coagulopathy, thrombocytopenia, hypovolemia.
- When time permits, epidural anesthesia is preferred over spinal in cases of uncertain volume status because onset of blockade is more gradual.

CHECKLIST
- Check vital signs, electrolytes.
- Assess potential for thrombocytopenia, coagulopathy & hypovolemia.

VARICELLA ZOSTER

SISSELA PARK, MD
LAURA RILEY, MD

FUNDAMENTAL KNOWLEDGE

Basics

- Varicella zoster is a herpes virus.
- Varicella: primary disease
  - Seen in antibody-negative individual
  - Febrile systemic illness characterized by generalized pruritic vesicles
- Zoster: recurrent disease
  - Painful vesicles limited to a unilateral dermatome
  - Uncommon in setting of normal immunity
- Approx. 90% of women of child-bearing age have antibodies & are immune.
- About 5–10% of pregnant women are susceptible.
- Incidence of varicella during pregnancy has been estimated at 1 to 5 per 10,000 pregnancies.

Clinical manifestations

- Incubation period 10–21 days
- First signs are usually fever, coryza & rhinorrhea.
- Skin lesions
  - Appear about 2 days after onset of systemic symptoms
  - Typically pruritic
  - Evolve from erythematous macules to vesicles, papules or pustules
  - Vesicles usually occur in clusters & can be found in all stages of crusting.
- Other systemic illnesses like pneumonia & encephalitis can occur.

Varicella pneumonia

- Reported rates as high as 20–25%
- Pregnant women may be at increased risk.
- Mortality 25–44% from varicella pneumonia during pregnancy
- Increased mortality noted during 3rd trimester vs. other trimesters
- Tends to present at the same time or a few days after the onset of the rash
- Common symptoms
  - Shortness of breath

- ➤ Cough
- ➤ Chest pain
- ■ Rapid respiratory failure occurs occasionally.
- ■ Typical x-ray findings
  - ➤ Diffuse interstitial infiltrates, often bilateral
  - ➤ Underlying slightly nodular appearance
- ■ Treatment
  - ➤ IV acyclovir
  - ➤ Respiratory support as needed

Complications

After maternal varicella during pregnancy

- ■ Spontaneous abortion
- ■ Preterm labor
- ■ Incidence of in utero varicella appears to be low (<2%).

Congenital varicella syndrome

- ■ Seen w/ maternal varicella (primary) btwn 8 & 20 weeks of gestation
- ■ Syndrome includes:
  - ➤ Characteristic skin scarring
  - ➤ Cicatricial scars in a typical unilateral dermatomal distribution
  - ➤ Hypoplastic limbs
  - ➤ Nasal hypoplasia
  - ➤ Microphthalmia
  - ➤ Microcephaly
  - ➤ Hydrocephaly
  - ➤ IUGR

Neonatal varicella syndrome

- ■ Result of transmission of 3rd-trimester maternal varicella to fetus
- ■ Incidence greatest w/ delivery btwn 2 days before & 5 days after onset of maternal varicella
- ■ Mortality rate 30%

STUDIES

- ■ Diagnosis is usually clinical.
- ■ Lab verification usually by antibody detection techniques
  - ➤ ELISA
  - ➤ Fluorescent antibody
  - ➤ Hemagglutination inhibition

MANAGEMENT/INTERVENTIONS

Obstetric

- Varicella zoster immunoglobulin (VZIG) is given following exposure to varicella.
  - ➤ Can prevent or modify infection in some pregnant women
  - ➤ To be protective, must be administered within 96 hours of exposure
  - ➤ For neonates, usually given shortly after delivery
    - Reduces rate of severe neonatal varicella to 15%
    - Death rate decreased to zero
- If primary varicella, consider acyclovir to shorten outbreak of lesions & duration of fever.
- Use proper infection-control measures.

Anesthetic mgt

- Avoid regional for 2 weeks after onset of cutaneous varicella because pt may still be viremic.
- Varicella pneumonia
  - ➤ May need monitoring in ICU & intubation
  - ➤ Frequent chest x-rays
  - ➤ Monitor ABGs.
  - ➤ Manage w/ pulmonologist.
  - ➤ Try to avoid anesthetic intervention.
  - ➤ Adult respiratory distress syndrome could develop w/ general anesthesia.

CAVEATS & PEARLS

- About 5–10% of pregnant women are susceptible to varicella zoster.
- Pregnant women may be at increased risk for varicella pneumonia.
  - ➤ Mortality 25–44%
  - ➤ Increased mortality in 3rd trimester
- Complications of varicella during pregnancy include:
  - ➤ Spontaneous abortion
  - ➤ Preterm labor
  - ➤ Congenital varicella syndrome
  - ➤ Neonatal varicella syndrome

CHECKLIST

- Rapid respiratory failure can occur w/ varicella pneumonia.
- Avoid regional anesthesia for 2 weeks after onset of skin vesicles, as pt may still be viremic.
- Pts w/ varicella pneumonia may need ICU monitoring & possibly intubation.

VIRAL HEPATITIS, GENERAL

LAWRENCE WEINSTEIN, MD
DOUG RAINES, MD

FUNDAMENTAL KNOWLEDGE

- Hepatitis is a general term for inflammation of the liver. It has multiple etiologies, including viral, autoimmune & alcoholic. Regardless of etiology, anesthetic mgt is based on symptoms & pathophysiologic manifestations at the time of labor & delivery. Subsequent sections will review basics of viral, autoimmune & alcoholic hepatitis & include discussion of the physiologic effects of hepatitis as they relate to anesthesia.

- Acute viral hepatitis is the most common cause of jaundice in the parturient. >80% of cases of viral hepatitis during pregnancy are caused by hepatitis viruses A, B & C. Less common causes of hepatitis include hepatitis viruses D, E, F & G, as well as the Epstein-Barr virus, cytomegalovirus, herpes simplex & rubella. This section will focus on the various hepatitis viruses & the clinical manifestations involved.

Symptoms

- Symptoms & physical exam findings can be similar among the various hepatitis viruses. The patterns & severity of such symptoms can vary between individuals & have variable courses for different viral strains.

STUDIES

Acute Viral Hepatitis

- Incubation period: the period of time between exposure to the virus & presentation of clinical signs or symptoms
- Symptomatic pre-icteric phase
  - Nonspecific constitutional symptoms such as malaise, fatigue, nausea, anorexia, arthralgias, myalgias, headaches, low-grade fever
  - Mild RUQ abdominal pain
  - About 10% of pts, usually those w/ the Hep B virus, develop a serum sickness type of illness w/ fever, rash & arthralgias; this is thought to be due to circulating immune complexes.
  - Elevated serum aminotransferases are seen; can be in the range 10–100× above normal values.
  - Elevated GGT
  - Alkaline phosphatase near normal

- Icteric phase: jaundice generally appears several days after the onset of prodromal symptoms but may coincide w/ presenting symptoms. This is due mostly to a direct bilirubinemia.
  - ➣ Yellow-hued or jaundiced appearance of skin, sclerae & soft palate
  - ➣ Pt can have pruritus from retention of bile salts.
  - ➣ Urine is dark from conjugated bilirubin excretion.
  - ➣ Constitutional symptoms initially worsen w/ the onset of jaundice but then start to abate soon after.
- Convalescence: constitutional symptoms & jaundice start to disappear
  - ➣ Acute viral hepatitis usually subsides over 2–3 weeks.
  - ➣ <1% will have a fulminant course.
  - ➣ Hep B, C & D have the potential to become chronic hepatitis.

Chronic Hepatitis

Chronic hepatitis consists of symptomatic, biochemical or serologic evidence of continuing or relapsing liver disease for >6 months, w/ histologically documented inflammation & necrosis.

- Most cases are due to the viral hepatitis, but other causes can include Wilson's disease, chronic alcohol abuse & autoimmune disease.
- Hep C has a high tendency to become chronic.
- Clinical features are variable. Most common symptom is fatigue. Other symptoms can include malaise, anorexia & jaundice.
- Physical findings can include hepatomegaly, spider angiomas, palmar erythema & splenomegaly.

MANAGEMENT/INTERVENTIONS
N/A

CAVEATS/PEARLS
See specific type of viral hepatitis.

CHECKLIST
See specific type of viral hepatitis.

VOLUME EXPANSION FOR THE NEONATE

RICHARD ARCHULETA, MD
SANDRA WEINREB, MD

FUNDAMENTAL KNOWLEDGE

- Resuscitative measures beyond effective oxygenation are rarely required in neonates.

- When required in neonatal resuscitation, the administration of epinephrine & volume expansion are the most effective measures.
- Indications for volume expansion
  - Little response to effective ventilation & other resuscitative measures
  - Neonate pale despite effective ventilation & good oxygenation
  - Faint pulses despite heart rate >100

STUDIES
Continue to evaluate neonate's respiration, heart rate & color at least every 30 seconds until neonate's respiratory status has stabilized.

MANAGEMENT/INTERVENTIONS
- Ensure that you have acquired a reliable route of IV access.
  - Umbilical vein catheterization w/ return of blood
  - IV access w/o local swelling of skin w/ administration of small bolus (0.5 cc) Difficult in neonates; extremities & scalp most often used
- Infuse 10 cc/kg of LR or NS IV *over 5–10 minutes*
  - Use a burette or syringes to ensure that only the desired amount of fluid is infused.
- May instead infuse 10 cc/kg O-negative blood.
  - If the neonate is stable enough for the delay, the blood should be cross-matched w/ the mother's blood.
  - If the blood is needed immediately, O-negative un-cross-matched blood may be used.
- May repeat bolus once if neonate displays some response to first bolus & in clinician's judgment neonate requires further volume resuscitation
  - Caution is advised because volume overload predisposes to intracranial hemorrhage in the neonate.

CAVEATS & PEARLS
Albumin is not recommended for acute neonatal volume expansion because it is associated w/ increased mortality & the chance of infection.

CHECKLIST
- Ensure that acute volume expansion is indicated.
- Ensure that you have reliable IV access.
- Ensure that crystalloid (LR or NS) or O-negative blood is infused in the proper quantity at the appropriate speed.
  - 10 cc/kg

➤ *Over 5–10 minutes*
- May repeat bolus once if indicated
- Continue other resuscitative measure as indicated.

VON HIPPEL-LINDAU DISEASE (VHL)

MEREDITH ALBRECHT, MD
MICHELE SZABO, MD

FUNDAMENTAL KNOWLEDGE

Definition
- Rare, multiorgan system disease characterized by hemangiomas involving retina, adrenal glands, kidneys, spinal cord (usually cervical or thoracic but can involve lumbosacral region) & cerebellum. May be enlarged during pregnancy.

Epidemiology
- Autosomal dominant w/ variable expression

Pathophysiology
- Angioblastic lesions can affect retina, cerebellum & spinal cord.
- Associated features include cysts (renal & pancreatic), renal carcinomas & pheochromocytoma.

Clinical Manifestations
- Includes dysarthrias & ataxia

Effect of Pregnancy on VHL/Effects of VHL on Pregnancy & Fetus
- Course of disease in pregnancy is not well established, but several published case reports exist.
- Some case reports suggest that pregnancy may adversely affect pt (ie, that these highly vascularized tumors may enlarge during pregnancy), but the majority suggest favorable outcome for mother & fetus.

STUDIES
- Careful history/physical exam focusing on the presence of symptomatic lesions
- Consider CT/MRI of brain & spinal cord to rule out CNS hemangiomas.

MANAGEMENT/INTERVENTIONS
- Both regional anesthesia & general anesthesia have been successfully used for delivery of pts w/ VHL.
- Primary concern is the disruption of vascular malformations (intracranial & spinal hemangioblastomas) during delivery or during the placement of spinal or epidural anesthesia.
- Several case reports describe successful epidural anesthesia (including in a pt w/ spinal hemangiomas).

CAVEATS/PEARLS
- Lesions (intracranial & spinal cord) can be asymptomatic or present w/ symptoms such as dysesthesias & ataxia.
- Rare associated features include cysts (renal & pancreatic) & pheochromocytoma.
- Both regional anesthesia & general anesthesia has been used successfully in pts w/ VHL.
- Anecdotal evidence exists that these highly vascularized lesions may grow during pregnancy, but overall, case report literature suggests that pregnancy outcomes are good for parturient & fetus.
- Consult multidisciplinary team, including neurosurgeon & OB, when considering delivery & anesthetic options for pts w/ CNS lesions.

CHECKLIST
- Consult multidisciplinary team, including neurosurgeon & OB, when considering delivery & anesthetic options for pts w/ CNS lesions.
- Both regional anesthesia & general anesthesia have been successfully used for delivery of pts w/ VHL.

VON WILLEBRAND DISEASE

JEANNA VIOLA, MD
JANE BALLANTYNE, MD

FUNDAMENTAL KNOWLEDGE
- The most common inherited platelet disorder; occurs in 1–3% of the population
- Autosomal dominant deficiency or defect in a factor (VW) that is required for platelet adherence to endothelium
- Three types
  - ➤ Types I & III are caused by a reduced amount of von Willebrand factor.

➤ Types IIa & IIb are caused by dysfunctional factor that is present in normal amounts.

➤ Type II can also be associated w/ a thrombocytopenia because the abnormal von Willebrand factor binds to platelets & encourages their uptake by the RE system.

■ Most pts have presented w/ this disease prior to pregnancy, manifesting as recurrent epistaxis, menorrhagia, prior history of profound surgical or dental bleeding.

■ Pregnant pts w/ this disease often experience a remission of their disease, due to increased levels of vWF during pregnancy, & may therefore require no treatment.

STUDIES

■ Elicit bleeding history, including response to major bleeding challenges such as surgery, childbirth, prior regional anesthetics.

■ Testing for the vWF antigen level determines the amount of vWF present (>50% is normal, used to diagnose types I & III).

■ The ristocetin cofactor activity (RICOF) level is then assessed, which is a measurement of platelet functional activity (>50% is normal, used to diagnose type II).

■ If the first round of tests are inconclusive:

➤ Factor VIII level can be sent (vWF protects factor VIII from degradation & prolongs its half-life as well as facilitates the secretion of factor VIII).

➤ Tests may be repeated on a separate occasion.

■ Prolonged BT (although significant intra-operator variation has been shown)

■ PTT elevated in severe disease

■ Platelet count normal or decreased (type IIb)

MANAGEMENT/INTERVENTIONS

■ When feasible, consult a hematologist.

■ Most parturients w/ VWD have type I & will experience a remission during pregnancy & require no treatment.

■ Type I: Desmopressin 0.3 mcg/kg IV (max 20 mcg) will effect an immediate release of vWF from the endothelial wall; it will also increase factor VIII 2–3 fold. Some hematologists recommend giving a dose 30 min before placing a spinal or epidural & a second dose 30 min before discontinuing an epidural if it has been >4–6 hours since the initial dose was given.

- Type II: Desmopressin not effective; treatment is platelet transfusion. A RICOF level of >30% in pts w/ type II indicates that regional anesthesia is safe.
- Type III severe vWF deficiency: cryoprecipitate or Humate C, an inactive viral product derived from plasma, which contain both factor VIIIc & active vWF.
- Pts w/ type I or III may be given desmopressin prophylactically prior to a C-section. Watch for side effects of desmopressin such as hyponatremia-induced seizures.
- Single-shot spinal anesthesia may be preferable to epidural anesthesia for C-section due to the smaller size of the needle, or consider GETA.

CAVEATS AND PEARLS
- Consult hematologist before delivery.
- Most parturients w/ VWD will experience a remission during pregnancy & require no treatment.
- The treatment for VWD depends on which subtype the pt has, as the pathophysiology is different.
- Most pts w/ this disease will present prior to pregnancy w/ epistaxis, menorrhagia or other dysfunctional bleeding.
- Regional anesthesia may be safe in a subset of pts; however, it may result in epidural hematoma, esp. in homozygotes.

CHECKLIST
- Determine the type of VW disease & obtain a history of the severity.
- Determine whether the pt has experienced any episodes of excessive bleeding during pregnancy.
- Consider checking VW factor antigen or RICOF levels to determine the extent of remission.
- Check consultant's recommendations.
- Discuss OB delivery plan.
- Obtain blood type & cross for possible transfusion of blood components.
- Careful airway exam, as GETA may be indicated
- Careful lower extremity neuro exam postop if regional anesthesia has been used

PART TWO

Obstetric Anesthesia Formulary

ACETAMINOPHEN (TYLENOL)

INDICATIONS
- Antipyretic & analgesic

DOSING
- 325–650 mg PO q4–6h or 1,000 mg 3 or 4 times/day; max 4 g/day

MATERNAL SIDE EFFECTS & IMPACT ON ANESTHESIA
- Used during pregnancy & appears safe for short-term use at therapeutic doses

FETAL & NEONATAL EFFECTS
- Pregnancy Category B (for definition, see the "*Pregnancy Categories*" section). No adverse effects have been reported. Compatible w/ breast-feeding.

COMMENT
- Use w/ care in pts w/ impaired liver function.

ACTIQ (FENTANYL)

INDICATIONS
- Potent narcotic analgesic w/ much shorter half-life than morphine sulfate. Drug of choice for conscious sedation & analgesia. Used as adjunct in spinals & epidurals. Reversed by naloxone.

DOSING
- Analgesia: 0.5–1 mcg/kg/dose IV/IM q30–60min
- Transdermal: Apply a 25-mcg/h system q48–72h.
- Neuraxial dosing varies depending on obstetric indication & regional anesthetic technique.

MATERNAL SIDE EFFECTS & IMPACT ON ANESTHESIA
- Used routinely in epidural infusions (w/ bupivacaine) for labor analgesia; may allow the reduction of local anesthetic dose.

FETAL & NEONATAL EFFECTS
- Pregnancy Category C; Category D if used for prolonged periods or in high doses at term (for definitions, see the "*Pregnancy Categories*" section). Readily crosses placenta & may cause neonatal depression. There appears to be no fetal accumulation of either drug during epidural infusion, however, & no adverse fetal effects have been

observed from epidural fentanyl administration in routine doses. Opioids may result in decreased beat-to-beat variability of the fetal heart rate (FHR) w/o fetal hypoxia. Fentanyl is excreted in breast milk; it is compatible w/ breast-feeding due to low oral bioavailability.

COMMENT
- May result in hypotension, respiratory depression, constipation, nausea, emesis, urinary retention; idiosyncratic reaction, known as chest wall rigidity syndrome, may require neuromuscular blockade to increase ventilation.

ACYCLOVIR (ZOVIRAX)

INDICATIONS
- Active against HSV-1 & HSV-2 (primary & recurrent genital herpes)

DOSING
- Acyclovir: 5 mg/kg IV q8h for 5 days for severe infection & 200 mg PO 5×/day for 10 days.
- Valacyclovir: 500 mg PO bid for 5 days

MATERNAL SIDE EFFECTS & IMPACT ON ANESTHESIA
- Maternal effects can include thrombocytopenia, renal impairment, encephalopathic changes (lethargy, obtundation, tremors, confusion).

FETAL & NEONATAL EFFECTS
- Pregnancy Category B (for definition, see the "*Pregnancy Categories*" section). Rapidly crosses the placenta. Acyclovir is considered safe during breast-feeding; safety of valacyclovir has not been determined.

COMMENT
- In rat studies, high levels of acyclovir were associated w/ fetal head & tail abnormalities & maternal toxicity.

ADENOCARD (ADENOSINE)

INDICATIONS
- Adenosine is used for terminating & differentiating supraventricular tachydysrhythmias by transiently slowing atrioventricular (AV) node conduction & the sinus rate. It acts upon adenosine receptors.

DOSING

- 6 mg rapid IV push, followed by 10 cc saline flush. If no response in 2 min, 12 mg IV push followed by 10 cc saline flush.

MATERNAL SIDE EFFECTS & IMPACT ON ANESTHESIA

- Ventricular tissue is unaffected. Adverse effects include headache, chest pressure, shortness of breath, flushing & lightheadedness/ dizziness. Of note, there is a characteristic cardiac pause after adenosine administration. It has an ultrashort half-life of a few seconds & is given as a rapid IV bolus. The effects of adenosine are antagonized by methylxanthines (eg, theophylline, caffeine) & potentiated by dipyridamole & carbamazepine.

FETAL & NEONATAL EFFECTS

- Pregnancy Category C (for definition, see the "*Pregnancy Categories*" section). Since adenosine has a half-life of about 10 seconds, in theory very little is distributed to the placenta & breast milk.

COMMENT

- Several contraindications & cautions are associated w/ adenosine (eg, sick sinus syndrome, 2nd-degree AVB, 3rd-degree AVB). Be cautious in pts w/ asthma or history of wheezing &/or bronchoconstriction because inhaled adenosine may cause bronchospasm.

ADENOSINE (ADENOCARD)

INDICATIONS

- Adenosine is used for terminating & differentiating supraventricular tachydysrhythmias by transiently slowing atrioventricular (AV) node conduction & the sinus rate. It acts upon adenosine receptors.

DOSING

- 6 mg rapid IV push, followed by 10 cc saline flush. If no response in 2 min, 12 mg IV push followed by 10 cc saline flush.

MATERNAL SIDE EFFECTS & IMPACT ON ANESTHESIA

- Ventricular tissue is unaffected. Adverse effects include headache, chest pressure, shortness of breath, flushing & lightheadedness/ dizziness. Of note, there is a characteristic cardiac pause after adenosine administration. It has an ultrashort half-life of a few seconds & is given as a rapid IV bolus. The effects of adenosine are antagonized by methylxanthines (eg, theophylline, caffeine) & potentiated by dipyridamole & carbamazepine.

FETAL & NEONATAL EFFECTS
- Pregnancy Category C (for definition, see the "*Pregnancy Categories*" section). Since adenosine has a half-life of about 10 seconds, in theory very little is distributed to the placenta & breast milk.

COMMENT
- Several contraindications & cautions are associated w/ adenosine (eg, sick sinus syndrome, 2nd-degree AVB, 3rd-degree AVB). Be cautious in pts w/ asthma or history of wheezing &/or bronchoconstriction because inhaled adenosine may cause bronchospasm.

ADVIL (IBUPROFEN)

INDICATIONS
- Ibuprofen is a nonsteroidal, anti-inflammatory, antipyretic analgesic agent. It inhibits the synthesis of prostaglandins.

DOSING
- 400 mg/dose PO q4–6h, max 1.2 g/day

MATERNAL SIDE EFFECTS & IMPACT ON ANESTHESIA
- Safe to administer regional anesthesia in women taking ibuprofen

FETAL & NEONATAL EFFECTS
- Pregnancy Category B; Category D in 3rd trimester (for definitions, see the "*Pregnancy Categories*" section). Known effects on fetus during 3rd trimester include constriction of ductus arteriosus prenatally, tricuspid insufficiency & pulmonary hypertension; nonclosure of the ductus arteriosus postnatally; bleeding. Ibuprofen is safe during breast-feeding; amounts are difficult to detect in breast milk after dosages of up to 1.6 g/day PO.

COMMENT
- Use w/ care in pts w/ peptic ulceration or a history of such ulceration, bleeding disorders or cardiovascular disease & pts on oral anticoagulants. Do not use routinely in pts who are allergic to aspirin. Use w/ care in pts w/ asthma, especially those who have developed bronchospasm w/ other nonsteroidal agents.

ALBUTEROL ORAL INHALED AEROSOL (PROVENTIL, VENTOLIN)

INDICATIONS
- Albuterol is a stimulant of the beta-2 receptors in the bronchi & thus is a potent bronchodilator used in allergic asthma; exercise-induced asthma; acute, subacute & chronic bronchitis; & emphysema. Useful as a tocolytic. Can be used to treat hyperkalemia.

DOSING
- 1 or 2 metered-dose inhalations q4–6h

MATERNAL SIDE EFFECTS & IMPACT ON ANESTHESIA
- Like all beta-2 mimetics, may cause tachycardia, hyperglycemia & hypotension. May also result in hypokalemia; it is useful in treating hyperkalemia.

FETAL & NEONATAL EFFECTS
- Pregnancy Category C (for definition, see the "*Pregnancy Categories*" section). Crosses the placenta & may cause tachycardia & hyperglycemia in the fetus. May cause retinal ischemia. Albuterol is an effective tocolytic similar to ritodrine. Like ritodrine, it is considered safe during breast-feeding.

COMMENT
Excessive inhalation may result in hypertension, hypoglycemia, hypokalemia & hypocalcemia. Concurrent administration w/ oxytocic drugs (including ergonovine) may cause hypotension. May decrease serum digoxin levels.

ALUMINUM HYDROXIDE (MAALOX)

INDICATIONS
- Increases gastric pH > 4 & inhibits proteolytic activity of pepsin, reducing acid indigestion. Antacids initially can be used in mild cases. No effect on frequency of reflux but decreases its acidity.

DOSING
- 5–15 mL/dose PO qd/qid

MATERNAL SIDE EFFECTS & IMPACT ON ANESTHESIA
- Decreases effects of tetracyclines, ranitidine, ketoconazole, benzodiazepines, penicillamine, phenothiazines, digoxin, indomethacin, isoniazid; corticosteroids decrease effects of aluminum in hyperphosphatemia

FETAL & NEONATAL EFFECTS
- Pregnancy Category B (for definition, see the "*Pregnancy Categories*" section). Usually safe but benefits must outweigh risks.

COMMENT
Use caution in pts w/ recent massive upper GI hemorrhage; renal failure may cause aluminum toxicity; can cause constipation.

AMIDATE (ETOMIDATE)

INDICATIONS
- Imidazole-containing hypnotic used to induce general anesthesia

DOSING
- 0.2–0.3 mg/kg IV

MATERNAL SIDE EFFECTS & IMPACT ON ANESTHESIA
- Adrenal suppression for up to 24 hours, myoclonus, PONV, venous irritation

FETAL & NEONATAL EFFECTS
- Pregnancy Category C (for definition, see the "*Pregnancy Categories*" section). Suppresses neonatal cortisol production, though this is of unclear clinical significance. Fetal/maternal ratio: 0.5.

COMMENT
- Produces minimal cardiorespiratory effects at low doses. May produce adrenal suppression after a single dose. When learning about these drugs in obstetrics, it is important to be familiar w/ the approximate fetal:maternal (F/M) ratios of drug concentrations at the time of delivery of the infant. Generally, the umbilical vein blood concentrations represent the fetal blood concentrations. An early high ratio indicates rapid placental transfer of the drug.

AMIODARONE (CORDARONE, PACERONE)

INDICATIONS
- Refractory or recurrent ventricular tachycardia or ventricular fibrillation, supraventricular arrhythmias

DOSING
- PO load 800–1,600 mg/day for 1–3 weeks, then 600–800 mg/day for 4 weeks, maintenance 100–400 mg/day, IV load 150–300 mg over 10 minutes, 360 mg over next 6 hours (1 mg/min), then 540 mg next 18 hours (0.5 mg/min). With liver disease, dosage adjustment may be required, but specific guidelines are unavailable.

MATERNAL SIDE EFFECTS & IMPACT ON ANESTHESIA
- Depresses SA node; prolongs PR, QRS, QT intervals; produces alpha & beta adrenergic blockade. May cause severe sinus bradycardia, ventricular arrhythmias, hepatitis & cirrhosis. Pulmonary fibrosis reported from acute & long-term use. Thyroid abnormality. Can increase serum levels of digoxin, oral anticoagulants, diltiazem, quinidine, procainamide & phenytoin.

FETAL & NEONATAL EFFECTS
- Pregnancy Category D (for definition, see the "*Pregnancy Categories*" section). Several case reports of side effects, including neonatal hypothyroidism.

COMMENT
N/A

AMITRIPTYLINE (ELAVIL)

INDICATIONS
- Tricyclic antidepressants (TCAs) are effective for the treatment of major depressive disorders; also sometimes prescribed for chronic pain or polyneuropathy.

DOSING
- For depression in outpatients, 75 mg/day divided in 1–3 doses, up to 200 mg/day

MATERNAL SIDE EFFECTS & IMPACT ON ANESTHESIA
- Common side effects include anticholinergic symptoms (drying of secretions, dilated pupils, sedation). Concomitant use of

TCAs & amphetamines has been reported to result in enhanced amphetamine effects from the release of norepinephrine. Ephedrine should be given cautiously to patients on TCAs.

FETAL & NEONATAL EFFECTS
■ Pregnancy Category NR (for definition, see the "*Pregnancy Categories*" section). Breast-feeding effects are unknown; only very minute amounts are found in the infant's serum.

COMMENT
■ Do not use w/ MAO inhibitors.

AMLODIPINE (NORVASC)

INDICATIONS
■ Amlodipine is a calcium channel blocker used to treat chronic hypertension.

DOSING
■ 5–10 mg PO qd

MATERNAL SIDE EFFECTS & IMPACT ON ANESTHESIA
■ Common side effects include dizziness, fatigue, flushing, headache & palpitations.

FETAL & NEONATAL EFFECTS
■ Pregnancy Category C (for definition, see the "*Pregnancy Categories*" section). Unknown effects on breast-feeding infants.

COMMENT
■ Avoid in pts w/ aortic stenosis, CHF, angina & liver impairment.

AMPICILLIN

INDICATIONS
■ Active against a wide range of gram-positive & gram-negative bacteria

DOSING
■ 100–200 mg/kg/day IV in 4–6 divided doses

MATERNAL SIDE EFFECTS & IMPACT ON ANESTHESIA
- May interact w/ anticoagulants, including heparin, & may increase risk of bleeding. Adjust dose in pts w/ renal failure.

FETAL & NEONATAL EFFECTS
- Pregnancy Category B (for definition, see the "*Pregnancy Categories*" section). Crosses placenta rapidly; fetal serum levels of ampicillin are detected within 30 minutes. Excreted in breast milk in low concentrations. May alter infant intestinal flora, resulting in diarrhea, candidiasis or allergic response. Can interfere w/ neonatal fever workup.

COMMENT
- Generally considered safe during pregnancy, but risks & benefits must be seriously considered before using meds in nursing mothers. Either nursing or ampicillin should be discontinued to prevent sensitization of the infant.

ANCEF (CEFAZOLIN)

INDICATIONS
- Active against various gram-positive skin organisms

DOSING
- 0.5–2 g IV q6–8h

MATERNAL SIDE EFFECTS & IMPACT ON ANESTHESIA
- May need dose adjustment in pts w/ renal failure. Avoid in pts severely allergic to penicillins. Can potentiate aminoglycoside-mediated nephrotoxicity. May induce acute alcohol intolerance by inhibiting aldehyde dehydrogenase, w/ a reaction similar to disulfiram administration. May increase hypoprothrombinemic effects of anticoagulations, thereby increasing the risk of bleeding.

FETAL & NEONATAL EFFECTS
- Pregnancy Category B (for definition, see the "*Pregnancy Categories*" section). Crosses placenta & is found in breast milk in low concentrations; American Academy of Pediatrics considers cefazolin safe during breast-feeding.

COMMENT
- Generally considered safe in pregnancy

ANECTINE (SUCCINYLCHOLINE)

INDICATIONS
- Depolarizing neuromuscular blocking drug (NMBD) to facilitate muscle paralysis for intubation

DOSING
- 1–1.5 mg/kg IV (onset 45 sec)

MATERNAL SIDE EFFECTS & IMPACT ON ANESTHESIA
- Can precipitate malignant hyperthermia, trismus, cardiac dysrhythmias, hyperkalemia, myalgias, myoglobinuria; increases intragastric pressure; increases intraocular pressure. Despite a decrease in plasma cholinesterase in parturients, intubating dose is not reduced.

FETAL & NEONATAL EFFECTS
- Pregnancy Category C (for definition, see the "*Pregnancy Categories*" section). Only small amounts cross placenta, since it is highly ionized & water-soluble.

COMMENT
- No depressant effects on neonatal ventilation w/ intubating dose. Despite decreased plasma cholinesterase levels in pregnant pts, metabolism is not prolonged due to increased volume of distribution.

APRESOLINE (HYDRALAZINE)

INDICATIONS
- Hypertension

DOSING
- 2.5–20 mg IV q4h prn; in pre-eclampsia/eclampsia 5–10 mg IV q20min up to 20 mg

MATERNAL SIDE EFFECTS & IMPACT ON ANESTHESIA
- May cause hypotension, reflex tachycardia, SLE syndrome

FETAL & NEONATAL EFFECTS
- Pregnancy Category C (for definition, see the "*Pregnancy Categories*" section). Studies suggest no increased incidence of fetal anomalies & no adverse effects on uterine blood flow. Report of transient neonatal

thrombocytopenia w/ daily 3rd-trimester use (w/ petechial bleeding & hematomas), lupus-like syndrome in neonate. American Academy of Pediatrics states hydralazine is compatible w/ breast-feeding.

COMMENT
- Animal studies have demonstrated teratogenic effects, including cleft palate & facial & cranial bone malformations.

ASPIRIN

INDICATIONS
- Used for analgesia. Inhibits platelet aggregation by inactivation of platelet cyclo-oxygenase, the enzyme that produces the cyclic endoperoxide precursor of thromboxane A2. Low-dose aspirin may be prescribed for pregnant women at risk for IUGR or pre-eclampsia. The CLASP study, which evaluated >9,000 women, concluded low-dose aspirin had no significant effect on either IUGR or pre-eclamptic conditions.

DOSING
- 325–1,000 mg q4–6h up to 4 g/day

MATERNAL SIDE EFFECTS & IMPACT ON ANESTHESIA
- There is no evidence of teratogenesis if used in the 1st trimester. Contraindicated in pts w/ peptic or duodenal ulcers, hemophilia, thrombocytopenia or other bleeding tendencies. There is no contraindication to regional anesthesia in pts taking aspirin.

FETAL & NEONATAL EFFECTS
- Pregnancy Category C in the first 2 trimesters; Pregnancy Category D in 3rd (for definitions, see the "*Pregnancy Categories*" section). Aspirin is associated w/ increased risk of intracranial hemorrhage in premature infants when used in the last week of pregnancy. Aspirin is transferred to breast milk; should be used cautiously during breast-feeding.

COMMENT
- Some persons, especially asthmatics, exhibit notable sensitivity to aspirin. Hypersensitivity reactions including skin eruptions, urticaria, angioedema, paroxysmal bronchospasm & dyspnea may be present in some pts, particularly asthmatics. Use w/ caution to pts w/ impaired renal function, in pts w/ severe liver disease, in pts w/ a

history of GI disorders such as peptic ulcers, ulcerative colitis & Crohn's disease, dyspepsia, anemia & when the pt is dehydrated. Aspirin may enhance the activity of warfarin, anticoagulants, methotrexate, oral antidiabetic preparations, valproic acid & sulfonamides. Suspect aspirin sensitivity if pt has an allergy to other nonsteroidal drugs.

ASTRAMORPH (MORPHINE)

INDICATIONS
■ No longer used as primary analgesic for pain in labor in the U.S. because of neonatal respiratory depression. Earliest anesthetic used for treatment of labor pain. Analgesia, intraoperative anesthesia, post-op analgesia.

DOSING
■ Usual dose for maternal analgesia is 2–5 mg IV or 5–10 mg IM. Onset of analgesia is 3–5 minutes after the IV administration & within 20–40 minutes after the IM dose. For post-op analgesia, morphine can be used in PCA or neuraxially (0.1–0.25 mg intrathecally or 2.0–5.0 mg epidurally). Use preservative-free preparation if neuraxial.

MATERNAL SIDE EFFECTS & IMPACT ON ANESTHESIA
■ Infrequently used during labor because of its greater respiratory depression in the neonate than w/ meperidine. As w/ other opiates, has antitussive, constipating, sedating & emetic potential.

FETAL & NEONATAL EFFECTS
■ Pregnancy Category C (for definition, see the "*Pregnancy Categories*" section). Readily crosses placenta & may cause neonatal respiratory depression. Opioids in general may result in decreased beat-to-beat variability of the fetal heart rate (FHR). Likelihood of neonatal respiratory depression depends on the dose & timing of administration.

COMMENT
■ Studies have suggested that that systematically administered morphine does not relieve the visceral pain of labor. Epidural morphine may have diminished efficacy if 3-chloroprocaine has been given epidurally previously.

ATENOLOL (TENORMIN)

INDICATIONS
■ Angina pectoris & hypertension. Atenolol is a cardioselective beta-1 adrenoceptor blocking agent.

DOSING
■ 25–100 mg PO qd

MATERNAL SIDE EFFECTS & IMPACT ON ANESTHESIA
■ May cause maternal bradycardia, bronchospasm in asthmatics, dizziness & hypotension

FETAL & NEONATAL EFFECTS
■ Pregnancy Category D (for definition, see the "*Pregnancy Categories*" section). Crosses placenta & may result in newborn infants w/ hypotonia & hypoglycemia & infants that are small for gestational age. Produces steady-state fetal levels that are approximately equal to those in the maternal serum. Atenolol is excreted into breast milk; generally should be avoided during lactation.

COMMENT
■ Contraindicated in the presence of 2nd- or 3rd-degree heart block & metabolic acidosis. Use particular caution in pts w/ asthma, bronchitis, chronic respiratory diseases, bradycardia <50 per minute, peripheral vascular diseases & Raynaud's phenomenon.

ATIVAN (LORAZEPAM)

INDICATIONS
■ Benzodiazepine indicated for anxiety disorders, preanesthesia sedation, status epilepticus. Non-label uses include alcohol withdrawal, antiemetic, insomnia.

DOSING
■ Anxiety disorders: initial, 2–3 mg/day PO divided into 2 or 3 daily doses

MATERNAL SIDE EFFECTS & IMPACT ON ANESTHESIA
- May interact w/ other meds, including other CNS drugs such as phenothiazines, narcotic analgesics, barbiturates, antidepressants, scopolamine, MAO inhibitors.

FETAL & NEONATAL EFFECTS
- Pregnancy Category D (for definition, see the "*Pregnancy Categories*" section). High IV doses may produce floppy infant syndrome. A higher incidence of respiratory depression (not statistically significant) occurred among infants whose mothers received lorazepam to potentiate the effects of narcotic analgesics. Preterm neonates whose mothers had been given lorazepam PO or IV had a high incidence of low Apgar scores, need for ventilation, hypothermia & poor suckling. Unknown effects on breast-feeding infants but may be of concern.

COMMENT
- N/A

ATORVASTATIN (LIPITOR)

INDICATION
- Adjunct to diet for reduction of elevated total cholesterol, LDL cholesterol, apolipoprotein B & triglyceride levels in pts w/ primary hypercholesterolemia, mixed dyslipidemia & heterozygous familial hypercholesterolemia

DOSING
- 10–40 mg PO qd

MATERNAL SIDE EFFECTS & IMPACT ON ANESTHESIA
- Contraindicated in pregnancy, in breast-feeding mothers & in women of childbearing potential not using adequate contraceptive measures. An interval of 1 month should be allowed from stopping atorvastatin treatment to conception in the event of planning a pregnancy.

FETAL & NEONATAL EFFECTS
- Pregnancy Category X (for definition, see the "*Pregnancy Categories*" section)

COMMENT
- May cause elevation of creatine phosphokinase & dose-related increases in transaminase levels

---

ATROPINE

INDICATIONS
- Vagolytic; treatment of life-threatening bradycardias. Competitive antagonism to ACh (acetylcholine) & other muscarinic agonists.

DOSING
- 0.5–1 mg IV q5min, not to exceed a total of 2 mg

MATERNAL SIDE EFFECTS & IMPACT ON ANESTHESIA
- Side effects include dryness of oral mucosa, thirst, reduced bronchial secretions, mydriasis w/ loss of accommodation (cycloplegia) & photophobia, flushing & dryness of the skin, transient bradycardia, tachycardia, arrhythmias, difficult micturition, reduction of tone & mobility of the GI tract, constipation. Anticholinergic effects may be exacerbated by concurrent use of tricyclic antidepressants.

FETAL & NEONATAL EFFECTS
- Pregnancy Category C (for definition, see the "*Pregnancy Categories*" section). Crosses the placenta & is excreted in breast milk. Can suppress fetal respiration without causing hypoxia or adverse effects on fetal heart rate. Not recommended for treating fetal & newborn bradycardias in the setting of hypoxemia. Compatible w/ breast-feeding but may reduce milk production.

COMMENT
- Crosses the blood-brain barrier. Watch for paradoxical bradycardia at lower doses.

ATROVENT (IPRATROPIUM)

INDICATIONS
- Bronchodilator. Used for bronchospasm associated w/ COPD, asthma (re: asthma–FDA off-label use), rhinorrhea w/ cold, seasonal allergy, etc.

DOSING

- Inhaler 2 puffs (36 mcg) $4 \times$/day up to 12 puffs/day
- Nebulizer 500 mcg 3 or 4 times/day

MATERNAL SIDE EFFECTS & IMPACT ON ANESTHESIA

- May be associated w/ dry cough, bitter taste. Contraindicated w/ narrow-angle glaucoma, bladder neck obstruction.

FETAL & NEONATAL EFFECTS

- Pregnancy Category B (for definition, see the "*Pregnancy Categories*" section). Use in pregnancy is indicated where there are maternal benefits. It is thought that very little drug passes into breast milk.

COMMENT

- May be contraindicated in pts w/ sensitivity to soya lecithin or related food products such as soybeans or peanuts.

AZITHROMYCIN (ZITHROMAX)

INDICATIONS

- Active against a wide range of gram-positive & gram-negative bacteria

DOSING

- 1,200–1,500 mg/week PO, w/ divided doses of tablets of 250–500 mg/day orally

MATERNAL SIDE EFFECTS & IMPACT ON ANESTHESIA

- Very rare allergic reactions have been reported, including Stevens-Johnson syndrome & toxic epidermal necrolysis. Use w/ caution in pts w/ impaired liver function. Do not administer concomitantly w/ ergot derivatives.

FETAL & NEONATAL EFFECTS

- Pregnancy Category B (for definition, see the "*Pregnancy Categories*" section). Crosses placenta. It is not known if transmission via breast milk is clinically significant.

COMMENT

- Should be taken at least 1 hour before or 2 hours after antacids

AZT (ZIDOVUDINE)

INDICATIONS
- Inhibits HIV replication

DOSING
- 300–600 mg/day PO in 3–5 divided doses

MATERNAL SIDE EFFECTS & IMPACT ON ANESTHESIA
- Women in the 1st trimester may consider delaying or discontinuing therapy until after 10–12 weeks gestation. Recommended component of the peri- & post-partum regimen for mother & neonate whenever possible.

FETAL & NEONATAL EFFECTS
- Pregnancy Category C (for definition, see the "*Pregnancy Categories*" section). Significantly reduces transmission of HIV to the fetus. There are conflicting data on perinatal exposure to antiretrovirals associated w/ significant (often fatal) mitochondrial disease in infants. Babies exposed to antiretrovirals in utero should receive long-term follow-up for potential mitochondrial dysfunction.

COMMENT
- Breast-feeding is not recommended in mothers w/ HIV due to presence of virus in breast milk & potential for transmission to HIV-negative child.

BACTRIM (CO-TRIMOXAZOLE/SULFAMETHOXAZOLE)

INDICATIONS
- Bacteriocidal agent often used in combination w/ trimethoprim (Proloprim, Trimpex). Effective against a wide variety of gram-positive & gram-negative bacteria, though high rates of resistance are common.

DOSING
- PO: 80–160 mg TMP/400–800 mg SMX depending on indication dosed 1–4 times/d
- IV: 80 mg TMP/400 mg SMX per 10 cc. Good penetration in CSF.

MATERNAL SIDE EFFECTS & IMPACT ON ANESTHESIA

■ Common side effects include nausea, vomiting, skin eruptions/rash, Steven-Johnson syndrome, pruritus. HIV-positive pts are likely to have more severe reactions.

FETAL & NEONATAL EFFECTS

■ Crosses placenta in all stages of gestation; fetal blood levels are 70–90% of maternal levels within 2–3 hours. Pregnancy Category D (for definition, see the "*Pregnancy Categories*" section) if given near term. When given immediately prior to delivery, toxic neonatal levels can persist for days, causing jaundice & hemolytic anemia. Excreted in low levels in breast milk; American Academy of Pediatrics states compatible w/ breast-feeding for term infants. Use w/ extreme caution when nursing premature infants or those w/ hyperbilirubinemia & G6PD deficiency.

COMMENTS

■ Though associated w/ tracheo-esophageal fistulas & cataracts in animals, teratogenicity has not been demonstrated in humans. SMX-TMP combo may have a slightly increased risk of cardiovascular congenital defects.

BENADRYL (DIPHENHYDRAMINE) ORAL/INJECTABLE

INDICATIONS

■ Anxiety, insomnia, varicella, insect bites, allergic rhinitis, generalized pruritus, urticaria

DOSING

■ 25–50 mg PO q4–6h or 10–50 mg IM/IV q2–3h; maximum parenteral dose 400 mg/day

MATERNAL SIDE EFFECTS & IMPACT ON ANESTHESIA

■ Concomitant use of antidepressants w/ strong anticholinergic effects (eg, amitriptyline, trimipramine, amoxapine, doxepin, imipramine, nortriptyline, maprotiline) may increase potential for adynamic ileus & urinary retention. Increases CNS depression when taken w/ barbiturates, narcotics, hypnotics, tricyclic antidepressants, MAO inhibitors, alcohol. Decreases effect of oral anticoagulants, including heparin.

FETAL & NEONATAL EFFECTS

■ Pregnancy Category B (for definition, see the "*Pregnancy Categories*" section). Crosses placenta & passes freely into breast milk. Relatively contraindicated during breast-feeding due to potential sedating effects on newborn.

COMMENT

■ While antihistamines are sometimes used to treat narcotic-induced pruritus, this condition is more directly & appropriately managed w/ a partial agonist-antagonist agent such as Nubain (nalbuphine) 5–10 mg IV w/ less risk of increased sedation.

BENZOCAINE 20% (CETACAINE, HURRICAINE)

INDICATIONS

■ Topical anesthetic can be applied as a cream or a spray. Many vaginitis creams incorporate benzocaine as the primary anesthetic. Lozenges/sprays are also available for oral sores or pharyngitis. Used in the setting of awake intubations, benzocaine blunts the gag reflex & allows for direct or fiberoptic laryngoscopy.

DOSING

■ Topical spray: Recommended dose is 1 second of continuous spray (average expulsion rate is 200 mg/sec). Exceeding this duration may be hazardous & may result in methemoglobinemia. Onset within 15–30 seconds.

MATERNAL SIDE EFFECTS & IMPACT ON ANESTHESIA

■ Pregnancy Category C (for definition, see the "*Pregnancy Categories*" section). One of its metabolites (orthotoluidine) has been associated w/ methemoglobinemia.

FETAL & NEONATAL EFFECTS

■ Pregnancy Category C. Methemoglobinemia can be problematic in the fetus, as it lacks the enzymes to metabolize it. Not expected to accumulate significantly in breast milk.

COMMENT

N/A

BETAMETHASONE

INDICATIONS
■ Prenatal treatment in pregnancies at risk of preterm delivery (24–34 weeks gestation) reduces neonatal mortality, respiratory distress syndrome & intraventricular hemorrhage. Single courses are as effective & safer than weekly courses in preventing composite neonatal morbidity (bronchopulmonary dysplasia, severe respiratory distress syndrome, severe intraventricular hemorrhage, sepsis, necrotizing enterocolitis, perinatal death). Also used in adrenal insufficiency, arthritis, dermatoses, inflammatory conditions & as an immuno-suppressive agent.

DOSING
■ 12 mg given 24 hours apart for 2 doses

MATERNAL SIDE EFFECTS & IMPACT ON ANESTHESIA
■ Corticosteroids do not appear to cause congenital anomalies in the infant. Common side effects include euphoria/depression, GI distress, growth depression, hypertension, impaired wound healing, increased risk of infection & skin atrophy. Serious side effects include osteoporosis, hyperglycemia, Cushing syndrome, cataracts/glaucoma & adrenocortical insufficiency.

FETAL & NEONATAL EFFECTS
■ Pregnancy Category C (for definition, see the "*Pregnancy Categories*" section). Corticosteroids do not appear to cause congenital anomalies in the infant. Neonatal adrenal insufficiency appears to be rare. Systemically administered corticosteroids are secreted into breast milk in quantities not likely to have an adverse effect on the infant.

COMMENT
■ Contraindicated in pts w/ active fungal infections. Use precaution in pts w/ liver failure, myasthenia gravis, ocular herpes simplex, osteoporosis, renal insufficiency & untreated systemic infections.

BICITRA (SODIUM CITRATE)

INDICATIONS
■ Used prior to anesthesia induction as a pre-op antacid to prevent aspiration pneumonitis

DOSING
- 15–30 mL of a 0.3-molar solution, administered 10–30 minutes prior to induction of anesthesia

MATERNAL SIDE EFFECTS & IMPACT ON ANESTHESIA
- Potassium citrate & sodium citrate are absorbed & metabolized to potassium bicarbonate & sodium bicarbonate, thus acting as systemic alkalizers. Oxidation is virtually complete; <5% of the citrates are excreted in the urine unchanged.

FETAL & NEONATAL EFFECTS
- Pregnancy Category NR (for definition, see the "*Pregnancy Categories*" section). The drug crosses the placenta & enters the fetus, & its delayed, long-term effects on the exposed offspring have not been investigated.

COMMENT
- Use special care in the pt w/ pre-eclampsia or toxemia of pregnancy, as the sodium in sodium-containing citrates may cause the body to retain water.

BUPIVACAINE (MARCAINE, SENSORCAINE)

INDICATIONS
- Epidural infusion for labor analgesia in low concentrations 0.125–0.04%; spinal injection for labor analgesia or cesarean delivery

DOSING
- 8–10 mL of 0.25–0.5% provides approx. 2 hours of epidural analgesia. When dilute solutions are used, bupivacaine produces excellent sensory analgesia w/ minimal motor blockade; tachyphylaxis occurs rarely. For labor spinals, 2.5 mg can provide at least 60 minutes of analgesia (adjuncts can be added to prolong effect); for cesarean delivery, spinal bupivacaine 12–15 mg (usually 0.75% bupivacaine w/ dextrose) is adequate (adjuncts can be added to improve effect).

MATERNAL SIDE EFFECTS & IMPACT ON ANESTHESIA
- High-dose (0.75%) bupivacaine is not recommended for use in epidurals in obstetrics due to the profound maternal & neonatal myocardial depression & difficult resuscitation associated w/ accidental intravascular injection.

FETAL & NEONATAL SIDE EFFECTS

■ Pregnancy Category C (for definition, see the "*Pregnancy Categories*" section). Highly protein-bound, which limits transplacental transfer. Any drug that reaches the fetus undergoes metabolism & excretion. The newborn has the hepatic enzymes necessary for the biotransformation of amide local anesthetics. Elimination half-life is longer in neonates than adults. Bupivacaine is considered safe for breast-feeding.

COMMENT

■ There is no association btwn local anesthetic use & fetal malformations during the first 4 months of pregnancy.

BUTORPHANOL (STADOL)

INDICATIONS

■ An opioid w/ agonist-antagonist properties, used for the relief of mild to moderate, deep or visceral pain & for chronic pain. Butorphanol is a synthetic opioid agonist-antagonist analgesic.

DOSING

■ Typical dose: 1–2 mg IV/IM; can be given as frequently as q1–2h

MATERNAL SIDE EFFECTS & IMPACT ON ANESTHESIA

■ Use w/ caution w/ other sedative or analgesic drugs, as these are likely to produce additive effects. As w/ nalbuphine, it has a ceiling effect on respiratory depression.

FETAL & NEONATAL EFFECTS

■ Pregnancy Category C; Category D if used for prolonged periods or in high doses at term (for definitions, see the "*Pregnancy Categories*" section). Although butorphanol may pass into the breast milk, it is not expected to cause problems in nursing babies. May cause a sinusoidal fetal heart rate pattern during labor that is not associated w/ hypoxia.

COMMENT

■ Overdose signs include cold, clammy skin; confusion; convulsions (seizures); dizziness (severe); drowsiness (severe); nervousness, restlessness, or weakness (severe); small pupils; slow heartbeat; slow or troubled breathing.

CAFFEINE (NO-DOZ, VIVARIN)

INDICATIONS
- A CNS vasoconstrictor, useful for mild post-dural puncture headaches. One of the most popular drugs in the world!

DOSING
- 300–500 mg PO/IV q12–24h

MATERNAL SIDE EFFECTS & IMPACT ON ANESTHESIA
- Causes tachycardia & nervousness. Avoid in pts w/ preexisting arrhythmias.

FETAL & NEONATAL EFFECTS
- Pregnancy Category C (for definition, see the "*Pregnancy Categories*" section). Caffeine crosses the placenta. Caffeine intake >300 mg/day is not recommended. Considered compatible w/ breast-feeding within recommended dosing guidelines.

COMMENT
- A cup of coffee contains about 40–100 mg of caffeine; soft drinks contain 10–55 mg.

CALCIUM CHLORIDE/CALCIUM GLUCONATE

INDICATIONS
- Cardiac life support, hyperphosphatemia, hypocalcemia, hypermagnesemia

DOSING
- Varies depending on treatment & indication
- For cardiac life support, calcium chloride 2–4 mg/kg (10% solution) IV repeated at 10-min intervals or calcium chloride 500 mg-1 g IV; or calcium gluconate 500 mg-2 g IV (10% solution) at 2–4 mL/min
- For hypocalcemia, calcium carbonate 500 mg-1 g PO 2 or 3 times/day

MATERNAL SIDE EFFECTS & IMPACT ON ANESTHESIA
- Excessive calcium can result in kidney stones, abdominal pain, bone pain, abdominal pain ("stones, moans, bones, groans").

FETAL & NEONATAL EFFECTS
■ Pregnancy Category NR (for definition, see the "*Pregnancy Categories*" section). Calcium is necessary for organogenesis of the heart, nerves & muscles & for development of normal heart rhythm & blood-clotting abilities. Complications such as neonatal hypocalcemia, w/ seizure activity, have been reported w/ maternal overdose.

COMMENT
■ TUMS is a common over-the-counter calcium supplement used by parturients. Hypercalcemia produces QT shortening, but this is very difficult to recognize clinically. Calcium is sometimes used to manage overdose of magnesium (as in eclampsia or pre-eclampsia).

CARBAMAZEPINE (TEGRETOL)

INDICATIONS
■ Carbamazepine, a tricyclic, is both an anticonvulsant & psychotropic. Typically used for epilepsy w/ motor & psychic manifestations. Also used in the treatment of trigeminal neuralgia.

DOSING
■ 1,600 mg/day PO

MATERNAL SIDE EFFECTS & IMPACT ON ANESTHESIA
■ Contraindicated in expectant or nursing mothers or pts w/ liver disease. Induction of hepatic enzymes in response to carbamazepine may have the effect of diminishing the activity of certain drugs that are metabolized in the liver. In obstetrics, its use is limited to cases where maternal benefit is greater than potential fetal harm.

FETAL & NEONATAL EFFECTS
■ Pregnancy Category D (for definition, see the "*Pregnancy Categories*" section). The active substance of carbamazepine passes into the breast milk. It is considered incompatible w/ breast-feeding.

COMMENT
■ Abnormalities of liver function & jaundice have been associated w/ long-term treatment. Overall, pregnant women should be advised of the multiple potential adverse outcomes of the drug, but it should not routinely be withheld as the benefits of preventing seizures may outweigh the potential fetal harm.

CARBOCAINE (MEPIVACAINE)

INDICATIONS
■ Spinal anesthesia for short OB procedures

DOSING
■ Varies depending on procedure, but similar to lidocaine (20% more potent)
■ Spinal: 50 mg for short OB procedures (cerclage, cerclage removal, etc.) Adjuvant: Sodium bicarbonate may be added w/ a 1:10 ratio.
■ Metabolism is via hydroxylation & N-demethylation in the liver. Elimination half-life is 2–3 hours.

MATERNAL SIDE EFFECTS & IMPACT ON ANESTHESIA
■ Intravascular administration may lead to lightheadedness, seizures, disorientation, heart block, hypotension.

FETAL SIDE EFFECTS
■ Pregnancy Category C (for definition, see the "*Pregnancy Categories*" section). Not recommended for epidural use, paracervical or pudendal blocks as the fetus cannot metabolize this drug. Safety in breastfeeding is unknown, but local anesthetics are not expected to accumulate significantly in breast milk.

COMMENTS
■ Use preservative-free solutions for intrathecal administration. Use hyperbaric preparations for wider spread of block.

CARBOPROST TROMETHAMINE (PROSTAGLANDIN F2α; HEMABATE)

INDICATIONS
■ Prostaglandin is similar to F2-alpha (dinoprost), but it has a longer duration & produces myometrial contractions that induce hemostasis at placentation site, which reduces post-partum bleeding. Hemabate is used to treat post-partum hemorrhage & causes of uterine atony (overdistended uterus, rapid or prolonged labor, chorioamnionitis, high parity).

DOSING

- Treatment of postpartum hemorrhage: 0.25mg (250 mcg/mL) IM q15–90min, up to 2 mg

MATERNAL SIDE EFFECTS & IMPACT ON ANESTHESIA

- Administration can cause marked pulmonary arteriolar muscle constriction, severe pulmonary hypertension & bronchoconstriction. Can cause hypertension, but not as severe as the ergotamines.

FETAL & NEONATAL EFFECTS

- Pregnancy Category C (for definition, see the "*Pregnancy Categories*" section). Hemabate can induce labor & can even be used to abort the fetus in early stages of pregnancy. Hemabate is found in breast milk, but it is unknown if this is of clinical significance.

COMMENT

- Avoid in pts w/ pre-existing asthma or reactive airway disorders.

CARDIZEM (DILTIAZEM)

INDICATIONS

- Angina, hypertension, arrhythmias (atrial fib/atrial flutter), paroxysmal supraventricular tachycardia; has been used as a tocolytic

DOSING

- Depends on indication
- Available in oral immediate-release, extended-release (qd) & sustained-release (bid) tabs & capsules for angina & hypertension
- IV forms are used to treat arrhythmias. Initial bolus 0.25 mg/kg over 2 min, repeat 0.35-mg/kg bolus in 15 min for inadequate response.
- Continuous infusion starts at 10 mg/hr, may be increased at 5-mg/hr intervals for therapeutic effect. Infusions lasting >24 hours are not recommended.

MATERNAL SIDE EFFECTS & IMPACT ON ANESTHESIA

- Most common side effects are edema, 1st-degree AV block, headache, hypotension. Concomitant use w/ beta-blockers, digoxin & amiodarone can lead to severe conduction disturbances, bradycardia & hypotension. Can increase plasma concentration of alfentanil, fentanyl & benzodiazepines.

FETAL & NEONATAL EFFECTS
- Pregnancy Category C (for definition, see the "*Pregnancy Categories*" section). Diffuses freely into breast milk, though no adverse effects reported. American Academy of Pediatrics says compatible w/ breast-feeding.

COMMENTS
- Do not use in pts w/ ventricular dysfunction, acute MI, pulmonary congestion, sick sinus syndrome or 2nd- or 3rd-degree AV block w/o pacer.

CATAPRES (CLONIDINE)

INDICATIONS
- Antihypertensive & analgesic. Clonidine has both central & peripheral action on alpha-2-adrenergic receptors. It reduces vascular responses to vasoconstrictor as well as vasodilator stimuli.

DOSING
- Initial dose: 0.1 mg twice daily
- Usual maintenance dose: 0.2–1.2 mg/day in divided doses 2–4× daily; maximum recommended dose 2.4 mg/day

MATERNAL SIDE EFFECTS & IMPACT ON ANESTHESIA
- Clonidine is not recommended for obstetrical, post-partum or perioperative pain mgt because of the risk of hemodynamic instability, especially hypotension & bradycardia. "Black Box" category for spinal & epidural use in parturients due to excessive sedation.

FETAL & NEONATAL EFFECTS
- Pregnancy Category C (for definition, see the "*Pregnancy Categories*" section). Crosses placenta easily, but no evidence of teratogenicity. Clonidine is excreted in human milk & levels quickly achieve those of the mother. The clinical significance is unknown.

COMMENT
- Withdrawal of clonidine therapy should be gradual as sudden discontinuation may cause rebound hypertension, sometimes severe. Contraindicated in pts w/ porphyria.

CEFAZOLIN (ANCEF)

INDICATIONS
■ Active against various gram-positive skin organisms

DOSING
■ 0.5–2 g IV q6–8h

MATERNAL SIDE EFFECTS & IMPACT ON ANESTHESIA
■ May need dose adjustment in pts w/ renal failure. Avoid in pts severely allergic to penicillins. Can potentiate aminoglycoside-mediated nephrotoxicity. May induce acute alcohol intolerance by inhibiting aldehyde dehydrogenase, w/ a reaction similar to disulfiram administration. May increase hypoprothrombinemic effects of anticoagulations, thereby increasing the risk of bleeding.

FETAL & NEONATAL EFFECTS
■ Pregnancy Category B (for definition, see the *"Pregnancy Categories"* section). Crosses placenta & is found in breast milk in low concentrations; American Academy of Pediatrics considers cefazolin safe during breast-feeding.

COMMENT
■ Generally considered safe in pregnancy

CEFTRIAXONE (ROCEPHIN)

INDICATIONS
■ Active against various gram-positive & gram-negative bacteria

DOSING
■ 1–2 g IV q12–24h depending on organism, location & severity of infection

MATERNAL SIDE EFFECTS & IMPACT ON ANESTHESIA
■ May need dose adjustment in pts w/ renal failure. May be associated w/ decreased prothrombin activity. Can be associated w/ urinary cast formation.

FETAL & NEONATAL EFFECTS
■ Pregnancy Category B (for definition, see the *"Pregnancy Categories"* section). Crosses placenta & is found in breast milk in low

concentrations. May displace bilirubin from albumin binding sites. Avoid in mothers of premature or hyperbilirubinemic neonates.

COMMENT
- Generally considered safe in pregnancy

CETACAINE (BENZOCAINE 20%)

INDICATIONS
- Topical anesthetic can be applied as a cream or a spray. Many vaginitis creams incorporate benzocaine as the primary anesthetic. Lozenges/sprays are also available for oral sores or pharyngitis. Used in the setting of awake intubations, benzocaine blunts the gag reflex & allows for direct or fiberoptic laryngoscopy.

DOSING
- Topical spray: Recommended dose is 1 second of continuous spray (average expulsion rate is 200 mg/sec). Exceeding this duration may be hazardous & may result in methemoglobinemia. Onset within 15–30 seconds.

MATERNAL SIDE EFFECTS & IMPACT ON ANESTHESIA
- Pregnancy Category C (for definition, see the "*Pregnancy Categories*" section). One of its metabolites (orthotoluidine) has been associated w/ methemoglobinemia.

FETAL & NEONATAL EFFECTS
- Pregnancy Category C. Methemoglobinemia can be problematic in the fetus, as it lacks the enzymes to metabolize it. Not expected to accumulate significantly in breast milk.

COMMENT
- N/A

CHIROCAINE (LEVO-BUPIVACAINE)

INDICATIONS
- Epidural analgesia

DOSING
- Epidural labor analgesia: 10–20 mL of 0.25% (25–50 mg)

- Epidural for cesarean delivery: 20–30 cc of 0.5% (100–150 mg)
- Epidural for post-op analgesia: 4–10 cc/hr of 0.125–0.25% (5–25 mg/hr)

MATERNAL SIDE EFFECTS & IMPACT ON ANESTHESIA

- May have a better cardiac safety profile than bupivacaine in higher doses, but higher cost & safe use of low concentrations of bupivacaine for epidural analgesia limit its utility.

FETAL & NEONATAL SIDE EFFECTS

- Pregnancy Category C (for definition, see the "*Pregnancy Categories*" section). Safety in breast-feeding is unknown, but local anesthetics are not expected to accumulate significantly in breast milk.

COMMENT

- N/A

CHLOROPROCAINE, 3% (NESACAINE)

INDICATIONS

- Used widely via epidural (in bolus form) for C-section

DOSING

- 20–30 cc (pH adjusted) given in 4 or 5 divided doses for a final dermatome level of T4–T5 bilaterally for C-section. 10 cc via epidural (T10 level) may be used to provide analgesia for instrument delivery or tubal ligation.

MATERNAL SIDE EFFECTS & IMPACT ON ANESTHESIA

- Even when injected IV, there are rare adverse effects. Metabolized by pseudocholinesterases, which are decreased in pregnancy.

FETAL & NEONATAL SIDE EFFECTS

- Pregnancy Category C (for definition, see the "*Pregnancy Categories*" section). Minimal effects. Drug that reaches the fetus undergoes metabolism & excretion. Elimination half-life is longer in neonates than adults. Not expected to accumulate significantly in breast milk.

COMMENT

- Always use bisulfite-free & EDTA-free preparations for regional anesthesia procedures. It is the local anesthetic of choice for epidural anesthesia in the setting of fetal acidosis.

CIPRO (CIPROFLOXACIN)

INDICATIONS
■ Active against a wide range of gram-positive & gram-negative bacteria

DOSING
■ 250–750 IV mg q12h, depending on severity of infection & susceptibility

MATERNAL SIDE EFFECTS & IMPACT ON ANESTHESIA
■ Can exacerbate respiratory muscle weakness in pts w/ MS. May decrease clearance & increase plasma levels of theophylline & caffeine.

FETAL & NEONATAL EFFECTS
■ Pregnancy Category C (for definition, see the "*Pregnancy Categories*" section) Crosses placenta. Causal relationship of some birth defects cannot be excluded, though not embryotoxic or teratogenic in rats at high doses. Not recommended during breast-feeding due to documented arthropathy in animals.

CIPROFLOXACIN (CIPRO)

INDICATIONS
■ Active against a wide range of gram-positive & gram-negative bacteria

DOSING
■ 250–750 IV mg q12h, depending on severity of infection & susceptibility

MATERNAL SIDE EFFECTS & IMPACT ON ANESTHESIA
■ Can exacerbate respiratory muscle weakness in pts w/ MS. May decrease clearance & increase plasma levels of theophylline & caffeine.

FETAL & NEONATAL EFFECTS
■ Pregnancy Category C (for definition, see the "*Pregnancy Categories*" section). Crosses placenta. Causal relationship of some birth defects cannot be excluded, though not embryotoxic or teratogenic in rats

at high doses. Not recommended during breast-feeding due to documented arthropathy in animals.

CIS-ATRACURIUM (NIMBEX)

INDICATIONS
■ Non-depolarizing neuromuscular blocking drug (NMBD) used to facilitate intubation & maintain neuromuscular blockade

DOSING
■ 0.2 mg/kg IV (onset 2–8 min)

MATERNAL SIDE EFFECTS & IMPACT ON ANESTHESIA
■ Action may be prolonged in pts receiving IV magnesium.

FETAL & NEONATAL EFFECTS
■ Pregnancy Category B (for definition, see the "*Pregnancy Categories*" section). No adverse effects w/ intubating dose.

COMMENT
■ Presumed safe in pregnant pts. Long onset of action makes it less desirable for rapid sequence induction.

CLEOCIN (CLINDAMYCIN)

INDICATIONS
■ Second-line for the treatment & prevention of neonatal group B streptococcal infection. Typically given after cesarean section delivery for skin incision prophylaxis in PCN-allergic women. Active against most gram-positive organisms & anaerobes.

DOSING
■ 150–450 mg/dose q6–8h orally; 600 mg-2.7 g/day in 4–6 divided doses IM or IV

MATERNAL SIDE EFFECTS & IMPACT ON ANESTHESIA
■ May enhance the effect of non-depolarizing muscle relaxants

FETAL & NEONATAL EFFECTS
■ Pregnancy Category B (for definition, see the "*Pregnancy Categories*" section). Crosses placenta. American Academy of Pediatrics

considers clindamycin compatible w/ breast-feeding, but it may alter the intestinal flora of the infant.

COMMENT
- Use w/ caution in pts w/ renal or hepatic impairment.

CLINDAMYCIN (CLEOCIN)

INDICATIONS
- Second-line for the treatment & prevention of neonatal group B streptococcal infection. Typically given after cesarean section delivery for skin incision prophylaxis in PCN-allergic women. Active against most gram-positive organisms & anaerobes.

DOSING
- 150–450 mg/dose q6–8h orally; 600 mg-2.7 g/day in 4–6 divided doses IM or IV

MATERNAL SIDE EFFECTS & IMPACT ON ANESTHESIA
- May enhance the effect of non-depolarizing muscle relaxants

FETAL & NEONATAL EFFECTS
- Pregnancy Category B (for definition, see the "*Pregnancy Categories*" section). Crosses placenta. American Academy of Pediatrics considers clindamycin compatible w/ breast-feeding, but it may alter the intestinal flora of the infant.

COMMENT
- Use w/ caution in pts w/ renal or hepatic impairment.

CLONIDINE (CATAPRES)

INDICATIONS
- Antihypertensive & analgesic. Clonidine has both central & peripheral action on alpha-2-adrenergic receptors. It reduces vascular responses to vasoconstrictor as well as vasodilator stimuli.

DOSING
- Initial dose: 0.1 mg twice daily
- Usual maintenance dose: 0.2–1.2 mg/day in divided doses 2–4× daily; maximum recommended dose 2.4 mg/day

MATERNAL SIDE EFFECTS & IMPACT ON ANESTHESIA
- Clonidine is not recommended for obstetrical, post-partum or peri-operative pain mgt because of the risk of hemodynamic instability, especially hypotension & bradycardia. "Black Box" category for spinal & epidural use in parturients due to excessive sedation.

FETAL & NEONATAL EFFECTS
- Pregnancy Category C (for definition, see the "*Pregnancy Categories*" section). Crosses placenta easily, but no evidence of teratogenicity. Clonidine is excreted in human milk & levels quickly achieve those of the mother. The clinical significance is unknown.

COMMENT
- Withdrawal of clonidine therapy should be gradual as sudden discontinuation may cause rebound hypertension, sometimes severe. Contraindicated in pts w/ porphyria.

COMPAZINE (PROCHLORPERAZINE)

INDICATIONS
- May relieve nausea & vomiting by blocking postsynaptic mesolimbic dopamine receptors through anticholinergic effects & depressing reticular activating system. In a placebo-controlled study, 69% of pts given prochlorperazine reported significant symptom relief, compared to 40% of pts in the placebo group.

DOSING
- PO: 5–10 mg tid/qid, max 40 mg/d
- IV: 2.5–10 mg q3–4h prn, max 10 mg/dose or 40 mg/d
- IM: 5–10 mg q3–4h
- PR: 25 mg bid

MATERNAL SIDE EFFECTS & IMPACT ON ANESTHESIA
- Co-administration w/ other CNS depressants or anticonvulsants may cause additive effects; w/ epinephrine, may cause hypotension.

FETAL & NEONATAL EFFECTS
- Pregnancy Category C (for definition, see the "*Pregnancy Categories*" section)

COMMENT

■ Drug-induced Parkinson syndrome or pseudoparkinsonism occurs quite frequently. Akathisia is most common extrapyramidal reaction in elderly pts. Lowers seizure threshold; may lower convulsive threshold. Adverse effects can include hypotension, sedation & extrapyramidal & anticholinergic symptoms. Data are conflicting regarding teratogenicity. Crosses placenta & appears in breast milk.

CORDARONE (AMIODARONE)

INDICATIONS

■ Refractory or recurrent ventricular tachycardia or ventricular fibrillation, supraventricular arrhythmias

DOSING

■ PO load 800–1,600 mg/day for 1–3 weeks, then 600–800 mg/day for 4 weeks, maintenance 100–400 mg/day, IV load 150–300 mg over 10 minutes, 360 mg over next 6 hours (1 mg/min), then 540 mg next 18 hours (0.5 mg/min). With liver disease, dosage adjustment may be required, but specific guidelines are unavailable.

MATERNAL SIDE EFFECTS & IMPACT ON ANESTHESIA

■ Depresses SA node; prolongs PR, QRS, QT intervals; produces alpha & beta adrenergic blockade. May cause severe sinus bradycardia, ventricular arrhythmias, hepatitis & cirrhosis. Pulmonary fibrosis reported from acute & long-term use. Thyroid abnormality. Can increase serum levels of digoxin, oral anticoagulants, diltiazem, quinidine, procainamide & phenytoin.

FETAL & NEONATAL EFFECTS

■ Pregnancy Category D (for definition, see the "*Pregnancy Categories*" section). Several case reports of side effects, including neonatal hypothyroidism.

COMMENT

■ N/A

CO-TRIMOXAZOLE/SULFAMETHOXAZOLE (BACTRIM)

INDICATIONS

■ Bacteriocidal agent often used in combination w/ trimethoprim (Proloprim, Trimpex). Effective against a wide variety of gram-positive & gram-negative bacteria, though high rates of resistance are common.

DOSING
- PO: 80–160 mg TMP/400–800 mg SMX depending on indication dosed 1–4 times/d
- IV: 80 mg TMP/400 mg SMX per 10 cc. Good penetration in CSF.

MATERNAL SIDE EFFECTS & IMPACT ON ANESTHESIA
- Common side effects include nausea, vomiting, skin eruptions/rash, Steven-Johnson syndrome, pruritus. HIV-positive pts are likely to have more severe reactions.

FETAL & NEONATAL EFFECTS
- Crosses placenta in all stages of gestation; fetal blood levels are 70–90% of maternal levels within 2–3 hours. Pregnancy Category D (for definition, see the *"Pregnancy Categories"* section) if given near term. When given immediately prior to delivery, toxic neonatal levels can persist for days, causing jaundice & hemolytic anemia. Excreted in low levels in breast milk; American Academy of Pediatrics states compatible w/ breast-feeding for term infants. Use w/ extreme caution when nursing premature infants or those w/ hyperbilirubinemia & G6PD deficiency.

COMMENTS
- Though associated w/ tracheo-esophageal fistulas & cataracts in animals, teratogenicity has not been demonstrated in humans. SMX-TMP combo may have a slightly increased risk of cardiovascular congenital defects.

COUMADIN (WARFARIN)

INDICATIONS
- Prevention & mgt of deep venous thrombosis & pulmonary embolism in non-pregnant pts. Warfarin is contraindicated in pregnancy.

DOSING
- Contraindicated in pregnancy.

MATERNAL SIDE EFFECTS & IMPACT ON ANESTHESIA
- N/A

FETAL & NEONATAL EFFECTS

■ Pregnancy Category D (for definition, see the "*Pregnancy Categories*" section). Warfarin should be avoided in pregnancy. Skeletal & CNS defects as well as fetal hemorrhage have been reported.

COMMENT

■ Warfarin is excreted in breast milk in an inactive form. Its ionic, non-lipophilic structure & high protein-binding affinity decrease the likelihood of breast milk excretion. There is no evidence of detectable warfarin levels, altered coagulation, bleeding or other adverse effects in exposed infants. However, some experts recommend monitoring coagulation status in infants at risk for vitamin K deficiency.

CYTOTEC (MISOPROSTOL)

ANTHONY HAPGOOD, MD; JASMIN FIELD, MD; YUKI KOICHI, MD; WILTON LEVINE, MD; TODD JEN, MD; ADRIAN HAMBURGER, MD; LISA LEFFERT, MD; ZHONGCONG XIE, MD; MAY PIAN-SMITH, MD; AND JOAN SPIEGEL, MD

INDICATIONS

■ A synthetic prostaglandin E1 analog commonly used to prevent gastric ulcers during concomitant NSAID use. Used for cervical ripening for term pregnancies & for pregnancy termination. A 3rd important use is to treat uterine hypotonia.

DOSING

■ For excessive uterine hypotonia: 1 mg PR or PV. Loss of non-term pregnancy may result w/ doses of 200–400 mcg orally.

MATERNAL SIDE EFFECTS & IMPACT ON ANESTHESIA

■ Common side effects include abdominal pain, diarrhea, dyspepsia & nausea.

FETAL & NEONATAL EFFECTS

■ Pregnancy Category X (for definition, see the "*Pregnancy Categories*" section). Abortion (at times incomplete), premature labor or teratogenicity may occur after administration during pregnancy; congenital anomalies & fetal death have occurred after unsuccessful use as an abortifacient. Use of misoprostol during the 1st trimester has been associated w/ skull defects, cranial nerve palsies, facial malformations & limb defects. The drug should not be used during pregnancy to reduce the risk of NSAID-induced ulcers. It is unknown if misoprostol is excreted in breast milk.

DALTEPARIN (FRAGMIN)

INDICATIONS
■ Anticoagulant, inhibits factor Xa & factor IIa. Used for prophylaxis of deep venous thrombosis & treatment of acute coronary syndrome, deep vein thrombosis, pulmonary embolus.

DOSING
■ DVT prophylaxis: 2,500–5,000 units SQ qd
■ Acute coronary syndrome: 120 units/kg (max. 10,000 units) SQ q12h for 5–8 days
■ DVT & PE treatment (FDA off-label use): 100 units/kg SQ bid, or 200 units/kg SQ qd

MATERNAL SIDE EFFECTS & IMPACT ON ANESTHESIA
■ Should be stopped at least 24 hours prior to regional anesthesia at treatment doses & at least 12 hours after prophylaxis doses. Monitor for evidence of bleeding or excessive anticoagulation. Use of a shorter-acting anticoagulant (eg, heparin) should be considered as delivery approaches. Hemorrhage can occur at any site & may lead to death of mother &/or fetus. Consider checking factor Xa levels to assess anticoagulation status prior to regional anesthesia in pts taking large doses. Conflicting data on maternal osteoporosis.

FETAL & NEONATAL EFFECTS
■ Pregnancy Category B (for definition, see the "*Pregnancy Categories*" section). Does not cross the placenta.

COMMENT
■ The dosages of dalteparin given for unstable angina or non-Q-wave MI are contraindicated for regional anesthesia.

DANTRIUM (DANTROLENE)

INDICATIONS
■ Chronic muscle spasticity & malignant hyperthermia

DOSING

■ 1 mg/kg IV by continuous rapid IV push & continue until symptoms subside or to a max cumulative dose of 10 mg/kg; discontinue all anesthetic agents & administer 100% oxygen (recommended).

MATERNAL SIDE EFFECTS & IMPACT ON ANESTHESIA

■ Oral drug has produced no adverse fetal or neonatal effects when given as prophylaxis to pregnant women who were susceptible to malignant hyperthermia. Dantrolene crosses the placenta. Common side effects: constipation, diarrhea, lightheadedness & weakness. Serious side effects: aplastic anemia, fatal & non-fatal liver disorders & tachycardia, erratic BP. There has been one reported case of post-partum uterine atony after dantrolene was given after a C-section.

FETAL & NEONATAL EFFECTS

■ Pregnancy Category C (for definition, see the "*Pregnancy Categories*" section). Secreted in breast milk. Best to avoid breast-feeding for at least 48 hours after discontinuation of dantrolene. Obviously, its urgent & life-saving role during MH crisis supports its use in pregnancy.

COMMENT

■ There are a number of drug interactions that may prolong their clearance. Avoid in pts w/ active liver disease, amyotrophic lateral sclerosis, impaired cardiac function, pulmonary function or chronic obstructive pulmonary disease, & in women & pts >35 years of age (greater likelihood of drug-induced, potentially fatal, hepatocellular disease).

DANTROLENE (DANTRIUM)

INDICATIONS

■ Chronic muscle spasticity & malignant hyperthermia

DOSING

■ 1 mg/kg IV by continuous rapid IV push & continue until symptoms subside or to a max cumulative dose of 10 mg/kg; discontinue all anesthetic agents & administer 100% oxygen (recommended).

MATERNAL SIDE EFFECTS & IMPACT ON ANESTHESIA

■ Oral drug has produced no adverse fetal or neonatal effects when given as prophylaxis to pregnant women who were susceptible to malignant hyperthermia. Dantrolene crosses the placenta. Common side effects: constipation, diarrhea, lightheadedness & weakness. Serious side effects: aplastic anemia, fatal & non-fatal liver disorders & tachycardia, erratic BP. There has been one reported case of post-partum uterine atony after dantrolene was given after a C-section.

FETAL & NEONATAL EFFECTS

■ Pregnancy Category C (for definition, see the "*Pregnancy Categories*" section). Secreted in breast milk. Best to avoid breast-feeding for at least 48 hours after discontinuation of dantrolene. Obviously, its urgent & life-saving role during MH crisis supports its use in pregnancy.

COMMENT

■ There are a number of drug interactions that may prolong their clearance. Avoid in pts w/ active liver disease, amyotrophic lateral sclerosis, impaired cardiac function, pulmonary function or chronic obstructive pulmonary disease, & in women & pts >35 years of age (greater likelihood of drug-induced, potentially fatal, hepatocellular disease).

DDAVP (DESMOPRESSIN)

INDICATIONS

■ Improves coagulation in pts w/ hemophilia A, renal failure & certain types of von Willebrand's disease. Can also be used as an antidiuretic. Prophylactic treatment for patients w/ type I or III von Willebrand's prior to C-section & neuraxial anesthesia. Single-shot spinal anesthesia may be preferable to epidural anesthesia due to the smaller size of the needle. For C-section consider GETA.

DOSING

■ 0.3 mcg/kg IV (dilute in 50 cc NS) up to a max of 20 mcg. Infuse over 15–30 minutes. Some hematologists have recommended giving a dose 30 minutes prior to placing a spinal or epidural & a second dose 30 minutes prior to discontinuing an epidural if it has been >4–6 hours since the initial dose was given. For ongoing epidural treatment of labor pain, redose DDAVP q6h.

MATERNAL SIDE EFFECTS & IMPACT ON ANESTHESIA

■ Causes immediate release of vWF from endothelial cell wall & increases factor VIII 2–3×. Increases renal water reabsorption. Watch for side effects such as hyponatremia-induced seizures. Antidiuretic doses have no uterotonic action.

FETAL & NEONATAL EFFECTS
■ Pregnancy category B (for definition, see the "*Pregnancy Categories*" section). Excretion in breast milk unknown.

COMMENT
■ In type II von Willebrand's, desmopressin is not effective; treatment is platelet transfusion. A RICOF level of >30% in pts w/ type II indicates that regional anesthesia is safe. Additional treatment for type III severe vWF deficiency should include cryoprecipitate or Humate-C, which contains both factor VIIIc & active vWF.

DEMEROL (MEPERIDINE)

INDICATIONS
■ Short-acting analgesic, potent respiratory depressant, cumulative effect w/ large doses over time. Widely used opioid worldwide due to its familiarity & low cost. Often used in combination w/ phenothiazines to diminish nausea & vomiting. Often used parenterally to decrease perioperative shivering.

DOSING
■ Usual dose is 25–50 mg IV or 50–100 mg IM q2–4h, w/ the onset of analgesia within 5 minutes of IV administration & 45 minutes after IM injection. Half-life is 2.5–3 hours in the mother & 18–23 hours in the neonate. A major metabolite is normeperidine, which acts as a potent respiratory depressant in both mother & neonate.

MATERNAL SIDE EFFECTS & IMPACT ON ANESTHESIA
■ Easily crosses the placenta by passive diffusion & equilibrates btwn the maternal & fetal compartments. Maximal fetal uptake occurs within 2–3 hours of maternal administration; therefore, the best time for delivery of the fetus is within 1 hour of last administered dose or >4 hours after the single IV dose.

FETAL & NEONATAL EFFECTS
■ Pregnancy Category B; Category D if used for prolonged periods or in high doses at term (for definitions, see the "*Pregnancy Categories*"

section). Readily crosses placenta & may cause neonatal depression. Opioids in general may result in decreased beat-to-beat variability of the fetal heart rate (FHR). Likelihood of neonatal respiratory depression depends on the dose & timing of administration. Meperidine is compatible w/ breast-feeding.

COMMENT

■ Meperidine has structural similarities to that of local anesthetics & has been used as a sole spinal anesthetic for cesarean delivery. Parenteral administration of both a single dose as well as multiple doses was shown to have subtle effects of the neonate. Single dose was thought to account for an alteration of infant breast-feeding behavior; whereas multiple doses, as would be administered during a prolonged labor, were thought to contribute to various neurobehavioral changes: decreased duration of wakefulness, decreased attentiveness & decreased duration of non-REM sleep.

DEPAKENE (VALPROIC ACID)

INDICATIONS

■ Anticonvulsant

DOSING

■ Usual starting dose is 500–750 mg/day divided 2 or 3 times/day. The dose is increased every several days to achieve blood levels in the range of 50–100 mcg/mL, which is typically achieved at a dosage of 1,000–2,500 mg/day.

MATERNAL SIDE EFFECTS & IMPACT ON ANESTHESIA

■ The use of valproic acid during pregnancy has been associated w/ fetal teratogenicity, most commonly neural tube defects. May cause thrombocytopenia, inhibition of platelets, low fibrinogen & other clotting abnormalities, lethargy, coma, fatal hepatic failure.

FETAL & NEONATAL EFFECTS

■ Pregnancy Category D (for definition, see the "*Pregnancy Categories*" section). The most frequently associated major malformations are neural tube defects, congenital heart disease, oral clefts, genital abnormalities, limb abnormalities. May cause clotting abnormalities & fatal hepatic failure. Valproate is compatible w/ breast-feeding; breast milk concentrations are 1–10% of serum. Children <2 years are at increased risk of toxicity.

COMMENT

■ Anticonvulsant meds should not be discontinued abruptly as seizures are also a threat to the patient & fetus. Children exposed to valproate during organogenesis should likely be tested or monitored for congenital defects.

DEPAKOTE (VALPROIC ACID)

INDICATIONS

■ Anticonvulsant

DOSING

■ Usual starting dose is 500–750 mg/day divided 2 or 3 times/day. The dose is increased every several days to achieve blood levels in the range of 50–100 mcg/mL, which is typically achieved at a dosage of 1,000–2,500 mg/day.

MATERNAL SIDE EFFECTS & IMPACT ON ANESTHESIA

■ The use of valproic acid during pregnancy has been associated w/ fetal teratogenicity, most commonly neural tube defects. May cause thrombocytopenia, inhibition of platelets, low fibrinogen & other clotting abnormalities, lethargy, coma, fatal hepatic failure.

FETAL & NEONATAL EFFECTS

■ Pregnancy Category D (for definition, see the "*Pregnancy Categories*" section). The most frequently associated major malformations are neural tube defects, congenital heart disease, oral clefts, genital abnormalities, limb abnormalities. May cause clotting abnormalities & fatal hepatic failure. Valproate is compatible w/ breast-feeding; breast milk concentrations are 1–10% of serum. Children <2 years are at increased risk of toxicity.

COMMENT

■ Anticonvulsant meds should not be discontinued abruptly as seizures are also a threat to the patient & fetus. Children exposed to valproate during organogenesis should likely be tested or monitored for congenital defects.

DESFLURANE (SUPRANE)

INDICATIONS
- Maintenance of general anesthesia

DOSING
- MAC for Desflurane is 6–7% in the non-pregnant patient, 30–40% less for parturient. Use 0.25–0.5 MAC until delivery of baby to avoid hypotension.

MATERNAL SIDE EFFECTS & IMPACT ON ANESTHESIA
- Causes dose-dependent uterine atony & hypotension due to peripheral vasodilation, decreases hepatic blood flow, increases cerebral vasodilation, can increase plasma catecholamines w/ abrupt increases in inspired concentration. Rapid onset & emergence.

FETAL & NEONATAL EFFECTS
- Pregnancy Category B (for definition, see the "*Pregnancy Categories*" section). Crosses the placenta & may cause temporary neonatal depression in large doses. Not thought to be a problem for breast-feeding.

COMMENT
- Pungent odor causes increased risk of coughing, laryngospasm, breath holding & increased pulmonary secretions. When used as the sole anesthetic agent for general anesthesia, awareness results in 12–26% of cases.

DESIPRAMINE (NORPRAMIN)

INDICATIONS
- Tricyclic antidepressant (TCAs) are effective for the treatment of major depressive disorders; also sometimes prescribed for chronic pain or polyneuropathy.

DOSING
- For depression, 100–200 mg/day in single or divided doses, up to max 300 mg/day

MATERNAL SIDE EFFECTS & IMPACT ON ANESTHESIA
- Common side effects include anticholinergic symptoms (drying of secretions, dilated pupils, sedation). Concomitant use of TCAs &

amphetamines has been reported to result in enhanced amphetamine effects from the release of norepinephrine. Ephedrine should be given cautiously to patients on TCAs.

FETAL & NEONATAL EFFECTS

■ Pregnancy Category NR (for definition, see the "*Pregnancy Categories*" section). Breast-feeding effects are unknown; only very minute amounts are found in the infant's serum.

COMMENT

■ Do not use w/ MAO inhibitors.

DESMOPRESSIN (DDAVP, STIMATE)

INDICATIONS

■ Improves coagulation in pts w/ hemophilia A, renal failure & certain types of von Willebrand's disease. Can also be used as an antidiuretic. Prophylactic treatment for patients w/ type I or III von Willebrand's prior to C-section & neuraxial anesthesia. Single-shot spinal anesthesia may be preferable to epidural anesthesia due to the smaller size of the needle. For C-section consider GETA.

DOSING

■ 0.3 mcg/kg IV (dilute in 50 cc NS) up to a max of 20 mcg. Infuse over 15–30 minutes. Some hematologists have recommended giving a dose 30 minutes prior to placing a spinal or epidural & a second dose 30 minutes prior to discontinuing an epidural if it has been >4–6 hours since the initial dose was given. For ongoing epidural treatment of labor pain, redose DDAVP q6h.

MATERNAL SIDE EFFECTS & IMPACT ON ANESTHESIA

■ Causes immediate release of vWF from endothelial cell wall & increases factor VIII 2–3×. Increases renal water reabsorption. Watch for side effects such as hyponatremia-induced seizures. Antidiuretic doses have no uterotonic action.

FETAL & NEONATAL EFFECTS

■ Pregnancy category B (for definition, see the "*Pregnancy Categories*" section). Excretion in breast milk unknown.

COMMENT
- In type II von Willebrand's, desmopressin is not effective; treatment is platelet transfusion. A RICOF level of >30% in pts w/ type II indicates that regional anesthesia is safe. Additional treatment for type III severe vWF deficiency should include cryoprecipitate or Humate-C, which contains both factor VIIIc & active vWF.

DIABETA (GLYBURIDE)

INDICATIONS
- Glyburide stimulates the secretion of insulin by the beta cells of the pancreas. In addition to this pancreatic action, glipizide administration may improve the metabolic utilization of glucose at a peripheral level.

DOSING
- Initial dose: 1.25–5 mg qd

MATERNAL SIDE EFFECTS & IMPACT ON ANESTHESIA
- Do not use in the 1st trimester, as safety in pregnancy has not been established. Do not use in pts w/ ketoacidosis or severe renal, hepatic, adrenal or thyroid dysfunction.

FETAL & NEONATAL EFFECTS
- Pregnancy Category C (for definition, see the "*Pregnancy Categories*" section). Do not use in the 1st trimester, as safety in pregnancy has not been established. The degree to which it affects newborns via transmission in breast milk is unknown.

COMMENT
- Insulin therapy is advocated by most specialists during pregnancy to enable tight blood glucose control.

DIAZEPAM (VALIUM)

INDICATIONS
- Acute alcohol withdrawal, anxiety, cardioversion, skeletal muscle spasms & seizures

DOSING
- 2–15 mg PO, rectally, IM or IV; can repeat as needed

MATERNAL SIDE EFFECTS & IMPACT ON ANESTHESIA
- The effects of diazepam on pregnancy have not been assessed. However, it has been suggested that diazepam be used w/ precaution in pregnancy. Contraindications include acute narrow-angle & untreated open-angle glaucoma & age <6 months.

FETAL & NEONATAL EFFECTS
- Pregnancy Category NR (for definition, see the *"Pregnancy Categories"* section). Safety in breast-feeding is controversial. Safety & effectiveness have not been established in children <6 months of age.

COMMENT
- Adverse effects include ataxia, drowsiness, fatigue, hypotension, respiratory depression & sedation. Diazepam should be gradually tapered after extended therapy; abrupt discontinuation should generally be avoided.

DIGITEK (DIGOXIN)

INDICATIONS
- A cardiac glycoside that increases cardiac inotropy & decreases conduction at the AV node & Purkinje fibers

DOSING
- Total digitalizing dose (TDD) to be administered over 24 h; 1st dose is one-half the TDD; 2nd dose is one-fourth the TDD, administered 8 h later; 3rd dose is one-fourth the TDD, administered 8 h after the second TDD: 0.75–1.5 mg PO in divided doses over 1 d; alternatively 0.5–1 mg IV/IM in divided doses over 1 d; maintenance dose: 0.125–0.5 mg PO qd or 0.1–0.4 mg IV/IM qd

MATERNAL SIDE EFFECTS & IMPACT ON ANESTHESIA
- Digoxin has a narrow therapeutic index. Serum levels must be closely followed. Toxicity may be potentiated by hypercalcemia, hypomagnesemia & hypokalemia. It also interacts w/ a large number of meds. Additional side effects of digoxin include GI upset & visual disturbances.

FETAL & NEONATAL EFFECTS
- Pregnancy Category C (for definition, see the *"Pregnancy Categories"* section). There have been no reports linking digoxin to congenital

defects, & animal studies have failed to show teratogenicity. Overdoses of digoxin may result in neonatal asphyxia & death. Considered safe during breast-feeding due to high maternal protein-binding.

COMMENT
■ Documented hypersensitivity; beriberi heart disease; idiopathic hypertrophic subaortic stenosis; constrictive pericarditis; carotid sinus syndrome

DIGOXIN (LANOXIN, DIGITEK)

INDICATIONS
■ A cardiac glycoside that increases cardiac inotropy & decreases conduction at the AV node & Purkinje fibers

DOSING
■ Total digitalizing dose (TDD) to be administered over 24 h; 1st dose is one-half the TDD; 2nd dose is one-fourth the TDD, administered 8 h later; 3rd dose is one-fourth the TDD, administered 8 h after the second TDD: 0.75–1.5 mg PO in divided doses over 1 d; alternatively 0.5–1 mg IV/IM in divided doses over 1 d; maintenance dose: 0.125–0.5 mg PO qd or 0.1–0.4 mg IV/IM qd

MATERNAL SIDE EFFECTS & IMPACT ON ANESTHESIA
■ Digoxin has a narrow therapeutic index. Serum levels must be closely followed. Toxicity may be potentiated by hypercalcemia, hypomagnesemia & hypokalemia. It also interacts w/ a large number of meds. Additional side effects of digoxin include GI upset & visual disturbances.

FETAL & NEONATAL EFFECTS
■ Pregnancy Category C (for definition, see the "*Pregnancy Categories*" section). There have been no reports linking digoxin to congenital defects, & animal studies have failed to show teratogenicity. Overdoses of digoxin may result in neonatal asphyxia & death. Considered safe during breast-feeding due to high maternal protein-binding.

COMMENT
■ Documented hypersensitivity; beriberi heart disease; idiopathic hypertrophic subaortic stenosis; constrictive pericarditis; carotid sinus syndrome

DILACOR (DILTIAZEM)

INDICATIONS
■ Angina, hypertension, arrhythmias (atrial fib/atrial flutter), paroxysmal supraventricular tachycardia; has been used as a tocolytic

DOSING
■ Depends on indication
■ Available in oral immediate-release, extended-release (qd) & sustained-release (bid) tabs & capsules for angina & hypertension
■ IV forms are used to treat arrhythmias. Initial bolus 0.25 mg/kg over 2 min, repeat 0.35-mg/kg bolus in 15 min for inadequate response.
■ Continuous infusion starts at 10 mg/hr, may be increased at 5-mg/hr intervals for therapeutic effect. Infusions lasting >24 hours are not recommended.

MATERNAL SIDE EFFECTS & IMPACT ON ANESTHESIA
■ Most common side effects are edema, 1st-degree AV block, headache, hypotension. Concomitant use w/ beta-blockers, digoxin & amiodarone can lead to severe conduction disturbances, bradycardia & hypotension. Can increase plasma concentration of alfentanil, fentanyl & benzodiazepines.

FETAL & NEONATAL EFFECTS
■ Pregnancy Category C (for definition, see the *"Pregnancy Categories"* section). Diffuses freely into breast milk, though no adverse effects reported. American Academy of Pediatrics says compatible w/ breast-feeding.

COMMENT
■ Do not use in pts w/ ventricular dysfunction, acute MI, pulmonary congestion, sick sinus syndrome or 2nd- or 3rd-degree AV block w/o pacer.

DILANTIN (PHENYTOIN)

INDICATIONS
■ Generalized tonic-clonic & complex partial seizures; seizures during or after neurosurgery; antiarrhythmic; antineuralgic; seizures secondary to eclampsia or pre-eclampsia

DOSING

- IV: 50–100 mg q10–15min, max 15 mg/kg, max rate 50 mg/minute
- PO: 400 mg, then 300 mg in 2h r & 4 hr
- Maintenance: 5 mg/kg or 300 mg PO once per day or divided tid

MATERNAL SIDE EFFECTS & IMPACT ON ANESTHESIA

- The effects of phenytoin on pregnancy have not been assessed. Some studies suggest that there is risk in certain maternal circumstances.

FETAL & NEONATAL EFFECTS

- Pregnancy Category NR (for definition, see the "*Pregnancy Categories*" section). Phenytoin is considered safe in breast-feeding.

COMMENT

- Phenytoin requirements are greater during pregnancy, requiring increases in doses in some pts. After delivery, the dose should be decreased to avoid toxicity.

DILAUDID (HYDROMORPHONE)

INDICATIONS

- Pain, moderate or severe. In obstetrics, primarily as a post-op analgesic (PCA).

DOSING

- 1–2 mg IM/SC/IV q4–6h; 2.5–10 mg PO or rectally q3–6h as needed

MATERNAL SIDE EFFECTS & IMPACT ON ANESTHESIA

- Dilaudid is relatively contraindicated in obstetrical anesthesia. Avoid in pts w/ depressed ventilatory dysfunction, intracranial lesion associated w/ increased ICP. May need dosing adjustment in pts w/ renal failure or liver disease & in geriatrics. Use precaution during concomitant administration of general anesthetics or phenothiazines.

FETAL & NEONATAL EFFECTS

- Pregnancy Category C (for definition, see the "*Pregnancy Categories*" section). Dilaudid is not FDA-approved in pediatric pts; it can cause apnea, respiratory depression, circulatory depression, hypotension, confusion, myoclonus & seizures.

COMMENT

- Dilaudid contains sodium bisulfite, a sulfite that may cause allergic-type reactions in certain susceptible people.

DILTIAZEM (CARDIZEM, DILACOR, TIAZAC)

INDICATIONS
■ Angina, hypertension, arrhythmias (atrial fib/atrial flutter), paroxysmal supraventricular tachycardia; has been used as a tocolytic

DOSING
■ Depends on indication
■ Available in oral immediate-release, extended-release (qd) & sustained-release (bid) tabs & capsules for angina & hypertension
■ IV forms are used to treat arrhythmias. Initial bolus 0.25 mg/kg over 2 min, repeat 0.35-mg/kg bolus in 15 min for inadequate response.
■ Continuous infusion starts at 10 mg/hr, may be increased at 5-mg/hr intervals for therapeutic effect. Infusions lasting >24 hours are not recommended.

MATERNAL SIDE EFFECTS & IMPACT ON ANESTHESIA
■ Most common side effects are edema, 1st-degree AV block, headache, hypotension. Concomitant use w/ beta-blockers, digoxin & amiodarone can lead to severe conduction disturbances, bradycardia & hypotension. Can increase plasma concentration of alfentanil, fentanyl & benzodiazepines.

FETAL & NEONATAL EFFECTS
■ Pregnancy Category C (for definition, see the "*Pregnancy Categories*" section). Diffuses freely into breast milk, though no adverse effects reported. American Academy of Pediatrics says compatible w/ breast-feeding.

COMMENT
■ Do not use in pts w/ ventricular dysfunction, acute MI, pulmonary congestion, sick sinus syndrome or 2nd- or 3rd-degree AV block w/o pacer.

DIPHENHYDRAMINE (BENADRYL) ORAL/INJECTABLE

INDICATIONS
■ Anxiety, insomnia, varicella, insect bites, allergic rhinitis, generalized pruritus, urticaria

DOSING

- 25–50 mg PO q4–6h or 10–50 mg IM/IV q2–3h; maximum parenteral dose 400 mg/day

MATERNAL SIDE EFFECTS & IMPACT ON ANESTHESIA

- Concomitant use of antidepressants w/ strong anticholinergic effects (eg, amitriptyline, trimipramine, amoxapine, doxepin, imipramine, nortriptyline, maprotiline) may increase potential for adynamic ileus & urinary retention. Increases CNS depression when taken w/ barbiturates, narcotics, hypnotics, tricyclic antidepressants, MAO inhibitors, alcohol. Decreases effect of oral anticoagulants, including heparin.

FETAL & NEONATAL EFFECTS

- Pregnancy Category B (for definition, see the "*Pregnancy Categories*" section). Crosses placenta & passes freely into breast milk. Relatively contraindicated during breast-feeding due to potential sedating effects on newborn.

COMMENT

- While antihistamines are sometimes used to treat narcotic-induced pruritus, this condition is more directly & appropriately managed w/ a partial agonist-antagonist agent such as Nubain (nalbuphine) 5–10 mg IV w/ less risk of increased sedation.

DIPRIVAN (PROPOFOL)

INDICATIONS

- 2, 6-diisopropylphenol, prepared in 1% isotonic oil-in-water emulsion; rapidly produces unconsciousness (onset approx. 30–45 sec) followed by rapid reawakening due to redistribution

DOSING

- 2–2.5 mg/kg IV for induction, 50–150 mcg/kg/min for maintenance

MATERNAL SIDE EFFECTS & IMPACT ON ANESTHESIA

- Venous irritation; greater drop in systolic BP than w/ thiopental

FETAL & NEONATAL EFFECTS

- Pregnancy Category B (for definition, see the "*Pregnancy Categories*" section). Rapidly crosses placenta. Higher doses for IV maintenance of GA (150 mcg/kg/min) may cause neonatal depression. Infants exposed to a maternal propofol dose of 2.8 mg/kg had significantly lower Apgar scores than infants whose mothers were given 5 mg/kg thiopental. A dose of 2 mg/kg IV results in an fetal/maternal ratio of 0.5. Oral bioavailability low; minimal breast milk transfer.

COMMENT
■ When learning about these drugs in obstetrics, it is important to be familiar w/ the approximate fetal:maternal (F/M) ratios of drug concentrations at the time of delivery of the infant. Generally, the umbilical vein blood concentrations represent the fetal blood concentrations. An early high ratio indicates rapid placental transfer of the drug.

DURAGESIC (FENTANYL)

INDICATIONS
■ Potent narcotic analgesic w/ much shorter half-life than morphine sulfate. Drug of choice for conscious sedation & analgesia. Used as adjunct in spinals & epidurals. Reversed by naloxone.

DOSING
■ Analgesia: 0.5–1 mcg/kg/dose IV/IM q30–60min
■ Transdermal: Apply a 25-mcg/h system q48–72h.
■ Neuraxial dosing varies depending on obstetric indication & regional anesthetic technique.

MATERNAL SIDE EFFECTS & IMPACT ON ANESTHESIA
■ Used routinely in epidural infusions (w/ bupivacaine) for labor analgesia; may allow the reduction of local anesthetic dose.

FETAL & NEONATAL EFFECTS
■ Pregnancy Category C; Category D if used for prolonged periods or in high doses at term (for definitions, see the "*Pregnancy Categories*" section). Readily crosses placenta & may cause neonatal depression. There appears to be no fetal accumulation of either drug during epidural infusion, however, & no adverse fetal effects have been observed from epidural fentanyl administration in routine doses. Opioids may result in decreased beat-to-beat variability of the fetal heart rate (FHR) w/o fetal hypoxia. Fentanyl is excreted in breast milk; it is compatible w/ breast-feeding due to low oral bioavailability.

COMMENT

■ May result in hypotension, respiratory depression, constipation, nausea, emesis, urinary retention; idiosyncratic reaction, known as chest wall rigidity syndrome, may require neuromuscular blockade to increase ventilation.

DURAMORPH (MORPHINE)

INDICATIONS

■ No longer used as primary analgesic for pain in labor in the U.S. because of neonatal respiratory depression. Earliest anesthetic used for treatment of labor pain. Analgesia, intraoperative anesthesia, post-op analgesia.

DOSING

■ Usual dose for maternal analgesia is 2–5 mg IV or 5–10 mg IM. Onset of analgesia is 3–5 minutes after the IV administration & within 20–40 minutes after the IM dose. For post-op analgesia, morphine can be used in PCA or neuraxially (0.1–0.25 mg intrathecally or 2.0–5.0 mg epidurally). Use preservative-free preparation if neuraxial.

MATERNAL SIDE EFFECTS & IMPACT ON ANESTHESIA

■ Infrequently used during labor because of its greater respiratory depression in the neonate than w/ meperidine. As w/ other opiates, has antitussive, constipating, sedating & emetic potential.

FETAL & NEONATAL EFFECTS

■ Pregnancy Category C (for definition, see the "*Pregnancy Categories*" section). Readily crosses placenta & may cause neonatal respiratory depression. Opioids in general may result in decreased beat-to-beat variability of the fetal heart rate (FHR). Likelihood of neonatal respiratory depression depends on the dose & timing of administration.

COMMENT

■ Studies have suggested that that systematically administered morphine does not relieve the visceral pain of labor. Epidural morphine may have diminished efficacy if 3-chloroprocaine has been given epidurally previously.

DURANEST (ETIDOCAINE)

INDICATIONS
- Can be used for peripheral nerve block, epidural & caudal anesthesia, though rarely used in obstetrics

DOSING
- Epidural: 0.5–1.5% concentration w/ 20–30 cc in 70-kg normal adults (parturient dose would be decreased by 30%, but the medication is rarely used for labor epidural)

MATERNAL SIDE EFFECTS & IMPACT ON ANESTHESIA
- Motor > sensory blockade, thereby decreasing its utility for labor

FETAL & NEONATAL EFFECTS
- Pregnancy Category C (for definition, see the "*Pregnancy Categories*" section). High protein-binding capacity inhibits placental transfer.

COMMENT
- Rapid onset, very long duration, high potency w/ moderate level of toxicity

---

EFFEXOR (VENLAFAXINE)

INDICATIONS
- SSRI typically used to treat depression, anxiety, obsessive-compulsive disorder, bulimia, panic disorder, posttraumatic stress disorder

DOSING
- Depression: initially 75 mg/day PO in 2 or 3 divided doses, with increases up to 225 mg/day PO for outpatients and 375 mg/day PO for inpatients
- Anxiety disorder: initially 37.5–75 mg/day PO, with increases up to 225 mg/day
- Dosing adjustments are appropriate if there is hepatic or renal insufficiency.

MATERNAL SIDE EFFECTS & IMPACT ON ANESTHESIA
- Common side effects include anorexia, constipation or diarrhea, paradoxical anxiety, dizziness, dry mouth. More serious complications can include abnormal bleeding (particularly when used

w/ other meds that can inhibit platelet function), hypertension, hyponatremia, seizures.

FETAL & NEONATAL EFFECTS

■ Pregnancy Category C (for definition, see the "*Pregnancy Categories*" section). An increased risk for CNS serotonergic symptoms was observed during the first 4 days of life in infants of mothers taking SSRIs during the 3rd trimester of pregnancy. Infants exposed prenatally to fluoxetine or a tricyclic antidepressant did NOT show differences in IQ, language or behavioral development compared to children w/o prenatal exposure to these drugs. SSRIs have unknown effects that may be of concern during breast-feeding.

COMMENT

■ Do not use concomitantly w/ MAO inhibitors.

ELAVIL (AMITRIPTYLINE)

INDICATIONS

■ Tricyclic antidepressants (TCAs) are effective for the treatment of major depressive disorders; also sometimes prescribed for chronic pain or polyneuropathy.

DOSING

■ For depression in outpatients, 75 mg/day divided in 1–3 doses, up to 200 mg/day

MATERNAL SIDE EFFECTS & IMPACT ON ANESTHESIA

■ Common side effects include anticholinergic symptoms (drying of secretions, dilated pupils, sedation). Concomitant use of TCAs & amphetamines has been reported to result in enhanced amphetamine effects from the release of norepinephrine. Ephedrine should be given cautiously to patients on TCAs.

FETAL & NEONATAL EFFECTS

■ Pregnancy Category NR (for definition, see the "*Pregnancy Categories*" section). Breast-feeding effects are unknown; only very minute amounts are found in the infant's serum.

COMMENT

■ Do not use w/ MAO inhibitors.

ENDOCET (OXYCODONE/ACETAMINOPHEN)

INDICATIONS
- Pain, moderate & severe

DOSING
- Contains 5 mg oxycodone & 325 mg acetaminophen. Usually, 1 tab or 1 teaspoon PO q6h as needed. Immediately post-op, as much as 1 or 2 tabs q4h prn. Total daily dosage of acetaminophen/oxycodone should not exceed 4,000 mg/60 mg.

MATERNAL SIDE EFFECTS & IMPACT ON ANESTHESIA
- Effects on pregnancy have not been assessed. Use w/ precaution in labor & delivery or w/ concomitant use of other CNS depressants. May need dosing adjustment in pts w/ liver disease.

FETAL & NEONATAL EFFECTS
- Pregnancy Category NR (for definition, see the *"Pregnancy Categories"* section). Safety in breast-feeding is unclear; however, it is used commonly as a post-cesarean analgesic at a time when there is not much milk production yet.

COMMENT
- Adverse effects include respiratory depression, constipation, nausea & vomiting, dizziness, dysphoria, lightheadedness, sedation, skin rash, pruritus.

ENOXAPARIN (LOVENOX)

INDICATIONS
- Treatment of deep vein thrombosis (DVT) w/ or w/o pulmonary embolism (PE) or thrombopenic disorders during pregnancy

DOSING
- DVT or PE treatment doses: 1 mg/kg q12h SC
- DVT prophylaxis dose: 30 mg SC BID

MATERNAL SIDE EFFECTS & IMPACT ON ANESTHESIA
- Enoxaparin should be stopped at least 24 hours prior to regional anesthesia at treatment doses & at least 12 hours after prophylaxis

doses. Monitor for evidence of bleeding or excessive anticoagulation. Use of a shorter-acting anticoagulant (eg, heparin) should be considered as delivery approaches. Hemorrhage can occur at any site & may lead to death of mother &/or fetus. Consider checking factor Xa levels to assess anticoagulation status prior to regional anesthesia in pts taking large doses.

FETAL & NEONATAL EFFECTS
- Pregnancy Category B (for definition, see the "*Pregnancy Categories*" section). Enoxaparin does not cross the placenta or present a direct risk to the embryo or fetus due to its large molecular weight. There is also no known risk to the nursing infant. There have been post-marketing reports of fetal death when pregnant women received enoxaparin, but causality for these cases has not been determined.

COMMENT
- Contraindicated in pts w/ major bleeding or thrombocytopenia. Low-molecular-weight heparins cannot be reversed w/ FFP, but possibly w/ protamine.

EPHEDRINE

INDICATIONS
- Hypotension

DOSING
- 10–25 mg/dose slow IVP, repeated q5–10min; max 150 mg/day

MATERNAL SIDE EFFECTS & IMPACT ON ANESTHESIA
- Adverse side effects include anxiety, hypertension, palpitations & tremor.

FETAL & NEONATAL EFFECTS
- Pregnancy Category C (for definition, see the "*Pregnancy Categories*" section). Fetal hyperactivity, irritability & tachycardia may follow maternal ingestion of ephedrine. Ephedrine use should be avoided when there is poor fetal reserve. Ephedrine should also be avoided in pts w/ essential hypertension or toxemia since it will enhance the

hypertensive effect. Its use should be limited to maternal hypotension unresponsive to rapid fluid infusion & left lateral uterine displacement following spinal or epidural anesthesia.

COMMENT
- Avoid in patients on MAO inhibitors, amphetamines, anesthesia w/ halothane, hypertension or other cardiovascular disorders, thyrotoxicosis or angina pectoris. Lower doses (2.5–5.0 mg) are appropriate in pre-eclamptic pts. Can be associated w/ significant hypertension when given concurrently w/ oxytocics.

EPINEPHRINE

INDICATIONS
- Epinephrine is a useful adjunct to local anesthetics. Primarily used to vasoconstrict surrounding blood vessels & thus delay systemic absorption of deposited/injected local anesthetics. It is also a useful diagnostic tool in the detection of intravascular placement of an epidural catheter. Alpha & beta agonist used for bronchospasm, anaphylaxis, hypotension, heart failure, cardiac arrest.

DOSING
- Test dosing w/ epinephrine requires a minimum of 15 mcg, or 3 cc of 1:200,000.
- As an additive, the same concentration of 1:200,000 (5 mcg/cc) can be used.
- For bronchospasm/anaphylaxis, 0.1–0.5mg SC, 0.1–0.25 mg IV, or 0.25–1.5 mcg/min IV continuous
- For hypotension, heart failure, cardiac arrest: 0.1–1 mg IV or 1 mg intratracheal q5min prn

MATERNAL SIDE EFFECTS & IMPACT ON ANESTHESIA
- Epinephrine will increase both BP & cardiac output & may also decrease uterine blood flow. In parturients who are pre-eclamptic or who have other underlying metabolic/adrenergic disorders (ie, pheochromocytoma) or who have been chronically on MAO inhibitors, very small doses of epinephrine can have significant hypertensive effects. May cause hypertension, arrhythmias, myocardial ischemia. Arrhythmias potentiated by concurrent halothane or digoxin. Do not use w/ local anesthetics in finger/toes. May decrease

uterine blood flow. At low doses, may decrease uterine contractility; at high doses, may increase uterine contractility.

FETAL & NEONATAL EFFECTS
■ Pregnancy Category C (for definition, see the "*Pregnancy Categories*" section). Epinephrine at high doses (25× the human dose) has been shown to be teratogenic to small animals. In labor, epinephrine given to the mother accelerates fetal heart rate & confounds its interpretation.

COMMENT
■ N/A

ERGOTAMINE

INDICATIONS
■ Cluster headache; migraine headache

DOSING
■ 1–2 mg PO or sublingually, then 1–2 mg q30–60min, max 6 mg/day

MATERNAL SIDE EFFECTS & IMPACT ON ANESTHESIA
■ Adequate well-controlled or observational studies in animals or pregnant women have demonstrated positive evidence of fetal abnormalities or risks. Contraindicated in women who are or may become pregnant. Common adverse effects: ergotism (vasoconstriction, vascular spasm, cyanosis, numbness of the extremities, possible gangrene), nausea, vomiting, dizziness, drowsiness, nausea, vomiting, flatulence.

FETAL & NEONATAL EFFECTS
■ Pregnancy Category X (for definition, see the "*Pregnancy Categories*" section). While there are no specific teratogenic effects, ergot use in the mother has been related to restricted fetal growth, increased intrauterine death & resorption in animals, presumably from drug-induced uterine motility & increased vasoconstriction in the placental bed. Unsafe in breast-feeding: infants may experience vomiting & diarrhea. Excessive doses may inhibit lactation.

COMMENT
■ Contraindications: CAD, glaucoma, uncontrolled hypertension, hepatic disease, hypersensitivity to ergot derivatives or components,

peripheral vascular disease, gastric ulcer, renal impairment, sepsis, stroke, severe pruritus

ESKALITH (LITHIUM CARBONATE)

INDICATIONS
■ Classified as a tranquilizer to treat mania, but may be used to treat cluster headaches & Graves disease

DOSING
■ Varies for specific indication
■ Mania (acute): 1,800 mg/day PO in 2 or 3 divided doses, w/ desired serum level 1–1.5 mEq/L
■ Mania (maintenance): 900–1,200 mg/day PO in 2 or 3 divided doses, w/ desired serum level 0.6–1.2 mEq/L
■ Cluster headache: 300–900 mg/day PO in divided doses, w/ desired serum level <1.2 mEq/L
■ Graves disease: 900 mg/day PO for 8 days, starting on day of radioiodine administration

MATERNAL SIDE EFFECTS & IMPACT ON ANESTHESIA
■ Administration of lithium throughout pregnancy can produce complications in the neonate since lithium passes readily across the placental barrier. Cases of cardiac arrhythmia, hypotonia, hypothyroidism & polyhydramnios have been reported.

FETAL & NEONATAL EFFECTS
■ Pregnancy Category D (for definition, see the "*Pregnancy Categories*" section). Lithium readily crosses the placenta & can cause hypothyroidism in the newborn.

COMMENT
■ Dosage needs to be adjusted in pts w/ renal dysfunction. May cause central or nephrogenic diabetes insipidus.

ETIDOCAINE (DURANEST)

INDICATIONS
■ Can be used for peripheral nerve block, epidural & caudal anesthesia, though rarely used in obstetrics

DOSING
■ Epidural: 0.5–1.5% concentration w/ 20–30 cc in 70-kg normal adults (parturient dose would be decreased by 30%, but the medication is rarely used for labor epidural)

MATERNAL SIDE EFFECTS & IMPACT ON ANESTHESIA
■ Motor > sensory blockade, thereby decreasing its utility for labor

FETAL & NEONATAL EFFECTS
■ Pregnancy Category C (for definition, see the "*Pregnancy Categories*" section). High protein-binding capacity inhibits placental transfer.

COMMENT
■ Rapid onset, very long duration, high potency w/ moderate level of toxicity

---

ETOMIDATE (AMIDATE)

INDICATIONS
■ Imidazole-containing hypnotic used to induce general anesthesia

DOSING
■ 0.2–0.3 mg/kg IV

MATERNAL SIDE EFFECTS & IMPACT ON ANESTHESIA
■ Adrenal suppression for up to 24 hours, myoclonus, PONV, venous irritation

FETAL & NEONATAL EFFECTS
■ Pregnancy Category C (for definition, see the "*Pregnancy Categories*" section). Suppresses neonatal cortisol production, though this is of unclear clinical significance. Fetal/maternal ratio: 0.5.

COMMENT
■ Produces minimal cardiorespiratory effects at low doses. May produce adrenal suppression after a single dose. When learning about these drugs in obstetrics, it is important to be familiar w/ the approximate fetal:maternal (F/M) ratios of drug concentrations at the time of delivery of the infant. Generally, the umbilical vein blood concentrations represent the fetal blood concentrations. An early high ratio indicates rapid placental transfer of the drug.

FAMOTIDINE (PEPCID)

INDICATIONS
■ Competitively inhibits histamine at the H2 receptor of gastric parietal cells, resulting in reduced gastric acid secretion, gastric volume & hydrogen ion concentrations

DOSING
■ 10 mg PO bid

MATERNAL SIDE EFFECTS & IMPACT ON ANESTHESIA
■ May decrease effects of ketoconazole & itraconazole; levels may increase w/ hydrochlorothiazide; fluconazole levels may decrease w/ long-term co-administration of rifampin; may increase concentrations of theophylline, phenytoin, tolbutamide, cyclosporine, glyburide, glipizide; effects of anticoagulants may increase w/ fluconazole co-administration

FETAL & NEONATAL EFFECTS
■ Pregnancy Category B (for definition, see the "*Pregnancy Categories*" section). The degree to which it passes into breast milk & affects the newborn is unknown.

COMMENT
N/A

FENTANYL (SUBLIMAZE, ACTIQ, DURAGESIC)

INDICATIONS
■ Potent narcotic analgesic w/ much shorter half-life than morphine sulfate. Drug of choice for conscious sedation & analgesia. Used as adjunct in spinals & epidurals. Reversed by naloxone.

DOSING
■ Analgesia: 0.5–1 mcg/kg/dose IV/IM q30–60min
■ Transdermal: Apply a 25-mcg/h system q48–72h.
■ Neuraxial dosing varies depending on obstetric indication & regional anesthetic technique.

MATERNAL SIDE EFFECTS & IMPACT ON ANESTHESIA
■ Used routinely in epidural infusions (w/ bupivacaine) for labor analgesia; may allow the reduction of local anesthetic dose.

FETAL & NEONATAL EFFECTS
- Pregnancy Category C; Category D if used for prolonged periods or in high doses at term (for definitions, see the *"Pregnancy Categories"* section). Readily crosses placenta & may cause neonatal depression. There appears to be no fetal accumulation of either drug during epidural infusion, however, & no adverse fetal effects have been observed from epidural fentanyl administration in routine doses. Opioids may result in decreased beat-to-beat variability of the fetal heart rate (FHR) w/o fetal hypoxia. Fentanyl is excreted in breast milk; it is compatible w/ breast-feeding due to low oral bioavailability.

COMMENT
- May result in hypotension, respiratory depression, constipation, nausea, emesis, urinary retention; idiosyncratic reaction, known as chest wall rigidity syndrome, may require neuromuscular blockade to increase ventilation.

FERROUS SULFATE

INDICATIONS
- Iron is indicated in pregnancy for the prevention & treatment of iron deficiency anemia.

DOSING
- 300 mg PO twice daily up to 300 mg 4 times/day (or 30 mg/day of elemental iron). IV form is available.

MATERNAL SIDE EFFECTS & IMPACT ON ANESTHESIA
- Contraindicated in women w/ hemochromatosis, hemolytic anemia & known hypersensitivity to iron salts. May cause constipation, nausea & black stools.

FETAL & NEONATAL EFFECTS
- Iron is secreted in breast milk.

COMMENT
- The iron requirement is approximately twice that of a non-pregnant woman because of an expanding blood volume & the demands of the fetus & placenta. Magnesium, food & antacids may inhibit the absorption of iron.

FIORICET (ACETAMINOPHEN/BUTALBITAL/CAFFEINE)

INDICATIONS
- Headache, complex tension or muscle contraction

DOSING
- 1 or 2 tablets PO q4h as needed; max 6 tablets per day

MATERNAL SIDE EFFECTS & IMPACT ON ANESTHESIA
- Effects on pregnancy have not been assessed. Common adverse effects: abdominal pain, nausea & vomiting, drowsiness, lightheadedness, dizziness, sedation & shortness of breath.

FETAL & NEONATAL EFFECTS
- Pregnancy Category NR (for definition, see the "*Pregnancy Categories*" section). Unknown if administration is safe in breast-feeding.

COMMENT
- Contraindications: porphyria & hypersensitivity to acetaminophen/butalbital/caffeine. Often a part of conservative medical mgt of postdural puncture headache.

FIORINAL (ASPIRIN/BUTALBITAL/CAFFEINE)

INDICATIONS
- Tension headache

DOSING
- 1 or 2 tablets or capsules PO q4h prn; max 6 tablets or capsules per day

MATERNAL SIDE EFFECTS & IMPACT ON ANESTHESIA
- Adequate well-controlled or observational studies in pregnant women have demonstrated a risk to the fetus. However, the benefits of therapy may outweigh the potential risk. Common adverse effects: dizziness, drowsiness, nausea, vomiting, flatulence.

FETAL & NEONATAL EFFECTS
- Pregnancy Category D (for definition, see the "*Pregnancy Categories*" section). Unknown whether administration is safe in breast-feeding.

COMMENT
- Contraindications: porphyria; hypersensitivity to aspirin, butalbital, caffeine; bleeding disorder; GI ulceration; syndrome of nasal polyps; angioedema & bronchospastic reactivity to aspirin or other NSAIDs. Fiorinal has interactions w/ many other drugs.

FLAGYL (METRONIDAZOLE)

INDICATIONS
- Active against a variety of anaerobic bacteria, particularly *B. fragilis*

DOSING
- 500–750 mg IV q8–12h

MATERNAL SIDE EFFECTS & IMPACT ON ANESTHESIA
- May potentiate the effects of anticoagulants. Can cause disulfiram-like reaction w/ ethanol consumption. Concurrent barbiturates may inhibit the therapeutic effectiveness of metronidazole. May decrease clearance of phenytoin & may increase serum levels of lithium.

FETAL & NEONATAL EFFECTS
- Pregnancy Category B (for definition, see the "*Pregnancy Categories*" section). The use of metronidazole during pregnancy is controversial & should be avoided if possible. Secreted in breast milk. Breast-feeding mothers should discard all breast milk for 24–48 hours to allow excretion of the drug.

COMMENT
- Occasional phlebitis at the IV infusion site

FLUOXETINE (PROZAC)

INDICATIONS
- SSRI typically used to treat depression, anxiety, obsessive-compulsive disorder, bulimia, panic disorder, posttraumatic stress disorder

DOSING
- Depression: initially 20 mg/day PO, up to 80 mg/day
- Bulimia: 20 mg/day PO, increasing to 60 mg/day over several days

- Obsessive-compulsive disorder: initially 20 mg/day PO; maintenance dose 20–80 mg/day PO
- Panic disorder: 10–60 mg/day PO; most common dosage is 20 mg/day
- Dosing adjustments are appropriate if there is hepatic insufficiency.

MATERNAL SIDE EFFECTS & IMPACT ON ANESTHESIA
- Common side effects include anorexia, dry mouth, nausea. More serious complications can include activation of mania or hypomania, hyponatremia, QT interval prolongation, seizure.

FETAL & NEONATAL EFFECTS
- Pregnancy Category C (for definition, see the "*Pregnancy Categories*" section). An increased risk for CNS serotonergic symptoms was observed during the first 4 days of life in infants of mothers taking SSRIs during the 3rd trimester of pregnancy. Infants exposed prenatally to fluoxetine or a tricyclic antidepressant did NOT show differences in IQ, language or behavioral development compared to children w/o prenatal exposure to these drugs. SSRIs have unknown effects that may be of concern during breast-feeding.

COMMENT
- Do not use concomitantly w/ MAO inhibitors.

FORANE (ISOFLURANE)

INDICATIONS
- Maintenance of general anesthesia

DOSING
- Isoflurane MAC is 1.2% in normal adults, decreased by 30–40% in the parturient. In the parturient, use 0.25–0.5 MAC until delivery of baby to limit hypotension & uterine atony.

MATERNAL SIDE EFFECTS & IMPACT ON ANESTHESIA
- Causes dose-dependent uterine atony, hypotension via peripheral vasodilation, myocardial depression, reflex tachycardia, respiratory depression or arrest, N/V, shivering

FETAL & NEONATAL EFFECTS
- Pregnancy Category C (for definition, see the "*Pregnancy Categories*" section). Distributes rapidly across the placenta during C-section w/

a fetal/maternal ratio of 0.7. May cause temporary neonatal depression in large doses. No evidence of long-term adverse effects. Not thought to be a problem for breast-feeding.

COMMENT
- When used as the sole anesthetic agent for general anesthesia, awareness results in 12–26% of cases.

FRAGMIN (DALTEPARIN)

INDICATIONS
- Anticoagulant, inhibits factor Xa & factor IIa. Used for prophylaxis of deep venous thrombosis & treatment of acute coronary syndrome, deep vein thrombosis, pulmonary embolus.

DOSING
- DVT prophylaxis: 2,500–5,000 units SQ qd
- Acute coronary syndrome: 120 units/kg (max. 10,000 units) SQ q12h for 5–8 days
- DVT & PE treatment (FDA off-label use): 100 units/kg SQ bid, or 200 units/kg SQ qd

MATERNAL SIDE EFFECTS & IMPACT ON ANESTHESIA
- Should be stopped at least 24 hours prior to regional anesthesia at treatment doses & at least 12 hours after prophylaxis doses. Monitor for evidence of bleeding or excessive anticoagulation. Use of a shorter-acting anticoagulant (eg, heparin) should be considered as delivery approaches. Hemorrhage can occur at any site & may lead to death of mother &/or fetus. Consider checking factor Xa levels to assess anticoagulation status prior to regional anesthesia in pts taking large doses. Conflicting data on maternal osteoporosis.

FETAL & NEONATAL EFFECTS
- Pregnancy Category B (for definition, see the "*Pregnancy Categories*" section). Does not cross the placenta.

COMMENT
- The dosages of dalteparin given for unstable angina or non-Q-wave MI are contraindicated for regional anesthesia.

FUROSEMIDE (LASIX)

INDICATIONS
- Not commonly used to treat hypertension during pregnancy. Can be used to treat pulmonary edema associated w/ pre-eclampsia. Increases excretion of water by interfering w/ chloride-binding cotransport system, which in turn inhibits sodium & chloride reabsorption in ascending loop of Henle & distal renal tubule.

DOSING
- 10 mg IV initial dose, 20–80 mg/d PO/IV/IM; titrate up to 600 mg/d for severe edematous states

MATERNAL SIDE EFFECTS & IMPACT ON ANESTHESIA
- Prevents normal physiologic volume expansion that occurs in pregnancy & may reduce uterine blood flow; restrict use to women w/ volume-overload states (eg, renal or cardiac disease)

FETAL & NEONATAL EFFECTS
- Pregnancy Category C; Category D if used for pregnancy-induced hypertension (for definitions, see the "*Pregnancy Categories*" section). Safety during pregnancy has not been established. Effects in breast-feeding are unknown.

COMMENT
- N/A

GABAPENTIN (NEURONTIN)

INDICATIONS
- Anticonvulsant. Used as an antiepileptic & in the treatment of neuropathic pain & postherpetic neuralgia. Gabapentin is structurally related to the neurotransmitter GABA (gamma-aminobutyric acid).

DOSING
- 900–1,800 mg/day PO

MATERNAL SIDE EFFECTS & IMPACT ON ANESTHESIA
- Safety & efficacy have not been established in children, pregnancy & lactation.

FETAL & NEONATAL EFFECTS
■ Pregnancy Category C (for definition, see the "*Pregnancy Categories*" section). It is not known if gabapentin is excreted in human breast milk; its low molecular weight suggests transfer does occur. No other data available.

COMMENT
■ The most frequent clinical adverse events occurring in all clinical studies were somnolence, dizziness, ataxia, headache, nystagmus, tremor, fatigue, diplopia, nausea and/or vomiting, rhinitis.

GARAMYCIN (GENTAMICIN)

INDICATIONS
■ Second-line agent in the treatment & prevention of neonatal group B streptococcal infection

DOSING
■ IV 3–5 mg/kg/day in divided doses q8h

MATERNAL SIDE EFFECTS & IMPACT ON ANESTHESIA
■ Most common side effect is allergic reaction. Neuromuscular blocking agents (rocuronium, vecuronium) may have enhanced potency when administered w/ aminoglycosides. Concurrent administration of magnesium & an aminoglycoside may further potentiate neuromuscular blockade during general anesthesia.

FETAL & NEONATAL EFFECTS
■ Pregnancy Category C (for definition, see the "*Pregnancy Categories*" section). Potentiation of MgSO4-induced neuromuscular weakness has been reported in infants of mothers given MgSO4 prior to delivery.

COMMENT
■ Studies have not been conducted w/ pregnant women on gentamycin.

GENTAMICIN (GARAMYCIN)

INDICATIONS
■ Second-line agent in the treatment & prevention of neonatal group B streptococcal infection

DOSING
- IV 3–5 mg/kg/day in divided doses q8h

MATERNAL SIDE EFFECTS & IMPACT ON ANESTHESIA
- Most common side effect is allergic reaction. Neuromuscular blocking agents (rocuronium, vecuronium) may have enhanced potency when administered w/ aminoglycosides. Concurrent administration of magnesium & an aminoglycoside may further potentiate neuromuscular blockade during general anesthesia.

FETAL & NEONATAL EFFECTS
- Pregnancy Category C (for definition, see the "*Pregnancy Categories*" section). Potentiation of MgSO4-induced neuromuscular weakness has been reported in infants of mothers given MgSO4 prior to delivery.

COMMENT
- Studies have not been conducted w/ pregnant women on gentamycin.

GLUCOPHAGE (METFORMIN)

INDICATIONS
- A biguanide oral anti-hyperglycemic agent, its mode of action is thought to be multifactorial & includes delayed uptake of glucose from the GI tract, increased peripheral glucose utilization mediated by increased insulin sensitivity & inhibition of increased hepatic & renal gluconeogenesis.

DOSING
- Initial dosage 850 mg qd or 500 mg bid

MATERNAL SIDE EFFECTS & IMPACT ON ANESTHESIA
- Use during pregnancy is not advised. There is no information available concerning safety during lactation.

FETAL & NEONATAL EFFECTS
- Pregnancy Category B (for definition, see the "*Pregnancy Categories*" section). Abnormal blood glucose levels during pregnancy have been associated w/ a higher incidence of congenital abnormalities than expected.

COMMENT

■ May cause ketoacidosis in children after exercise. Insulin therapy is advocated by most specialists during pregnancy to enable tight blood glucose control.

GLYBURIDE (MICRONASE, DIABETA, GLYNASE)

INDICATIONS

■ Glyburide stimulates the secretion of insulin by the beta cells of the pancreas. In addition to this pancreatic action, glipizide administration may improve the metabolic utilization of glucose at a peripheral level.

DOSING

■ Initial dose: 1.25–5 mg qd

MATERNAL SIDE EFFECTS & IMPACT ON ANESTHESIA

■ Do not use in the 1st trimester, as safety in pregnancy has not been established. Do not use in pts w/ ketoacidosis or severe renal, hepatic, adrenal or thyroid dysfunction.

FETAL & NEONATAL EFFECTS

■ Pregnancy Category C (for definition, see the "*Pregnancy Categories*" section). Do not use in the 1st trimester, as safety in pregnancy has not been established. The degree to which it affects newborns via transmission in breast milk is unknown.

COMMENT

■ Insulin therapy is advocated by most specialists during pregnancy to enable tight blood glucose control.

GLYCOPYRROLATE

INDICATIONS

■ Parasympatholytic, bradycardia, antimuscarinic; may be used to counteract the bradycardic effects of neostigmine when used in neuromuscular blockade reversal

DOSING

■ 0.1–0.2 mg IV for each 1 mg of neostigmine

MATERNAL SIDE EFFECTS & IMPACT ON ANESTHESIA

■ Pregnancy Category B (for definition, see the "*Pregnancy Categories*" section). Has been used before C-section to reduce gastric secretions. Has been advocated as the anticholinergic drug of choice during anesthesia for ECT in pregnant pts. Increases maternal heart rate but not BP.

FETAL & NEONATAL EFFECTS

■ Pregnancy Category B. Crosses the placenta, but considerably less than atropine. No data available for breast feeding, but similar to atropine (safe).

COMMENT

■ N/A

GLYNASE (GLYBURIDE)

INDICATIONS

■ Glyburide stimulates the secretion of insulin by the beta cells of the pancreas. In addition to this pancreatic action, glipizide administration may improve the metabolic utilization of glucose at a peripheral level.

DOSING

■ Initial dose: 1.25–5 mg qd

MATERNAL SIDE EFFECTS & IMPACT ON ANESTHESIA

■ Do not use in the 1st trimester, as safety in pregnancy has not been established. Do not use in pts w/ ketoacidosis or severe renal, hepatic, adrenal or thyroid dysfunction.

FETAL & NEONATAL EFFECTS

■ Pregnancy Category C (for definition, see the "*Pregnancy Categories*" section). Do not use in the 1st trimester, as safety in pregnancy has not been established. The degree to which it affects newborns via transmission in breast milk is unknown.

COMMENT

■ Insulin therapy is advocated by most specialists during pregnancy to enable tight blood glucose control.

HALDOL (HALOPERIDOL)

INDICATIONS
- Haloperidol is an antipsychotic agent that is structurally related to the piperazine phenothiazines. Haloperidol is an effective antipsychotic for the treatment of schizophrenia. Also used for the treatment of acute psychosis, schizoaffective disorders, paranoid syndrome & Tourette's syndrome. Also used as an antiemetic.

DOSING
- Varies depending on the indication
- Psychotic disorders w/ moderate symptomatology: 0.5–2 mg PO 2 or 3 times/day, max 100 mg/day
- Tourette's: 6–15 mg/day PO
- Antiemetic: 1–4 mg IM or PO

MATERNAL SIDE EFFECTS & IMPACT ON ANESTHESIA
- May be useful in the setting of awake fiberoptic intubation for C-section

FETAL & NEONATAL EFFECTS
- Pregnancy Category C (for definition, see the "*Pregnancy Categories*" section). Although there are isolated cases of teratogenicity associated w/ haloperidol, no cause-effect relationship has been established. Haloperidol crosses the placenta. It is suggested that haloperidol use during pregnancy be limited to psychotic pts requiring long-term therapy. Found in breast milk; use during breast-feeding may be of concern.

COMMENT
- Adverse reactions attributed to continuous infusion of haloperidol include intermittent 3rd-degree heart block & prolonged QT interval w/ torsades de pointes occurred during the highest rate of infusion (40 mg/hour).

HALOPERIDOL (HALDOL)

INDICATIONS
- Haloperidol is an antipsychotic agent that is structurally related to the piperazine phenothiazines. Haloperidol is an effective antipsychotic for the treatment of schizophrenia. Also used for the treatment

of acute psychosis, schizoaffective disorders, paranoid syndrome & Tourette's syndrome. Also used as an antiemetic.

DOSING
- Varies depending on the indication
- Psychotic disorders w/ moderate symptomatology: 0.5–2 mg PO 2 or 3 times/day, max 100 mg/day
- Tourette's: 6–15 mg/day PO
- Antiemetic: 1–4 mg IM or PO

MATERNAL SIDE EFFECTS & IMPACT ON ANESTHESIA
- May be useful in the setting of awake fiberoptic intubation for C-section

FETAL & NEONATAL EFFECTS
- Pregnancy Category C (for definition, see the "*Pregnancy Categories*" section). Although there are isolated cases of teratogenicity associated w/ haloperidol, no cause-effect relationship has been established. Haloperidol crosses the placenta. It is suggested that haloperidol use during pregnancy be limited to psychotic pts requiring long-term therapy. Found in breast milk; use during breast-feeding may be of concern.

COMMENT
- Adverse reactions attributed to continuous infusion of haloperidol include intermittent 3rd-degree heart block & prolonged QT interval w/ torsades de pointes occurred during the highest rate of infusion (40 mg/hour).

HEMABATE (PROSTAGLANDIN F2α, CARBOPROST TROMETHAMINE)

INDICATIONS
- Prostaglandin is similar to F2-alpha (dinoprost), but it has a longer duration & produces myometrial contractions that induce hemostasis at placentation site, which reduces post-partum bleeding. Hemabate is used to treat post-partum hemorrhage & causes of uterine atony (overdistended uterus, rapid or prolonged labor, chorioamnionitis, high parity).

DOSING

■ Treatment of postpartum hemorrhage: 0.25mg (250 mcg/mL) IM q15–90min, up to 2 mg

MATERNAL SIDE EFFECTS & IMPACT ON ANESTHESIA

■ Administration can cause marked pulmonary arteriolar muscle constriction, severe pulmonary hypertension & bronchoconstriction. Can cause hypertension, but not as severe as the ergotamines.

FETAL & NEONATAL EFFECTS

■ Pregnancy Category C (for definition, see the "*Pregnancy Categories*" section). Hemabate can induce labor & can even be used to abort the fetus in early stages of pregnancy. Hemabate is found in breast milk, but it is unknown if this is of clinical significance.

COMMENT

■ Avoid in pts w/ pre-existing asthma or reactive airway disorders.

HEPARIN SODIUM

INDICATIONS

■ May be used when pt has stopped previous anticoagulant such as enoxaparin. Used for tight control of anticoagulation profile in high-risk (for life-threatening embolism) pts, such as those w/ prosthetic valves, concurrent DVT or PE or other underlying embolic states.

DOSING

■ Aim for PTT of 1.5–2.0× control. 5,000 units SQ BID is administered as a prophylaxis dose.

MATERNAL SIDE EFFECTS & IMPACT ON ANESTHESIA

■ The major side effect of heparin is hemorrhage. Careful lab monitoring is necessary in pts receiving higher, therapeutic doses. Monitoring PTT prior to regional anesthesia in patients receiving prophylaxis doses is generally not needed, but a normal PTT ensures safety against epidural hematoma during regional anesthesia.

FETAL & NEONATAL EFFECTS

■ Pregnancy Category C (for definition, see the "*Pregnancy Categories*" section). Heparin does not cross the placenta or present a direct risk to the embryo or fetus. There is also no risk to the nursing infant, because transfer into milk is inhibited by the drug's molecular size.

COMMENT
- Pregnant women on long-term heparin therapy are at risk of maternal heparin-induced osteopenia & should receive active vitamin D (calcitriol) supplements. Contraindicated in pts w/ a history of heparin-induced thrombocytopenia (HIT).

HUMALOG (INSULIN)

INDICATIONS
- Drug of choice for all types of diabetes mellitus during pregnancy. Stimulates proper utilization of glucose by cells & reduces blood glucose levels. Therapy is largely empiric, w/ multiple choices available to achieve glycemic control.

DOSING
- 0.5–1 U/kg/d SC in divided doses. Base dose on IBW; titrate dose to maintain a pre-meal & bedtime glucose level of 80–110 mg/dL. Combine short-acting & longer-acting insulins to maintain blood glucose within target.

MATERNAL SIDE EFFECTS & IMPACT ON ANESTHESIA
- Calcium channel blockers may inhibit pancreatic insulin release & block free fatty acid uptake & utilization by the myocardium, which is needed for myocardial work & contractility. High-dose insulin may change myocardial energy consumption from free fatty acids to carbohydrates. Does not cross the placenta but may cause hypoglycemia in mother, which can result in hypoglycemia in newborn.

FETAL & NEONATAL EFFECTS
- Pregnancy Category B (for definition, see the "*Pregnancy Categories*" section). Insulin does not cross the placenta but may cause maternal hypoglycemia, which can result in hypoglycemia in newborn.

COMMENT
- Monitor glucose levels in both newborn & mother post-delivery.

HUMULIN (INSULIN)

INDICATIONS
- Drug of choice for all types of diabetes mellitus during pregnancy. Stimulates proper utilization of glucose by cells & reduces blood

glucose levels. Therapy is largely empiric, w/ multiple choices available to achieve glycemic control.

DOSING
- 0.5–1 U/kg/d SC in divided doses. Base dose on IBW; titrate dose to maintain a pre-meal & bedtime glucose level of 80–110 mg/dL. Combine short-acting & longer-acting insulins to maintain blood glucose within target.

MATERNAL SIDE EFFECTS & IMPACT ON ANESTHESIA
- Calcium channel blockers may inhibit pancreatic insulin release & block free fatty acid uptake & utilization by the myocardium, which is needed for myocardial work & contractility. High-dose insulin may change myocardial energy consumption from free fatty acids to carbohydrates. Does not cross the placenta but may cause hypoglycemia in mother, which can result in hypoglycemia in newborn.

FETAL & NEONATAL EFFECTS
- Pregnancy Category B (for definition, see the "*Pregnancy Categories*" section). Insulin does not cross the placenta but may cause maternal hypoglycemia, which can result in hypoglycemia in newborn.

COMMENT
- Monitor glucose levels in both newborn & mother post-delivery.

HURRICAINE (BENZOCAINE 20%)

INDICATIONS
- Topical anesthetic can be applied as a cream or a spray. Many vaginitis creams incorporate benzocaine as the primary anesthetic. Lozenges/sprays are also available for oral sores or pharyngitis. Used in the setting of awake intubations, benzocaine blunts the gag reflex & allows for direct or fiberoptic laryngoscopy.

DOSING
- Topical spray: Recommended dose is 1 second of continuous spray (average expulsion rate is 200 mg/sec). Exceeding this duration may be hazardous & may result in methemoglobinemia. Onset within 15–30 seconds.

MATERNAL SIDE EFFECTS & IMPACT ON ANESTHESIA
- Pregnancy Category C (for definition, see the "*Pregnancy Categories*" section). One of its metabolites (orthotoluidine) has been associated w/ methemoglobinemia.

FETAL & NEONATAL EFFECTS
- Pregnancy Category C (for definition, see the "*Pregnancy Categories*" section). Methemoglobinemia can be problematic in the fetus, as it lacks the enzymes to metabolize it. Not expected to accumulate significantly in breast milk.

COMMENT
- N/A

HYDRALAZINE (APRESOLINE)

INDICATIONS
- Hypertension

DOSING
- 2.5–20 mg IV q4h prn; in pre-eclampsia/eclampsia 5–10 mg IV q20min up to 20 mg

MATERNAL SIDE EFFECTS & IMPACT ON ANESTHESIA
- May cause hypotension, reflex tachycardia, SLE syndrome

FETAL & NEONATAL EFFECTS
- Pregnancy Category C (for definition, see the "*Pregnancy Categories*" section). Studies suggest no increased incidence of fetal anomalies & no adverse effects on uterine blood flow. Report of transient neonatal thrombocytopenia w/ daily 3rd-trimester use (w/ petechial bleeding & hematomas), lupus-like syndrome in neonate. American Academy of Pediatrics states hydralazine is compatible w/ breast-feeding.

COMMENT
- Animal studies have demonstrated teratogenic effects, including cleft palate & facial & cranial bone malformations.

HYDROCHLOROTHIAZIDE

INDICATIONS
- Not commonly used to treat hypertension during pregnancy. May have a transient effect on intravascular volume. Inhibits reabsorption of sodium in distal tubules, causing increased excretion of sodium & water, as well as potassium & hydrogen ions.

DOSING
- 25–100 mg PO qd, max 200 mg/kg/d

MATERNAL SIDE EFFECTS & IMPACT ON ANESTHESIA
- Prevents normal physiologic volume expansion that occurs in pregnancy & may reduce uterine blood flow; restrict use to women w/ true volume-overload states (eg, renal or cardiac disease)

FETAL & NEONATAL EFFECTS
- Pregnancy Category B (for definition, see the "*Pregnancy Categories*" section). Potential hazards include fetal or neonatal jaundice, thrombocytopenia, hemolytic anemia, electrolyte imbalance & hypoglycemia. Thiazides pass into breast milk; use is indicated when importance of the drug for the mother is clear.

COMMENT
- Thiazides may decrease the effects of anticoagulants, antigout agents & sulfonylureas; may increase toxicity of allopurinol, anesthetics, antineoplastics, calcium salts, loop diuretics, lithium, diazoxide, digitalis, amphotericin B & nondepolarizing muscle relaxants.

HYDROCORTISONE

INDICATIONS
- Endocrine disorders, inflammatory conditions, including those of the lower bowel & rectum, multiple sclerosis exacerbations, nephrotic syndrome & minor skin irritations

DOSING
- Varies depending on the disorder

MATERNAL SIDE EFFECTS & IMPACT ON ANESTHESIA
- Corticosteroids do not appear to cause congenital anomalies in the infant. During periods of stress such as surgery, the steroid dose

should be increased before, during & after the stressful situation. Adrenocortical insufficiency may persist for months after stopping the corticosteroid; therefore, replacement therapy may be needed during periods of stress. Common side effects include euphoria/depression, GI distress, growth depression, hypertension, impaired wound healing, increased risk of infection & skin atrophy. Serious side effects include Cushing syndrome, fluid & electrolyte disturbances, HPA axis suppression/adrenal insufficiency & hyperglycemia.

FETAL & NEONATAL EFFECTS
■ Pregnancy Category NR (for definition, see the "*Pregnancy Categories*" section). Corticosteroids do not appear to cause congenital anomalies in the infant. Neonatal adrenal insufficiency appears to be rare. Systemically administered corticosteroids are secreted into breast milk in quantities not likely to have an adverse effect on the infant.

COMMENT
■ Contraindicated in pts w/ active fungal infections. Use precaution in pts w/ liver failure, myasthenia gravis, ocular herpes simplex, osteoporosis, renal insufficiency & untreated systemic infections.

HYDROMORPHONE (DILAUDID)

INDICATIONS
■ Pain, moderate or severe. In obstetrics, primarily as a post-op analgesic (PCA).

DOSING
■ 1–2 mg IM/SC/IV q4–6h; 2.5–10 mg PO or rectally q3–6h as needed

MATERNAL SIDE EFFECTS & IMPACT ON ANESTHESIA
■ Dilaudid is relatively contraindicated in obstetrical anesthesia. Avoid in pts w/ depressed ventilatory dysfunction, intracranial lesion associated w/ increased ICP. May need dosing adjustment in pts w/ renal failure or liver disease & in geriatrics. Use precaution during concomitant administration of general anesthetics or phenothiazines.

FETAL & NEONATAL EFFECTS
■ Pregnancy Category C (for definition, see the "*Pregnancy Categories*" section). Dilaudid is not FDA-approved in pediatric pts; it can cause

apnea, respiratory depression, circulatory depression, hypotension, confusion, myoclonus & seizures.

COMMENT
- Dilaudid contains sodium bisulfite, a sulfite that may cause allergic-type reactions in certain susceptible people.

IBUPROFEN (MOTRIN, ADVIL)

INDICATIONS
- Ibuprofen is a nonsteroidal, anti-inflammatory, antipyretic analgesic agent. It inhibits the synthesis of prostaglandins.

DOSING
- 400 mg/dose PO q4–6h, max 1.2 g/day

MATERNAL SIDE EFFECTS & IMPACT ON ANESTHESIA
- Safe to administer regional anesthesia in women taking ibuprofen

FETAL & NEONATAL EFFECTS
- Pregnancy Category B; Category D in 3rd trimester (for definitions, see the "*Pregnancy Categories*" section). Known effects on fetus during 3rd trimester include constriction of ductus arteriosus prenatally, tricuspid insufficiency & pulmonary hypertension; nonclosure of the ductus arteriosus postnatally; bleeding. Ibuprofen is safe during breast-feeding; amounts are difficult to detect in breast milk after dosages of up to 1.6 g/day PO.

COMMENT
- Use w/ care in pts w/ peptic ulceration or a history of such ulceration, bleeding disorders or cardiovascular disease & pts on oral anticoagulants. Do not use routinely in pts who are allergic to aspirin. Use w/ care in pts w/ asthma, especially those who have developed bronchospasm w/ other nonsteroidal agents.

ILETIN (INSULIN)

INDICATIONS
- Drug of choice for all types of diabetes mellitus during pregnancy. Stimulates proper utilization of glucose by cells & reduces blood

glucose levels. Therapy is largely empiric, w/ multiple choices available to achieve glycemic control.

DOSING

■ 0.5–1 U/kg/d SC in divided doses. Base dose on IBW; titrate dose to maintain a pre-meal & bedtime glucose level of 80–110 mg/dL. Combine short-acting & longer-acting insulins to maintain blood glucose within target.

MATERNAL SIDE EFFECTS & IMPACT ON ANESTHESIA

■ Calcium channel blockers may inhibit pancreatic insulin release & block free fatty acid uptake & utilization by the myocardium, which is needed for myocardial work & contractility. High-dose insulin may change myocardial energy consumption from free fatty acids to carbohydrates. Does not cross the placenta but may cause hypoglycemia in mother, which can result in hypoglycemia in newborn.

FETAL & NEONATAL EFFECTS

■ Pregnancy Category B (for definition, see the "*Pregnancy Categories*" section). Insulin does not cross the placenta but may cause maternal hypoglycemia, which can result in hypoglycemia in newborn.

COMMENT

■ Monitor glucose levels in both newborn & mother post-delivery.

IMIPRAMINE (TOFRANIL)

INDICATIONS

■ Tricyclic antidepressants (TCAs) are effective for the treatment of major depressive disorders; also sometimes prescribed for chronic pain or polyneuropathy.

DOSING

■ For depression in outpatients, 75 mg/day divided in 1–3 doses, up to 200 mg/day

MATERNAL SIDE EFFECTS & IMPACT ON ANESTHESIA

■ Common side effects include anticholinergic symptoms (drying of secretions, dilated pupils, sedation). Concomitant use of TCAs & amphetamines has been reported to result in enhanced amphetamine effects from the release of norepinephrine. Ephedrine should be given cautiously to patients on TCAs.

FETAL & NEONATAL EFFECTS
- Pregnancy Category NR (for definition, see the "*Pregnancy Catego-ries*" section). Breast-feeding effects are unknown; only very minute amounts are found in the infant's serum.

COMMENT
- Do not use w/MAO inhibitors.

IMITREX (SUMATRIPTAN)

INDICATIONS
- Vascular 5-hydroxytryptamine receptor subtype agonist used for treating acute migraines

DOSING
- Oral tablet or injection. Initial dose 25–100 mg, may be repeated after 2 hours if headache is still present. Max daily dose 200 mg.

MATERNAL SIDE EFFECTS & IMPACT ON ANESTHESIA
- May cause vasospasm. Rare but serious cardiac events in pts w/o cardiac risk factors have been reported within 1 hour of adminis-tration. Hypertensive crisis in pts w/o history of hypertension also reported. May lower seizure threshold.

FETAL & NEONATAL EFFECTS
- Pregnancy Category C (for definition, see the "*Pregnancy Categories*" section). Evidence of teratogenicity, impaired fertility & embry-olethality in animal studies. Excreted freely in breast milk. No testing in pts <12 years old.

COMMENT
- Careful exclusion of other causes of headache should be made prior to administration. Contraindicated w/ MAO-A inhibitors (reduces clearancc of Imitrex). Use w/ caution in pts on SSRIs.

INDOCIN (INDOMETHACIN)

INDICATIONS
- Acute gouty arthritis, acute painful shoulder (bursitis & tendo-nitis), ankylosing spondylitis, closure of patent ductus arteriosus, osteoarthritis, rheumatoid arthritis

DOSING
- 25–150 mg PO or rectally every day in divided doses; max parenteral dose 200 mg/day

MATERNAL SIDE EFFECTS & IMPACT ON ANESTHESIA
- The effects of indomethacin on pregnancy have not been assessed, but it has been suggested that indomethacin be avoided in later pregnancy. Indomethacin has not been suggested to have an impact on anesthetics, but use precautions in the following pts: liver dysfunction; renal disease; hypertension or CHF; history of GI ulceration, bleeding or perforation; dehydration; asthma; coagulation defects; anemia; epilepsy; parkinsonism; depression; psychiatric conditions.

FETAL & NEONATAL EFFECTS
- Pregnancy Category Not Rated (for definition, see the "*Pregnancy Categories*" section). Indomethacin has been generally regarded as unsafe in breast-feeding. Neonates w/ active bleeding, infection, necrotizing enterocolitis, severe renal failure, thrombocytopenia or coagulation defects should not be given indomethacin.

COMMENT
- Indomethacin is primarily metabolized in the liver. Pts w/ a history of recent rectal bleeding or proctitis should not be given indomethacin.

INDOMETHACIN (INDOCIN)

INDICATIONS
- Acute gouty arthritis, acute painful shoulder (bursitis & tendonitis), ankylosing spondylitis, closure of patent ductus arteriosus, osteoarthritis, rheumatoid arthritis

DOSING
- 25–150 mg PO or rectally every day in divided doses; max parenteral dose 200 mg/day

MATERNAL SIDE EFFECTS & IMPACT ON ANESTHESIA
- The effects of indomethacin on pregnancy have not been assessed, but it has been suggested that indomethacin be avoided in later pregnancy. Indomethacin has not been suggested to have an impact on anesthetics, but use precautions in the following pts: liver dysfunction; renal disease; hypertension or CHF; history of GI

ulceration, bleeding or perforation; dehydration; asthma; coagulation defects; anemia; epilepsy; parkinsonism; depression; psychiatric conditions.

FETAL & NEONATAL EFFECTS
■ Pregnancy Category Not Rated (for definition, see the "*Pregnancy Categories*" section). Indomethacin has been generally regarded as unsafe in breast-feeding. Neonates w/ active bleeding, infection, necrotizing enterocolitis, severe renal failure, thrombocytopenia or coagulation defects should not be given indomethacin.

COMMENT
■ Indomethacin is primarily metabolized in the liver. Pts w/ a history of recent rectal bleeding or proctitis should not be given indomethacin.

INSULIN (NOVOLIN, HUMULIN, HUMALOG, LENTE, ILETIN, NPH)

INDICATIONS
■ Drug of choice for all types of diabetes mellitus during pregnancy. Stimulates proper utilization of glucose by cells & reduces blood glucose levels. Therapy is largely empiric, w/ multiple choices available to achieve glycemic control.

DOSING
■ 0.5–1 U/kg/d SC in divided doses. Base dose on IBW; titrate dose to maintain a pre-meal & bedtime glucose level of 80–110 mg/dL. Combine short-acting & longer-acting insulins to maintain blood glucose within target.

MATERNAL SIDE EFFECTS & IMPACT ON ANESTHESIA
■ Calcium channel blockers may inhibit pancreatic insulin release & block free fatty acid uptake & utilization by the myocardium, which is needed for myocardial work & contractility. High-dose insulin may change myocardial energy consumption from free fatty acids to carbohydrates. Does not cross the placenta but may cause hypoglycemia in mother, which can result in hypoglycemia in newborn.

FETAL & NEONATAL EFFECTS
■ Pregnancy Category B (for definition, see the "*Pregnancy Categories*" section). Insulin does not cross the placenta but may cause maternal hypoglycemia, which can result in hypoglycemia in newborn.

COMMENT
- Monitor glucose levels in both newborn & mother post-delivery.

IPRATROPIUM (ATROVENT)

INDICATIONS
- Bronchodilator. Used for bronchospasm associated w/ COPD, asthma (re: asthma–FDA off-label use), rhinorrhea w/ cold, seasonal allergy, etc.

DOSING
- Inhaler 2 puffs (36 mcg) 4x/day up to 12 puffs/day
- Nebulizer 500 mcg 3 or 4 times/day

MATERNAL SIDE EFFECTS & IMPACT ON ANESTHESIA
- May be associated w/ dry cough, bitter taste. Contraindicated w/ narrow-angle glaucoma, bladder neck obstruction.

FETAL & NEONATAL EFFECTS
- Pregnancy Category B (for definition, see the "*Pregnancy Categories*" section). Use in pregnancy is indicated where there are maternal benefits. It is thought that very little drug passes into breast milk.

COMMENT
- May be contraindicated in pts w/ sensitivity to soya lecithin or related food products such as soybeans or peanuts.

ISOFLURANE (FORANE)

INDICATIONS
- Maintenance of general anesthesia

DOSING
- Isoflurane MAC is 1.2% in normal adults, decreased by 30–40% in the parturient. In the parturient, use 0.25–0.5 MAC until delivery of baby to limit hypotension & uterine atony.

MATERNAL SIDE EFFECTS & IMPACT ON ANESTHESIA
- Causes dose-dependent uterine atony, hypotension via peripheral vasodilation, myocardial depression, reflex tachycardia, respiratory depression or arrest, N/V, shivering

FETAL & NEONATAL EFFECTS
- Pregnancy Category C (for definition, see the "*Pregnancy Categories*" section). Distributes rapidly across the placenta during C-section w/ a fetal/maternal ratio of 0.7. May cause temporary neonatal depression in large doses. No evidence of long-term adverse effects. Not thought to be a problem for breast-feeding.

COMMENT
- When used as the sole anesthetic agent for general anesthesia, awareness results in 12–26% of cases.

KETALAR (KETAMINE)

INDICATIONS
- An aryl-cyclohexylamine & congener of phencyclidine (PCP). IV induction agent. Useful in parturients w/ unstable hypovolemia or asthma.

DOSING
- IV: 1–2 mg/kg
- IM: 3–5 mg/kg

MATERNAL SIDE EFFECTS & IMPACT ON ANESTHESIA
- Avoid in pts w/ hypertension. Increases oral secretions. May cause hallucinations & nightmares (may be reduced if co-administered w/ benzodiazepine), myoclonus, increases in ICP, nystagmus, diplopia. Effects may be attenuated by pretreatment w/ midazolam.

FETAL & NEONATAL EFFECTS
- Pregnancy Category NR (for definition, see the "*Pregnancy Categories*" section). Doses of 1 mg/kg do not cause neonatal depression. Doses of 2 mg/kg IV have been associated w/ excessive neonatal muscle tone & apnea, & difficulty w/ endotracheal intubation was noted. Although the drug is less soluble than thiopental, its fetal/maternal ratio is 1.26 after 90 seconds after a dose of 2 mg/kg for general anesthesia.

COMMENT
- Produces minimal respiratory depression. Increases systolic BP 10–40%. When learning about these drugs in obstetrics, it is important to

be familiar w/ the approximate fetal:maternal (F/M) ratios of drug concentrations at the time of delivery of the infant. Generally, the umbilical vein blood concentrations represent the fetal blood concentrations. An early high ratio indicates rapid placental transfer of the drug.

KETAMINE (KETALAR)

INDICATIONS
- An aryl-cyclohexylamine & congener of phencyclidine (PCP). IV induction agent. Useful in parturients w/ unstable hypovolemia or asthma.

DOSING
- IV: 1–2 mg/kg
- IM: 3–5 mg/kg

MATERNAL SIDE EFFECTS & IMPACT ON ANESTHESIA
- Avoid in pts w/ hypertension. Increases oral secretions. May cause hallucinations & nightmares (may be reduced if co-administered w/ benzodiazepine), myoclonus, increases in ICP, nystagmus, diplopia. Effects may be attenuated by pretreatment w/ midazolam.

FETAL & NEONATAL EFFECTS
- Pregnancy Category NR (for definition, see the "*Pregnancy Categories*" section). Doses of 1 mg/kg do not cause neonatal depression. Doses of 2 mg/kg IV have been associated w/ excessive neonatal muscle tone & apnea, & difficulty w/ endotracheal intubation was noted. Although the drug is less soluble than thiopental, its fetal/maternal ratio is 1.26 after 90 seconds after a dose of 2 mg/kg for general anesthesia.

COMMENT
- Produces minimal respiratory depression. Increases systolic BP 10–40%. When learning about these drugs in obstetrics, it is important to be familiar w/ the approximate fetal:maternal (F/M) ratios of drug concentrations at the time of delivery of the infant. Generally, the umbilical vein blood concentrations represent the fetal blood concentrations. An early high ratio indicates rapid placental transfer of the drug.

KETOROLAC (TORADOL)

INDICATIONS
- Ketorolac is a nonsteroidal, anti-inflammatory, analgesic, antipyretic agent that inhibits prostaglandin synthetase.

DOSING
- PO: 15–30 mg q6h, max 40 mg/day for max of 5 days
- IV: 30 mg q6h for max of 5 days

MATERNAL SIDE EFFECTS & IMPACT ON ANESTHESIA
- Excellent analgesic adjunct for post-op pain after C-section in women receiving intrathecal morphine. Do not use in women considering pregnancy, since these agents block blastocyst implantation.

FETAL & NEONATAL EFFECTS
- Pregnancy Category C, but Category D in 3rd trimester (for definitions, see the "*Pregnancy Categories*" section). Crosses the placenta. Ketorolac, like all prostaglandin synthesis inhibitors during pregnancy, constricts the ductus arteriosis. Persistent pulmonary hypertension of the newborn can occur if administered close to the time of delivery. See "*Ibuprofen.*"

COMMENT
- The most frequent adverse effects are GI disturbances, reactions ranging from abdominal discomfort, nausea & vomiting & abdominal pain to serious GI bleeding or activation of peptic ulcer.

LABETALOL (NORMODYNE, TRANDATE)

INDICATIONS
- Hypertension

DOSING
- A wide therapeutic range. Titrate to effect. 5–10 mg IV, over 2 minutes. May repeat up to 200 mg total. For oral dosing, 100–400 mg PO BID.

MATERNAL SIDE EFFECTS & IMPACT ON ANESTHESIA
- May cause bradycardia, bronchospasm in asthmatics, postural hypotension, dizziness. Not thought to affect the usual course of labor & delivery when given to pregnant hypertensive pts.

FETAL & NEONATAL EFFECTS
■ Pregnancy Category C (for definition, see the "*Pregnancy Categories*" section). Crosses the placenta & may cause fetal bradycardia, hypoglycemia, respiratory depression, hypotension. Considered compatible w/ breast-feeding.

COMMENT
■ Has an alpha to beta blockade action of 1:7

LANOXIN (DIGOXIN)

INDICATIONS
■ A cardiac glycoside that increases cardiac inotropy & decreases conduction at the AV node & Purkinje fibers

DOSING
■ Total digitalizing dose (TDD) to be administered over 24 h; 1st dose is one-half the TDD; 2nd dose is one-fourth the TDD, administered 8 h later; 3rd dose is one-fourth the TDD, administered 8 h after the second TDD: 0.75–1.5 mg PO in divided doses over 1 d; alternatively 0.5–1 mg IV/IM in divided doses over 1 d; maintenance dose: 0.125–0.5 mg PO qd or 0.1–0.4 mg IV/IM qd

MATERNAL SIDE EFFECTS & IMPACT ON ANESTHESIA
■ Digoxin has a narrow therapeutic index. Serum levels must be closely followed. Toxicity may be potentiated by hypercalcemia, hypomagnesemia & hypokalemia. It also interacts w/ a large number of meds. Additional side effects of digoxin include GI upset & visual disturbances.

FETAL & NEONATAL EFFECTS
■ Pregnancy Category C (for definition, see the "*Pregnancy Categories*" section). There have been no reports linking digoxin to congenital defects, & animal studies have failed to show teratogenicity. Overdoses of digoxin may result in neonatal asphyxia & death. Considered safe during breast-feeding due to high maternal protein-binding.

COMMENT
■ Documented hypersensitivity; beriberi heart disease; idiopathic hypertrophic subaortic stenosis; constrictive pericarditis; carotid sinus syndrome

LASIX (FUROSEMIDE)

INDICATIONS
- Not commonly used to treat hypertension during pregnancy. Can be used to treat pulmonary edema associated w/ pre-eclampsia. Increases excretion of water by interfering w/ chloride-binding cotransport system, which in turn inhibits sodium & chloride reabsorption in ascending loop of Henle & distal renal tubule.

DOSING
- 10 mg IV initial dose, 20–80 mg/d PO/IV/IM; titrate up to 600 mg/d for severe edematous states

MATERNAL SIDE EFFECTS & IMPACT ON ANESTHESIA
- Prevents normal physiologic volume expansion that occurs in pregnancy & may reduce uterine blood flow; restrict use to women w/ volume-overload states (eg, renal or cardiac disease)

FETAL & NEONATAL EFFECTS
- Pregnancy Category C; Category D if used for pregnancy-induced hypertension (for definitions, see the "*Pregnancy Categories*" section). Safety during pregnancy has not been established. Effects in breast-feeding are unknown.

COMMENT
- N/A

LENTE (INSULIN)

INDICATIONS
- Drug of choice for all types of diabetes mellitus during pregnancy. Stimulates proper utilization of glucose by cells & reduces blood glucose levels. Therapy is largely empiric, w/ multiple choices available to achieve glycemic control.

DOSING
- 0.5–1 U/kg/d SC in divided doses. Base dose on IBW; titrate dose to maintain a pre-meal & bedtime glucose level of 80–110 mg/dL. Combine short-acting & longer-acting insulins to maintain blood glucose within target.

MATERNAL SIDE EFFECTS & IMPACT ON ANESTHESIA
- Calcium channel blockers may inhibit pancreatic insulin release & block free fatty acid uptake & utilization by the myocardium, which is needed for myocardial work & contractility. High-dose insulin may change myocardial energy consumption from free fatty acids to carbohydrates. Does not cross the placenta but may cause hypoglycemia in mother, which can result in hypoglycemia in newborn.

FETAL & NEONATAL EFFECTS
- Pregnancy Category B (for definition, see the "*Pregnancy Categories*" section). Insulin does not cross the placenta but may cause maternal hypoglycemia, which can result in hypoglycemia in newborn.

COMMENT
- Monitor glucose levels in both newborn & mother post-delivery.

LEVO-BUPIVACAINE (CHIROCAINE)

INDICATIONS
- Epidural analgesia

DOSING
- Epidural labor analgesia: 10–20 mL of 0.25% (25–50 mg)
- Epidural for cesarean delivery: 20–30 cc of 0.5% (100–150 mg)
- Epidural for post-op analgesia: 4–10 cc/hr of 0.125–0.25% (5–25 mg/hr)

MATERNAL SIDE EFFECTS & IMPACT ON ANESTHESIA
- May have a better cardiac safety profile than bupivacaine in higher doses, but higher cost & safe use of low concentrations of bupivacaine for epidural analgesia limit its utility.

FETAL & NEONATAL SIDE EFFECTS
- Pregnancy Category C (for definition, see the "*Pregnancy Categories*" section). Safety in breast-feeding is unknown, but local anesthetics are not expected to accumulate significantly in breast milk.

COMMENT
- N/A

LEVOPHED (NOREPINEPHRINE)

INDICATIONS
■ Alpha & beta adrenergic agonist. Alpha activity is dominant. Used for hypotension.

DOSING
■ Start w/ 1–8 mcg/min & titrate to desired effects.

MATERNAL SIDE EFFECTS & IMPACT ON ANESTHESIA
■ May cause hypertension, arrhythmia, myocardia ischemia, increased uterine contractility, frequency of contractions, CNS stimulation. Halogenated vapor anesthetics may sensitize the myocardium to the effects of catecholamines. When given in combination w/ oxytocic agents, may cause severe hypertension.

FETAL & NEONATAL EFFECTS
■ Pregnancy category C (for definition, see the "*Pregnancy Categories*" section). It is unknown if norepinephrine causes fetal harm or the degree to which it is excreted in breast milk.

COMMENT
■ N/A

LEVOTHROID (LEVOTHYROXINE)

INDICATIONS
■ A synthetically prepared hormone identical to T4 used in the treatment of hypothyroidism

DOSING
■ 1.6–1.8 mcg/kg lean body weight/d PO qd

MATERNAL SIDE EFFECTS & IMPACT ON ANESTHESIA
■ Hypothyroid women have a lower fertility rate than euthyroid women. The required dose of thyroid replacement often increases during pregnancy by 20–50%. A large goiter may produce dysphagia, hoarseness & stridor from extrinsic obstruction to airflow; consider evaluating pts w/ these symptoms w/ a barium swallow study & pulmonary function tests, including flow volume loops. Use w/ caution in angina pectoris or cardiovascular disease. Monitor thyroid status

periodically. Use caution in pts w/ adrenocortical insufficiency, in whom steroid replacement should precede levothyroxine replacement.

FETAL & NEONATAL EFFECTS
■ Pregnancy Category A (for definition, see the "*Pregnancy Categories*" section). Negligible transplacental passage of the drug. T4 is excreted into breast milk in low concentrations.

COMMENT
■ TSH is the most accurate measure of the euthyroid state. In most instances, neonatal thyroid development is independent of maternal thyroid function. No contraindications to levothyroxine replacement therapy except in pts w/ uncorrected adrenal insufficiency.

LEVOTHYROXINE (SYNTHROID, LEVOXYL, LEVOTHROID)

INDICATIONS
■ A synthetically prepared hormone identical to T4 used in the treatment of hypothyroidism

DOSING
■ 1.6–1.8 mcg/kg lean body weight/d PO qd

MATERNAL SIDE EFFECTS & IMPACT ON ANESTHESIA
■ Hypothyroid women have a lower fertility rate than euthyroid women. The required dose of thyroid replacement often increases during pregnancy by 20–50%. A large goiter may produce dysphagia, hoarseness & stridor from extrinsic obstruction to airflow; consider evaluating pts w/ these symptoms w/ a barium swallow study & pulmonary function tests, including flow volume loops. Use w/ caution in angina pectoris or cardiovascular disease. Monitor thyroid status periodically. Use caution in pts w/ adrenocortical insufficiency, in whom steroid replacement should precede levothyroxine replacement.

FETAL & NEONATAL EFFECTS
■ Pregnancy Category A (for definition, see the "*Pregnancy Categories*" section). Negligible transplacental passage of the drug. T4 is excreted into breast milk in low concentrations.

COMMENT

■ TSH is the most accurate measure of the euthyroid state. In most instances, neonatal thyroid development is independent of maternal thyroid function. No contraindications to levothyroxine replacement therapy except in pts w/ uncorrected adrenal insufficiency.

LEVOXYL (LEVOTHYROXINE)

INDICATIONS

■ A synthetically prepared hormone identical to T4 used in the treatment of hypothyroidism

DOSING

■ 1.6–1.8 mcg/kg lean body weight/d PO qd

MATERNAL SIDE EFFECTS & IMPACT ON ANESTHESIA

■ Hypothyroid women have a lower fertility rate than euthyroid women. The required dose of thyroid replacement often increases during pregnancy by 20–50%. A large goiter may produce dysphagia, hoarseness & stridor from extrinsic obstruction to airflow; consider evaluating pts w/ these symptoms w/ a barium swallow study & pulmonary function tests, including flow volume loops. Use w/ caution in angina pectoris or cardiovascular disease. Monitor thyroid status periodically. Use caution in pts w/ adrenocortical insufficiency, in whom steroid replacement should precede levothyroxine replacement.

FETAL & NEONATAL EFFECTS

■ Pregnancy Category A (for definition, see the "*Pregnancy Categories*" section). Negligible transplacental passage of the drug. T4 is excreted into breast milk in low concentrations.

COMMENT

■ TSH is the most accurate measure of the euthyroid state. In most instances, neonatal thyroid development is independent of maternal thyroid function. No contraindications to levothyroxine replacement therapy except in pts w/ uncorrected adrenal insufficiency.

LIDOCAINE (XYLOCAINE)

INDICATIONS
■ pH-adjusted 2% lidocaine is useful for C-section under epidural. 1.5% lidocaine (45mg) w/ 1:200,000 epinephrine is useful to rule out intrathecal or intravascular placement of the epidural catheter. May also be used for the treatment of ventricular tachycardias. Lidocaine patch may be used for localized chronic pain treatment.

DOSE
■ Depends on procedure. 20 cc of 2% lidocaine epidurally in divided doses for C-section. Intrathecal doses vary depending on procedure length.

MATERNAL SIDE EFFECTS & IMPACT ON ANESTHESIA
■ Rapidly crosses the placenta. Intravascular administration may lead to lightheadedness, seizures, disorientation, heart block, hypotension. Acidosis in the fetus predisposes to ion trapping of the lidocaine.

FETAL & NEONATAL SIDE EFFECTS
■ Pregnancy Category B (for definition, see the "*Pregnancy Categories*" section). Rapidly crosses the placenta. Lidocaine injected into fetal scalp accidentally (as during paracervical block) may cause toxicity. Acidosis in the fetus predisposes to ion trapping of the lidocaine. Compatible w/ breast-feeding.

COMMENT
■ Lidocaine administered intrathecally has been associated w/ transient radicular irritation.

LIPITOR (ATORVASTATIN)

INDICATION
■ Adjunct to diet for reduction of elevated total cholesterol, LDL cholesterol, apolipoprotein-B & triglyceride levels in pts w/ primary hypercholesterolemia, mixed dyslipidemia & heterozygous familial hypercholesterolemia

DOSING
- 10–40 mg PO qd

MATERNAL SIDE EFFECTS & IMPACT ON ANESTHESIA
- Contraindicated in pregnancy, in breast-feeding mothers & in women of childbearing potential not using adequate contraceptive measures. An interval of 1 month should be allowed from stopping atorvastatin treatment to conception in the event of planning a pregnancy.

FETAL & NEONATAL EFFECTS
- Pregnancy Category X (for definition, see the "*Pregnancy Categories*" section)

COMMENT
- May cause elevation of creatine phosphokinase & dose-related increases in transaminase levels

---

LITHIUM CARBONATE (ESKALITH, LITHOBID)

INDICATIONS
- Classified as a tranquilizer to treat mania, but may be used to treat cluster headaches & Graves' disease

DOSING
- Varies for specific indication
- Mania (acute): 1,800 mg/day PO in 2 or 3 divided doses, w/ desired serum level 1–1.5 mEq/L
- Mania (maintenance): 900–1,200 mg/day PO in 2 or 3 divided doses, w/ desired serum level 0.6–1.2 mEq/L
- Cluster headache: 300–900 mg/day PO in divided doses, w/ desired serum level <1.2 mEq/L
- Graves disease: 900 mg/day PO for 8 days, starting on day of radioiodine administration

MATERNAL SIDE EFFECTS & IMPACT ON ANESTHESIA
- Administration of lithium throughout pregnancy can produce complications in the neonate since lithium passes readily across the placental barrier. Cases of cardiac arrhythmia, hypotonia, hypothyroidism & polyhydramnios have been reported.

FETAL & NEONATAL EFFECTS
- Pregnancy Category D (for definition, see the "*Pregnancy Categories*" section). Lithium readily crosses the placenta & can cause hypothyroidism in the newborn.

COMMENT
- Dosage needs to be adjusted in pts w/ renal dysfunction. May cause central or nephrogenic diabetes insipidus.

LITHOBID (LITHIUM CARBONATE)

INDICATIONS
- Classified as a tranquilizer to treat mania, but may be used to treat cluster headaches & Graves disease

DOSING
- Varies for specific indication
- Mania (acute): 1,800 mg/day PO in 2 or 3 divided doses, w/ desired serum level 1–1.5 mEq/L
- Mania (maintenance): 900–1,200 mg/day PO in 2 or 3 divided doses, w/ desired serum level 0.6–1.2 mEq/L
- Cluster headache: 300–900 mg/day PO in divided doses, w/ desired serum level <1.2 mEq/L
- Graves disease: 900 mg/day PO for 8 days, starting on day of radioiodine administration

MATERNAL SIDE EFFECTS & IMPACT ON ANESTHESIA
- Administration of lithium throughout pregnancy can produce complications in the neonate since lithium passes readily across the placental barrier. Cases of cardiac arrhythmia, hypotonia, hypothyroidism & polyhydramnios have been reported.

FETAL & NEONATAL EFFECTS
- Pregnancy Category D (for definition, see the "*Pregnancy Categories*" section). Lithium readily crosses the placenta & can cause hypothyroidism in the newborn.

COMMENT
- Dosage needs to be adjusted in pts w/ renal dysfunction. May cause central or nephrogenic diabetes insipidus.

LOPRESSOR (METOPROLOL)

INDICATIONS
- Beta-1 adrenergic blockade. Commonly used for hypertension, angina pectoris, arrhythmias, myocardial infarction, hypertrophic cardiomyopathy.

DOSING
- 50–100 mg PO q6–24h, 2.5- to 5-mg IV boluses q2min, prn

MATERNAL SIDE EFFECTS & IMPACT ON ANESTHESIA
- May cause bradycardia, clinically significant bronchoconstriction (with doses >100 mg/day), dizziness. Increased risk of heart block.

FETAL & NEONATAL EFFECTS
- Pregnancy Category C (for definition, see the "*Pregnancy Categories*" section). Crosses the placenta. May cause fetal or neonatal bradycardia, neonatal hypoglycemia & delayed spontaneous breathing of the newborn.

COMMENT
- N/A

LORAZEPAM (ATIVAN)

INDICATIONS
- Benzodiazepine indicated for anxiety disorders, preanesthesia sedation, status epilepticus. Non-label uses include alcohol withdrawal, antiemetic, insomnia.

DOSING
- Anxiety disorders: initial, 2–3 mg/day PO divided into 2 or 3 daily doses

MATERNAL SIDE EFFECTS & IMPACT ON ANESTHESIA
- May interact w/ other meds, including other CNS drugs such as phenothiazines, narcotic analgesics, barbiturates, antidepressants, scopolamine, MAO inhibitors.

FETAL & NEONATAL EFFECTS

■ Pregnancy Category D (for definition, see the "*Pregnancy Categories*" section). High IV doses may produce floppy infant syndrome. A higher incidence of respiratory depression (not statistically significant) occurred among infants whose mothers received lorazepam to potentiate the effects of narcotic analgesics. Preterm neonates whose mothers had been given lorazepam PO or IV had a high incidence of low Apgar scores, need for ventilation, hypothermia & poor suckling. Unknown effects on breast-feeding infants but may be of concern.

COMMENT

■ N/A

LOVENOX (ENOXAPARIN)

INDICATIONS

■ Treatment of deep vein thrombosis (DVT) w/ or w/o pulmonary embolism (PE) or thrombopenic disorders during pregnancy

DOSING

■ DVT or PE treatment doses: 1 mg/kg q12h SC
■ DVT prophylaxis dose: 30 mg SC BID

MATERNAL SIDE EFFECTS & IMPACT ON ANESTHESIA

■ Enoxaparin should be stopped at least 24 hours prior to regional anesthesia at treatment doses & at least 12 hours after prophylaxis doses. Monitor for evidence of bleeding or excessive anticoagulation. Use of a shorter-acting anticoagulant (eg, heparin) should be considered as delivery approaches. Hemorrhage can occur at any site & may lead to death of mother &/or fetus. Consider checking factor Xa levels to assess anticoagulation status prior to regional anesthesia in pts taking large doses.

FETAL & NEONATAL EFFECTS

■ Pregnancy Category B (for definition, see the "*Pregnancy Categories*" section). Enoxaparin does not cross the placenta or present a direct risk to the embryo or fetus due to its large molecular weight. There is also no known risk to the nursing infant. There have been post-marketing reports of fetal death when pregnant women received enoxaparin, but causality for these cases has not been determined.

COMMENT

■ Contraindicated in pts w/ major bleeding or thrombocytopenia. Low-molecular-weight heparins cannot be reversed w/ FFP, but possibly w/ protamine.

LYPHOCIN (VANCOMYCIN)

INDICATIONS

■ Active against various (methicillin-resistant) gram-positive bacteria. May be used for vaginal delivery in PCN-allergic women needing endocarditis prophylaxis w/ mitral valve prolapse.

DOSING

■ 20–30 mg/kg/day IV in 2–4 divided doses over 1–2 hours

MATERNAL EFFECTS & IMPACT ON ANESTHESIA

■ Nephrotoxicity has been associated w/ co-administration of vancomycin & an aminoglycoside. May potentiate neuromuscular blockade; the dose of the neuromuscular blocking agent must carefully be titrated to effect. Potential respiratory paralysis & post-op ventilation requirements may occur secondary to prolonged neuromuscular blockade. Rapid administration causes histamine release, w/ redness of the face & neck & potential transient hypotension ("Red Man syndrome").

FETAL SIDE EFFECTS

■ Pregnancy Category B (for definition, see the "*Pregnancy Categories*" section). Likely does not cause renal toxicity & ototoxicity in the fetus, but data are limited.

COMMENT

■ Administer by slow infusion only.

MAALOX (ALUMINUM HYDROXIDE)

INDICATIONS

■ Increases gastric pH > 4 & inhibits proteolytic activity of pepsin, reducing acid indigestion. Antacids initially can be used in mild cases. No effect on frequency of reflux but decreases its acidity.

DOSING
- 5–15 mL/dose PO qd/qid

MATERNAL SIDE EFFECTS & IMPACT ON ANESTHESIA
- Decreases effects of tetracyclines, ranitidine, ketoconazole, benzodiazepines, penicillamine, phenothiazines, digoxin, indomethacin, isoniazid; corticosteroids decrease effects of aluminum in hyperphosphatemia

FETAL & NEONATAL EFFECTS
- Pregnancy Category B (for definition, see the "*Pregnancy Categories*" section). Usually safe but benefits must outweigh risks.

COMMENT
- Use caution in pts w/ recent massive upper GI hemorrhage; renal failure may cause aluminum toxicity; can cause constipation.

MAGNESIUM HYDROXIDE (MILK OF MAGNESIA, ROLAIDS)

INDICATIONS
- Increases gastric pH > 4 & inhibits proteolytic activity of pepsin, reducing acid indigestion. Antacids initially can be used in mild cases. No effect on frequency of reflux but decreases its acidity.

DOSING
- 5–15 mL/dose PO qd/qid

MATERNAL SIDE EFFECTS & IMPACT ON ANESTHESIA
- Decreases effects of tetracyclines, ranitidine, ketoconazole, benzodiazepines, penicillamine, phenothiazines, digoxin, indomethacin, isoniazid; corticosteroids decrease effects of aluminum in hyperphosphatemia

FETAL & NEONATAL EFFECTS
- Pregnancy Category B (for definition, see the "*Pregnancy Categories*" section). Usually safe but benefits must outweigh risks.

COMMENT
- Use caution in pts w/ recent massive upper GI hemorrhage; renal failure may cause aluminum toxicity; can cause constipation.

MAGNESIUM SULFATE

INDICATIONS
- Magnesium sulfate is used to prevent or halt seizures (eclampsia) during pregnancy. It is usually given IV or IM. Treatment to prevent seizures is usually continued for 24 hours after delivery. The action of magnesium in preventing or stopping seizures during pregnancy is unknown. Also used for tocolysis in preterm labor.

DOSING
- 1 g q6h for 4 doses or IV 250 mg/kg over a 4-hour period or 8–12 g magnesium sulfate/24 hours in divided doses

MATERNAL SIDE EFFECTS & IMPACT ON ANESTHESIA
- There is an increase in the effects of neuromuscular blocking agents when given together w/ magnesium. There is a profound prolongation of neuromuscular blockers in conjunction w/ magnesium.

FETAL & NEONATAL EFFECTS
- Pregnancy Category A (for definition, see the "*Pregnancy Categories*" section). Magnesium has not been shown to increase the risk of fetal abnormalities if administered during all trimesters. Affects the CNS of the fetus. If this medication has been given to the mother in large doses & the baby is born before the drug has had time to clear the mother's body, the baby may have temporary problems w/ breathing right after birth. Rare side effects of magnesium sulfate that may affect the fetus include low Apgar scores at birth, low BP & pulmonary edema.

COMMENT
- Do not use magnesium sulfate & nifedipine together because this combination can cause dangerously low BP. Side effects of magnesium include nausea, muscle weakness & loss of reflexes.

MARCAINE (BUPIVACAINE)

INDICATIONS
- Epidural infusion for labor analgesia in low concentrations 0.125–0.04%; spinal injection for labor analgesia or cesarean delivery

DOSING

■ 8–10 mL of 0.25–0.5% provides approx. 2 hours of epidural analgesia. When dilute solutions are used, bupivacaine produces excellent sensory analgesia w/ minimal motor blockade; tachyphylaxis occurs rarely. For labor spinals, 2.5 mg can provide at least 60 minutes of analgesia (adjuncts can be added to prolong effect); for cesarean delivery, spinal bupivacaine 12–15 mg (usually 0.75% bupivacaine w/ dextrose) is adequate (adjuncts can be added to improve effect).

MATERNAL SIDE EFFECTS & IMPACT ON ANESTHESIA

■ High-dose (0.75%) bupivacaine is not recommended for use in epidurals in obstetrics due to the profound maternal & neonatal myocardial depression & difficult resuscitation associated w/ accidental intravascular injection.

FETAL & NEONATAL SIDE EFFECTS

■ Pregnancy Category C (for definition, see the "*Pregnancy Categories*" section). Highly protein-bound, which limits transplacental transfer. Any drug that reaches the fetus undergoes metabolism & excretion. The newborn has the hepatic enzymes necessary for the biotransformation of amide local anesthetics. Elimination half-life is longer in neonates than adults. Bupivacaine is considered safe for breast-feeding.

COMMENT

■ There is no association btwn local anesthetic use & fetal malformations during the first 4 months of pregnancy.

MEPERIDINE (DEMEROL)

INDICATIONS

■ Short-acting analgesic, potent respiratory depressant, cumulative effect w/ large doses over time. Widely used opioid worldwide due to its familiarity & low cost. Often used in combination w/ phenothiazines to diminish nausea & vomiting. Often used parenterally to decrease perioperative shivering.

DOSING

■ Usual dose is 25–50 mg IV or 50–100 mg IM q2–4h, w/ the onset of analgesia within 5 minutes of IV administration & 45 minutes after IM injection. Half-life is 2.5–3 hours in the mother & 18–23 hours in the neonate. A major metabolite is normeperidine, which acts as a potent respiratory depressant in both mother & neonate.

MATERNAL SIDE EFFECTS & IMPACT ON ANESTHESIA
■ Easily crosses the placenta by passive diffusion & equilibrates btwn the maternal & fetal compartments. Maximal fetal uptake occurs within 2–3 hours of maternal administration; therefore, the best time for delivery of the fetus is within 1 hour of last administered dose or >4 hours after the single IV dose.

FETAL & NEONATAL EFFECTS
■ Pregnancy Category B; Category D if used for prolonged periods or in high doses at term (for definitions, see the "*Pregnancy Categories*" section). Readily crosses placenta & may cause neonatal depression. Opioids in general may result in decreased beat-to-beat variability of the fetal heart rate (FHR). Likelihood of neonatal respiratory depression depends on the dose & timing of administration. Meperidine is compatible w/ breast-feeding.

COMMENT
■ Meperidine has structural similarities to that of local anesthetics & has been used as a sole spinal anesthetic for cesarean delivery. Parenteral administration of both a single dose as well as multiple doses was shown to have subtle effects of the neonate. Single dose was thought to account for an alteration of infant breast-feeding behavior; whereas multiple doses, as would be administered during a prolonged labor, were thought to contribute to various neurobehavioral changes: decreased duration of wakefulness, decreased attentiveness & decreased duration of non-REM sleep.

MEPIVACAINE (CARBOCAINE, POLOCAINE)

INDICATIONS
■ Spinal anesthesia for short OB procedures

DOSING
■ Varies depending on procedure, but similar to lidocaine (20% more potent)
■ Spinal: 50 mg for short OB procedures (cerclage, cerclage removal, etc.) Adjuvant: Sodium bicarbonate may be added w/ a 1:10 ratio.

- Metabolism is via hydroxylation & N-demethylation in the liver. Elimination half-life is 2–3 hours.

MATERNAL SIDE EFFECTS & IMPACT ON ANESTHESIA
- Intravascular administration may lead to lightheadedness, seizures, disorientation, heart block, hypotension.

FETAL SIDE EFFECTS
- Pregnancy Category C (for definition, see the "*Pregnancy Categories*" section). Not recommended for epidural use, paracervical or pudendal blocks as the fetus cannot metabolize this drug. Safety in breast-feeding is unknown, but local anesthetics are not expected to accumulate significantly in breast milk.

COMMENTS
- Use preservative-free solutions for intrathecal administration. Use hyperbaric preparations for wider spread of block.

METFORMIN (GLUCOPHAGE)

INDICATIONS
- A biguanide oral anti-hyperglycemic agent, its mode of action is thought to be multifactorial & includes delayed uptake of glucose from the GI tract, increased peripheral glucose utilization mediated by increased insulin sensitivity & inhibition of increased hepatic & renal gluconeogenesis.

DOSING
- Initial dosage 850 mg qd or 500 mg bid

MATERNAL SIDE EFFECTS & IMPACT ON ANESTHESIA
- Use during pregnancy is not advised. There is no information available concerning safety during lactation.

FETAL & NEONATAL EFFECTS
- Pregnancy Category B (for definition, see the "*Pregnancy Categories*" section). Abnormal blood glucose levels during pregnancy have been associated w/ a higher incidence of congenital abnormalities than expected.

COMMENT

- May cause ketoacidosis in children after exercise. Insulin therapy is advocated by most specialists during pregnancy to enable tight blood glucose control.

METHERGINE (METHYLERGONOVINE; ERGOTAMINE)

INDICATIONS

- Ergotamine stimulates smooth muscle, especially that of the uterus, arteries & veins, producing contraction or constriction. Indicated to control bleeding & maintain uterine contraction post-partum & post-abortion.

DOSING

- Post-partum hemorrhage: 0.2 mg unit dose IM. Repeat within 2–4 hours if necessary. May be given IV (0.2 mg) over 10 minutes, but can precipitate severe maternal hypertension.

MATERNAL SIDE EFFECTS & IMPACT ON ANESTHESIA

- Relative contraindications to use include pregnancy, during the 1st & 2nd stages of labor; in severe or persistent sepsis, obstetric pts w/ cardiovascular disease, chronic anemia, toxemia of pregnancy or eclampsia; impaired hepatic, renal or respiratory function.

FETAL & NEONATAL EFFECTS

- Pregnancy Category C (for definition, see the "*Pregnancy Categories*" section). Ergotamine is distributed into breast milk. May cause feto-toxicity by reducing uterine blood flow. It is one of the most commonly prescribed drugs within the 1st week post-partum; no adverse effects have been reported in nursing infants.

COMMENT

- Avoid in pts w/ pre-existing hypertension, pre-eclampsia or other hypertensive disorders. Ergotamines can inhibit lactation.

METHYLERGONOVINE (METHERGINE; ERGOTAMINE)

INDICATIONS

- Ergotamine stimulates smooth muscle, especially that of the uterus, arteries & veins, producing contraction or constriction. Indicated to control bleeding & maintain uterine contraction post-partum & post-abortion.

DOSING
- Post-partum hemorrhage: 0.2 mg unit dose IM. Repeat within 2–4 hours if necessary. May be given IV (0.2 mg) over 10 minutes, but can precipitate severe maternal hypertension.

MATERNAL SIDE EFFECTS & IMPACT ON ANESTHESIA
- Relative contraindications to use include pregnancy, during the 1st & 2nd stages of labor; in severe or persistent sepsis, obstetric pts w/ cardiovascular disease, chronic anemia, toxemia of pregnancy or eclampsia; impaired hepatic, renal or respiratory function.

FETAL & NEONATAL EFFECTS
- Pregnancy Category C (for definition, see the "*Pregnancy Categories*" section). Ergotamine is distributed into breast milk. May cause feto-toxicity by reducing uterine blood flow. It is one of the most commonly prescribed drugs within the 1st week post-partum; no adverse effects have been reported in nursing infants.

COMMENT
- Avoid in pts w/ pre-existing hypertension, pre-eclampsia or other hypertensive disorders. Ergotamines can inhibit lactation.

METOCLOPRAMIDE (REGLAN)

INDICATIONS
- Dopaminergic antagonist that works by increasing lower esophageal sphincter tone & gastric emptying. Stimulates muscular activity, leading to decrease in reflux.

DOSING
- 10–15 mg PO or IV qid

MATERNAL SIDE EFFECTS & IMPACT ON ANESTHESIA
- No adverse effects on mother or fetus have been reported when administered during the 1st trimester. Rare extrapyramidal side effects have been reported.

FETAL & NEONATAL EFFECTS
- Pregnancy Category B (for definition, see the "*Pregnancy Categories*" section). Metoclopramide has not been found to increase the

incidence of abnormalities in infants born to mothers who received the drug at various times up to the 28th week of pregnancy. Compatible w/ breast-feeding.

METOPROLOL (LOPRESSOR, TOPROL XL)

INDICATIONS
■ Beta-1 adrenergic blockade. Commonly used for hypertension, angina pectoris, arrhythmias, myocardial infarction, hypertrophic cardiomyopathy.

DOSING
■ 50–100 mg PO q6–24h, 2.5- to 5-mg IV boluses q2min, prn

MATERNAL SIDE EFFECTS & IMPACT ON ANESTHESIA
■ May cause bradycardia, clinically significant bronchoconstriction (with doses >100 mg/day), dizziness. Increased risk of heart block.

FETAL & NEONATAL EFFECTS
■ Pregnancy Category C (for definition, see the "*Pregnancy Categories*" section). Crosses the placenta. May cause fetal or neonatal bradycardia, neonatal hypoglycemia & delayed spontaneous breathing of the newborn.

COMMENT
■ NA

METRONIDAZOLE (FLAGYL, METRO)

INDICATIONS
■ Active against a variety of anaerobic bacteria, particularly *B. fragilis*

DOSING
■ 500–750 mg IV q8–12h

MATERNAL SIDE EFFECTS & IMPACT ON ANESTHESIA
■ May potentiate the effects of anticoagulants. Can cause disulfiram-like reaction w/ ethanol consumption. Concurrent barbiturates may inhibit the therapeutic effectiveness of metronidazole. May decrease clearance of phenytoin & may increase serum levels of lithium.

FETAL & NEONATAL EFFECTS

- Pregnancy Category B (for definition, see the "*Pregnancy Categories*" section). The use of metronidazole during pregnancy is controversial & should be avoided if possible. Secreted in breast milk. Breast-feeding mothers should discard all breast milk for 24–48 hours to allow excretion of the drug.

COMMENT

- Occasional phlebitis at the IV infusion site

MICONAZOLE

INDICATIONS

- Localized treatment of vulvovaginal candidiasis caused by certain species of *Candida*. Also treats Dermatomycoses (tinea pedis, tinea cruris, tinea corporis).

DOSING

- Varies for cream, powder, suppository & ovule route.

MATERNAL SIDE EFFECTS & IMPACT ON ANESTHESIA

- Azoles inhibit CYP3A4, & marked QTc prolongation may result from interactions w/ drugs metabolized by that system. Increased sedative effect of midazolam may also occur due to inhibition of CYP3A4.

FETAL & NEONATAL EFFECTS

- Pregnancy Category C (for definition, see the "*Pregnancy Categories*" section). Absorbed in trace amounts from the vagina & should be used in the 1st trimester of pregnancy only when considered essential to the pt's welfare. Excretion into breast milk unknown, but problems in humans have not been documented.

COMMENT

- N/A

MICRONASE (GLYBURIDE)

INDICATIONS

- Glyburide stimulates the secretion of insulin by the beta cells of the pancreas. In addition to this pancreatic action, glipizide administration may improve the metabolic utilization of glucose at a peripheral level.

DOSING
- Initial dose: 1.25–5 mg qd

MATERNAL SIDE EFFECTS & IMPACT ON ANESTHESIA
- Do not use in the 1st trimester, as safety in pregnancy has not been established. Do not use in pts w/ ketoacidosis or severe renal, hepatic, adrenal or thyroid dysfunction.

FETAL & NEONATAL EFFECTS
- Pregnancy Category C (for definition, see the "*Pregnancy Categories*" section). Do not use in the 1st trimester, as safety in pregnancy has not been established. The degree to which it affects newborns via transmission in breast milk is unknown.

COMMENT
- Insulin therapy is advocated by most specialists during pregnancy to enable tight blood glucose control.

MIDAZOLAM (VERSED)

INDICATIONS
- Benzodiazepine used for anesthesia induction, sedation, anxiolysis

DOSING
- 1–5 mg IV until desired effect

MATERNAL SIDE EFFECTS & IMPACT ON ANESTHESIA
- Not recommended in high doses (0.2 mg/kg) for induction of general anesthesia since there is a high risk of neonatal respiratory depression requiring intubation

FETAL & NEONATAL EFFECTS
- Pregnancy Category D (for definition, see the "*Pregnancy Categories*" section). The use of midazolam before C-section has a depressant effect on the newborn that is greater than that observed w/ thiopental. Its use is indicated where maternal benefit warrants it. Found in breast milk; use during breast-feeding may be of concern.

COMMENT
- N/A

MILK OF MAGNESIA (MAGNESIUM HYDROXIDE)

INDICATIONS
■ Increases gastric pH > 4 & inhibits proteolytic activity of pepsin, reducing acid indigestion. Antacids initially can be used in mild cases. No effect on frequency of reflux but decreases its acidity.

DOSING
■ 5–15 mL/dose PO qd/qid

MATERNAL SIDE EFFECTS & IMPACT ON ANESTHESIA
■ Decreases effects of tetracyclines, ranitidine, ketoconazole, benzodiazepines, penicillamine, phenothiazines, digoxin, indomethacin, isoniazid; corticosteroids decrease effects of aluminum in hyperphosphatemia

FETAL & NEONATAL EFFECTS
■ Pregnancy Category B (for definition, see the "*Pregnancy Categories*" section). Usually safe but benefits must outweigh risks.

COMMENT
■ Use caution in pts w/ recent massive upper GI hemorrhage; renal failure may cause aluminum toxicity; can cause constipation.

MISOPROSTOL (CYTOTEC)

INDICATIONS
■ A synthetic prostaglandin E1 analog commonly used to prevent gastric ulcers during concomitant NSAID use. Used for cervical ripening for term pregnancies & for pregnancy termination. A 3rd important use is to treat uterine hypotonia.

DOSING
■ For excessive uterine hypotonia: 1 mg PR or PV. Loss of non-term pregnancy may result w/ doses of 200–400 mcg orally.

MATERNAL SIDE EFFECTS & IMPACT ON ANESTHESIA
■ Common side effects include abdominal pain, diarrhea, dyspepsia & nausea.

FETAL & NEONATAL EFFECTS
■ Pregnancy Category X (for definition, see the "*Pregnancy Categories*" section). Abortion (at times incomplete), premature labor or

teratogenicity may occur after administration during pregnancy; congenital anomalies & fetal death have occurred after unsuccessful use as an abortifacient. Use of misoprostol during the 1st trimester has been associated w/ skull defects, cranial nerve palsies, facial malformations & limb defects. The drug should not be used during pregnancy to reduce the risk of NSAID-induced ulcers. It is unknown if misoprostol is excreted in breast milk.

MORPHINE (ASTRAMORPH, DURAMORPH)

INDICATIONS
■ No longer used as primary analgesic for pain in labor in the U.S. because of neonatal respiratory depression. Earliest anesthetic used for treatment of labor pain. Analgesia, intraoperative anesthesia, post-op analgesia.

DOSING
■ Usual dose for maternal analgesia is 2–5 mg IV or 5–10 mg IM. Onset of analgesia is 3–5 minutes after the IV administration & within 20–40 minutes after the IM dose. For post-op analgesia, morphine can be used in PCA or neuraxially (0.1–0.25 mg intrathecally or 2.0–5.0 mg epidurally). Use preservative-free preparation if neuraxial.

MATERNAL SIDE EFFECTS & IMPACT ON ANESTHESIA
■ Infrequently used during labor because of its greater respiratory depression in the neonate than w/ meperidine. As w/ other opiates, has antitussive, constipating, sedating & emetic potential.

FETAL & NEONATAL EFFECTS
■ Pregnancy Category C (for definition, see the "*Pregnancy Categories*" section). Readily crosses placenta & may cause neonatal respiratory depression. Opioids in general may result in decreased beat-to-beat variability of the fetal heart rate (FHR). Likelihood of neonatal respiratory depression depends on the dose & timing of administration.

COMMENT
■ Studies have suggested that that systematically administered morphine does not relieve the visceral pain of labor. Epidural morphine may have diminished efficacy if 3-chloroprocaine has been given epidurally previously.

MOTRIN (IBUPROFEN)

INDICATIONS
- Ibuprofen is a nonsteroidal, anti-inflammatory, antipyretic analgesic agent. It inhibits the synthesis of prostaglandins.

DOSING
- 400 mg/dose PO q4–6h, max 1.2 g/day

MATERNAL SIDE EFFECTS & IMPACT ON ANESTHESIA
- Safe to administer regional anesthesia in women taking ibuprofen

FETAL & NEONATAL EFFECTS
- Pregnancy Category B; Category D in 3rd trimester (for definitions, see the "*Pregnancy Categories*" section). Known effects on fetus during 3rd trimester include constriction of ductus arteriosus prenatally, tricuspid insufficiency & pulmonary hypertension; nonclosure of the ductus arteriosus postnatally; bleeding. Ibuprofen is safe during breast-feeding; amounts are difficult to detect in breast milk after dosages of up to 1.6 g/day PO.

COMMENT
- Use w/ care in pts w/ peptic ulceration or a history of such ulceration, bleeding disorders or cardiovascular disease & pts on oral anticoagulants. Do not use routinely in pts who are allergic to aspirin. Use w/ care in pts w/ asthma, especially those who have developed bronchospasm w/ other nonsteroidal agents.

NALBUPHINE (NUBAIN)

INDICATIONS
- An opioid w/ agonist-antagonist properties, used for the relief of mild to moderate, deep or visceral pain & for chronic pain. However, nalbuphine demonstrates a ceiling effect w/ increasing doses & results in no further respiratory depression w/ doses >30 mg. Can also be used to counteract side effects of pure narcotic agonists.

DOSING
- Usual analgesic dose: 10–20 mg q4–6h IV, SC or IM. Onset of analgesia is within 2–3 minutes of IV dose & within 15 minutes of SC/IM dose. Duration of the effect is 3–6 hours. For reversal of narcotic-induced

side effects (eg, pruritus or emesis from neuraxially administered morphine), 5 mg nalbuphine IV is effective.

MATERNAL SIDE EFFECTS & IMPACT ON ANESTHESIA

■ Effects on breast milk are unknown. May be used as an alternative to Narcan to relieve itching & other effects associated w/ IV, epidural or spinal narcotics (usually give 5 mg IV).

FETAL & NEONATAL EFFECTS

■ Pregnancy Category B; Category D if used for prolonged periods or given in high doses at term (for definitions, see the "*Pregnancy Categories*" section). High degree of placental transfer, resulting in increased incidence of decreased FHR variability compared to meperidine. Respiratory depression in the neonate can occur w/ administration during labor. Fetal & neonatal adverse effects that have been reported when nalbuphine was used during labor include fetal bradycardia, respiratory depression at birth, apnea, cyanosis & hypotonia. Maternal administration of naloxone has reversed these effects in some cases. Severe & prolonged fetal bradycardia has been reported & permanent neurologic damage due to fetal bradycardia has occurred. Nalbuphine is considered safe for breast-feeding.

COMMENT

■ RCTs comparing nalbuphine w/ meperidine found no difference in efficacy of analgesia, but nalbuphine resulted in less nausea & vomiting.

NALOXONE (NARCAN)

INDICATIONS

■ Reversal of opioid side effects, particularly respiratory depression & pruritus. Naloxone hydrochloride is a competitive antagonist at opioid receptors. May be used to reverse neonatal respiratory depression secondary to the administration of opioids to the mother.

DOSING

■ Severe narcotic overdose (coma): 0.4–2.0 mg IV q2–3h prn
■ Respiratory depression: 80–100 mcg IV repeated prn
■ Pruritus: 40–80 mcg IV repeated prn or as a continuous infusion

MATERNAL SIDE EFFECTS & IMPACT ON ANESTHESIA
- Nausea & vomiting, hypertension, cardiac arrhythmias, pulmonary edema, seizures

FETAL & NEONATAL EFFECTS
- Pregnancy Category B (for definition, see the "*Pregnancy Categories*" section). Does cross placenta to reverse fetal bradycardia. There are no embryotoxic or teratogenic effects due to naloxone. It is not known whether naloxone is excreted in human milk.

COMMENT
- Use caution when administering to neonates of mothers previously dependent on opioids; a withdrawal syndrome may be precipitated.

NARCAN (NALOXONE)

INDICATIONS
- Reversal of opioid side effects, particularly respiratory depression & pruritus. Naloxone hydrochloride is a competitive antagonist at opioid receptors. May be used to reverse neonatal respiratory depression secondary to the administration of opioids to the mother.

DOSING
- Severe narcotic overdose (coma): 0.4–2.0 mg IV q2–3h prn
- Respiratory depression: 80–100 mcg IV repeated prn
- Pruritus: 40–80 mcg IV repeated prn or as a continuous infusion

MATERNAL SIDE EFFECTS & IMPACT ON ANESTHESIA
- Nausea & vomiting, hypertension, cardiac arrhythmias, pulmonary edema, seizures

FETAL & NEONATAL EFFECTS
- Pregnancy Category B (for definition, see the "*Pregnancy Categories*" section). Does cross placenta to reverse fetal bradycardia. There are no embryotoxic or teratogenic effects due to naloxone. It is not known whether naloxone is excreted in human milk.

COMMENT
- Use caution when administering to neonates of mothers previously dependent on opioids; a withdrawal syndrome may be precipitated.

NAROPIN (ROPIVACAINE)

INDICATIONS
- Epidural infusion for labor analgesia. Intrathecal injection for procedures lasting <2 hours. When dilute solutions are used, ropivacaine produces excellent sensory anesthesia w/ minimal motor blockade, & tachyphylaxis occurs rarely.

DOSING
- Spinal: 15–20 mg (3 cc of 0.75%) for C-section
- Epidural dosing for C-section: 0.5% up to 30 cc, or 0.75% up to 25 cc
- Epidural dosing for labor infusion: 10–30 mg/hr
- Adjuvant: Sodium bicarbonate may be added w/ a ratio of 0.5 to 20 cc for epidural injection (do not use if there is any precipitation).

MATERNAL SIDE EFFECTS & IMPACT ON ANESTHESIA
- Intravascular administration may result in cardiac arrhythmias & cardiac arrest. Ropivacaine reportedly has a lower incidence of cardiac arrhythmias & cardiac arrest than bupivacaine.

NEONATAL SIDE EFFECTS
- Minimal. Very safe. Any drug that reaches the fetus undergoes metabolism & excretion. The newborn has the hepatic enzymes necessary for the biotransformation of amide local anesthetics. Elimination half-life is longer in neonates than in adults. Can be safely used in breast-feeding.

COMMENT
- Intrathecal use of ropivacaine is not approved by the FDA. Ropivacaine is commercially available preservative-free. Boluses should be limited 3–5 cc at a time, so as to detect intravascular or intrathecal administration.

NEOSTIGMINE

INDICATIONS
- Reversal of muscle relaxants, myasthenia gravis

DOSING
- 0.03–0.06 mg/kg (up to 5 mg) for muscle relaxant reversal
- 0.5–2 mg IV & repeat as needed for myasthenia gravis

MATERNAL SIDE EFFECTS & IMPACT ON ANESTHESIA
- Increases ACh, causing both muscarinic & nicotinic side effects such as salivation, bradycardia, tearing, miosis & bronchoconstriction. Reversal should not be attempted unless at least 1 response to train-of-four stimulation is present. Attempts to reverse a deep or resistant block w/ a large dose of neostigmine may increase the phase I block residual weakness.

FETAL & NEONATAL EFFECTS
- Pregnancy category C (for definition, see the "*Pregnancy Categories*" section). Transient muscle weakness occurs in 20% of infants born to mothers treated w/ anticholinesterases in pregnancy. May cause uterine irritability & induce preterm labor. Because it is ionized at physiologic pH, neostigmine does not pass significantly into breast milk.

COMMENT
- Magnesium for pre-eclamptic therapy may antagonize the effects of neostigmine.

NEO-SYNEPHRINE (PHENYLEPHRINE)

INDICATIONS
- Hypotension, Post postsynaptic alpha-receptor agonist w/little effect on beta receptors of the heart

DOSING
- IV bolus 40–100 mcg/dose, or 10 mcg/min initially, then titrated to response

MATERNAL SIDE EFFECTS & IMPACT ON ANESTHESIA
- May cause hypertension, reflex bradycardia. The pressor effect is potentiated w/ the concurrent use of oxytocic drugs. Phenylephrine effects can be potentiated by bretylium, guanethidine, halogenated vapor anesthetics, MAO inhibitors.

FETAL & NEONATAL EFFECTS
- Pregnancy Category C (for definition, see the "*Pregnancy Categories*" section). Studies of healthy parturients undergoing C-section w/ regional anesthesia showed no adverse effects compared w/ ephedrine. The degree to which it passes into breast milk is unknown.

COMMENT
■ Potent postsynaptic alpha-receptor agonist w/ little effect on beta receptors of the heart

---

NESACAINE (3% 2-CHLOROPROCAINE)

INDICATIONS
■ Used widely via epidural (in bolus form) for C-section

DOSING
■ 20–30 cc (pH adjusted) given in 4 or 5 divided doses for a final dermatome level of T4–T5 bilaterally for C-section. 10 cc via epidural (T10 level) may be used to provide analgesia for instrument delivery or tubal ligation.

MATERNAL SIDE EFFECTS & IMPACT ON ANESTHESIA
■ Even when injected IV, there are rare adverse effects. Metabolized by pseudocholinesterases, which are decreased in pregnancy.

FETAL & NEONATAL SIDE EFFECTS
■ Pregnancy Category C (for definition, see the "*Pregnancy Categories*" section). Minimal effects. Drug that reaches the fetus undergoes metabolism & excretion. Elimination half-life is longer in neonates than adults. Not expected to accumulate significantly in breast milk.

COMMENT
■ Always use bisulfite-free & EDTA-free preparations for regional anesthesia procedures. It is the local anesthetic of choice for epidural anesthesia in the setting of fetal acidosis.

NEURONTIN (GABAPENTIN)

INDICATIONS
■ Anticonvulsant. Used as an antiepileptic & in the treatment of neuropathic pain & postherpetic neuralgia. Gabapentin is structurally related to the neurotransmitter GABA (gamma-aminobutyric acid).

DOSING
■ 900–1,800 mg/day PO

MATERNAL SIDE EFFECTS & IMPACT ON ANESTHESIA
- Safety & efficacy have not been established in children, pregnancy & lactation.

FETAL & NEONATAL EFFECTS
- Pregnancy Category C (for definition, see the "*Pregnancy Categories*" section). It is not known if gabapentin is excreted in human breast milk; its low molecular weight suggests transfer does occur. No other data available.

COMMENT
- The most frequent clinical adverse events occurring in all clinical studies were somnolence, dizziness, ataxia, headache, nystagmus, tremor, fatigue, diplopia, nausea and/or vomiting, rhinitis.

NIMBEX (CIS-ATRACURIUM)

INDICATIONS
- Non-depolarizing neuromuscular blocking drug (NMBD) used to facilitate intubation & maintain neuromuscular blockade

DOSING
- 0.2 mg/kg IV (onset 2–8 min)

MATERNAL SIDE EFFECTS & IMPACT ON ANESTHESIA
- Action may be prolonged in pts receiving IV magnesium.

FETAL & NEONATAL EFFECTS
- Pregnancy Category B (for definition, see the "*Pregnancy Categories*" section). No adverse effects w/ intubating dose.

COMMENT
- Presumed safe in pregnant pts. Long onset of action makes it less desirable for rapid sequence induction.

NITRO-BID (NITROGLYCERIN)

INDICATIONS
- Nitroglycerin can be used for transient uterine relaxation during removal of retained placental tissue. It is also used in angina.

DOSING

■ Start w/ 40-mcg (0.04 mg) boluses until desired effect is achieved. Careful & continuous hemodynamic monitoring is necessary.

MATERNAL SIDE EFFECTS & IMPACT ON ANESTHESIA

■ Documented headache, hypersensitivity, severe anemia, shock, postural hypotension, head trauma, closed-angle glaucoma, cerebral hemorrhage

FETAL & NEONATAL EFFECTS

■ Pregnancy Category C (for definition, see the "*Pregnancy Categories*" section).

COMMENT

■ Exercise caution w/ coronary artery disease & low systolic BP.

NITROGLYCERIN IV (TRIDIL, NITRO-BID)

INDICATIONS

■ Nitroglycerin can be used for transient uterine relaxation during removal of retained placental tissue. It is also used in angina.

DOSING

■ Start w/ 40-mcg (0.04 mg) boluses until desired effect is achieved. Careful & continuous hemodynamic monitoring is necessary.

MATERNAL SIDE EFFECTS & IMPACT ON ANESTHESIA

■ Documented headache, hypersensitivity, severe anemia, shock, postural hypotension, head trauma, closed-angle glaucoma, cerebral hemorrhage

FETAL & NEONATAL EFFECTS

■ Pregnancy Category C (for definition, see the "*Pregnancy Categories*" section).

COMMENT

■ Exercise caution w/ coronary artery disease & low systolic BP.

NITROPRESS (SODIUM NITROPRUSSIDE)

INDICATIONS
- Direct NO donor. Used for hypertension, controlled hypotension, congestive heart failure.

DOSING
- Start w/ 0.1 mcg/kg/min, then titrate to patient response to maximum 10 mcg/kg/min.

MATERNAL SIDE EFFECTS & IMPACT ON ANESTHESIA
- May cause excessive hypotension, reflex tachycardia, tachyphylaxis. Accumulation of cyanide w/ liver dysfunction leading to cyanide toxicity, thiocyanate w/ kidney dysfunction resulting in thiocyanate toxicity. Also impairs hypoxic pulmonary vasoconstriction, leading to hypoxia.

FETAL & NEONATAL EFFECTS
- Pregnancy Category C (for definition, see the "*Pregnancy Categories*" section). Fetal cyanide toxicity of nitroprusside has been described in animal models. It is not known if nitroprusside or its metabolites are excreted in significant amounts in breast milk.

COMMENT
- Thiocyanate toxicity may become life-threatening at serum concentration of 200 mg/L. Nitroprusside infusion >2 mcg/kg/min generates cyanide ion faster than the body can normally eliminate it. The capacity of methemoglobin to buffer cyanide is exhausted after approximately 500 mcg/kg nitroprusside. Concurrent administration of sodium thiosulfate may reduce the risk of cyanide toxicity by increasing the rate of cyanide conversion.

NITROUS OXIDE

INDICATIONS
- CNS depressant that causes surgical sedation & analgesia; adjunct for maintenance of general anesthesia; reduces MAC of other inhalational agents at high concentrations (>70%)

DOSING

- MAC decreases in pregnancy 30–40%. A common practice is to give 30% nitrous oxide & 0.5 MAC of an inhalational anesthetic for urgent C-section. Following delivery of the neonate, nitrous oxide concentrations may be increased & the inhalational agent may be reduced or discontinued to avoid uterine hypotonia. Low concentrations (25–50%) are used in the parturient to avoid hypoxemia. Rapid onset & recovery w/ low blood/gas partition coefficient.

MATERNAL SIDE EFFECTS & IMPACT ON ANESTHESIA

- PONV common; hypoxia, bone marrow suppression & neuropathy in immunologically or nutritionally compromised patients. Minimal changes in BP & cardiac output. Controversial: Some studies indicate it may increase ICP/CBF as well as CRMO2.

FETAL & NEONATAL EFFECTS

- Pregnancy Category NR (for definition, see the "*Pregnancy Categories*" section). Fetal/maternal ratio of 0.3 within 3 minutes. Prolonged delivery times may result in neonatal depression. Supplemental oxygen is recommended for neonates who have been exposed prior to delivery. Some studies suggest teratogenicity in humans, possibly due to its inhibition of hepatic methionine synthase activity & thus vitamin B12/folate deficiencies (however, this requires prolonged exposure, >2 hours). There are many reports of short-term use of nitrous oxide in the 2nd & 3rd trimesters w/o adverse effect.

COMMENT

- Can decrease fertility of female personnel exposed to unscavenged gas. Personnel exposed also have an increased risk of renal & hepatic disease & peripheral neuropathy. When used as the sole anesthetic agent for general anesthesia, awareness results in 12–26% of cases.

NO-DOZ (CAFFEINE)

INDICATIONS

- A CNS vasoconstrictor, useful for mild post-dural puncture headaches. One of the most popular drugs in the world!

DOSING

- 300–500 mg PO/IV q12–24h

MATERNAL SIDE EFFECTS & IMPACT ON ANESTHESIA
■ Causes tachycardia & nervousness. Avoid in pts w/ preexisting arrhythmias.

FETAL & NEONATAL EFFECTS
■ Pregnancy Category C (for definition, see the "*Pregnancy Categories*" section). Caffeine crosses the placenta. Caffeine intake >300 mg/day is not recommended. Considered compatible w/ breast-feeding within recommended dosing guidelines.

COMMENT
■ A cup of coffee contains about 40–100 mg of caffeine; soft drinks contain 10–55 mg.

NORCURON (VECURONIUM)

INDICATIONS
■ Nondepolarizing neuromuscular blocking drug (NMBD) used to facilitate intubation & maintain neuromuscular blockade

DOSING
■ 0.2 mg/kg IV (onset 175 sec)

MATERNAL SIDE EFFECTS & IMPACT ON ANESTHESIA
■ Action may be prolonged in pts w/ renal insufficiency & IV magnesium.

FETAL & NEONATAL EFFECTS
■ Pregnancy Category C (for definition, see the "*Pregnancy Categories*" section). No adverse effects w/ intubating dose.

COMMENT
■ Avoid in pts w/ liver disease. Long onset to action makes it less desirable for rapid sequence intubation.

NOREPINEPHRINE (LEVOPHED)

INDICATIONS
■ Alpha & beta adrenergic agonist. Alpha activity is dominant. Used for hypotension.

DOSING
- Start w/ 1–8 mcg/min & titrate to desired effects.

MATERNAL SIDE EFFECTS & IMPACT ON ANESTHESIA
- May cause hypertension, arrhythmia, myocardia ischemia, increased uterine contractility, frequency of contractions, CNS stimulation. Halogenated vapor anesthetics may sensitize the myocardium to the effects of catecholamines. When given in combination w/ oxytocic agents, may cause severe hypertension.

FETAL & NEONATAL EFFECTS
- Pregnancy category C (for definition, see the "*Pregnancy Categories*" section). It is unknown if norepinephrine causes fetal harm or the degree to which it is excreted in breast milk.

COMMENT
- N/A

NORMODYNE (LABETALOL)

INDICATIONS
- Hypertension

DOSING
- A wide therapeutic range. Titrate to effect. 5–10 mg IV, over 2 minutes. May repeat up to 200 mg total. For oral dosing, 100–400 mg PO BID.

MATERNAL SIDE EFFECTS & IMPACT ON ANESTHESIA
- May cause bradycardia, bronchospasm in asthmatics, postural hypotension, dizziness. Not thought to affect the usual course of labor & delivery when given to pregnant hypertensive pts.

FETAL & NEONATAL EFFECTS
- Pregnancy Category C (for definition, see the "*Pregnancy Categories*" section). Crosses the placenta & may cause fetal bradycardia, hypoglycemia, respiratory depression, hypotension. Considered compatible w/ breast-feeding.

COMMENT
- Has an alpha to beta blockade action of 1:7

NORPRAMIN (DESIPRAMINE)

INDICATIONS
- Tricyclic antidepressants (TCAs) are effective for the treatment of major depressive disorders; also sometimes prescribed for chronic pain or polyneuropathy.

DOSING
- For depression, 100–200 mg/day in single or divided doses, up to max 300 mg/day

MATERNAL SIDE EFFECTS & IMPACT ON ANESTHESIA
- Common side effects include anticholinergic symptoms (drying of secretions, dilated pupils, sedation). Concomitant use of TCAs & amphetamines has been reported to result in enhanced amphetamine effects from the release of norepinephrine. Ephedrine should be given cautiously to patients on TCAs.

FETAL & NEONATAL EFFECTS
- Pregnancy Category NR (for definition, see the "*Pregnancy Categories*" section). Breast-feeding effects are unknown; only very minute amounts are found in the infant's serum.

COMMENT
- Do not use w/ MAO inhibitors.

NORVASC (AMLODIPINE)

INDICATIONS
- Amlodipine is a calcium channel blocker used to treat chronic hypertension.

DOSING
- 5–10 mg PO qd

MATERNAL SIDE EFFECTS & IMPACT ON ANESTHESIA
- Common side effects include dizziness, fatigue, flushing, headache & palpitations.

FETAL & NEONATAL EFFECTS
- Pregnancy Category C (for definition, see the "*Pregnancy Categories*" section). Unknown effects on breast-feeding infants.

COMMENT
- Avoid in pts w/ aortic stenosis, CHF, angina & liver impairment.

NOVOCAINE (PROCAINE)

INDICATIONS
- Low potency, lower toxicity, short-acting local anesthetic w/ rapid onset (3–5 min), used for infiltration, nerve block & spinal anesthesia. Frequently used in dentistry & for intractable pain associated w/ malignancy or neuralgia. Poor topical effect.

DOSING
- Infiltration: 350–600 mg single total dose
- Peripheral nerve block: total dose should not exceed 1 g.
- Spinal anesthesia: 50–75 mg for perineal surgery, 100–125 mg for lower abdomen, 200 mg for anesthesia to costal margin
- Anesthetic doses are reduced by 30% in parturients.

MATERNAL SIDE EFFECTS & IMPACT ON ANESTHESIA
- Toxicity profile similar to other local anesthetics. Metabolite para-aminobenzoic acid causes allergic reactions. Preservative sodium bisulfite also causes severe allergic reactions & anaphylaxis in those sensitive to it.

FETAL & NEONATAL EFFECTS
- Pregnancy Category C (for definition, see the "*Pregnancy Categories*" section). Not expected to accumulate significantly in breast milk.

COMMENT
- Epinephrine 1:200,000 or 1:100,000 can be added for vasoconstriction, which prolongs action from 45 to 60 minutes.

NOVOLIN (INSULIN)

INDICATIONS
- Drug of choice for all types of diabetes mellitus during pregnancy. Stimulates proper utilization of glucose by cells & reduces blood glucose levels. Therapy is largely empiric, w/ multiple choices available to achieve glycemic control.

DOSING

- 0.5–1 U/kg/d SC in divided doses. Base dose on IBW; titrate dose to maintain a pre-meal & bedtime glucose level of 80–110 mg/dL. Combine short-acting & longer-acting insulins to maintain blood glucose within target.

MATERNAL SIDE EFFECTS & IMPACT ON ANESTHESIA

- Calcium channel blockers may inhibit pancreatic insulin release & block free fatty acid uptake & utilization by the myocardium, which is needed for myocardial work & contractility. High-dose insulin may change myocardial energy consumption from free fatty acids to carbohydrates. Does not cross the placenta but may cause hypoglycemia in mother, which can result in hypoglycemia in newborn.

FETAL & NEONATAL EFFECTS

- Pregnancy Category B (for definition, see the "*Pregnancy Categories*" section). Insulin does not cross the placenta but may cause maternal hypoglycemia, which can result in hypoglycemia in newborn.

COMMENT

- Monitor glucose levels in both newborn & mother post-delivery.

NPH (INSULIN)

INDICATIONS

- Drug of choice for all types of diabetes mellitus during pregnancy. Stimulates proper utilization of glucose by cells & reduces blood glucose levels. Therapy is largely empiric, w/ multiple choices available to achieve glycemic control.

DOSING

- 0.5–1 U/kg/d SC in divided doses. Base dose on IBW; titrate dose to maintain a pre-meal & bedtime glucose level of 80–110 mg/dL. Combine short-acting & longer-acting insulins to maintain blood glucose within target.

MATERNAL SIDE EFFECTS & IMPACT ON ANESTHESIA

- Calcium channel blockers may inhibit pancreatic insulin release & block free fatty acid uptake & utilization by the myocardium, which is needed for myocardial work & contractility. High-dose insulin may change myocardial energy consumption from free fatty acids to carbohydrates. Does not cross the placenta but may cause hypoglycemia in mother, which can result in hypoglycemia in newborn.

FETAL & NEONATAL EFFECTS

■ Pregnancy Category B (for definition, see the "*Pregnancy Categories*" section). Insulin does not cross the placenta but may cause maternal hypoglycemia, which can result in hypoglycemia in newborn.

COMMENT

■ Monitor glucose levels in both newborn & mother post-delivery.

NUBAIN (NALBUPHINE)

INDICATIONS

■ An opioid w/ agonist-antagonist properties, used for the relief of mild to moderate, deep or visceral pain & for chronic pain. However, nalbuphine demonstrates a ceiling effect w/ increasing doses & results in no further respiratory depression w/ doses >30 mg. Can also be used to counteract side effects of pure narcotic agonists.

DOSING

■ Usual analgesic dose: 10–20 mg q4–6h IV, SC or IM. Onset of analgesia is within 2–3 minutes of IV dose & within 15 minutes of SC/IM dose. Duration of the effect is 3–6 hours. For reversal of narcotic-induced side effects (eg, pruritus or emesis from neuraxially administered morphine), 5 mg nalbuphine IV is effective.

MATERNAL SIDE EFFECTS & IMPACT ON ANESTHESIA

■ Effects on breast milk are unknown. May be used as an alternative to Narcan to relieve itching & other effects associated w/ IV, epidural or spinal narcotics (usually give 5 mg IV).

FETAL & NEONATAL EFFECTS

■ Pregnancy Category B; Category D if used for prolonged periods or given in high doses at term (for definitions, see the "*Pregnancy Categories*" section). High degree of placental transfer, resulting in increased incidence of decreased FHR variability compared to meperidine. Respiratory depression in the neonate can occur w/ administration during labor. Fetal & neonatal adverse effects that have been reported when nalbuphine was used during labor include fetal bradycardia, respiratory depression at birth, apnea, cyanosis & hypotonia. Maternal administration of naloxone has reversed these effects in some cases. Severe & prolonged fetal bradycardia has been reported & permanent neurologic damage due to fetal bradycardia has occurred. Nalbuphine is considered safe for breast-feeding.

COMMENT
- RCTs comparing nalbuphine w/ meperidine found no difference in efficacy of analgesia, but nalbuphine resulted in less nausea & vomiting.

NYSTATIN

INDICATIONS
- Acne vulgaris & various Candida infections (keratitis, oral, vaginal, pneumonia, skin infections)

DOSING
- Varies for cream, powder, vaginal or systemic route

MATERNAL SIDE EFFECTS & IMPACT ON ANESTHESIA
- An increased sedative effect of midazolam may be noted, because azoles inhibit CYP3A4. Marked QTc prolongation may also result from interactions w/ drugs metabolized by CYP3A4.

FETAL & NEONATAL EFFECTS
- Pregnancy Category A (for definition, see the "*Pregnancy Categories*" section)

COMMENT
N/A

OMEPRAZOLE (PRILOSEC)

INDICATIONS
- Decreases gastric acid secretion by inhibiting the parietal cell H^+/K^+ ATPase pump. Used for short-term & long-term treatment (4–8 wks to 12 months) of GERD.

DOSING
- GERD: 20 mg PO qd

MATERNAL SIDE EFFECTS & IMPACT ON ANESTHESIA
- May decrease effects of itraconazole & ketoconazole; may increase toxicity of warfarin, digoxin, phenytoin

FETAL & NEONATAL EFFECTS
- Pregnancy Category C (for definition, see the "*Pregnancy Categories*" section). Safety during pregnancy has not been established. The extent to which it passes into the breast milk &/or affects newborns is unknown.

COMMENT
- Bioavailability may increase in elderly pts. Adverse effects include headache, rash, diarrhea, hypergastrinemia, polyps.

ONDANSETRON (ZOFRAN)

INDICATIONS
- Selective 5-HT3-receptor antagonist that blocks serotonin both peripherally & centrally, used in the prevention of nausea & vomiting. Metabolized in the liver via the P-450 mechanism.

DOSING
- 2–4 mg IV q6–8h

MATERNAL SIDE EFFECTS & IMPACT ON ANESTHESIA
- Safely used in the treatment of hyperemesis gravidarum. Very rare extrapyramidal side effects.

FETAL & NEONATAL EFFECTS
- Pregnancy Category B (for definition, see the "*Pregnancy Categories*" section)

COMMENT
- Best used for prevention & prophylaxis of nausea & vomiting. Off-label use for peri-operative pruritus: 8 mg IVP.

OXYCODONE/ACETAMINOPHEN (PERCOCET, ROXICET, ENDOCET, TYLOX)

INDICATIONS
- Pain, moderate & severe

DOSING

■ Contains 5 mg oxycodone & 325 mg acetaminophen. Usually, 1 tab or 1 teaspoon PO q6h as needed. Immediately post-op, as much as 1 or 2 tabs q4h prn. Total daily dosage of acetaminophen/oxycodone should not exceed 4,000 mg/60 mg.

MATERNAL SIDE EFFECTS & IMPACT ON ANESTHESIA

■ Effects of Percocet on pregnancy have not been assessed. Use w/ precaution in labor & delivery or w/ concomitant use of other CNS depressants. May need dosing adjustment in pts w/ liver disease.

FETAL & NEONATAL EFFECTS

■ Pregnancy Category NR (for definition, see the "*Pregnancy Categories*" section). Safety of Percocet in breast-feeding is unclear; however, it is used commonly as a post-cesarean analgesic at a time when there is not much milk production yet.

COMMENT

■ Adverse effects of Percocet include respiratory depression, constipation, nausea & vomiting, dizziness, dysphoria, lightheadedness, sedation, skin rash, pruritus.

OXYTOCIN (PITOCIN, SYNTOCINON)

INDICATIONS

■ Oxytocin is a hormone used to help start or continue labor & to control bleeding after delivery. It is also sometimes used to help milk secretion in breast-feeding.

DOSING

■ IV infusion (drip method) for post-partum bleeding: 10–40 units of oxytocin may be added to 1,000 mL of a non-hydrating diluent & run at a rate necessary to control uterine atony

■ IM: 1 mL (10 units) of oxytocin can be given after delivery of the placenta.

MATERNAL SIDE EFFECTS & IMPACT ON ANESTHESIA

■ Before delivery, the fetal heart, resting uterine tone & the frequency, duration & force of contractions should be monitored. Oxytocin should be discontinued immediately in the event of uterine hyperactivity or fetal distress. During C-section, oxytocin may be given following cord clamping to encourage separation of the placenta from the uterus. Uterine hypotonia may be treated w/ 2 units IVP. Cardiovascular collapse & death have been reported in hypovolemic women given 10 units IVP of oxytocin for uterine bleeding undergoing C-section. A rare complication is severe water intoxication.

FETAL & NEONATAL EFFECTS
■ Pregnancy Category C (for definition, see the "*Pregnancy Categories*" section). The risk of neonatal jaundice may be 1.6× that of neonates whose mothers did not receive oxytocin-induced labors. Other poor outcomes may be associated w/ uterine hyperstimulation. No known complications from Pitocin via breast milk after normal doses.

COMMENT
■ Rapid bolus may cause hypotension, tachycardia, myocardial arrhythmias, coronary vasospasm, cardiac arrest, headache & confusion.

PACERONE (AMIODARONE)

INDICATIONS
■ Refractory or recurrent ventricular tachycardia or ventricular fibrillation, supraventricular arrhythmias

DOSING
■ PO load 800–1,600 mg/day for 1–3 weeks, then 600–800 mg/day for 4 weeks, maintenance 100–400 mg/day, IV load 150–300 mg over 10 minutes, 360 mg over next 6 hours (1 mg/min), then 540 mg next 18 hours (0.5 mg/min). With liver disease, dosage adjustment may be required, but specific guidelines are unavailable.

MATERNAL SIDE EFFECTS & IMPACT ON ANESTHESIA
■ Depresses SA node; prolongs PR, QRS, QT intervals; produces alpha & beta adrenergic blockade. May cause severe sinus bradycardia, ventricular arrhythmias, hepatitis & cirrhosis. Pulmonary fibrosis reported from acute & long-term use. Thyroid abnormality. Can increase serum levels of digoxin, oral anticoagulants, diltiazem, quinidine, procainamide & phenytoin.

FETAL & NEONATAL EFFECTS
■ Pregnancy Category D (for definition, see the "*Pregnancy Categories*" section). Several case reports of side effects, including neonatal hypothyroidism.

COMMENT
N/A

PAROXETINE (PAXIL)

INDICATIONS
- SSRI typically used to treat depression, anxiety, obsessive-compulsive disorder, bulimia, panic disorder, posttraumatic stress disorder

DOSING
- Depression: 20 mg/day PO, may increase gradually to 50 mg/day PO
- Obsessive-compulsive disorder: 20 mg/day PO, up to 60 mg/day PO
- Anxiety disorder: 20 mg/day PO
- Panic disorder: 10–75 mg/day PO
- Dosages may be decreased in cases of renal or hepatic insufficiency.

MATERNAL SIDE EFFECTS & IMPACT ON ANESTHESIA
- Anorexia, diarrhea or constipation, anxiety, abnormal bleeding (particularly when used w/ other drugs that can affect platelet function), hyponatremia, seizures

FETAL & NEONATAL EFFECTS
- Pregnancy Category C (for definition, see the "*Pregnancy Categories*" section). An increased risk for CNS serotonergic symptoms was observed during the first 4 days of life in infants of mothers taking SSRIs during the 3rd trimester of pregnancy. Infants exposed prenatally to fluoxetine or a tricyclic antidepressant did NOT show differences in IQ, language or behavioral development compared to children w/o prenatal exposure to these drugs. SSRIs have unknown effects that may be of concern during breast-feeding.

COMMENT
- Sometimes used for compulsive gambling. Do not use w/ MAO inhibitors.

PAXIL (PAROXETINE)

INDICATIONS
- SSRI typically used to treat depression, anxiety, obsessive-compulsive disorder, bulimia, panic disorder, posttraumatic stress disorder

DOSING

- Depression: 20 mg/day PO, may increase gradually to 50 mg/day PO
- Obsessive-compulsive disorder: 20 mg/day PO, up to 60 mg/day PO
- Anxiety disorder: 20 mg/day PO
- Panic disorder: 10–75 mg/day PO Dosages may be decreased in cases of renal or hepatic insufficiency.

MATERNAL SIDE EFFECTS & IMPACT ON ANESTHESIA

- Anorexia, diarrhea or constipation, anxiety, abnormal bleeding (particularly when used w/ other drugs that can affect platelet function), hyponatremia, seizures

FETAL & NEONATAL EFFECTS

- Pregnancy Category C (for definition, see the "*Pregnancy Categories*" section). An increased risk for CNS serotonergic symptoms was observed during the first 4 days of life in infants of mothers taking SSRIs during the 3rd trimester of pregnancy. Infants exposed prenatally to fluoxetine or a tricyclic antidepressant did NOT show differences in IQ, language or behavioral development compared to children w/o prenatal exposure to these drugs. SSRIs have unknown effects that may be of concern during breast-feeding.

COMMENT

- Sometimes used for compulsive gambling. Do not use w/ MAO inhibitors.

PENICILLIN G

INDICATIONS

- Active against a wide range of gram-positive & gram-negative bacteria. First-line for the treatment & prevention of neonatal group B streptococcal infection.

DOSING

- 0.6–4.8 million units/day IM or IV in divided doses

MATERNAL SIDE EFFECTS & IMPACT ON ANESTHESIA

- May interact w/ anticoagulants, including heparin, & may increase risk of bleeding. Pen G contains procaine & may cause allergic reactions in pts sensitive to the local anesthetic.

FETAL & NEONATAL EFFECTS
- Pregnancy Category B (for definition, see the "*Pregnancy Categories*" section). Crosses placenta rapidly. Can cause diarrhea, candidiasis or allergic reaction in the infant.

COMMENT
- Penicillin G Procaine is for IM administration only. Penicillin VK is very painful on rapid infusion. The pain can be attenuated w/ 3–5 cc of 1% lidocaine placed into the antibiotic solution.

PENTOTHAL (THIOPENTAL SODIUM)

INDICATIONS
- Barbiturate induction agent that rapidly produces unconsciousness (onset approx. 30–45 sec) followed by rapid reawakening due to redistribution

DOSING
- 3–5 mg/kg IV

MATERNAL SIDE EFFECTS & IMPACT ON ANESTHESIA
- Rapid induction & redistribution, typically w/ minimal effect on fetus. Hemodynamic effects not as pronounced as propofol.

FETAL & NEONATAL EFFECTS
- Pregnancy Category C (for definition, see the "*Pregnancy Categories*" section). Minimal effects if dose <4 mg/kg, due to rapid maternal redistribution & clearing by fetal liver. (See "*Propofol*" for comparison.) Fetal/maternal ratio 0.4–1.1. Considered safe for breastfeeding.

COMMENT
- Absolutely contraindicated in certain porphyrias (acute intermittent porphyria, variant porphyria, hereditary co-porphyria). When learning about these drugs in obstetrics, it is important to be familiar w/ the approximate fetal:maternal (F/M) ratios of drug concentrations at the time of delivery of the infant. Generally, the umbilical vein blood concentrations represent the fetal blood concentrations. An early high ratio indicates rapid placental transfer of the drug.

PEPCID (FAMOTIDINE)

INDICATIONS
- Competitively inhibits histamine at the H2 receptor of gastric parietal cells, resulting in reduced gastric acid secretion, gastric volume & hydrogen ion concentrations

DOSING
- 10 mg PO bid

MATERNAL SIDE EFFECTS & IMPACT ON ANESTHESIA
- May decrease effects of ketoconazole & itraconazole; levels may increase w/ hydrochlorothiazide; fluconazole levels may decrease w/ long-term co-administration of rifampin; may increase concentrations of theophylline, phenytoin, tolbutamide, cyclosporine, glyburide, glipizide; effects of anticoagulants may increase w/ fluconazole co-administration

FETAL & NEONATAL EFFECTS
- Pregnancy Category B (for definition, see the "*Pregnancy Categories*" section). The degree to which it passes into breast milk & affects the newborn is unknown.

COMMENT
- N/A

PERCOCET (OXYCODONE/ACETAMINOPHEN)

INDICATIONS
- Pain, moderate & severe

DOSING
- Contains 5 mg oxycodone & 325 mg acetaminophen. Usually, 1 tab or 1 teaspoon PO q6h as needed. Immediately post-op, as much as 1 or 2 tabs q4h prn. Total daily dosage of acetaminophen/oxycodone should not exceed 4,000 mg/60 mg.

MATERNAL SIDE EFFECTS & IMPACT ON ANESTHESIA
- Effects of Percocet on pregnancy have not been assessed. Use w/ precaution in labor & delivery or w/ concomitant use of other CNS depressants. May need dosing adjustment in pts w/ liver disease.

FETAL & NEONATAL EFFECTS

■ Pregnancy Category NR (for definition, see the *"Pregnancy Categories"* section). Safety of Percocet in breast-feeding is unclear; however, it is used commonly as a post-cesarean analgesic at a time when there is not much milk production yet.

COMMENT

■ Adverse effects of Percocet include respiratory depression, constipation, nausea & vomiting, dizziness, dysphoria, lightheadedness, sedation, skin rash, pruritus.

PHENERGAN (PROMETHAZINE)

INDICATIONS

■ Symptomatic treatment of nausea in vestibular dysfunction. Antidopaminergic agent effective in treating emesis. Blocks postsynaptic mesolimbic dopaminergic receptors in brain & reduces stimuli to brain stem reticular system. Often used in combination w/ opioids to reduce nausea & vomiting & produce sedation; may potentiate the analgesic effects of the opioids.

DOSING

■ PO: 12.5–25 mg q4–6h prn (syr or tab)
■ PR: 12.5–25 mg q4–6h prn
■ IV/IM: 12.5–25 mg q4–6h; use caution w/ IV administration, concentration not to exceed 25 mg/mL, rate not to exceed 25 mg/min. IV dose of 25–50 mg rapidly produces effective sedation.
■ Do not administer SC or intra-arterially.

MATERNAL SIDE EFFECTS & IMPACT ON ANESTHESIA

■ May have additive effects when used concurrently w/ other CNS depressants or anticonvulsants; co-administration w/ epinephrine may cause hypotension

FETAL & NEONATAL EFFECTS

■ Pregnancy Category C (for definition, see the *"Pregnancy Categories"* section). Rapidly crosses the placenta & may result in decreased beat-to-beat variability. Does not result in neonatal respiratory depression. Safety in breast-feeding is unknown.

COMMENT
- Use w/ caution in pts w/ cardiovascular disease, impaired liver function, seizures, sleep apnea, asthma. Moderate respiratory stimulant resulting in an increase in minute ventilation & ventilatory response to CO_2, thus counteracting the respiratory depressant qualities of narcotics.

PHENOBARBITAL SODIUM

INDICATIONS
- Seizure, anxiety, insomnia. Treatment of alcohol withdrawal seizure, hyperbilirubinemia, narcotic withdrawal symptoms.

DOSING
- Loading dose: 200–600 mg IV at rate of <60 mg/minute up to total dose of 20 mg/kg
- Maintenance dose: 100–300 mg/day PO
- Pediatric dose: 3–5 mg/kg/day PO

MATERNAL SIDE EFFECTS & IMPACT ON ANESTHESIA
- Adequate well-controlled or observational studies in pregnant women have demonstrated a risk to the fetus. However, the benefits of therapy may outweigh the potential risk.

FETAL & NEONATAL EFFECTS
- Pregnancy Category D (for definition, see the "*Pregnancy Categories*" section). Phenobarbital sodium has been generally regarded as unsafe in breast-feeding, but it has been used in neonates for the treatment of hyperbilirubinemia & febrile seizure.

COMMENT
- Dose adjustments are required in geriatrics, dialysis pts & pts w/ renal & liver disease. Avoid abrupt discontinuation in pts w/ prolonged exposure. Phenobarbital sodium interacts w/ many drugs.

PHENYLEPHRINE (NEO-SYNEPHRINE)

INDICATIONS
- Hypotension, potent postsynaptic alpha-receptor agonist w/little effect on beta receptors of the heart

DOSING

- IV bolus 40–100 mcg/dose, or 10 mcg/min initially, then titrated to response

MATERNAL SIDE EFFECTS & IMPACT ON ANESTHESIA

- May cause hypertension, reflex bradycardia. The pressor effect is potentiated w/ the concurrent use of oxytocic drugs. Phenylephrine effects can be potentiated by bretylium, guanethidine, halogenated vapor anesthetics, MAO inhibitors.

FETAL & NEONATAL EFFECTS

- Pregnancy Category C (for definition, see the "*Pregnancy Categories*" section). Studies of healthy parturients undergoing C-section w/ regional anesthesia showed no adverse effects compared w/ ephedrine. The degree to which it passes into breast milk is unknown.

COMMENT

- Potent postsynaptic alpha-receptor agonist w/ little effect on beta receptors of the heart

---

PHENYTOIN (DILANTIN)

INDICATIONS

- Generalized tonic-clonic & complex partial seizures; seizures during or after neurosurgery; antiarrhythmic; antineuralgic; seizures secondary to eclampsia or pre-eclampsia

DOSING

- IV: 50–100 mg q10–15min, max 15 mg/kg, max rate 50 mg/minute
- PO: 400 mg, then 300 mg in 2h r & 4 hr
- Maintenance: 5 mg/kg or 300 mg PO once per day or divided tid

MATERNAL SIDE EFFECTS & IMPACT ON ANESTHESIA

- The effects of phenytoin on pregnancy have not been assessed. Some studies suggest that there is risk in certain maternal circumstances.

FETAL & NEONATAL EFFECTS

- Pregnancy Category NR (for definition, see the "*Pregnancy Categories*" section). Phenytoin is considered safe in breast-feeding.

COMMENT

■ Phenytoin requirements are greater during pregnancy, requiring increases in doses in some pts. After delivery, the dose should be decreased to avoid toxicity.

PITOCIN (OXYTOCIN)

INDICATIONS

■ Oxytocin is a hormone used to help start or continue labor & to control bleeding after delivery. It is also sometimes used to help milk secretion in breast-feeding.

DOSING

■ IV infusion (drip method) for post-partum bleeding: 10–40 units of oxytocin may be added to 1,000 mL of a non-hydrating diluent & run at a rate necessary to control uterine atony

■ IM: 1 mL (10 units) of oxytocin can be given after delivery of the placenta.

MATERNAL SIDE EFFECTS & IMPACT ON ANESTHESIA

■ Before delivery, the fetal heart, resting uterine tone & the frequency, duration & force of contractions should be monitored. Oxytocin should be discontinued immediately in the event of uterine hyper-activity or fetal distress. During C-section, oxytocin may be given following cord clamping to encourage separation of the placenta from the uterus. Uterine hypotonia may be treated w/ 2 units IVP. Cardiovascular collapse & death have been reported in hypovolemic women given 10 units IVP of oxytocin for uterine bleeding undergo-ing C-section. A rare complication is severe water intoxication.

FETAL & NEONATAL EFFECTS

■ Pregnancy Category C (for definition, see the "*Pregnancy Categories*" section). The risk of neonatal jaundice may be 1.6× that of neonates whose mothers did not receive oxytocin-induced labors. Other poor outcomes may be associated w/ uterine hyperstimulation. No known complications from Pitocin via breast milk after normal doses.

COMMENT

■ Rapid bolus may cause hypotension, tachycardia, myocardial ar-rhythmias, coronary vasospasm, cardiac arrest, headache & confu-sion.

POLOCAINE (MEPIVACAINE)

INDICATIONS
- Spinal anesthesia for short OB procedures

DOSING
- Varies depending on procedure, but similar to lidocaine (20% more potent)
- Spinal: 50 mg for short OB procedures (cerclage, cerclage removal, etc.) Adjuvant: Sodium bicarbonate may be added w/ a 1:10 ratio.
- Metabolism is via hydroxylation & N-demethylation in the liver. Elimination half-life is 2–3 hours.

MATERNAL SIDE EFFECTS & IMPACT ON ANESTHESIA
- Intravascular administration may lead to lightheadedness, seizures, disorientation, heart block, hypotension.

FETAL SIDE EFFECTS
- Pregnancy Category C (for definition, see the "*Pregnancy Categories*" section). Not recommended for epidural use, paracervical or pudendal blocks as the fetus cannot metabolize this drug. Safety in breastfeeding is unknown, but local anesthetics are not expected to accumulate significantly in breast milk.

COMMENTS
- Use preservative-free solutions for intrathecal administration. Use hyperbaric preparations for wider spread of block.

PONTOCAINE (TETRACAINE)

INDICATIONS
- Spinal anesthesia for surgical procedures

DOSING
- Hyperbaric solution (1% solution in 10% glucose) for spinal for C-section: usually 7–10 mg

MATERNAL SIDE EFFECTS & IMPACT ON ANESTHESIA
- Hypotension common w/ spinal administration. Toxicity profile similar to all other local anesthetics; CNS, cardiovascular toxicity dose-dependent.

FETAL & NEONATAL EFFECTS

- Pregnancy Category C (for definition, see the "*Pregnancy Categories*" section). Limited information available about its use in pregnancy. Not expected to accumulate significantly in breast milk.

COMMENT

- High potency w/ long duration of action 90–120 minutes plain, 120–240 min w/ epinephrine. Tetracaine produces more motor blockade than similar dose of bupivacaine at same sensory levels.

PREDNISONE

INDICATIONS

- Prednisone is a corticosteroid used in chronic asthma, Addison's disease & autoimmune diseases (rheumatoid, lupus).

DOSING

- Varies depending on the disorder

MATERNAL SIDE EFFECTS & IMPACT ON ANESTHESIA

- No evidence of increased congenital anomalies in infants after maternal treatment w/ corticosteroids. Cushing syndrome is always a concern for any pt on long-term steroids. Pts develop central obesity, moon facies & a buffalo hump; these effects are caused by redistribution of fat. Many pts also develop psychiatric symptoms, edema, delayed wound healing, glaucoma & subcapsular cataracts.

FETAL & NEONATAL EFFECTS

- Pregnancy Category B (for definition, see the "*Pregnancy Categories*" section). The amount of corticosteroid found in breast milk is negligible when the mother receives prednisone 20 mg/day or less. The dose received by the infant can be minimized by avoiding breastfeeding for 3–4 hours after a dose.

COMMENT

- Corticosteroids cause an increase in the absolute granulocyte count & decreases in the lymphocyte & monocyte count. Corticosteroids also raise plasma glucose levels. Most pts can continue taking the corticosteroid w/ treatment of hyperglycemia.

PREGNANCY CATEGORIES

INDICATIONS
- N/A

DOSING
- N/A

MATERNAL SIDE EFFECTS
- N/A

FETAL & NEONATAL EFFECTS
A: Adequate, well-controlled studies in pregnant women have not shown an increased risk of fetal abnormalities to the fetus in any trimester of pregnancy.

B: Animal studies have revealed no evidence of harm to the fetus; however, there are no adequate & well-controlled studies in pregnant women OR Animal studies have shown an adverse effect, but adequate & well-controlled studies in pregnant women have failed to demonstrate a risk to the fetus in any trimester.

C: Animal studies have shown an adverse effect & there are no adequate & well-controlled studies in pregnant women OR No animal studies have been conducted & there are no adequate & well-controlled studies in pregnant women.

D: Adequate well-controlled or observational studies in pregnant women have demonstrated a risk to the fetus.

However, the benefits of therapy may outweigh the potential risk. For example, the drug may be acceptable if needed in a life-threatening situation or serious disease for which safer drugs cannot be used or are ineffective.

X: Adequate well-controlled or observational studies in animals or pregnant women have demonstrated positive evidence of fetal abnormalities or risks.

The use of the product is contraindicated in women who are or may become pregnant.

NR: Drug Not Rated

COMMENT
- N/A

PRILOSEC (OMEPRAZOLE)

INDICATIONS
■ Decreases gastric acid secretion by inhibiting the parietal cell H^+/K^+ ATPase pump. Used for short-term & long-term treatment (4–8 wks to 12 months) of GERD.

DOSING
■ GERD: 20 mg PO qd

MATERNAL SIDE EFFECTS & IMPACT ON ANESTHESIA
■ May decrease effects of itraconazole & ketoconazole; may increase toxicity of warfarin, digoxin, phenytoin

FETAL & NEONATAL EFFECTS
■ Pregnancy Category C (for definition, see the "*Pregnancy Categories*" section). Safety during pregnancy has not been established. The extent to which it passes into the breast milk &/or affects newborns is unknown.

COMMENT
■ Bioavailability may increase in elderly pts. Adverse effects include headache, rash, diarrhea, hypergastrinemia, polyps.

PROCAINE (NOVOCAINE)

INDICATIONS
■ Low potency, lower toxicity, short-acting local anesthetic w/ rapid onset (3–5 min), used for infiltration, nerve block & spinal anesthesia. Frequently used in dentistry & for intractable pain associated w/ malignancy or neuralgia. Poor topical effect.

DOSING
■ Infiltration: 350–600 mg single total dose
■ Peripheral nerve block: total dose should not exceed 1 g.
■ Spinal anesthesia: 50–75 mg for perineal surgery, 100–125 mg for lower abdomen, 200 mg for anesthesia to costal margin
■ Anesthetic doses are reduced by 30% in parturients.

MATERNAL SIDE EFFECTS & IMPACT ON ANESTHESIA
- Toxicity profile similar to other local anesthetics. Metabolite para-aminobenzoic acid causes allergic reactions. Preservative sodium bisulfite also causes severe allergic reactions & anaphylaxis in those sensitive to it.

FETAL & NEONATAL EFFECTS
- Pregnancy Category C (for definition, see the "*Pregnancy Categories*" section). Not expected to accumulate significantly in breast milk.

COMMENT
- Epinephrine 1:200,000 or 1:100,000 can be added for vasoconstriction, which prolongs action from 45 to 60 minutes.

PROCHLORPERAZINE (COMPAZINE)

INDICATIONS
- May relieve nausea & vomiting by blocking postsynaptic mesolimbic dopamine receptors through anticholinergic effects & depressing reticular activating system. In a placebo-controlled study, 69% of pts given prochlorperazine reported significant symptom relief, compared to 40% of pts in the placebo group.

DOSING
- PO: 5–10 mg tid/qid, max 40 mg/d
- IV: 2.5–10 mg q3–4h prn, max 10 mg/dose or 40 mg/d
- IM: 5–10 mg q3–4h
- PR: 25 mg bid

MATERNAL SIDE EFFECTS & IMPACT ON ANESTHESIA
- Co-administration w/ other CNS depressants or anticonvulsants may cause additive effects; w/ epinephrine, may cause hypotension.

FETAL & NEONATAL EFFECTS
- Pregnancy Category C (for definition, see the "*Pregnancy Categories*" section)

COMMENT
- Drug-induced Parkinson syndrome or pseudoparkinsonism occurs quite frequently. Akathisia is most common extrapyramidal reaction in elderly pts. Lowers seizure threshold; may lower convulsive

threshold. Adverse effects can include hypotension, sedation & extrapyramidal & anticholinergic symptoms. Data are conflicting regarding teratogenicity. Crosses placenta & appears in breast milk.

PROMETHAZINE (PHENERGAN)

INDICATIONS
- Symptomatic treatment of nausea in vestibular dysfunction. Antidopaminergic agent effective in treating emesis. Blocks postsynaptic mesolimbic dopaminergic receptors in brain & reduces stimuli to brain stem reticular system. Often used in combination w/ opioids to reduce nausea & vomiting & produce sedation; may potentiate the analgesic effects of the opioids.

DOSING
- PO: 12.5–25 mg q4–6h prn (syr or tab)
- PR: 12.5–25 mg q4–6h prn
- IV/IM: 12.5–25 mg q4–6h; use caution w/ IV administration, concentration not to exceed 25 mg/mL, rate not to exceed 25 mg/min. IV dose of 25–50 mg rapidly produces effective sedation.
- Do not administer SC or intra-arterially.

MATERNAL SIDE EFFECTS & IMPACT ON ANESTHESIA
- May have additive effects when used concurrently w/ other CNS depressants or anticonvulsants; co-administration w/ epinephrine may cause hypotension

FETAL & NEONATAL EFFECTS
- Pregnancy Category C (for definition, see the "*Pregnancy Categories*" section). Rapidly crosses the placenta & may result in decreased beat-to-beat variability. Does not result in neonatal respiratory depression. Safety in breast feeding is unknown.

COMMENT
- Use w/ caution in pts w/ cardiovascular disease, impaired liver function, seizures, sleep apnea, asthma. Moderate respiratory stimulant resulting in an increase in minute ventilation & ventilatory response to CO_2, thus counteracting the respiratory depressant qualities of narcotics.

PROPOFOL (DIPRIVAN)

INDICATIONS
■ 2, 6-diisopropylphenol, prepared in 1% isotonic oil-in-water emulsion; rapidly produces unconsciousness (onset approx. 30–45 sec) followed by rapid reawakening due to redistribution

DOSING
■ 2–2.5 mg/kg IV for induction, 50–150 mcg/kg/min for maintenance

MATERNAL SIDE EFFECTS & IMPACT ON ANESTHESIA
■ Venous irritation; greater drop in systolic BP than w/ thiopental

FETAL & NEONATAL EFFECTS
■ Pregnancy Category B (for definition, see the "*Pregnancy Categories*" section). Rapidly crosses placenta. Higher doses for IV maintenance of GA (150 mcg/kg/min) may cause neonatal depression. Infants exposed to a maternal propofol dose of 2.8 mg/kg had significantly lower Apgar scores than infants whose mothers were given 5 mg/kg thiopental. A dose of 2 mg/kg IV results in an fetal/maternal ratio of 0.5. Oral bioavailability low; minimal breast milk transfer.

COMMENT
■ When learning about these drugs in obstetrics, it is important to be familiar w/ the approximate fetal:maternal (F/M) ratios of drug concentrations at the time of delivery of the infant. Generally, the umbilical vein blood concentrations represent the fetal blood concentrations. An early high ratio indicates rapid placental transfer of the drug.

PROPYLTHIOURACIL (PTU)

INDICATIONS
■ Propylthiouracil is an antithyroid agent & is the first-line agent for treating hyperthyroidism, such as Graves' disease, multinodular goiter or toxic adenoma.

DOSING
■ 300 mg q8h until patient is euthyroid; then dose is reduced to one half to one third for a total dose of 100–300 mg/day

MATERNAL SIDE EFFECTS & IMPACT ON ANESTHESIA
- Readily crosses placenta & can cause fetal harm. Can induce goiter & cretinism in fetus. If PTU is needed to treat hyperthyroidism complicated by pregnancy, the dose must be sufficient but not excessive. Frequently thyroid dysfunction diminishes as pregnancy proceeds; therefore, a reduction of dosage may be possible. In some cases, propylthiouracil can be withdrawn 2 or 3 weeks before delivery.

FETAL & NEONATAL EFFECTS
- Pregnancy Category D (for definition, see the "*Pregnancy Categories*" section). According to the manufacturer, PTU is contraindicated while breast-feeding. However, some studies have not shown a detrimental effect during breast-feeding. Infants may present w/ transient hypothyroxinemia (slightly depressed free thyroxine w/ high TSH levels) & should be evaluated for hypothyroidism & hyperthyroidism in the newborn period.

COMMENT
- In planning the anesthetic mgt for the hyperthyroid patient for surgery, euthyroidism should be established pre-op if possible.

PROSTAGLANDIN F2α (CARBOPROST TROMETHAMINE; HEMABATE)

INDICATIONS
- Prostaglandin is similar to F2-alpha (dinoprost), but it has a longer duration & produces myometrial contractions that induce hemostasis at placentation site, which reduces post-partum bleeding. Hemabate is used to treat post-partum hemorrhage & causes of uterine atony (overdistended uterus, rapid or prolonged labor, chorioamnionitis, high parity).

DOSING
- Treatment of postpartum hemorrhage: 0.25 mg (250 mcg/mL) IM q15–90 min, up to 2 mg

MATERNAL SIDE EFFECTS & IMPACT ON ANESTHESIA
- Administration can cause marked pulmonary arteriolar muscle constriction, severe pulmonary hypertension & bronchoconstriction. Can cause hypertension, but not as severe as the ergotamines.

FETAL & NEONATAL EFFECTS
- Pregnancy Category C (for definition, see the "*Pregnancy Categories*" section). Hemabate can induce labor & can even be used to abort the fetus in early stages of pregnancy. Hemabate is found in breast milk, but it is unknown if this is of clinical significance.

COMMENT
- Avoid in pts w/ pre-existing asthma or reactive airway disorders.

PROTAMINE

INDICATIONS
- Reversal of the effects of heparin

DOSING
- Usually 1 mg for 100 units of heparin activity. IV at <5 mg/min.

MATERNAL SIDE EFFECTS & IMPACT ON ANESTHESIA
- May cause peripheral vasodilation w/ sudden hypotension, severe pulmonary hypertension. Transient reversal of heparin may be followed by rebound heparinization. Can cause anticoagulation if given in excess relative to amount of circulating heparin. Can monitor w/ aPTT or ACT. Avoid in pts w/ hypersensitivity to NPH or fish allergy.

FETAL & NEONATAL EFFECTS
- Pregnancy category C (for definition, see the "*Pregnancy Categories*" section). It is not known to what extent it is excreted in breast milk.

COMMENT
- Rapid administration may cause severe hypotension & anaphylactoid reactions, including pulmonary hypertension.

PROVENTIL (ALBUTEROL ORAL INHALED AEROSOL)

INDICATIONS
- Albuterol is a stimulant of the beta-2 receptors in the bronchi & thus is a potent bronchodilator used in allergic asthma; exercise-induced asthma; acute, subacute & chronic bronchitis; & emphysema. Useful as a tocolytic. Can be used to treat hyperkalemia.

DOSING
- 1 or 2 metered-dose inhalations q4–6h

MATERNAL SIDE EFFECTS & IMPACT ON ANESTHESIA
- Like all beta-2 mimetics, may cause tachycardia, hyperglycemia & hypotension. May also result in hypokalemia; it is useful in treating hyperkalemia.

FETAL & NEONATAL EFFECTS
- Pregnancy Category C (for definition, see the "*Pregnancy Categories*" section). Crosses the placenta & may cause tachycardia & hyperglycemia in the fetus. May cause retinal ischemia. Albuterol is an effective tocolytic similar to ritodrine. Like ritodrine, it is considered safe during breast-feeding.

COMMENT
- Excessive inhalation may result in hypertension, hypoglycemia, hypokalemia & hypocalcemia. Concurrent administration w/ oxytocic drugs (including ergonovine) may cause hypotension. May decrease serum digoxin levels.

PROZAC (FLUOXETINE)

INDICATIONS
- SSRI typically used to treat depression, anxiety, obsessive-compulsive disorder, bulimia, panic disorder, posttraumatic stress disorder

DOSING
- Depression: initially 20 mg/day PO, up to 80 mg/day
- Bulimia: 20 mg/day PO, increasing to 60 mg/day over several days
- Obsessive-compulsive disorder: initially 20 mg/day PO; maintenance dose 20–80 mg/day PO
- Panic disorder: 10–60 mg/day PO; most common dosage is 20 mg/day
- Dosing adjustments are appropriate if there is hepatic insufficiency.

MATERNAL SIDE EFFECTS & IMPACT ON ANESTHESIA
- Common side effects include anorexia, dry mouth, nausea. More serious complications can include activation of mania or hypomania, hyponatremia, QT interval prolongation, seizure.

DOSING
- Varies for the individual medication

MATERNAL SIDE EFFECTS & IMPACT ON ANESTHESIA
FETAL & NEONATAL EFFECTS
■ Pregnancy Category C (for definition, see the "*Pregnancy Categories*" section). An increased risk for CNS serotonergic symptoms was observed during the first 4 days of life in infants of mothers taking SSRIs during the 3rd trimester of pregnancy. Infants exposed prenatally to fluoxetine or a tricyclic antidepressant did NOT show differences in IQ, language or behavioral development compared to children w/o prenatal exposure to these drugs. SSRIs have unknown effects that may be of concern during breast-feeding.

COMMENT
■ Do not use concomitantly w/ MAO inhibitors.

PTU (PROPYLTHIOURACIL)

INDICATIONS
■ Propylthiouracil is an antithyroid agent & is the first-line agent for treating hyperthyroidism, such as Graves disease, multinodular goiter or toxic adenoma.

DOSING
■ 300 mg q8h until patient is euthyroid; then dose is reduced to one half to one third for a total dose of 100–300 mg/day

MATERNAL SIDE EFFECTS & IMPACT ON ANESTHESIA
■ Readily crosses placenta & can cause fetal harm. Can induce goiter & cretinism in fetus. If PTU is needed to treat hyperthyroidism complicated by pregnancy, the dose must be sufficient but not excessive. Frequently thyroid dysfunction diminishes as pregnancy proceeds; therefore, a reduction of dosage may be possible. In some cases, propylthiouracil can be withdrawn 2 or 3 weeks before delivery.

FETAL & NEONATAL EFFECTS
■ Pregnancy Category D (for definition, see the "*Pregnancy Categories*" section). According to the manufacturer, PTU is contraindicated while breast-feeding. However, some studies have not shown a detrimental effect during breast-feeding. Infants may present w/ transient hypothyroxinemia (slightly depressed free thyroxine w/ high TSH levels) & should be evaluated for hypothyroidism & hyperthyroidism in the newborn period.

COMMENT
- In planning the anesthetic mgt for the hyperthyroid patient for surgery, euthyroidism should be established pre-op if possible.

RANITIDINE (ZANTAC)

INDICATIONS
- Inhibits histamine stimulation of the H2 receptor in gastric parietal cells, which reduces gastric acid secretion, gastric volume & hydrogen ion concentrations

DOSING
- 3.5 mg/kg/dose PO bid/tid ac & hs; alternatively, 150 mg PO bid or 75 mg PO bid

MATERNAL SIDE EFFECTS & IMPACT ON ANESTHESIA
- May decrease effects of ketoconazole & itraconazole; may alter serum levels of ferrous sulfate, diazepam, nondepolarizing muscle relaxants & oxaprozin

FETAL & NEONATAL EFFECTS
- Pregnancy Category B (for definition, see the "*Pregnancy Categories*" section). Usually safe but benefits must outweigh risks.

COMMENT
- Use caution in pts w/ renal or liver impairment; if changes in renal function occur during therapy, consider adjusting dose or discontinuing treatment. Adverse effects include headache & malaise.

REGLAN (METOCLOPRAMIDE)

INDICATIONS
- Dopaminergic antagonist that works by increasing lower esophageal sphincter tone & gastric emptying. Stimulates muscular activity, leading to decrease in reflux.

DOSING
- 10–15 mg PO or IV qid

MATERNAL SIDE EFFECTS & IMPACT ON ANESTHESIA

■ No adverse effects on mother or fetus have been reported when administered during the 1st trimester. Rare extrapyramidal side effects have been reported.

FETAL & NEONATAL EFFECTS

■ Pregnancy Category B (for definition, see the "*Pregnancy Categories*" section). Metoclopramide has not been found to increase the incidence of abnormalities in infants born to mothers who received the drug at various times up to the 28th week of pregnancy. Compatible w/ breast-feeding.

REMIFENTANIL (ULTIVA)

INDICATIONS

■ Ultrashort-acting synthetic, opioid receptor agonist w/ rapid onset

DOSING

■ Doses may vary; usually 0.05–1 mcg/kg IV.

MATERNAL SIDE EFFECTS & IMPACT ON ANESTHESIA

■ Rapidly metabolized by plasma & tissue esterases & thus is cleared independently of the liver or kidneys; the context-sensitive half-life is 3.5 minutes independent of the mode of administration.

FETAL & NEONATAL EFFECTS

■ Pregnancy Category C (for definition, see the "*Pregnancy Categories*" section). Rapid transplacental transfer, but similar metabolism by the fetus ensures rapid drug clearance.

COMMENT

■ Multiple studies have evaluated its use for labor PCA. There is concern regarding the need for an initial large bolus, which results in significant maternal respiratory depression. In addition, studies have shown large individual variation in the initial dose required, as well as in increased dosages required as labor progresses. The best dosing regimen remains undiscovered. Remifentanil should not be administered into the same IV tubing w/ blood because of potential drug inactivation by nonspecific esterases in blood products.

RETROVIR (ZIDOVUDINE)

INDICATIONS
- Inhibits HIV replication

DOSING
- 300–600 mg/day PO in 3–5 divided doses

MATERNAL SIDE EFFECTS & IMPACT ON ANESTHESIA
- Women in the 1st trimester may consider delaying or discontinuing therapy until after 10–12 weeks gestation. Recommended component of the peri- & post-partum regimen for mother & neonate whenever possible.

FETAL & NEONATAL EFFECTS
- Pregnancy Category C (for definition, see the "*Pregnancy Categories*" section). Significantly reduces transmission of HIV to the fetus. There are conflicting data on perinatal exposure to antiretrovirals associated w/ significant (often fatal) mitochondrial disease in infants. Babies exposed to antiretrovirals in utero should receive long-term follow-up for potential mitochondrial dysfunction.

COMMENT
- Breast-feeding is not recommended in mothers w/ HIV due to presence of virus in breast milk & potential for transmission to HIV-negative child.

ROCEPHIN (CEFTRIAXONE)

INDICATIONS
- Active against various gram-positive & gram-negative bacteria

DOSING
- 1–2 g IV q12–24h depending on organism, location & severity of infection

MATERNAL SIDE EFFECTS & IMPACT ON ANESTHESIA
- May need dose adjustment in pts w/ renal failure. May be associated w/ decreased prothrombin activity. Can be associated w/ urinary cast formation.

FETAL & NEONATAL EFFECTS
- Pregnancy Category B (for definition, see the "*Pregnancy Categories*" section). Crosses placenta & is found in breast milk in low concentrations. May displace bilirubin from albumin binding sites. Avoid in mothers of premature or hyperbilirubinemic neonates.

COMMENT
- Generally considered safe in pregnancy

ROCURONIUM (ZEMURON)

INDICATIONS
- Nondepolarizing neuromuscular blocking drug (NMBD) used to facilitate rapid intubation & maintain neuromuscular blockade

DOSING
- 0.6 mg/kg IV (onset 98 sec)

MATERNAL SIDE EFFECTS & IMPACT ON ANESTHESIA
- Action may be prolonged in pts w/ renal insufficiency & IV magnesium.

FETAL & NEONATAL EFFECTS
- Pregnancy Category B (for definition, see the "*Pregnancy Categories*" section). No adverse effects w/ intubating dose.

COMMENT
- Safe in pregnancy

ROLAIDS (MAGNESIUM HYDROXIDE)

INDICATIONS
- Increases gastric pH > 4 & inhibits proteolytic activity of pepsin, reducing acid indigestion. Antacids initially can be used in mild cases. No effect on frequency of reflux but decreases its acidity.

DOSING
- 5–15 mL/dose PO qd/qid

MATERNAL SIDE EFFECTS & IMPACT ON ANESTHESIA
- Decreases effects of tetracyclines, ranitidine, ketoconazole, benzodiazepines, penicillamine, phenothiazines, digoxin, indomethacin,

isoniazid; corticosteroids decrease effects of aluminum in hyper-phosphatemia

FETAL & NEONATAL EFFECTS

- Pregnancy Category B (for definition, see the "*Pregnancy Categories*" section). Usually safe but benefits must outweigh risks.

COMMENT

- Use caution in pts w/ recent massive upper GI hemorrhage; renal failure may cause aluminum toxicity; can cause constipation.

ROPIVACAINE (NAROPIN)

INDICATIONS

- Epidural infusion for labor analgesia. Intrathecal injection for procedures lasting <2 hours. When dilute solutions are used, ropivacaine produces excellent sensory anesthesia w/ minimal motor blockade, & tachyphylaxis occurs rarely.

DOSING

- Spinal: 15–20 mg (3 cc of 0.75%) for C-section
- Epidural dosing for C-section: 0.5% up to 30 cc, or 0.75% up to 25 cc
- Epidural dosing for labor infusion: 10–30 mg/hr
- Adjuvant: Sodium bicarbonate may be added w/ a ratio of 0.5 to 20 cc for epidural injection (do not use if there is any precipitation).

MATERNAL SIDE EFFECTS & IMPACT ON ANESTHESIA

- Intravascular administration may result in cardiac arrhythmias & cardiac arrest. Ropivacaine reportedly has a lower incidence of cardiac arrhythmias & cardiac arrest than bupivacaine.

NEONATAL SIDE EFFECTS

- Minimal. Very safe. Any drug that reaches the fetus undergoes metabolism & excretion. The newborn has the hepatic enzymes necessary for the biotransformation of amide local anesthetics. Elimination half-life is longer in neonates than in adults. Can be safely used in breast-feeding.

COMMENT

- Intrathecal use of ropivacaine is not approved by the FDA. Ropivacaine is commercially available preservative-free. Boluses should be limited 3–5 cc at a time, so as to detect intravascular or intrathecal administration.

ROXICET (OXYCODONE/ACETAMINOPHEN)

INDICATIONS
■ Pain, moderate & severe

DOSING
■ Contains 5 mg oxycodone & 325 mg acetaminophen. Usually, 1 tab or 1 teaspoon PO q6h as needed. Immediately post-op, as much as 1 or 2 tabs q4h prn. Total daily dosage of acetaminophen/oxycodone should not exceed 4,000 mg/60 mg.

MATERNAL SIDE EFFECTS & IMPACT ON ANESTHESIA
■ Effects on pregnancy have not been assessed. Use w/ precaution in labor & delivery or w/ concomitant use of other CNS depressants. May need dosing adjustment in pts w/ liver disease.

FETAL & NEONATAL EFFECTS
■ Pregnancy Category NR (for definition, see the "*Pregnancy Categories*" section). Safety in breast-feeding is unclear; however, it is used commonly as a post-cesarean analgesic at a time when there is not much milk production yet.

COMMENT
■ Adverse effects include respiratory depression, constipation, nausea & vomiting, dizziness, dysphoria, lightheadedness, sedation, skin rash, pruritus.

SENSORCAINE (BUPIVACAINE)

INDICATIONS
■ Epidural infusion for labor analgesia in low concentrations 0.125–0.04%; spinal injection for labor analgesia or cesarean delivery

DOSING
■ 8–10 mL of 0.25–0.5% provides approx. 2 hours of epidural analgesia. When dilute solutions are used, bupivacaine produces excellent sensory analgesia w/ minimal motor blockade; tachyphylaxis occurs

rarely. For labor spinals, 2.5 mg can provide at least 60 minutes of analgesia (adjuncts can be added to prolong effect); for cesarean delivery, spinal bupivacaine 12–15 mg (usually 0.75% bupivacaine w/ dextrose) is adequate (adjuncts can be added to improve effect).

MATERNAL SIDE EFFECTS & IMPACT ON ANESTHESIA
- High-dose (0.75%) bupivacaine is not recommended for use in epidurals in obstetrics due to the profound maternal & neonatal myocardial depression & difficult resuscitation associated w/ accidental intravascular injection.

FETAL & NEONATAL SIDE EFFECTS
- Pregnancy Category C (for definition, see the "*Pregnancy Categories*" section). Highly protein-bound, which limits transplacental transfer. Any drug that reaches the fetus undergoes metabolism & excretion. The newborn has the hepatic enzymes necessary for the biotransformation of amide local anesthetics. Elimination half-life is longer in neonates than adults. Bupivacaine is considered safe for breastfeeding.

COMMENT
- There is no association btwn local anesthetic use & fetal malformations during the first 4 months of pregnancy.

SERTRALINE (ZOLOFT)

INDICATIONS
- SSRI typically used to treat depression, anxiety, obsessive-compulsive disorder, bulimia, panic disorder, posttraumatic stress disorder

DOSING
- Depression or obsessive-compulsive disorder: 50 mg/day PO, up to 200 mg/day PO
- Panic disorder: 25 mg/day PO initially, up to 200 mg/day PO
- Dosages should be decreased in pts w/ liver disease.

MATERNAL SIDE EFFECTS & IMPACT ON ANESTHESIA
- Potential for anorexia, dry mouth, constipation or diarrhea, abnormal bleeding (when taken w/ other platelet inhibitors), hyponatremia, seizures

FETAL & NEONATAL EFFECTS

- Pregnancy Category C (for definition, see the "*Pregnancy Categories*" section). An increased risk for CNS serotonergic symptoms was observed during the first 4 days of life in infants of mothers taking SSRIs during the 3rd trimester of pregnancy. Infants exposed prenatally to fluoxetine or a tricyclic antidepressant did NOT show differences in IQ, language or behavioral development compared to children w/o prenatal exposure to these drugs. SSRIs have unknown effects that may be of concern during breast-feeding.

COMMENT

- Do not take w/ MAO inhibitors.

SEVOFLURANE (ULTANE)

INDICATIONS

- Induction & maintenance of general anesthesia. Better for induction because less irritating to airway than other inhalational agents.

DOSING

- MAC for sevoflurane is 2.6%, decreased by 30–40% for the parturient. Use 0.25–0.5 MAC until delivery of baby to limit hypotension & uterine atony. Rapid onset (2 min) & recovery.

MATERNAL SIDE EFFECTS & IMPACT ON ANESTHESIA

- Causes dose-dependent uterine atony & hypotension. Can cause brady/tachycardia, hypertension, agitation, hypo/hyperthermia, nausea, vomiting, laryngospasm, shivering, etc. May increase risk of seizures.

FETAL & NEONATAL EFFECTS

- Pregnancy Category B (for definition, see the "*Pregnancy Categories*" section). Crosses the placenta & may cause temporary neonatal depression in large doses. Concentrations in breast milk are negligible 24 hours after anesthesia.

COMMENT

- Keep fresh gas flow >1–2 L/min as sevoflurane degradation product (compound A) has been shown to cause nephrotoxicity in rats. When used as the sole anesthetic agent for general anesthesia, awareness results in 12–26% of cases.

SODIUM CITRATE (BICITRA)

INDICATIONS
- Used prior to anesthesia induction as a pre-op antacid to prevent aspiration pneumonitis

DOSING
- 15–30 mL of a 0.3-molar solution, administered 10–30 minutes prior to induction of anesthesia

MATERNAL SIDE EFFECTS & IMPACT ON ANESTHESIA
- Potassium citrate & sodium citrate are absorbed & metabolized to potassium bicarbonate & sodium bicarbonate, thus acting as systemic alkalizers. Oxidation is virtually complete; <5% of the citrates are excreted in the urine unchanged.

FETAL & NEONATAL EFFECTS
- Pregnancy Category NR (for definition, see the "*Pregnancy Categories*" section). The drug crosses the placenta & enters the fetus, & its delayed, long-term effects on the exposed offspring have not been investigated.

COMMENT
- Use special care in the pt w/ pre-eclampsia or toxemia of pregnancy, as the sodium in sodium-containing citrates may cause the body to retain water.

SODIUM NITROPRUSSIDE (NITROPRESS)

INDICATIONS
- Direct NO donor. Used for hypertension, controlled hypotension, congestive heart failure.

DOSING
- Start w/ 0.1 mcg/kg/min, then titrate to patient response to maximum 10 mcg/kg/min.

MATERNAL SIDE EFFECTS & IMPACT ON ANESTHESIA
- May cause excessive hypotension, reflex tachycardia, tachyphylaxis. Accumulation of cyanide w/ liver dysfunction leading to cyanide toxicity, thiocyanate w/ kidney dysfunction resulting in thiocyanate

toxicity. Also impairs hypoxic pulmonary vasoconstriction, leading to hypoxia.

FETAL & NEONATAL EFFECTS
- Pregnancy Category C (for definition, see the "*Pregnancy Categories*" section). Fetal cyanide toxicity of nitroprusside has been described in animal models. It is not known if nitroprusside or its metabolites are excreted in significant amounts in breast milk.

COMMENT
- Thiocyanate toxicity may become life-threatening at serum concentration of 200 mg/L. Nitroprusside infusion >2 mcg/kg/min generates cyanide ion faster than the body can normally eliminate it. The capacity of methemoglobin to buffer cyanide is exhausted after approximately 500 mcg/kg nitroprusside. Concurrent administration of sodium thiosulfate may reduce the risk of cyanide toxicity by increasing the rate of cyanide conversion.

STADOL (BUTORPHANOL)

INDICATIONS
- An opioid w/ agonist-antagonist properties, used for the relief of mild to moderate, deep or visceral pain & for chronic pain. Butorphanol is a synthetic opioid agonist-antagonist analgesic.

DOSING
- Typical dose: 1–2 mg IV/IM; can be given as frequently as q1–2h

MATERNAL SIDE EFFECTS & IMPACT ON ANESTHESIA
- Use w/ caution w/ other sedative or analgesic drugs, as these are likely to produce additive effects. As w/ nalbuphine, it has a ceiling effect on respiratory depression.

FETAL & NEONATAL EFFECTS
- Pregnancy Category C; Category D if used for prolonged periods or in high doses at term (for definitions, see the "*Pregnancy Categories*" section). Although butorphanol may pass into the breast milk, it is not expected to cause problems in nursing babies. May cause a sinusoidal fetal heart rate pattern during labor that is not associated w/ hypoxia.

COMMENT

■ Overdose signs include cold, clammy skin; confusion; convulsions (seizures); dizziness (severe); drowsiness (severe); nervousness, restlessness, or weakness (severe); small pupils; slow heartbeat; slow or troubled breathing.

STIMATE (DESMOPRESSIN)

INDICATIONS

■ Improves coagulation in pts w/ hemophilia A, renal failure & certain types of von Willebrand's disease. Can also be used as an antidiuretic. Prophylactic treatment for patients w/ type I or III von Willebrand's prior to C-section & neuraxial anesthesia. Single-shot spinal anesthesia may be preferable to epidural anesthesia due to the smaller size of the needle. For C-section consider GETA.

DOSING

■ 0.3 mcg/kg IV (dilute in 50 cc NS) up to a max of 20 mcg. Infuse over 15–30 minutes. Some hematologists have recommended giving a dose 30 minutes prior to placing a spinal or epidural & a second dose 30 minutes prior to discontinuing an epidural if it has been >4–6 hours since the initial dose was given. For ongoing epidural treatment of labor pain, redose DDAVP q6h.

MATERNAL SIDE EFFECTS & IMPACT ON ANESTHESIA

■ Causes immediate release of vWF from endothelial cell wall & increases factor VIII 2–3×. Increases renal water reabsorption. Watch for side effects such as hyponatremia-induced seizures. Antidiuretic doses have no uterotonic action.

FETAL & NEONATAL EFFECTS

■ Pregnancy category B (for definition, see the "*Pregnancy Categories*" section). Excretion in breast milk unknown.

COMMENT

■ In type II von Willebrand's, desmopressin is not effective; treatment is platelet transfusion. A RICOF level of >30% in pts w/ type II indicates that regional anesthesia is safe. Additional treatment for type III severe vWF deficiency should include cryoprecipitate or Humate-C, which contains both factor VIIIc & active vWF.

SUBLIMAZE (FENTANYL)

INDICATIONS
- Potent narcotic analgesic w/ much shorter half-life than morphine sulfate. Drug of choice for conscious sedation & analgesia. Used as adjunct in spinals & epidurals. Reversed by naloxone.

DOSING
- Analgesia: 0.5–1 mcg/kg/dose IV/IM q30–60 min
- Transdermal: Apply a 25-mcg/h system q48–72 h.
- Neuraxial dosing varies depending on obstetric indication & regional anesthetic technique.

MATERNAL SIDE EFFECTS & IMPACT ON ANESTHESIA
- Used routinely in epidural infusions (w/ bupivacaine) for labor analgesia; may allow the reduction of local anesthetic dose.

FETAL & NEONATAL EFFECTS
- Pregnancy Category C; Category D if used for prolonged periods or in high doses at term (for definitions, see the "*Pregnancy Categories*" section). Readily crosses placenta & may cause neonatal depression. There appears to be no fetal accumulation of either drug during epidural infusion, however, & no adverse fetal effects have been observed from epidural fentanyl administration in routine doses. Opioids may result in decreased beat-to-beat variability of the fetal heart rate (FHR) w/o fetal hypoxia. Fentanyl is excreted in breast milk; it is compatible w/ breast-feeding due to low oral bioavailability.

COMMENT
- May result in hypotension, respiratory depression, constipation, nausea, emesis, urinary retention; idiosyncratic reaction, known as chest wall rigidity syndrome, may require neuromuscular blockade to increase ventilation.

SUCCINYLCHOLINE (ANECTINE)

INDICATIONS
- Depolarizing neuromuscular blocking drug (NMBD) to facilitate muscle paralysis for intubation

DOSING
- 1–1.5 mg/kg IV (onset 45 sec)

MATERNAL SIDE EFFECTS & IMPACT ON ANESTHESIA
- Can precipitate malignant hyperthermia, trismus, cardiac dysrhythmias, hyperkalemia, myalgias, myoglobinuria; increases intragastric pressure; increases intraocular pressure. Despite a decrease in plasma cholinesterase in parturients, intubating dose is not reduced.

FETAL & NEONATAL EFFECTS
- Pregnancy Category C (for definition, see the "*Pregnancy Categories*" section). Only small amounts cross placenta, since it is highly ionized & water-soluble.

COMMENT
- No depressant effects on neonatal ventilation w/ intubating dose. Despite decreased plasma cholinesterase levels in pregnant pts, metabolism is not prolonged due to increased volume of distribution.

SUFENTA (SUFENTANIL)

INDICATIONS
- Spinal & epidural anesthesia

DOSING
- 5 mcg w/ 1.25 mg isobaric bupivacaine may be used intrathecally (combined spinal-epidural) to provide a "walking" labor epidural. May be substituted for fentanyl for C-section spinal anesthetic; however, the high incidence of pruritus may limit its usefulness.

MATERNAL SIDE EFFECTS & IMPACT ON ANESTHESIA
- As w/ other opiates, there is a chance of drowsiness, nausea, vomiting, respiratory depression. In the perioperative setting, may be associated w/ chest wall rigidity. Can interact w/ other sedatives, including barbiturates, benzodiazepines & centrally acting muscle relaxants.

FETAL & NEONATAL EFFECTS
- Pregnancy Category C (for definition, see the "*Pregnancy Categories*" section). Thought to be safe for breast-feeding.

COMMENT
- Intrathecal sufentanil may reduce requirements for intraoperative antiemetics & post-op narcotics.

SUFENTANIL (SUFENTA)

INDICATIONS
- Spinal & epidural anesthesia

DOSING
- 5 mcg w/ 1.25 mg isobaric bupivacaine may be used intrathecally (combined spinal-epidural) to provide a "walking" labor epidural. May be substituted for fentanyl for C-section spinal anesthetic; however, the high incidence of pruritus may limit its usefulness.

MATERNAL SIDE EFFECTS & IMPACT ON ANESTHESIA
- As w/ other opiates, there is a chance of drowsiness, nausea, vomiting, respiratory depression. In the perioperative setting, may be associated w/ chest wall rigidity. Can interact w/ other sedatives, including barbiturates, benzodiazepines & centrally acting muscle relaxants.

FETAL & NEONATAL EFFECTS
- Pregnancy Category C (for definition, see the "*Pregnancy Categories*" section). Thought to be safe for breast-feeding.

COMMENT
- Intrathecal sufentanil may reduce requirements for intraoperative antiemetics & post-op narcotics.

SUMATRIPTAN (IMITREX)

INDICATIONS
- Vascular 5-hydroxytryptamine receptor subtype agonist used for treating acute migraines

DOSING
- Oral tablet or injection. Initial dose 25–100 mg, may be repeated after 2 hours if headache is still present. Max daily dose 200 mg.

MATERNAL SIDE EFFECTS & IMPACT ON ANESTHESIA
- May cause vasospasm. Rare but serious cardiac events in pts w/o cardiac risk factors have been reported within 1 hour of administration. Hypertensive crisis in pts w/o history of hypertension also reported. May lower seizure threshold.

FETAL & NEONATAL EFFECTS
- Pregnancy Category C (for definition, see the "*Pregnancy Categories*" section). Evidence of teratogenicity, impaired fertility & embryolethality in animal studies. Excreted freely in breast milk. No testing in pts <12 years old.

COMMENT
- Careful exclusion of other causes of headache should be made prior to administration. Contraindicated w/ MAO-A inhibitors (reduces clearance of Imitrex). Use w/ caution in pts on SSRIs.

SUPRANE (DESFLURANE)

INDICATIONS
- Maintenance of general anesthesia

DOSING
- MAC for Desflurane is 6–7% in the non-pregnant patient, 30–40% less for parturient. Use 0.25–0.5 MAC until delivery of baby to avoid hypotension.

MATERNAL SIDE EFFECTS & IMPACT ON ANESTHESIA
- Causes dose-dependent uterine atony & hypotension due to peripheral vasodilation, decreases hepatic blood flow, increases cerebral vasodilation, can increase plasma catecholamines w/ abrupt increases in inspired concentration. Rapid onset & emergence.

FETAL & NEONATAL EFFECTS
- Pregnancy Category B (for definition, see the "*Pregnancy Categories*" section). Crosses the placenta & may cause temporary neonatal depression in large doses. Not thought to be a problem for breastfeeding.

COMMENT
- Pungent odor causes increased risk of coughing, laryngospasm, breath holding & increased pulmonary secretions. When used as

the sole anesthetic agent for general anesthesia, awareness results in 12–26% of cases.

SYNTHROID (LEVOTHYROXINE)

INDICATIONS
■ A synthetically prepared hormone identical to T4 used in the treatment of hypothyroidism

DOSING
■ 1.6–1.8 mcg/kg lean body weight/d PO qd

MATERNAL SIDE EFFECTS & IMPACT ON ANESTHESIA
■ Hypothyroid women have a lower fertility rate than euthyroid women. The required dose of thyroid replacement often increases during pregnancy by 20–50%. A large goiter may produce dysphagia, hoarseness & stridor from extrinsic obstruction to airflow; consider evaluating pts w/ these symptoms w/ a barium swallow study & pulmonary function tests, including flow volume loops. Use w/ caution in angina pectoris or cardiovascular disease. Monitor thyroid status periodically. Use caution in pts w/ adrenocortical insufficiency, in whom steroid replacement should precede levothyroxine replacement.

FETAL & NEONATAL EFFECTS
■ Pregnancy Category A (for definition, see the "*Pregnancy Categories*" section). Negligible transplacental passage of the drug. T4 is excreted into breast milk in low concentrations.

COMMENT
■ TSH is the most accurate measure of the euthyroid state. In most instances, neonatal thyroid development is independent of maternal thyroid function. No contraindications to levothyroxine replacement therapy except in pts w/ uncorrected adrenal insufficiency.

SYNTOCINON (OXYTOCIN)

INDICATIONS
■ Oxytocin is a hormone used to help start or continue labor & to control bleeding after delivery. It is also sometimes used to help milk secretion in breast-feeding.

DOSING

- IV infusion (drip method) for post-partum bleeding: 10–40 units of oxytocin may be added to 1,000 mL of a non-hydrating diluent & run at a rate necessary to control uterine atony
- IM: 1 mL (10 units) of oxytocin can be given after delivery of the placenta.

MATERNAL SIDE EFFECTS & IMPACT ON ANESTHESIA

- Before delivery, the fetal heart, resting uterine tone & the frequency, duration & force of contractions should be monitored. Oxytocin should be discontinued immediately in the event of uterine hyperactivity or fetal distress. During C-section, oxytocin may be given following cord clamping to encourage separation of the placenta from the uterus. Uterine hypotonia may be treated w/ 2 units IVP. Cardiovascular collapse & death have been reported in hypovolemic women given 10 units IVP of oxytocin for uterine bleeding undergoing C-section. A rare complication is severe water intoxication.

FETAL & NEONATAL EFFECTS

- Pregnancy Category C (for definition, see the "*Pregnancy Categories*" section). The risk of neonatal jaundice may be 1.6× that of neonates whose mothers did not receive oxytocin-induced labors. Other poor outcomes may be associated w/ uterine hyperstimulation. No known complications from Pitocin via breast milk after normal doses.

COMMENT

- Rapid bolus may cause hypotension, tachycardia, myocardial arrhythmias, coronary vasospasm, cardiac arrest, headache & confusion.

TEGRETOL (CARBAMAZEPINE)

INDICATIONS

- Carbamazepine, a tricyclic, is both an anticonvulsant & psychotropic. Typically used for epilepsy w/ motor & psychic manifestations. Also used in the treatment of trigeminal neuralgia.

DOSING

- 1,600 mg/day PO

MATERNAL SIDE EFFECTS & IMPACT ON ANESTHESIA

- Contraindicated in expectant or nursing mothers or pts w/ liver disease. Induction of hepatic enzymes in response to carbamazepine may have the effect of diminishing the activity of certain drugs that are metabolized in the liver. In obstetrics, its use is limited to cases where maternal benefit is greater than potential fetal harm.

FETAL & NEONATAL EFFECTS
■ Pregnancy Category D (for definition, see the "*Pregnancy Categories*" section). The active substance of carbamazepine passes into the breast milk. It is considered incompatible w/ breast-feeding.

COMMENT
■ Abnormalities of liver function & jaundice have been associated w/ long-term treatment. Overall, pregnant women should be advised of the multiple potential adverse outcomes of the drug, but it should not routinely be withheld as the benefits of preventing seizures may outweigh the potential fetal harm.

TENORMIN (ATENOLOL)

INDICATIONS
■ Angina pectoris & hypertension. Atenolol is a cardioselective beta-1 adrenoceptor blocking agent.

DOSING
■ 25–100 mg PO qd

MATERNAL SIDE EFFECTS & IMPACT ON ANESTHESIA
■ May cause maternal bradycardia, bronchospasm in asthmatics, dizziness & hypotension

FETAL & NEONATAL EFFECTS
■ Pregnancy Category D (for definition, see the "*Pregnancy Categories*" section). Crosses placenta & may result in newborn infants w/ hypotonia & hypoglycemia & infants that are small for gestational age. Produces steady-state fetal levels that are approximately equal to those in the maternal serum. Atenolol is excreted into breast milk; generally should be avoided during lactation.

COMMENT
■ Contraindicated in the presence of 2nd- or 3rd-degree heart block & metabolic acidosis. Use particular caution in pts w/ asthma, bronchitis, chronic respiratory diseases, bradycardia <50 per minute, peripheral vascular diseases & Raynaud's phenomenon.

TERBUTALINE

INDICATIONS
- Short-acting beta-2 selective adrenergic agonist. Bronchospasm, tocolysis.

DOSING
- Bronchospasm: Inhaler, 2 metered-dose inhalations (400 mcg) q4–6h; tablets, 2.5–5 mg q6h 3x/day; SC, 250 mcg once, can repeat. Max 500 mcg in 4 hours.
- Tocolysis: SC, 250 mcg q1–6h; IV, 250 mcg once, or 10–25 mcg/min continuous. Or SC 250 mcg once. Adjust dosage w/ impaired renal function.

MATERNAL SIDE EFFECTS & IMPACT ON ANESTHESIA
- May cause ECG changes including sinus pause, atrial premature beats, AV block, ventricular premature beats, ST-T wave depression, T-wave inversion, sinus bradycardia & atrial escape beats w/ aberrant conduction. May cause muscle cramps, elevation of liver enzymes, seizures, pulmonary edema, hypokalemia, CNS excitement. May exacerbate preexisting diabetes mellitus & ketoacidosis.

FETAL & NEONATAL EFFECTS
- Pregnancy Category B (for definition, see the "*Pregnancy Categories*" section). No increased risk of fetal anomalies reported but few 1st-trimester data. Neonatal hypoglycemia. Neonatal/fetal tachycardia can be seen. Crosses into breast milk & decision to continue drug is based on importance of drug to the mother.

COMMENT
- May cause pain at injection site

TETRACAINE (PONTOCAINE)

INDICATIONS
- Spinal anesthesia for surgical procedures

DOSING
- Hyperbaric solution (1% solution in 10% glucose) for spinal for C-section: usually 7–10 mg

MATERNAL SIDE EFFECTS & IMPACT ON ANESTHESIA
- Hypotension common w/ spinal administration. Toxicity profile similar to all other local anesthetics; CNS, cardiovascular toxicity dose-dependent.

FETAL & NEONATAL EFFECTS
- Pregnancy Category C (for definition, see the "*Pregnancy Categories*" section). Limited information available about its use in pregnancy. Not expected to accumulate significantly in breast milk.

COMMENT
- High potency w/ long duration of action 90–120 minutes plain, 120–240 min w/ epinephrine. Tetracaine produces more motor blockade than similar dose of bupivacaine at same sensory levels.

THIOPENTAL SODIUM (PENTOTHAL)

INDICATIONS
- Barbiturate induction agent that rapidly produces unconsciousness (onset approx. 30–45 sec) followed by rapid reawakening due to redistribution

DOSING
- 3–5 mg/kg IV

MATERNAL SIDE EFFECTS & IMPACT ON ANESTHESIA
- Rapid induction & redistribution, typically w/ minimal effect on fetus. Hemodynamic effects not as pronounced as propofol.

FETAL & NEONATAL EFFECTS
- Pregnancy Category C (for definition, see the "*Pregnancy Categories*" section). Minimal effects if dose <4 mg/kg, due to rapid maternal redistribution & clearing by fetal liver. (See "*Propofol*" for comparison.) Fetal/maternal ratio 0.4–1.1. Considered safe for breast-feeding.

COMMENT
- Absolutely contraindicated in certain porphyrias (acute intermittent porphyria, variant porphyria, hereditary co-porphyria). When learning about these drugs in obstetrics, it is important to be familiar w/

the approximate fetal:maternal (F/M) ratios of drug concentrations at the time of delivery of the infant. Generally, the umbilical vein blood concentrations represent the fetal blood concentrations. An early high ratio indicates rapid placental transfer of the drug.

TIAZAC (DILTIAZEM)

INDICATIONS
- Angina, hypertension, arrhythmias (atrial fib/atrial flutter), paroxysmal supraventricular tachycardia; has been used as a tocolytic

DOSING
- Depends on indication
- Available in oral immediate-release, extended-release (qd) & sustained-release (bid) tabs & capsules for angina & hypertension
- IV forms are used to treat arrhythmias. Initial bolus 0.25 mg/kg over 2 min, repeat 0.35-mg/kg bolus in 15 min for inadequate response.
- Continuous infusion starts at 10 mg/hr, may be increased at 5-mg/hr intervals for therapeutic effect. Infusions lasting >24 hours are not recommended.

MATERNAL SIDE EFFECTS & IMPACT ON ANESTHESIA
- Most common side effects are edema, 1st-degree AV block, headache, hypotension. Concomitant use w/ beta-blockers, digoxin & amiodarone can lead to severe conduction disturbances, bradycardia & hypotension. Can increase plasma concentration of alfentanil, fentanyl & benzodiazepines.

FETAL & NEONATAL EFFECTS
- Pregnancy Category C (for definition, see the "*Pregnancy Categories*" section). Diffuses freely into breast milk, though no adverse effects reported. American Academy of Pediatrics says compatible w/ breast-feeding.

COMMENTS
- Do not use in pts w/ ventricular dysfunction, acute MI, pulmonary congestion, sick sinus syndrome or 2nd- or 3rd-degree AV block w/o pacer.

TOFRANIL (IMIPRAMINE)

INDICATIONS
- Tricyclic antidepressants (TCAs) are effective for the treatment of major depressive disorders; also sometimes prescribed for chronic pain or polyneuropathy.

DOSING
- For depression in outpatients, 75 mg/day divided in 1–3 doses, up to 200 mg/day

MATERNAL SIDE EFFECTS & IMPACT ON ANESTHESIA
- Common side effects include anticholinergic symptoms (drying of secretions, dilated pupils, sedation). Concomitant use of TCAs & amphetamines has been reported to result in enhanced amphetamine effects from the release of norepinephrine. Ephedrine should be given cautiously to patients on TCAs.

FETAL & NEONATAL EFFECTS
- Pregnancy Category NR (for definition, see the "*Pregnancy Categories*" section). Breast-feeding effects are unknown; only very minute amounts are found in the infant's serum.

COMMENT
- Do not use w/ MAO inhibitors.

TOPROL XL (METOPROLOL)

INDICATIONS
- Beta-1 adrenergic blockade. Commonly used for hypertension, angina pectoris, arrhythmias, myocardial infarction, hypertrophic cardiomyopathy.

DOSING
- 50–100 mg PO q6–24h, 2.5- to 5-mg IV boluses q2min, prn

MATERNAL SIDE EFFECTS & IMPACT ON ANESTHESIA
- May cause bradycardia, clinically significant bronchoconstriction (with doses >100 mg/day), dizziness. Increased risk of heart block.

FETAL & NEONATAL EFFECTS

■ Pregnancy Category C (for definition, see the "*Pregnancy Categories*" section). Crosses the placenta. May cause fetal or neonatal bradycardia, neonatal hypoglycemia & delayed spontaneous breathing of the newborn.

COMMENT

■ NA

TORADOL (KETOROLAC)

INDICATIONS

■ Ketorolac is a nonsteroidal, anti-inflammatory, analgesic, antipyretic agent that inhibits prostaglandin synthetase.

DOSING

■ PO: 15–30 mg q6h, max 40 mg/day for max of 5 days
■ IV: 30 mg q6h for max of 5 days

MATERNAL SIDE EFFECTS & IMPACT ON ANESTHESIA

■ Excellent analgesic adjunct for post-op pain after C-section in women receiving intrathecal morphine. Do not use in women considering pregnancy, since these agents block blastocyst implantation.

FETAL & NEONATAL EFFECTS

■ Pregnancy Category C, but Category D in 3rd trimester (for definitions, see the "*Pregnancy Categories*" section). Crosses the placenta. Ketorolac, like all prostaglandin synthesis inhibitors during pregnancy, constricts the ductus arteriosis. Persistent pulmonary hypertension of the newborn can occur if administered close to the time of delivery. See "*Ibuprofen.*"

COMMENT

■ The most frequent adverse effects are GI disturbances, reactions ranging from abdominal discomfort, nausea & vomiting & abdominal pain to serious GI bleeding or activation of peptic ulcer.

TRANDATE (LABETALOL)

INDICATIONS
- Hypertension

DOSING
- A wide therapeutic range. Titrate to effect. 5–10 mg IV, over 2 minutes. May repeat up to 200 mg total. For oral dosing, 100–400 mg PO BID.

MATERNAL SIDE EFFECTS & IMPACT ON ANESTHESIA
- May cause bradycardia, bronchospasm in asthmatics, postural hypotension, dizziness. Not thought to affect the usual course of labor & delivery when given to pregnant hypertensive pts.

FETAL & NEONATAL EFFECTS
- Pregnancy Category C (for definition, see the "*Pregnancy Categories*" section). Crosses the placenta & may cause fetal bradycardia, hypoglycemia, respiratory depression, hypotension. Considered compatible w/ breast-feeding.

COMMENT
- Has an alpha to beta blockade action of 1:7

TRIDIL (NITROGLYCERIN)

INDICATIONS
- Nitroglycerin can be used for transient uterine relaxation during removal of retained placental tissue. It is also used in angina.

DOSING
- Start w/ 40-mcg (0.04 mg) boluses until desired effect is achieved. Careful & continuous hemodynamic monitoring is necessary.

MATERNAL SIDE EFFECTS & IMPACT ON ANESTHESIA
- Documented headache, hypersensitivity, severe anemia, shock, postural hypotension, head trauma, closed-angle glaucoma, cerebral hemorrhage

FETAL & NEONATAL EFFECTS
- Pregnancy Category C (for definition, see the "*Pregnancy Categories*" section).

COMMENT

- Exercise caution w/ coronary artery disease & low systolic BP.

TYLENOL (ACETAMINOPHEN)

INDICATIONS

- Antipyretic & analgesic

DOSING

- 325–650 mg PO q4–6h or 1,000 mg 3 or 4 times/day; max 4 g/day

MATERNAL SIDE EFFECTS & IMPACT ON ANESTHESIA

- Used during pregnancy & appears safe for short-term use at therapeutic doses

FETAL & NEONATAL EFFECTS

- Pregnancy Category B (for definition, see the "*Pregnancy Categories*" section). No adverse effects have been reported. Compatible w/ breast-feeding.

COMMENT

- Use w/ care in pts w/ impaired liver function.

TYLOX (OXYCODONE/ACETAMINOPHEN)

INDICATIONS

- Pain, moderate & severe

DOSING

- Contains 5 mg oxycodone & 325 mg acetaminophen. Usually, 1 tab or 1 teaspoon PO q6h as needed. Immediately post-op, as much as 1 or 2 tabs q4h prn. Total daily dosage of acetaminophen/oxycodone should not exceed 4,000 mg/60 mg.

MATERNAL SIDE EFFECTS & IMPACT ON ANESTHESIA

- Effects on pregnancy have not been assessed. Use w/ precaution in labor & delivery or w/ concomitant use of other CNS depressants. May need dosing adjustment in pts w/ liver disease.

FETAL & NEONATAL EFFECTS

- Pregnancy Category NR (for definition, see the "*Pregnancy Categories*" section). Safety in breast-feeding is unclear; however, it is used commonly as a post-cesarean analgesic at a time when there is not much milk production yet.

COMMENT
- Adverse effects include respiratory depression, constipation, nausea & vomiting, dizziness, dysphoria, lightheadedness, sedation, skin rash, pruritus.

ULTANE (SEVOFLURANE)

INDICATIONS
- Induction & maintenance of general anesthesia. Better for induction because less irritating to airway than other inhalational agents.

DOSING
- MAC for sevoflurane is 2.6%, decreased by 30–40% for the parturient. Use 0.25–0.5 MAC until delivery of baby to limit hypotension & uterine atony. Rapid onset (2 min) & recovery.

MATERNAL SIDE EFFECTS & IMPACT ON ANESTHESIA
- Causes dose-dependent uterine atony & hypotension. Can cause brady/tachycardia, hypertension, agitation, hypo/hyperthermia, nausea, vomiting, laryngospasm, shivering, etc. May increase risk of seizures.

FETAL & NEONATAL EFFECTS
- Pregnancy Category B (for definition, see the "*Pregnancy Categories*" section). Crosses the placenta & may cause temporary neonatal depression in large doses. Concentrations in breast milk are negligible 24 hours after anesthesia.

COMMENT
- Keep fresh gas flow >1–2 L/min as sevoflurane degradation product (compound A) has been shown to cause nephrotoxicity in rats. When used as the sole anesthetic agent for general anesthesia, awareness results in 12–26% of cases.

ULTIVA (REMIFENTANIL)

INDICATIONS
- Ultrashort-acting synthetic, opioid receptor agonist w/ rapid onset

DOSING

■ Doses may vary; usually 0.05–1 mcg/kg IV.

MATERNAL SIDE EFFECTS & IMPACT ON ANESTHESIA

■ Rapidly metabolized by plasma & tissue esterases & thus is cleared independently of the liver or kidneys; the context-sensitive half-life is 3.5 minutes independent of the mode of administration.

FETAL & NEONATAL EFFECTS

■ Pregnancy Category C (for definition, see the "*Pregnancy Categories*" section). Rapid transplacental transfer, but similar metabolism by the fetus ensures rapid drug clearance.

COMMENT

■ Multiple studies have evaluated its use for labor PCA. There is concern regarding the need for an initial large bolus, which results in significant maternal respiratory depression. In addition, studies have shown large individual variation in the initial dose required, as well as in increased dosages required as labor progresses. The best dosing regimen remains undiscovered. Remifentanil should not be administered into the same IV tubing w/ blood because of potential drug inactivation by nonspecific esterases in blood products.

VALACYCLOVIR (VALTREX)

INDICATIONS

■ Active against HSV-1 & HSV-2 (primary & recurrent genital herpes)

DOSING

■ Acyclovir: 5 mg/kg IV q8h for 5 days for severe infection & 200 mg PO 5×/day for 10 days.
■ Valacyclovir: 500 mg PO bid for 5 days

MATERNAL SIDE EFFECTS & IMPACT ON ANESTHESIA

■ Maternal effects can include thrombocytopenia, renal impairment, encephalopathic changes (lethargy, obtundation, tremors, confusion).

FETAL & NEONATAL EFFECTS

■ Pregnancy Category B (for definition, see the "*Pregnancy Categories*" section). Rapidly crosses the placenta. Acyclovir is considered safe during breast-feeding; safety of valacyclovir has not been determined.

COMMENT
- In rat studies, high levels of acyclovir were associated w/ fetal head & tail abnormalities & maternal toxicity.

VALIUM (DIAZEPAM)

INDICATIONS
- Acute alcohol withdrawal, anxiety, cardioversion, skeletal muscle spasms & seizures

DOSING
- 2–15 mg PO, rectally, IM or IV; can repeat as needed

MATERNAL SIDE EFFECTS & IMPACT ON ANESTHESIA
- The effects of diazepam on pregnancy have not been assessed. However, it has been suggested that diazepam be used w/ precaution in pregnancy. Contraindications include acute narrow-angle & untreated open-angle glaucoma & age <6 months.

FETAL & NEONATAL EFFECTS
- Pregnancy Category NR (for definition, see the "*Pregnancy Categories*" section). Safety in breast-feeding is controversial. Safety & effectiveness have not been established in children <6 months of age.

COMMENT
- Adverse effects include ataxia, drowsiness, fatigue, hypotension, respiratory depression & sedation. Diazepam should be gradually tapered after extended therapy; abrupt discontinuation should generally be avoided.

VALPROIC ACID (DEPAKOTE, DEPAKENE)

INDICATIONS
- Anticonvulsant

DOSING
- Usual starting dose is 500–750 mg/day divided 2 or 3 times/day. The dose is increased every several days to achieve blood levels in the

range of 50–100 mcg/mL, which is typically achieved at a dosage of 1,000–2,500 mg/day.

MATERNAL SIDE EFFECTS & IMPACT ON ANESTHESIA
■ The use of valproic acid during pregnancy has been associated w/ fetal teratogenicity, most commonly neural tube defects. May cause thrombocytopenia, inhibition of platelets, low fibrinogen & other clotting abnormalities, lethargy, coma, fatal hepatic failure.

FETAL & NEONATAL EFFECTS
■ Pregnancy Category D (for definition, see the "*Pregnancy Categories*" section). The most frequently associated major malformations are neural tube defects, congenital heart disease, oral clefts, genital abnormalities, limb abnormalities. May cause clotting abnormalities & fatal hepatic failure. Valproate is compatible w/ breast-feeding; breast milk concentrations are 1–10% of serum. Children <2 years are at increased risk of toxicity.

COMMENT
■ Anticonvulsant meds should not be discontinued abruptly as seizures are also a threat to the patient & fetus. Children exposed to valproate during organogenesis should likely be tested or monitored for congenital defects.

VALTREX (VALACYCLOVIR)

INDICATIONS
■ Active against HSV-1 & HSV-2 (primary & recurrent genital herpes)

DOSING
■ Acyclovir: 5 mg/kg IV q8h for 5 days for severe infection & 200 mg PO 5×/day for 10 days.
■ Valacyclovir: 500 mg PO bid for 5 days

MATERNAL SIDE EFFECTS & IMPACT ON ANESTHESIA
■ Maternal effects can include thrombocytopenia, renal impairment, encephalopathic changes (lethargy, obtundation, tremors, confusion).

FETAL & NEONATAL EFFECTS
■ Pregnancy Category B (for definition, see the "*Pregnancy Categories*" section). Rapidly crosses the placenta. Acyclovir is considered safe

during breast-feeding; safety of valacyclovir has not been determined.

COMMENT
- In rat studies, high levels of acyclovir were associated w/ fetal head & tail abnormalities & maternal toxicity.

VANCOCIN (VANCOMYCIN)

INDICATIONS
- Active against various (methicillin-resistant) gram-positive bacteria. May be used for vaginal delivery in PCN-allergic women needing endocarditis prophylaxis w/ mitral valve prolapse.

DOSING
- 20–30 mg/kg/day IV in 2–4 divided doses over 1–2 hours

MATERNAL EFFECTS & IMPACT ON ANESTHESIA
- Nephrotoxicity has been associated w/ co-administration of vancomycin & an aminoglycoside. May potentiate neuromuscular blockade; the dose of the neuromuscular blocking agent must carefully be titrated to effect. Potential respiratory paralysis & post-op ventilation requirements may occur secondary to prolonged neuromuscular blockade. Rapid administration causes histamine release, w/ redness of the face & neck & potential transient hypotension ("Red Man syndrome").

FETAL SIDE EFFECTS
- Pregnancy Category B (for definition, see the "*Pregnancy Categories*" section). Likely does not cause renal toxicity & ototoxicity in the fetus, but data are limited.

COMMENT
- Administer by slow infusion only.

VANCOMYCIN (LYPHOCIN, VANCOCIN)

INDICATIONS
- Active against various (methicillin-resistant) gram-positive bacteria. May be used for vaginal delivery in PCN-allergic women needing endocarditis prophylaxis w/ mitral valve prolapse.

DOSING

- 20–30 mg/kg/day IV in 2–4 divided doses over 1–2 hours

MATERNAL EFFECTS & IMPACT ON ANESTHESIA

- Nephrotoxicity has been associated w/ co-administration of vancomycin & an aminoglycoside. May potentiate neuromuscular blockade; the dose of the neuromuscular blocking agent must carefully be titrated to effect. Potential respiratory paralysis & post-op ventilation requirements may occur secondary to prolonged neuromuscular blockade. Rapid administration causes histamine release, w/ redness of the face & neck & potential transient hypotension ("Red Man syndrome").

FETAL SIDE EFFECTS

- Pregnancy Category B (for definition, see the "*Pregnancy Categories*" section). Likely does not cause renal toxicity & ototoxicity in the fetus, but data are limited.

COMMENT

- Administer by slow infusion only.

VASOPRESSIN

INDICATIONS

- Diabetes insipidus; upper GI hemorrhage; pulseless ventricular tachycardia or ventricular fibrillation; shock refractory to fluid & vasopressor therapy

DOSING

- DI: 5–10 units IM/SC q8–12h
- Upper GI hemorrhage: 0.1–0.4 units/min IV infusion
- Pulseless ventricular tachycardia or ventricular fibrillation: 40 units IV bolus
- Shock: 0.04 units/min IV infusion

MATERNAL SIDE EFFECTS & IMPACT ON ANESTHESIA

- May cause oliguria, water intoxication, hypertension, pulmonary edema, hypertension, arrhythmias, myocardial ischemia

FETAL & NEONATAL EFFECTS

- Pregnancy category C (for definition, see the "*Pregnancy Categories*" section). Not known if it causes fetal harm. Doses sufficient for antidiuretic effect are not likely to produce tonic uterine contractions that could be harmful to the fetus or threaten the continuation of the pregnancy.

COMMENT
- Antidiuretic effect of vasopressin is inhibited by concurrent norepinephrine, lithium, heparin or alcohol. Pressor effects of vasopressin are potentiated by concurrent ganglionic blocking agents.

VECURONIUM (NORCURON)

INDICATIONS
- Nondepolarizing neuromuscular blocking drug (NMBD) used to facilitate intubation & maintain neuromuscular blockade

DOSING
- 0.2 mg/kg IV (onset 175 sec)

MATERNAL SIDE EFFECTS & IMPACT ON ANESTHESIA
- Action may be prolonged in pts w/ renal insufficiency & IV magnesium.

FETAL & NEONATAL EFFECTS
- Pregnancy Category C (for definition, see the "*Pregnancy Categories*" section). No adverse effects w/ intubating dose.

COMMENT
- Avoid in pts w/ liver disease. Long onset to action makes it less desirable for rapid sequence intubation.

VENLAFAXINE (EFFEXOR)

INDICATIONS
- SSRI typically used to treat depression, anxiety, obsessive-compulsive disorder, bulimia, panic disorder, posttraumatic stress disorder

DOSING
- Depression: initially 75 mg/day PO in 2 or 3 divided doses, with increases up to 225 mg/day PO for outpatients and 375 mg/day PO for inpatients

- Anxiety disorder: initially 37.5–75 mg/day PO, with increases up to 225 mg/day
- Dosing adjustments are appropriate if there is hepatic or renal insufficiency.

MATERNAL SIDE EFFECTS & IMPACT ON ANESTHESIA

- Common side effects include anorexia, constipation or diarrhea, paradoxical anxiety, dizziness, dry mouth. More serious complications can include abnormal bleeding (particularly when used w/ other meds that can inhibit platelet function), hypertension, hyponatremia, seizures.

FETAL & NEONATAL EFFECTS

- Pregnancy Category C (for definition, see the "*Pregnancy Categories*" section). An increased risk for CNS serotonergic symptoms was observed during the first 4 days of life in infants of mothers taking SSRIs during the 3rd trimester of pregnancy. Infants exposed prenatally to fluoxetine or a tricyclic antidepressant did NOT show differences in IQ, language or behavioral development compared to children w/o prenatal exposure to these drugs. SSRIs have unknown effects that may be of concern during breast-feeding.

COMMENT

- Do not use concomitantly w/ MAO inhibitors.

VENTOLIN (ALBUTEROL ORAL INHALED AEROSOL)

INDICATIONS

- Albuterol is a stimulant of the beta-2 receptors in the bronchi & thus is a potent bronchodilator used in allergic asthma; exercise-induced asthma; acute, subacute & chronic bronchitis; & emphysema. Useful as a tocolytic. Can be used to treat hyperkalemia.

DOSING

- 1 or 2 metered-dose inhalations q4–6h

MATERNAL SIDE EFFECTS & IMPACT ON ANESTHESIA

- Like all beta-2 mimetics, may cause tachycardia, hyperglycemia & hypotension. May also result in hypokalemia; it is useful in treating hyperkalemia.

FETAL & NEONATAL EFFECTS
- Pregnancy Category C (for definition, see the "*Pregnancy Categories*" section). Crosses the placenta & may cause tachycardia & hyperglycemia in the fetus. May cause retinal ischemia. Albuterol is an effective tocolytic similar to ritodrine. Like ritodrine, it is considered safe during breast-feeding.

COMMENT
- Excessive inhalation may result in hypertension, hypoglycemia, hypokalemia & hypocalcemia. Concurrent administration w/ oxytocic drugs (including ergonovine) may cause hypotension. May decrease serum digoxin levels.

VERSED (MIDAZOLAM)

INDICATIONS
- Benzodiazepine used for anesthesia induction, sedation, anxiolysis

DOSING
- 1–5 mg IV until desired effect

MATERNAL SIDE EFFECTS & IMPACT ON ANESTHESIA
- Not recommended in high doses (0.2 mg/kg) for induction of general anesthesia since there is a high risk of neonatal respiratory depression requiring intubation

FETAL & NEONATAL EFFECTS
- Pregnancy Category D (for definition, see the "*Pregnancy Categories*" section). The use of midazolam before C-section has a depressant effect on the newborn that is greater than that observed w/ thiopental. Its use is indicated where maternal benefit warrants it. Found in breast milk; use during breast-feeding may be of concern.

COMMENT
- N/A

VIVARIN (CAFFEINE)

INDICATIONS
- A CNS vasoconstrictor, useful for mild post-dural puncture headaches. One of the most popular drugs in the world!

DOSING
- 300–500 mg PO/IV q12–24h

MATERNAL SIDE EFFECTS & IMPACT ON ANESTHESIA
- Causes tachycardia & nervousness. Avoid in pts w/ preexisting arrhythmias.

FETAL & NEONATAL EFFECTS
- Pregnancy Category C (for definition, see the "*Pregnancy Categories*" section). Caffeine crosses the placenta. Caffeine intake >300 mg/day is not recommended. Considered compatible w/ breast-feeding within recommended dosing guidelines.

COMMENT
- A cup of coffee contains about 40–100 mg of caffeine; soft drinks contain 10–55 mg.

WARFARIN (COUMADIN)

INDICATIONS
- Prevention & mgt of deep venous thrombosis & pulmonary embolism in non-pregnant pts. Warfarin is contraindicated in pregnancy.

DOSING
- Contraindicated in pregnancy.

MATERNAL SIDE EFFECTS & IMPACT ON ANESTHESIA
N/A

FETAL & NEONATAL EFFECTS
- Pregnancy Category D (for definition, see the "*Pregnancy Categories*" section). Warfarin should be avoided in pregnancy. Skeletal & CNS defects as well as fetal hemorrhage have been reported.

COMMENT
- Warfarin is excreted in breast milk in an inactive form. Its ionic, non-lipophilic structure & high protein binding affinity decrease the likelihood of breast milk excretion. There is no evidence of detectable warfarin levels, altered coagulation, bleeding or other adverse effects in exposed infants. However, some experts recommend monitoring coagulation status in infants at risk for vitamin K deficiency.

XYLOCAINE (LIDOCAINE)

INDICATIONS
■ pH-adjusted 2% lidocaine is useful for C-section under epidural. 1.5% lidocaine (45mg) w/ 1:200,000 epinephrine is useful to rule out intrathecal or intravascular placement of the epidural catheter. May also be used for the treatment of ventricular tachycardias. Lidocaine patch may be used for localized chronic pain treatment.

DOSE
■ Depends on procedure. 20 cc of 2% lidocaine epidurally in divided doses for C-section. Intrathecal doses vary depending on procedure length.

MATERNAL SIDE EFFECTS & IMPACT ON ANESTHESIA
■ Rapidly crosses the placenta. Intravascular administration may lead to lightheadedness, seizures, disorientation, heart block, hypotension. Acidosis in the fetus predisposes to ion trapping of the lidocaine.

FETAL & NEONATAL SIDE EFFECTS
■ Pregnancy Category B (for definition, see the "*Pregnancy Categories*" section). Rapidly crosses the placenta. Lidocaine injected into fetal scalp accidentally (as during paracervical block) may cause toxicity. Acidosis in the fetus predisposes to ion trapping of the lidocaine. Compatible w/ breast-feeding.

COMMENT
■ Lidocaine administered intrathecally has been associated w/ transient radicular irritation.

ZANTAC (RANITIDINE)

INDICATIONS
■ Inhibits histamine stimulation of the H2 receptor in gastric parietal cells, which reduces gastric acid secretion, gastric volume & hydrogen ion concentrations

DOSING
■ 3.5 mg/kg/dose PO bid/tid ac & hs; alternatively, 150 mg PO bid or 75 mg PO bid

MATERNAL SIDE EFFECTS & IMPACT ON ANESTHESIA
- May decrease effects of ketoconazole & itraconazole; may alter serum levels of ferrous sulfate, diazepam, nondepolarizing muscle relaxants & oxaprozin

FETAL & NEONATAL EFFECTS
- Pregnancy Category B (for definition, see the "*Pregnancy Categories*" section). Usually safe but benefits must outweigh risks.

COMMENT
- Use caution in pts w/ renal or liver impairment; if changes in renal function occur during therapy, consider adjusting dose or discontinuing treatment. Adverse effects include headache & malaise.

ZEMURON (ROCURONIUM)

INDICATIONS
- Nondepolarizing neuromuscular blocking drug (NMBD) used to facilitate rapid intubation & maintain neuromuscular blockade

DOSING
- 0.6 mg/kg IV (onset 98 sec)

MATERNAL SIDE EFFECTS & IMPACT ON ANESTHESIA
- Action may be prolonged in pts w/ renal insufficiency & IV magnesium.

FETAL & NEONATAL EFFECTS
- Pregnancy Category B (for definition, see the "*Pregnancy Categories*" section). No adverse effects w/ intubating dose.

COMMENT
- Safe in pregnancy

ZIDOVUDINE (AZT, RETROVIR)

INDICATIONS
- Inhibits HIV replication

DOSING
- 300–600 mg/day PO in 3–5 divided doses

MATERNAL SIDE EFFECTS & IMPACT ON ANESTHESIA
- Women in the 1st trimester may consider delaying or discontinuing therapy until after 10–12 weeks gestation. Recommended component of the peri- & post-partum regimen for mother & neonate whenever possible.

FETAL & NEONATAL EFFECTS
- Pregnancy Category C (for definition, see the "*Pregnancy Categories*" section). Significantly reduces transmission of HIV to the fetus. There are conflicting data on perinatal exposure to antiretrovirals associated w/ significant (often fatal) mitochondrial disease in infants. Babies exposed to antiretrovirals in utero should receive long-term follow-up for potential mitochondrial dysfunction.

COMMENT
- Breast-feeding is not recommended in mothers w/ HIV due to presence of virus in breast milk & potential for transmission to HIV-negative child.

ZITHROMAX (AZITHROMYCIN)

INDICATIONS
- Active against a wide range of gram-positive & gram-negative bacteria

DOSING
- 1,200–1,500 mg/week PO, w/ divided doses of tablets of 250–500 mg/day orally

MATERNAL SIDE EFFECTS & IMPACT ON ANESTHESIA
- Very rare allergic reactions have been reported, including Stevens-Johnson syndrome & toxic epidermal necrolysis. Use w/ caution in pts w/ impaired liver function. Do not administer concomitantly w/ ergot derivatives.

FETAL & NEONATAL EFFECTS
- Pregnancy Category B (for definition, see the "*Pregnancy Categories*" section). Crosses placenta. It is not known if transmission via breast milk is clinically significant.

COMMENT
- Should be taken at least 1 hour before or 2 hours after antacids

ZOFRAN (ONDANSETRON)

INDICATIONS
- Selective 5-HT3-receptor antagonist that blocks serotonin both peripherally & centrally, used in the prevention of nausea & vomiting. Metabolized in the liver via the P-450 mechanism.

DOSING
- 2–4 mg IV q6–8h

MATERNAL SIDE EFFECTS & IMPACT ON ANESTHESIA
- Safely used in the treatment of hyperemesis gravidarum. Very rare extrapyramidal side effects.

FETAL & NEONATAL EFFECTS
- Pregnancy Category B (for definition, see the "*Pregnancy Categories*" section)

COMMENT
- Best used for prevention & prophylaxis of nausea & vomiting. Off-label use for peri-operative pruritus: 8 mg IVP.

ZOLOFT (SERTRALINE)

INDICATIONS
- SSRI typically used to treat depression, anxiety, obsessive-compulsive disorder, bulimia, panic disorder, posttraumatic stress disorder

DOSING
- Depression or obsessive-compulsive disorder: 50 mg/day PO, up to 200 mg/day PO
- Panic disorder: 25 mg/day PO initially, up to 200 mg/day PO
- Dosages should be decreased in pts w/ liver disease.

MATERNAL SIDE EFFECTS & IMPACT ON ANESTHESIA
- Potential for anorexia, dry mouth, constipation or diarrhea, abnormal bleeding (when taken w/ other platelet inhibitors), hyponatremia, seizures

MATERNAL SIDE EFFECTS & IMPACT ON ANESTHESIA
FETAL & NEONATAL EFFECTS

■ Pregnancy Category C (for definition, see the "*Pregnancy Categories*" section). An increased risk for CNS serotonergic symptoms was observed during the first 4 days of life in infants of mothers taking SSRIs during the 3rd trimester of pregnancy. Infants exposed prenatally to fluoxetine or a tricyclic antidepressant did NOT show differences in IQ, language or behavioral development compared to children w/o prenatal exposure to these drugs. SSRIs have unknown effects that may be of concern during breast-feeding.

COMMENT

■ Do not take w/ MAO inhibitors.

ZOVIRAX (ACYCLOVIR)

INDICATIONS

■ Active against HSV-1 & HSV-2 (primary & recurrent genital herpes)

DOSING

■ Acyclovir: 5 mg/kg IV q8h for 5 days for severe infection & 200 mg PO 5×/day for 10 days.
■ Valacyclovir: 500 mg PO bid for 5 days

MATERNAL SIDE EFFECTS & IMPACT ON ANESTHESIA

■ Maternal effects can include thrombocytopenia, renal impairment, encephalopathic changes (lethargy, obtundation, tremors, confusion).

FETAL & NEONATAL EFFECTS

■ Pregnancy Category B (for definition, see the "*Pregnancy Categories*" section). Rapidly crosses the placenta. Acyclovir is considered safe during breast-feeding; safety of valacyclovir has not been determined.

COMMENT

■ In rat studies, high levels of acyclovir were associated w/ fetal head & tail abnormalities & maternal toxicity.